First Principles
of Gastroenterology
THE BASIS OF DISEASE AND
AN APPROACH TO MANAGEMENT

SECOND EDITION

First Principles of Gastroenterology

THE BASIS OF DISEASE AND AN APPROACH TO MANAGEMENT

SECOND EDITION

A.B.R. THOMSON
and E.A. SHAFFER, editors

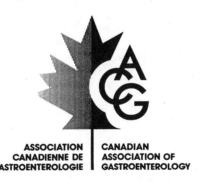

ASSOCIATION
CANADIENNE DE
GASTROENTEROLOGIE

CANADIAN
ASSOCIATION OF
GASTROENTEROLOGY

Sponsored by
the Canadian Association of Gastroenterology
and Astra Pharma Inc.

The publication of this book was sponsored by the Canadian Association of Gastroenterology and supported by an education grant from Astra Pharma Inc.

Publishers:

Canadian Association of Gastroenterology
c/o Dr. A.B.R. Thomson
University of Alberta
519 Newton Research Building
11315-87 Ave.
Edmonton, Alberta T6G 2C2

Astra Pharma Inc.
1004 Middlegate Road
Mississauga, Ontario
L4Y 1M4

Canadian Cataloguing in Publication Data

Main entry under title:

First principles of gastroenterology : the basis of disease and an approach to management
2nd ed.
Issued also in French under title: Principes fondamentaux de gastro-entérologie
Co-published by Astra Pharma Inc.
Includes bibliographical references and index.
ISBN 0-920163-12-2 (bound) ISBN 0-920163-10-6 (pbk.)

1. Gastrointestinal system – Diseases.
2. Gastrointestinal system – Diseases – Treatment.
3. Digestive organs – Diseases. 4. Digestive organs – Diseases – Treatment.
I. Thomson, A.B.R. (Alan Bryan Robert), 1943– . II. Shaffer, E.A. (Eldon A.),
1941– . III. Canadian Association of Gastroenterology. IV. Astra Pharma Inc.

RC801.F57 1994   616.3'3   C94-931939-2

Great care has been taken to ensure the accuracy of the contents of this publication. However, the publishers cannot be responsible for errors or any consequences arising from the information published herein.

Printed in Canada on recycled paper by the University of Toronto Press Incorporated.

Project Management by MacLean Communications, Mississauga, Ontario.
Tel: (905) 824-9745 Fax: (905) 824-1704

Dedication

We dedicate this textbook to the memory of Dr. Henry Shaffer, who was the inspiration and role model to many young physicians, by fulfilling the Oslerean Philosophy (*"The desire to take medicine is perhaps the greatest feature which distinguishes man from animals"*).

This work is also dedicated to Dr. I.T. Beck, a caring, thoughtful, stimulating and supportive role model who has been an inspiration and mentor for many younger and older gastroenterologists.

Without the caring support from our families for our academic work, the meaning of our accomplishments would diminish. We acknowledge and express our sincere thanks for the encouragement and loving support of Jeannette, James, Matthew, Jessica and Benjamin Thomson, and of Beryl, Andrea, Emily and Alexandra Shaffer.

A.B.R. Thomson
E.A. Shaffer

Contents

Preface

Growth in the field of gastroenterology and hepatology is exponential and inexorable. Not only has it provided the scientific basis for how we manage our patients, but it also has brought with it a problem: an ever-expanding wealth of information that needs clarification. There are several important large tomes dedicated to diseases of the gastrointestinal tract and hepatobiliary system. Information in these is encyclopedic and not readily synthesized into the practice of medicine or as a learning experience for trainees. To answer this need, a multi-authored text, *First Principles of Gastroenterology*, was brought out two years ago. It provided valuable information for students, residents and practicing physicians, be they internists, hepatologists or gastroenterologists. It was also unique, having both English and French contributors and being published in both languages. A first!

The text has been an overwhelming success, with extremely positive feedback from physicians and academic centers. Because of this and the opportunity to "do better," a second edition was born. This entailed extensive revision, the inclusion of an important section on pediatric gastroenterology and nutrition, greatly extended discussion of HIV disease and inflammatory bowel disease, a multi-authored approach to liver disease and, most important, an update. Many talented authorities from across Canada are involved in this edition.

The editors wish to acknowledge the generous sponsorship by Astra Pharma Inc., particularly Mr. Peter Dixon for his unstinting efforts. We also recognize the valued contributions by graduate medical students, fellows training in gastroenterology and members of the Canadian Association of Gastroenterology.

The renewal process is perpetual. The third edition is already in the gestational phase.

A.B.R. Thomson
E.A. Shaffer

First Principles of Gastroenterology

THE BASIS OF DISEASE AND AN APPROACH TO MANAGEMENT

SECOND EDITION

1
Common Symptoms and Signs in Gastroenterology

W.G. Thompson, M.C. Champion, R.R. Gillies,
S. Gregoire, S. Meban, D.G. Patel, L.J. Scully and A.S.C. Sekar

1. INTRODUCTION / W.G. Thompson

THE KEY to accurate diagnosis and effective management of gastrointestinal problems is flawless history-taking. Since up to 50% of gastrointestinal disorders are associated with no anatomical change, no physical findings and no positive test result, diagnosis and therapy must often be based on the medical interview. The gastrointestinal history must include an accurate description of the symptom itself, a past history of gastrointestinal disorders or surgery, a meticulous search for symptoms that might suggest organic disease (such as gastrointestinal hemorrhage, anemia or weight loss) and finally, a careful assessment of the patient's psychosocial state, with particular attention directed toward traumatic events or concerns associated with the onset of the patient's complaints.

The physician should determine the onset of the symptom, its occurrence in the past, its periodicity, its location and radiation if appropriate, its aggravating and relieving factors, and its relationship to other symptoms. A review of past history should include not only any previous gastrointestinal surgery or diseases, but also systemic illnesses (such as diabetes or severe cardiovascular disease) that might affect the gut. One should pay particular attention to such symptoms as gastrointestinal hemorrhage, profound weight loss, voluminous diarrhea or episodes of extreme abdominal pain, which might indicate organic disease. Similarly, such phenomena as anemia, fever or incapacity to work may indicate a more serious gastrointestinal disorder demanding treatment and follow-up. A family history of inflammatory bowel disease or bowel cancer may indicate a more careful investigation as well.

When considering a gastrointestinal complaint, the astute physician cannot ignore the patient's psyche. Many studies establish that those who bring gastrointestinal complaints to a physician, even if they are organic in nature, frequently have psychosocial disabilities. Failure to identify and manage the patient's reaction to his or her psychosocial environment (whether it be hostility toward a spouse, an abnormal fear of cancer or a profound loss) may lead to an unsatisfactory therapeutic outcome.

The following is a synopsis of the common gastrointestinal symptoms. These notes include a description of the symptom itself, a word about how the symptom is generated, the important historical features and associated physical findings, and a brief approach to diagnosis and management. These serve as introductory comments; greater detail can be found throughout the text in discussions of specific diseases.

2. GLOBUS / W.G. Thompson

2.1 Synonyms
Globus hystericus; lump in the throat.

2.2 Description
Globus is a lump in the throat or a perceived inability to swallow unassociated with meals. Nearly one out of every two persons experiences this symptom, often at the time of an intense emotional experience.

2.3 Mechanism
Globus is a "functional" disorder since no pathologic or pathophysiologic abnormality has been clearly identified. Many believe that globus is due to a dysmotility of the upper esophageal sphincter.

2.4 Important Historical Features
Generally speaking, patients with globus can swallow meals normally but feel an inability to swallow their saliva between meals. The tendency of globus to occur when the patient is experiencing intense emotion has led in the past to the use of the epithet "globus hystericus." Since one-half of the population experiences this symptom, the term *hystericus* hardly seems justified. Patients may have psychogenic features such as anxiety, but are not overt in displaying other conversion features. There are no physical findings.

2.5 Differential Diagnosis
Globus is easily distinguished from true dysphagia by its occurrence between

meals and by the lack of difficulty in swallowing such items as bread and meat. The sensation is continuous.

2.6 Management
There is no treatment beyond reassurance. Deep-seated emotional features may warrant a psychiatric opinion.

3. HEARTBURN / W.G. Thompson

3.1 Synonyms
Pyrosis.

3.2 Description
Heartburn is a burning sensation experienced behind the sternum. It characteristically occurs or is worsened when the subject is bending over, straining or lying down, especially after a meal. It is aggravated by certain foods (acidic drinks, chocolate, coffee), obesity or anxiety. Unlike angina, it is not usually worsened by exercise or exertion.

3.3 Related Symptoms
Heartburn may be associated with a sensation of reflux into the gullet, or even actual regurgitation into the mouth (with the risk of aspiration). It should be distinguished from rumination, in which the subject regurgitates meals routinely and then swallows them again, usually with no consequence beyond disgust in the observer.

3.4 Mechanism
Heartburn is associated with reflux of gastric contents (usually acidic) into the esophagus. The mechanism is complex. Decreased tone or inappropriate relaxation of the lower esophageal sphincter favors reflux. Anatomic disturbances such as obesity or hiatus hernia may also be important. In diseases in which peristalsis of the esophagus is disturbed (e.g., scleroderma) any acid that does reflux into the esophagus will not be adequately cleared.

Contrary to popular opinion, the presence of a hiatus hernia has little role in the genesis of heartburn (Figure 1). Both hiatus hernia and heartburn occur in approximately one-third of subjects (not necessarily the same third). Thus, individual cases may have heartburn without hiatus hernia and vice versa.

The mechanism of the pain is obscure. There appear to be no nerve endings for pain in the esophageal mucosa. Severe esophagitis may exist in the absence of heartburn or indeed of any symptoms. Conversely, individuals

GASTROESOPHAGEAL REFLUX

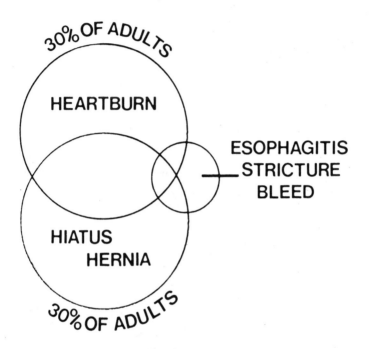

FIGURE 1. Heartburn and hiatus hernia each occurs in about 30% of adults, so some overlap is inevitable; a causal relationship has not been established. Complicated GERD may occur with heartburn, hiatus hernia, both or neither..

with heartburn may have an apparently normal esophagus. This gives rise to the suspicion that gastroesophageal reflux may be associated with a disturbance in esophageal motility; this may be responsible for the sensation of heartburn.

3.5 History and Physical
When heartburn is suspected, one should determine the effect of position, food, stress and exercise on the discomfort. The interviewer should carefully exclude such symptoms as dysphagia, odynophagia, weight loss, bleeding and anemia, which indicate complications of reflux or more serious esophageal disease.

There are no physical findings that can be associated with heartburn. The presence of substernal or costochondral tenderness suggests a musculoskeletal origin for the symptom.

3.6 Differential Diagnosis
The presence of heartburn implies that the individual has gastroesophageal reflux disease (GERD). If the burning retrosternal sensation is aggravated by bending and relieved by antacids, then no further investigation is necessary. Some, however, have a retrosternal sensation that cannot be distinguished from that of angina pectoris, particularly if it is in some way related to effort, relieved by nitroglycerin and associated with other features of heart disease. As discussed in the chapter on the esophagus, esophageal spasm may be responsible for chest pain. However, it is often difficult to prove this relationship even with sophisticated motility equipment. Musculoskeletal disturbances such as costochondritis may be responsible for chest pain; they are characterized by local tenderness.

3.7 Approach to Investigation and Management
One-third of adults have experienced heartburn and one in ten suffer heartburn at least once per week. If the heartburn is not incapacitating and is unaccompanied by dysphagia or anemia, then a trial of therapy is a reasonable first approach. Foods that delay gastric emptying (e.g., fat) or that weaken the lower esophageal sphincter (e.g., chocolate, onions) should be avoided. Antacids or alginate compounds such as Gaviscon® are usually successful in relieving the symptoms or even preventing them. Having small meals, fasting before bedtime, elevating the head of the bed and avoiding bending or exertion on a full stomach may be beneficial as well.

In the event that such simple management fails to relieve heartburn, or that dysphagia, anemia or bleeding occurs, then some investigation is necessary. An endoscopy provides the most information, since it allows the degree of inflammation of the esophagus to be assessed. If a stricture is present, it should be biopsied. If the stricture proves nonmalignant, dilation may be carried out. More vigorous pharmacologic therapy for resistant gastroesophageal reflux disease is discussed in Chapter 5, "The Esophagus."

4. WATERBRASH / W.G. Thompson

4.1 Description
Waterbrash is the spontaneous flooding of the mouth with a clear, slightly salty fluid, which may be of sufficient quantity to require expectoration.

4.2 Mechanism

The source of the fluid appears to be the salivary glands. It is believed to result from a vagal cholinergic reflex, with afferents originating in the upper gastrointestinal tract and efferents destined for the salivary glands.

4.3 Important Historical Points

The fluid, with a neutral or somewhat salty taste, is quite distinct from the acidic or bitter contents that are refluxed from the stomach. The symptom commonly accompanies upper gastrointestinal distress such as heartburn, peptic ulcer disease and even acute gastroenteritis. By itself, it has no pathologic significance.

4.4 Differential Diagnosis

Waterbrash must be distinguished from gastroesophageal reflux disease and rumination. Diagnosis and management depend upon the underlying upper gastrointestinal disorder.

5. DYSPHAGIA / A.S.C. Sekar

5.1 Description

Dysphagia means difficulty in swallowing. Some patients describe food sticking in the throat or retrosternally.

5.2 Important Historical Points and Differential Diagnosis

A careful history is important. Mechanical narrowing is a common cause; an inflammatory stricture must be distinguished from a carcinoma. If the dysphagia is relatively short in duration (e.g., only a few months) and is worsening, this suggests a progressive mechanical narrowing of the lumen such as may occur with an esophageal carcinoma. With benign disease, symptoms are often present for a longer period of time than with carcinoma. A previous history of heartburn or acid regurgitation in a patient with progressive dysphagia might point to an esophageal stricture secondary to gastroesophageal reflux disease. Not all patients with a benign esophageal stricture have a clear history of preceding heartburn or acid regurgitation. This is particularly true in the elderly patient. A history of ingestion of caustic agents such as lye suggests an esophageal stricture secondary to severe chemical esophagitis.

Infections of the esophagus can also cause difficult swallowing. Infections, usually due to Candida albicans or herpes virus, are often accompanied by significant pain on swallowing, termed *odynophagia*. Often the odynophagia is so severe that the patient even has difficulty swallowing his or her saliva.

Although herpes esophagitis can occur in relatively healthy patients, Candida esophagitis is associated with diabetes, an underlying malignancy or immunosuppression.

The patient may point to the site of obstruction, but this is not always reliable. A stricture of the lower esophagus may be experienced at the xiphoid area or as high as the throat. Upper esophageal obstruction is experienced high in the throat region, not low in the chest.

Dysphagia can also occur with motor disorders of the esophagus. These conditions include esophageal spasm and achalasia. With motor disorders of the esophagus, the dysphagia may be for both solids and liquids. The dysphagia is intermittent and may have a long history. Sometimes with esophageal spasm the dysphagia may be accompanied by pain (odynophagia), especially with extremely cold or hot liquids. These patients are usually able to wash down impacted particles of food, whereas patients with a mechanical cause (such as a stricture) may need to regurgitate impacted particles of food to obtain relief.

A common cause of intermittent dysphagia is a mucosal ring at the gastroesophageal junction (lower esophageal or Schatzki's ring). On occasion when a relatively large bolus of food is swallowed the ring can cause mechanical obstruction, producing a dramatic onset of acute dysphagia (sometimes associated with pain). Often such patients will have to leave the table and regurgitate. Patients with a Schatzki's ring usually have symptoms for many years before they seek medical attention. It is the most common cause of foreign-body impaction in the esophagus.

A rare cause of upper esophageal dysphagia is the Paterson-Kelly syndrome or Plummer-Vinson syndrome. Here a chronic iron deficiency anemia is associated with narrowing of the upper esophagus due to a web.

Cricopharyngeal dysphagia may be due to a cricopharyngeal or Zenker's diverticulum, which develops from an abnormality of the cricopharyngeal sphincter. Patients with a diverticulum often complain of regurgitating food that they swallowed a day or so earlier.

There are non-esophageal causes of dysphagia. Underlying neuromuscular disease may cause cricopharyngeal dysphagia, where patients have difficulty initiating a swallow. A large goiter or mediastinal tumor can cause extrinsic compression of the upper esophagus.

5.3 Approach to Diagnosis and Management

A barium swallow is the most important initial investigation in the diagnosis of dysphagia. It might reveal a Zenker's diverticulum, an esophageal stricture (benign or malignant) or a Schatzki's ring. If inflammation of the esophagus is suspected, endoscopy with biopsies is indicated. If a stricture is identified on a barium swallow, endoscopy with biopsies is necessary to determine whether this stricture is benign or malignant. Also, benign strictures can be dilated following the endoscopic diagnosis. A barium swallow may help diagnose motility disturbances such as esophageal spasm and achalasia. Esophageal manometry is often required to confirm such motility disturbances.

Once a cause of dysphagia has been established, management will depend on the cause. For example, reflux esophagitis will be managed with the usual antireflux measures, with or without prokinetic drugs such as domperidone, H_2-receptor antagonists such as ranitidine or a proton pump antagonist such as omeprazole. Esophageal strictures can be dilated following endoscopy. Esophageal carcinoma requires either surgery, radiation or palliative insertion of prosthesis. Esophageal motility disturbances can sometimes be managed medically with nitroglycerin or calcium channel blocking agents. Achalasia and esophageal spasm sometimes require surgical myotomy or pneumatic dilation.

6. DYSPEPSIA / W.G. Thompson

6.1 Synonyms
Indigestion.

6.2 Description
Dyspepsia is an imprecise term. It is best described as a chronic (over three months), recurrent, often meal-related epigastric discomfort, pain or fullness. The location of the pain and the relationship to meals resemble the classic description of peptic ulcer disease. Dyspepsia is usually a daily experience, yet is seldom disabling.

6.3 Mechanism
The mechanism of dyspepsia is uncertain. Even in those dyspeptic patients who have a peptic ulcer, the cause of the pain is uncertain. It is disputed whether the discomfort is related to (1) impaired gastric emptying, (2) a disorder of the basic electrical rhythm of the stomach or (3) pyloroduodenal dysmotility. None are proven.

Although many patients believe that specific foods are responsible for dyspepsia, only fat appears to be a consistent offender. Fat may induce dyspepsia by slowing gastric emptying or by releasing cholecystokinin, which is known to affect the smooth muscle of the upper gastrointestinal tract.

Other upper gastrointestinal symptoms relate to dyspepsia. These include nausea, vomiting (rarely), belching and a feeling of gaseous distention. Terms such as gallbladder dyspepsia, pancreatic dyspepsia, appendiceal dyspepsia and gaseous dyspepsia are misleading and serve no useful purpose. There should be no confusion between the episodic nature and severity of pain due to biliary colic or pancreatic disease and the more predictable and regular occurrence of dyspepsia. Indeed, dyspeptic symptoms are equally common in those who have and in those who do not have gallstones.

6.4 Important Historical Points

In an individual case it is almost impossible to distinguish ulcer from nonulcer dyspepsia. Large studies have shown that, statistically, epigastric pain occurring at night and relieved with antacids is more likely to be associated with peptic ulcer disease. The pain of dyspepsia is not incapacitating. Of course, evidence of complications such as bleeding, weight loss or vomiting would not be expected in nonulcer dyspepsia. The pain or discomfort of the irritable bowel syndrome may occur in the epigastrium. This is generally distinguished from discomfort originating in the upper gastrointestinal tract by its association with defecation and a coexistent alteration in bowel habit.

On physical examination any epigastric tenderness will not distinguish between ulcer and nonulcer dyspepsia. In the latter there should be no complications suggestive of peptic ulcer disease, such as peritoneal signs, a succussion splash or the presence of an epigastric mass.

6.5 Approach to Diagnosis and Management

Dyspepsia occurs in about 10% of the population, many of whom do not seek medical help. Of those who do, approximately one-third will not have a peptic ulcer. There is little evidence that those who have nonulcer dyspepsia will eventually develop an ulcer. Yet the symptoms usually persist for long periods in the patient's life.

Thus, investigation and management will depend upon the establishment of a clear diagnosis at the outset, the cost of investigation and the cost of treatment. Since anti-ulcer medication is very effective and seemingly safe, one attitude would be to treat all such individuals without investigation. In the United States, where x-ray and endoscopy are very expensive and the cost must be borne by the individual, indiscriminate therapy has achieved some currency. In such countries as Canada, where drug costs are similar but procedural costs are much less and are not borne by the individual, it seems more efficacious to establish the diagnosis at the outset before committing the patient to drug therapy. Cost and outcome analysis has not established which is the best approach. Although a carefully conducted upper gastrointestinal series will discover most ulcers, endoscopy is more accurate and will detect mucosal lesions as well.

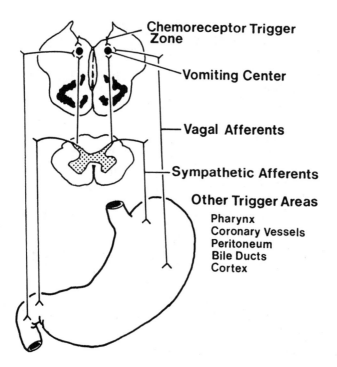

Chemoreceptor Trigger Zone

Vomiting Center

Vagal Afferents

Sympathetic Afferents

Other Trigger Areas
Pharynx
Coronary Vessels
Peritoneum
Bile Ducts
Cortex

FIGURE 2. The vomiting center and chemoreceptor trigger zone control vomiting. Peripheral trigger areas send visceral afferent impulses, which excite the vomiting center into action.

The advantage of early diagnosis is that if no ulcer is found then the chronic use of expensive, systemic drugs can be avoided. Further, the uncertainty factor in failing to establish a diagnosis compounds inappropriate therapy and aggravates patient unease.

7. NAUSEA AND VOMITING / M.C. Champion

7.1 Synonyms
Barf, upchuck, bring up.

7.2 Description
Nausea is a psychic as well as physical experience and defies precise definition. Vomiting is evacuation of the stomach contents through the mouth. Nausea normally precedes vomiting. There can be associated tachycardia, hypersalivation, waterbrash and excessive perspiration.

7.3 Mechanism (Figure 2)

A variety of stimuli may produce nausea (labyrinthine stimulation, pain, unpleasant memories). The neural pathways mediating nausea are not known. During nausea, gastric tone and peristalsis are reduced. The tone of the duodenum and proximal jejunum tends to be increased.

Vomiting occurs as the gastric contents are forcefully brought up to and out of the mouth. This occurs by forceful sustained contraction of the abdominal muscles at a time when the cardia of the stomach is raised and open and the pylorus is contracted. Elevation of the cardia eliminates the intra-abdominal portion of the esophagus and relaxes the lower esophageal sphincter. This allows the stomach contents to enter the esophagus. The act of vomiting is completed with rapid upward displacement of the diaphragm and reversal of thoracic pressure from negative to positive. The glottis closes, the soft palate rises, the mouth opens and the stomach contents are expelled. The control of vomiting consists of two anatomically and functionally separate units, a vomiting center and a chemoreceptor trigger zone. The vomiting center is in the reticular formation of the medulla and is excited directly by visceral afferent impulses (sympathetic and vagal) arising from the gastrointestinal tract and other peripheral trigger areas. These trigger areas are found in the pharynx, cardiac vessels, peritoneum, bile ducts, cortex and stomach. The chemoreceptor trigger zone is on the floor of the fourth ventricle, on the blood side of the blood–brain barrier. The chemoreceptor trigger zone is unable to cause vomiting without an intact vomiting center.

7.4 History and Physical

Patients may complain of nausea and hypersalivation. With gastrointestinal causes of the nausea (and vomiting) there may be associated symptoms of heartburn or epigastric pain. Prior to vomiting, patients may retch (spasmodic, abortive respiratory movements with the glottis closed).

History-taking should probe for precipitating factors, other symptoms that suggest the underlying cause, drug use and dietary habits. The history should also explore psychological trauma or disturbances of body image suggestive of anorexia nervosa.

Physical examination is often normal. An abdominal mass may point to an underlying cause (e.g., gastric carcinoma). Prolonged vomiting may cause dehydration.

7.5 Differential Diagnosis

Prolonged nausea, by itself, rarely has an organic origin. There are many causes of nausea and vomiting, including intracerebral problems (e.g., hydrocephalus, brain tumor), stimulation of the peripheral trigger areas (e.g., severe chest pain, pain from kidney stones), systemic disease (malignancy), medications and pregnancy. Upper gastrointestinal diseases (esophagitis, peptic ulcer disease, gastric carcinoma) are common. Early morning nausea and vomiting suggest pregnancy, alcohol withdrawal, a metabolic cause (e.g., uremia) or a psychogenic origin.

7.6 Approach to Diagnosis and Management

In approaching a patient with nausea and vomiting, one should look for and correct any underlying causes. Prolonged vomiting may cause dehydration and the patient may need to be rehydrated intravenously. Medications should be discontinued.

There are many drugs that have anti-emetic actions. Antihistamines act on the vestibular apparatus as well as on the chemoreceptor trigger zone. Phenothiazines also exert their action on the chemoreceptor trigger zone. Metoclopramide and domperidone are both anti-emetics and gastric prokinetics (which stimulate the stomach to empty). Domperidone exerts its action on the chemoreceptor trigger zone, whereas metoclopramide also crosses the blood–brain barrier and affects the vomiting center.

8. ANOREXIA / M.C. Champion

8.1 Description

Anorexia is the lack (or loss) of appetite. Anorexia is a common and important, but nonspecific, symptom. It can be a presenting feature in patients with organic or psychological disease. Anorexia and weight loss may be the early signs of malignancy.

8.2 Mechanism

The hypothalamus plays a major role in regulating the intake of food. There appear to be a "satiety center" and a "feeding center" in the hypothalamus, which exert the fundamental control of food intake. Stimulation of the satiety center inhibits the feeding center and gastric hunger contractions. The feeding center is an integrative station that coordinates complex reflexes associated with food intake.

8.3 History and Physical

The history should detect other symptoms that may suggest underlying organic or psychological disease. A calorie count is also helpful to assess the actual intake of food. The amount and duration of weight loss should also be documented.

Physical examination may be normal except for evidence of weight loss. It may point to the underlying organic problem, such as cardiac failure or malignancy.

8.4 Differential Diagnosis

Many (and perhaps most) illnesses feature a loss of appetite. These range from gastrointestinal disease to malignancy, chronic renal failure, congestive heart failure and many psychiatric diseases, such as depression and anorexia nervosa.

8.5 Approach to Investigation and Management

Investigation should exclude organic disease. The approach depends upon the patient's symptoms and signs. If no physical ailment is discovered, careful screening may be necessary to exclude psychiatric disease.

9. GAS AND BLOATING / W.G. Thompson

9.1 Synonyms

Burbulence, flatulence, burp, belch, borborygmi, gaseous distention, wind, flatus, fart.

9.2 Description

Gas within the intestinal tract is normal. Nonetheless, many patients have one or more symptoms that they associate with "excess" gas. Gas symptoms may constitute a primary complaint. A *belch* occurs, often after a large meal, when swallowed air displaced by food is released from the stomach. The lower esophageal sphincter relaxes, and gas enters from the stomach. Then the upper esophageal (cricopharyngeal) sphincter relaxes and the air exits via the mouth. Such a satisfied belch is a sign of respect to the host in some countries. A *burp* might be considered a mini-belch. Some describe it as a release of gas from the esophagus rather than from the stomach.

Borborygmi is the name given to intestinal noise. Gaseous *distention* is a feeling of abdominal fullness or even the need to loosen clothing, which the patient interprets as being due to excess gas in the intestinal tract. Bloating is not necessarily accompanied by belching or farting. It may force a patient to loosen clothing "as if pregnant" and is a common feature of the irritable bowel syndrome. A *fart* is the release of gas (flatus, wind) from the anus.

9.3 Mechanism

Gas enters the gastrointestinal tract by the following means: (1) Stomach gas is mainly nitrogen and is a result of swallowed air. Neonates have gasless stomachs, as do children with esophageal atresia and adults with achalasia. The source of the nitrogen is swallowed air, which enters with food, with dry swallows, or by the unconscious sucking of air into the chest. This latter mechanism is consciously used by patients with laryngectomy to generate esophageal speech. With many tummy troubles, belching and burping feel good; some patients unconsciously learn to belch by this mechanism. (2) The interaction of hydrochloric acid with bicarbonate in the duodenum releases carbon dioxide. The high diffusing capacity of CO_2 allows it to quickly enter the bloodstream. (3) Small amounts of any gas may enter the gut, depending upon the relative partial pressures between the lumen and the intravascular fluids. (4) The most important source of gas in the lower intestinal tract is the fermentation of unabsorbed nutrients (particularly glycoproteins) by colonic bacteria.

These gaseous symptoms by themselves are seldom hallmarks of organic disease. However, patients with acute enteritis, upper gastrointestinal hemorrhage or malabsorption may have peristaltic rushes, which exaggerate borborygmi and the feeling of distention and flatus. Increased solutes reaching the colon provide extra sources of gas.

Some individuals do produce excess flatus because of increased production of carbon dioxide and hydrogen, and some generate methane from the colon. Perhaps the colonic bacterial flora unique to each individual produces too much or consumes too little of these gases. We all recognize that vegetables containing certain carbohydrates (e.g., beans, cabbage) may result in increased gas production.

For most patients complaining of gaseous distention or bloating, the volume of gas in the gut is no greater than normal. The gas that is present, however, moves abnormally, suggesting that this is a manifestation of disordered gut motility. The exact origin of the symptom is unknown.

9.4 Important Historical Points and Physical Examination Features

People complaining of excessive belching are almost certainly repeatedly swallowing air. They may be able to belch on command. If this is the case the physician often can demonstrate how air sucked into the esophagus is then repeated. Such a demonstration may clinch the diagnosis and suggest remedial action to the patient.

Dietary history will identify those vegetables, or milk or other foods that will generate excess gas. One should look for evidence of intestinal disease such as weight loss, nutritional deficiencies and diarrhea.

9.5 Differential Diagnosis

Excess gas production is seldom a sign of serious organic disease unless there are major accompanying symptoms. Pyloric obstruction may lead to bacterial overgrowth in the stomach, which ferments food. This is a rare cause of belching and burping. Enteritis or malabsorption need be excluded only if other features of these diseases are present.

9.6 Approach to Management

The belcher or burper may be trained to resist the temptation to ingest air. Those with gaseous distention and borborygmi might respond to reassurance and the use of bran to regulate bowel habit. Bran sometimes increases gas production by providing more substrate for colonic bacteria.

Once suspicious foods have been eliminated, there is little that one can offer the excessively flatulent patient. Using antibiotics to alter the colonic flora is dangerous and unlikely to be successful. The ingestion of activated charcoal works in a few cases, but most patients do not tolerate the mess.

10. CONSTIPATION / W.G. Thompson

10.1 Synonyms

Costiveness, obstipation.

10.2 Description

Constipation defies accurate definition. What is "normal" frequency? Ninety-five percent or more of the population have between three movements per day and three movements per week. Some people consider that fewer than three movements a week without discomfort or dissatisfaction is normal. The effort needed to pass the stool and the consistency of the stool are probably of greater importance. Most would agree that hard bowel movements that are difficult to pass constitute constipation even if they occur as often as daily. One definition of constipation is the need to strain at stool on more than 25% of occasions. Thus constipation may be defined as persistent symptoms of difficult, infrequent or seemingly incomplete evacuation.

10.3 Mechanism

The causes of constipation are summarized in Table 1; organic causes are discussed elsewhere in this text. The commonest kind of constipation is that associated with the spastic colon type of irritable bowel. In this instance, the stool is hard, difficult to pass, and often scybalous (i.e., like rabbit stools or sheep stools). Frequently, passage of such stools is accompanied by abdominal pain.

TABLE 1. Causes of chronic constipation

Functional
Irritable bowel syndrome

Motility disorders of unknown mechanism
Atonic colon
Failure of defecation
    Obstruction by hyperactive anal sphincter
    Impaired rectoanal reflex

Pharmacologic
Opiates, antidepressants, calcium
Laxative abuse

Organic
Hypothyroidism
Depression
Hirschsprung's disease
Pseudo-obstruction
    Hollow viscera myopathy
    Hollow viscera neuropathy
Obstructing lesions (e.g., carcinoma, diverticulitis)

Some other functional causes of constipation are difficult to define. In simple atonic constipation, stool in the rectum fails to stimulate the defecation reflex. That is, a full rectum fails to initiate the evacuating response of the internal sphincter. In others, there is no gastrocolonic response to a meal. Still others are part of a generalized motility disorder called chronic idiopathic intestinal pseudo-obstruction. This disorder may be confined to the colon, but often affects other parts of the gastrointestinal tract. In this group must be included problems associated with long-standing use or abuse of laxatives. It is not certain whether the laxative use causes or results from the motility disorder.

10.4 Important Historical Points and Physical Examination Features
The physician's questions should elicit details about the nature of the stool. The presence of hard, pellet-like, difficult-to-pass stools, sometimes with a little bit of blood coating the edge, in an otherwise healthy young person strongly suggests the irritable bowel syndrome. On rectal examination or sigmoidoscopy the rectum is often empty or contains only scybala. This type of constipation is often interspersed with periods of normalcy or diarrhea.

The atonic type of constipation, on the other hand, is associated with a full colon and/or rectum. Often, examination of the abdomen reveals distention, and one may palpate large amounts of stool in the more proximal colon.

Various sensory or anorectal dysfunctions may also cause constipation.

Constipation and blood mixed with the stool raise the possibility of an obstructing lesion, such as a carcinoma. Hirschsprung's disease may present in adults, although usually there is a history of childhood disability. Other possibilities include a spinal lesion, hypothyroidism, hypercalcemia or drug use (e.g., opiates).

10.5 Approach to Diagnosis
Sigmoidoscopic examination using either the rigid or flexible instrument is necessary to rule out local diseases such as fissures, fistulas or distal proctitis. Many cancers are within the range of the sigmoidoscope. One might also detect melanosis coli, a pigment in the rectal mucosa that indicates chronic laxative use.

If the constipated patient is over 40, has blood or pus in the stool, or has had significant weight loss, a barium enema is indicated to rule out polyps, cancer or Crohn's disease of the colon.

A gut transit study may be revealing. Twenty radiopaque markers are ingested and daily plain abdominal x-rays are taken. If the markers have disappeared in five days, the transit time is said to be normal. In cases of longer transit, the position of the markers may help distinguish colonic inertia from anorectal disorder. More sophisticated studies are then required.

10.6 Approach to Management
Obviously, the best management of constipation is to treat any underlying disease. For the spastic type of irritable colon, a good response can be expected if sufficient bulk is added to the diet. It is best to avoid the chronic use of stimulant laxatives because of their potential to damage the myenteric plexus in the colon. If overused, laxatives may cause excessive loss of fluids and electrolytes. Colonic inertia or anorectal dysfunction causing severe constipation or obstipation requires specialist care.

11. DIARRHEA / W.G. Thompson

11.1 Synonyms
Lax bowels, the flux.

11.2 Description
Diarrhea is best described as too frequent passage of too loose (unformed)

stools. Diarrhea is frequently accompanied by urgency, and occasionally incontinence. When considering a patient with diarrhea the following must be considered: frequency (>3 movements/day), consistency (loose/watery), urgency, volume (>200 g/day) and whether the condition is continuous. Persistent, frequent, loose, urgent, large-volume stools are most likely to have a pathology. Lesser and intermittent symptoms are more likely to be functional.

11.3 Mechanism

Diarrhea is due to one or more of four mechanisms: osmotic attraction of water into the lumen of the gut, secretion of excess fluid into the gut (or decreased absorption), exudation of fluid from the inflamed surface of the gut, and rapid gastrointestinal transit.

Osmotic diarrhea results if the osmotic pressure of intestinal contents is higher than that of the serum. This may result from malabsorption of fat (e.g., in celiac disease) or of lactose (e.g., in intestinal lactase deficiency). Certain laxatives, such as lactulose and magnesium hydroxide, exert their cathartic effect largely through osmosis. Certain artificial sweeteners, such as sorbitol and mannitol, have a similar effect. Characteristically, osmotic diarrhea ceases when the patient fasts.

Secretory diarrhea occurs when there is a net secretion of water into the lumen. This may occur with bacterial toxins, such as those produced by E. coli or Vibrio cholerae, or with hormones, such as vasoactive intestinal polypeptide (VIP), which is produced by rare islet cell tumors (pancreatic cholera). These provoke adenylate cyclase activity in the enterocyte (intestinal epithelial cell), increase cyclic AMP and turn on intestinal secretion. A similar effect may occur as a result of excess bile salts in the colon (choleretic enteropathy) and from the cathartic affect of hydroxylated fatty acids resulting from the bacterial action on malabsorbed fat. Such a diarrhea does not diminish with fasting. Osmotic and secretory diarrhea result from abnormalities in the small intestine such that the flow of water through the ileocecal area overcomes the absorptive capacity of the colon.

Exudative diarrhea results from direct damage to the small or large intestinal mucosa. This interferes with the absorption of sodium salts and water and is complicated by exudation of serum proteins, blood and pus. Infectious or inflammatory disorders of the gut cause this kind of diarrhea.

Acceleration of intestinal transit may result in diarrhea (e.g., as a result of hyperthyroidism). The rapid flow-through impairs the ability of the gut to absorb water, resulting in diarrhea. In most instances of diarrhea two or more of these four mechanisms are at work.

11.4 Important Historical Points and Physical Examination Features

It is important to establish the frequency of defecation, the duration of the diarrhea, the nature of the stool and its volume. If diarrhea has been present for less than two weeks, it is most likely a result of an infection or toxin. A history of many previous attacks, on the other hand, may indicate a recurrence of inflammatory bowel disease. The frequency of the stool gives some idea of severity; one should establish whether incontinence is also present. To elicit the latter history may require direct or leading questions. Stool from malabsorption is often foul-smelling and contains oil droplets. A history of nutrient deficiency, anemia or weight loss also suggests malabsorption. Watery diarrhea, particularly when large in volume, supports a diagnosis of small bowel disease. A large villous adenoma of the distal colon may produce a watery diarrhea. The presence of blood or pus in the stool suggests an exudative diarrhea, a type of diarrhea that is often relatively small in volume. Loose bowel movements interspersed with normal or even constipated ones are evidence of the irritable bowel syndrome.

There are many causes of diarrhea (Table 2). The presence of profound weight loss and malnutrition in a young person points to a malabsorption syndrome due to small bowel or pancreatic disease or to inflammatory bowel disease. Metabolic conditions such as hyperthyroidism or the overuse of (magnesium-containing) antacids or laxatives might also be responsible for chronic diarrhea.

Travel to tropical countries can be marred by an attack of so-called traveler's diarrhea. The most common cause is toxigenic E. coli (it is known as toxigenic because a toxin is produced). However, a large variety of intestinal infestations can occur with travel. Pseudomembranous colitis may occur within weeks of the use of antibiotics. Campylobacter or cryptococcosis may be acquired from pets. Contaminated water may result in giardiasis, amebiasis or cryptococcosis. Chronic use of alcohol may damage the small intestinal mucosa. Diabetics frequently have diarrhea because of autonomic neuropathy, perhaps with bacterial overgrowth.

Finally, it is essential to establish if the patient has an alternative sexual preference. Almost any of the usual gastrointestinal pathogens can be spread by homosexual activity, including lymphogranuloma venereum and gonococcus. In addition to the "gay bowel syndrome," homosexuals are liable to the gastrointestinal complications of AIDS.

11.5 Differential Diagnosis and Management

The differential diagnosis is very complex. A careful history is often the most important diagnostic tool. Patients examined for the first time deserve at least

TABLE 2.   Anatomic approach to the causes of chronic diarrhea

Gastric
Dumping syndrome

Small intestine
Celiac disease
Lymphoma
Whipple's disease
Bacterial, viral or parasitic infection
Abnormal intestinal tract motility with bacterial overgrowth (scleroderma, amyloidosis, diabetes, hyperthyroidism)

Large bowel
Villous adenoma (adenocarcinoma)
Inflammatory bowel disease (ulcerative colitis, Crohn's disease)
Irritable bowel (diarrhea phase)
Functional diarrhea

Pancreatic
Chronic pancreatitis
Islet cell tumors
    Gastrin secretions
    VIP secretions

Drugs
Antacids
Antibiotics
Alcohol
Antimetabolites
Laxatives
Digitalis
Colchicine
Sorbitol, fructose
Many others

Metabolic
Hyperthyroidism
Hypoparathyroidism
Addison's disease
Diabetes
Carcinoid syndrome

a sigmoidoscopy to rule out local colon disease. If a small intestinal diarrhea is suspected, a three-day collection of stool to determine daily weight and fat content is necessary. If there is steatorrhea, or if stool weight exceeds 500 g per day, there is likely to be small intestinal or pancreatic disease. Smaller volumes, particularly if accompanied by blood, point to inflammation of the colon.

The recent onset of acute diarrhea requires careful examination of the stool for pus cells and culture for bacterial pathogens, or a study for ova and parasites in the case of suspected protozoa. Viral studies are important in infants, and special studies are required in AIDS.

12. MALNUTRITION / D.G. Patel

12.1 Description
Nutrition may be defined as the process by which an organism utilizes food. This complex process involves ingestion, digestion, absorption, transport, utilization and excretion. Any alteration in one or many of these factors can produce malnutrition. Globally, primary malnutrition due to lack of food is the most common cause of malnutrition. Malnutrition in the Western world is mainly due to inadequate intake of nutrients, malabsorption and/or the hypercatabolism accompanying a critical illness. Protein-energy undernutrition is increasingly recognized in eating disorders such as anorexia nervosa.

12.2 Mechanism
The malnutrition associated with gastrointestinal disorders is usually multifactorial and varies with the nature and activity of the disease.

1. Lack of food intake due to anorexia or food-related symptoms such as dysphagia, pain or vomiting.
2. Maldigestion due to pancreatic disease. Deficiency of bile salts due to cholestatic hepatobiliary disease or to ileal disease leads to maldigestion of triglyceride and lipid-soluble vitamins. Steatorrhea (fat malabsorption) produces negative caloric balance and deficiency of fat-soluble vitamins.
3. Malabsorption due to mucosal disease of the small intestine or loss of surface area due to intestinal bypass, fistula or resection.
4. Excessive loss of nutrients, as in protein-losing enteropathy and loss of zinc in diarrheal illness.
5. Therapeutic agents that may selectively affect nutrient utilization – e.g., cholestyramine use for bile acid–induced diarrhea can worsen steatorrhea.
6. Alcoholism – an extremely common cause of malnutrition in the Western

world. Social and economic status, behavior problems, isolation and depression cause reduced intake of nutrients. Alcoholics rarely consume a well-balanced diet and depend very heavily on "empty" calories from alcohol. Protein and vitamin deficiencies, particularly of the B-complex group, are extremely common. Alcohol is a toxic agent that even in the presence of adequate nutritional intake can produce damage to the pancreas, liver and small bowel mucosa, aggravating malnutrition.

12.3 Signs of Malnutrition

1. Weight loss in the absence of edema is a good indicator of energy deficiency.
2. Muscle wasting, particularly in the temporal area and dorsum of the hand between thumb and index finger, suggests protein-calorie deficiency.
3. Dry, scaly skin with pigmentation results from vitamin and trace metal deficiency.
4. Angular mouth fissure (cheilosis) is due to riboflavin deficiency.
5. Glossitis and depapillation of the tongue are due to B_{12}, folate or iron deficiency.
6. Hepatomegaly may be due to fatty liver, a common finding in protein malnutrition or alcoholism.
7. Peripheral neuropathy (decreased position sense), decreased vibration sense or ataxia may result from B_{12} deficiency.
8. Weakness and paresthesia of the legs are signs of nutritional polyneuropathy, especially in alcoholics (due to thiamine or pyridoxine deficiency).

13. ACUTE ABDOMEN / S. Meban

13.1 Description

The term *acute abdomen* describes an urgent situation in which abdominal symptoms onset suddenly and are sufficiently severe to suggest a potentially lethal condition. Pain is usually the predominant feature. Since many "acute abdomens" require prompt treatment, it is important to make a diagnosis as soon as possible.

13.2 Mechanism

Acute abdominal pain may be referred to the abdominal wall from the intra-abdominal organs or may involve direct stimulation of the somatic nerves in the abdominal wall. Less commonly, pain may be referred to the abdomen from extra-abdominal sites. On occasion, acute abdominal pain is a feature of systemic disease.

Visceral pain. This type of pain is carried by the sympathetic autonomic nerves and enters the spinal cord from T6 to L2. The parasympathetic system also carries pain sensation from the pelvic organs via S2, 3 and 4. The nerve supply to viscera arising from the primitive gut is bilateral, and pain is usually experienced in the midline. Foregut pain is epigastric in location. Midgut pain is umbilical, and hindgut pain is felt in the hypogastrium. Organs that are bilateral give rise to pain that is confined to one or the other side of the body.

Somatic pain. Somatic afferents supplying the abdominal wall enter the spinal cord between T5 and L2. Additionally, the undersurface of the diaphragm has innervation from the phrenic nerve (C3, 4 and 5). Thus, irritation of the diaphragm may refer pain to the shoulder.

The stimulus to pain may be chemical irritation from a perforated peptic ulcer or bacterial contamination from perforation of the colon. Other stimuli include ischemia and distention (or stretching) of the gut or parietal peritoneum. Direct pressure on a nerve by a prolapsed intervertebral disc or tumor may result in abdominal pain.

Pain perception may be altered by aberrant function of the pain-conducting pathways. There is also marked variation in the pain "threshold" of individuals.

13.3 History

Severe pain of sudden onset suggests a catastrophic event – e.g., perforation of an ulcer, mesenteric embolism or rupture of aortic aneurysm. The level of referral gives a clue to the organ in which the pain originates. Visceral pain is less precise in location than somatic pain.

Steady, severe pain is usually more ominous than colicky pain. Biliary colic is a misnomer, in that the pain is often steady (unlike the true colic of bowel obstruction or a ureteric stone). The latter corresponds to peristaltic waves and eases or disappears between waves.

Radiation patterns are important clues. Irritation of the diaphragm from blood in the peritoneal cavity may cause shoulder tip pain. Biliary pain may radiate to the right scapular region.

13.4 Associated Symptoms

Anorexia, nausea and vomiting are nonspecific but more common in disease of the GI tract. Abdominal distention and change in bowel habit suggest obstruction. Blood in the stool may come from ulceration, tumor or infarction. In women an accurate menstrual history aids the diagnosis of ovarian disease, ectopic pregnancy and pelvic inflammatory disease.

13.5 Physical Examination

Examination is carried out with the patient in the supine position. Preferably, analgesia should be delayed until a diagnosis is made to avoid masking physical signs.

Inspection should note any abdominal distention or local masses. The patient with peritonitis lies immobile, as any movement increases peritoneal irritation. With colic the patient may be restless, seeking a more comfortable position.

Gentle palpation may detect masses. It also detects tenderness and muscle guarding or rigidity, which might suggest peritoneal irritation.

Percussion is useful to assess the nature of abdominal distention or to outline masses. Percussion is also helpful as a "mini rebound" test that more accurately localizes the point of maximum tenderness. It is also much less distressing to the patient with peritonitis.

Auscultation may reveal a range of bowel sounds, from the silent abdomen of peritonitis to the hyperactive sounds of bowel obstruction. Bruits suggest vascular disease, but an epigastric bruit may also be found normally.

Rectal examination should be carried out and recorded by at least one examiner. Tenderness above the peritoneal reflection indicates pelvic peritonitis (e.g., appendicitis or diverticulitis).

Pelvic examination may be necessary to help exclude a gynecological cause of abdominal pain.

13.6 Differential Diagnosis

Apart from abdominal and extra-abdominal causes of abdominal pain, one should also consider nonsurgical causes such as diabetic ketoacidosis.

13.7 Approach to Diagnosis

In most cases a good history and a thorough physical examination provide the clinical diagnosis. Complete blood count (CBC) and urinalysis are standard, in addition to serum amylase and electrolytes when indicated. A serum lactate level should be done if bowel ischemia is suspected. Chest x-ray and views of the abdomen help narrow the differential diagnosis.

More sophisticated tests may be necessary. Ultrasound is very useful in the diagnosis of biliary tract disease. Plain films of the abdomen will show large bowel obstruction, but a barium enema may be required to show the level of obstruction and to exclude pseudo-obstruction. Intravenous pyelography can demonstrate kidney nonfunction or hydroureter in suspected renal pain. An opaque calculus may be seen on plain abdominal x-rays. In suspected bowel ischemia, mesenteric angiography is essential. In diverticulitis a Gastrografin®

enema can be helpful. Increasingly the abdominal CT scan is being used for diagnosis of the acute abdomen. The most appropriate investigation should be discussed with a radiologist.

13.8 Approach to Management
This will depend on diagnosis. In the early stages it may be impossible to distinguish the colic of acute enteritis from appendicitis. Only careful observation and repeated examination allow differentiation. Many abdominal pains settle without a confirmed diagnosis. Occasionally peritonitis requires laparotomy without a clear-cut preoperative diagnosis.

14. CHRONIC ABDOMEN / W.G. Thompson

14.1 Synonym
Recurrent abdominal pain in children.

14.2 Description
Ten percent of children suffer recurrent abdominal pain and approximately 20% of adults have abdominal pain at least six times per year unrelated to menstruation. The pain is chronic when it has been present for six months or more. It may be related to gastrointestinal functions such as eating and defecation. It is often a feature of dyspepsia or the irritable bowel syndrome. Occasionally, the pain has no relationship to bodily functions, and no gastrointestinal, hepatobiliary, genital or renal cause for the pain can be found.

14.3 Causes and Mechanism
The mechanisms of abdominal pain are discussed above, in Section 13 ("Acute Abdomen"). Of course, chronic abdominal pain may be caused by many organic diseases. *Peptic ulcer* generally produces pain after meals or on an empty stomach and is relieved by food or antacid. Abdominal pain awakening the patient at night is a particularly discriminating feature.

Biliary colic may be due to cystic or common bile duct obstruction by a stone. Characteristically this pain is significant enough to awaken the patient at night or require a visit to the emergency room for analgesia. It lasts from 1 hour to 12 hours; beyond 17 hours, consider acute cholecystitis or pancreatitis. Attacks are sporadic and at intervals, not continuous. Biliary pain is located in the epigastrium, the right upper quadrant and/or the right scapula. It leaves the patient shaken but well. Should the gallbladder become inflamed, cholecystitis results. Obstruction of the common bile duct with a stone results in pain, jaundice and sometimes fever.

Pancreatitis is a devastating illness, with steady epigastric pain radiating to the back and sometimes accompanied by shock. It almost always requires admission to hospital.

Ischemic bowel disease, subacute bowel obstruction caused by Crohn's disease, *neoplasm* or *volvulus* may present with recurrent bouts of abdominal pain, often related to eating. These conditions are usually progressive and accompanied by physical signs.

In a patient with *diverticular disease*, a peridiverticular abscess may develop, causing recurrent bouts of severe left lower quadrant abdominal pain and fever. Usually, diverticula are asymptomatic and symptoms that do occur are those of coincident irritable bowel syndrome.

Renal colic due to a stone in the ureter is rarely chronic but may be recurrent. It consists of severe flank pain radiating to the groin and testicle, and may be accompanied by hematuria. Typically, a patient smitten with renal colic is unable to lie still.

Gynecologic conditions ranging from mittelschmerz (ruptured ovarian cyst) to pelvic inflammatory disease may account for recurrent abdominal pain. Menstruation-related pain in a young woman suggests endometriosis. Chronic pelvic pain often relates to the irritable bowel syndrome.

Chronic appendicitis probably does not exist.

The organic abdominal pains are presented elsewhere under the discussion of the underlying illness. *Functional abdominal pain* may originate in any part of the gastrointestinal tract or biliary tree. It is unrelated to bodily function and may be continuous. It is uncertain whether the pain is due to a normal perception of abnormal gut motility or an abnormal perception of normal motility; there are frequently accompanying psychosocial difficulties.

14.4 Important Historical Points and Physical Examination Features

Pain, when related to a bodily function – defecation, eating, micturition or menstruation – focuses the investigation upon the involved system. Certain physical findings (such as an abdominal mass, or blood or mass upon rectal examination) point to specific organic diseases. Fever, weight loss, rectal bleeding and/or anemia indicate further tests.

14.5 Differential Diagnosis, Diagnosis and Management

Management of the organic causes of the chronic abdomen can be directed at the underlying disease process. In many instances, however, there is no organic basis. Here, the physician's responsibility is to reassure the patient that no serious disease exists, and help the patient coexist with the symptoms in the light of the patient's social background. One might improve digestion through regular and better eating habits, and treat bowel dysfunction, particularly constipation, with increased dietary bulk.

14.6 Pain and Emotion

There are patients who have severe recurrent abdominal pain unrelated to bodily function or organic disease. Such patients see many doctors without satisfaction; the genesis of the symptom is thought to be psychogenic. This pain is often given such descriptors as "illness behavior" and "pain proneness." Some have hypochondriasis and do not improve when organic disease has been disproved. An extreme example is the Münchausen syndrome, where the patient deliberately relates a tall tale of medical duress in order to precipitate treatment, perhaps even surgery.

Functional pain is frequent in those who have recent conflicts, have experienced a death in the family, or have become overly concerned with fatal illness. Depression and anxiety are frequent. Here, it is important not to carry out extensive investigation in a fruitless search for an elusive cause. This only reinforces the patient's belief that something is wrong and undermines the patient's confidence in the benign diagnosis.

Such pain may be an emotional expression, in which case regular visits are necessary to allow the patient to vent his or her problems. Drugs, especially narcotics, should be used with restraint, and the physician should strive to develop a strong doctor–patient relationship while dealing with the patient's depression, anxiety, frustration and often hostility. These patients test our skill in the art rather than the science of medicine.

15. JAUNDICE / L.J. Scully

15.1 Definition

A syndrome characterized by increased serum bilirubin levels and a yellow appearance due to deposition of bile pigment in the skin and mucus membranes.

15.2 Mechanism

Bilirubin is a waste product of hemoglobin metabolism. Interruption of the breakdown pathway at any of a number of steps, or a marked increase in load due to red cell destruction, results in an increase in serum bilirubin and (if high enough) clinical jaundice.

Under normal circumstances senescent red blood cells are taken up and destroyed in the reticuloendothelial system. Through a number of steps the heme molecule of hemoglobin is converted to bilirubin and, tightly bound to albumin, is transported in the plasma to the liver cells. Hepatocytes take up bilirubin, conjugate it to glucuronide and excrete the bilirubin diglucuronide in bile into the duodenum. In the bowel, bacteria break down bilirubin to urobilinogen, 80% of which is excreted in the feces, contributing to the normal stool color. The remaining 20% is reabsorbed and excreted in bile and urine (enterohepatic circulation of urobilinogen).

Functional or anatomic obstruction at almost any level in this pathway (from hemoglobin breakdown to uptake by the hepatocellular membrane to excretion into the biliary system) will result in jaundice, with an increase in serum bilirubin. A large increase in the breakdown products of hemoglobin alone (e.g., hemolytic anemia) will cause an increase in serum unconjugated bilirubin. If the problem lies after the uptake and conjugation step, the increase is in serum conjugated bilirubin. Causes of jaundice are usually classified as (1) hemolysis, (2) genetic defects in bilirubin handling, (3) hepatocellular disease and (4) obstruction.

15.3 Clinical Presentation
Clinical jaundice is detected when the serum bilirubin level reaches 2–4 mg/dL (40–80 µmol/L). It is usually preceded by a few days of pale stools (as excretion of bilirubin into the intestine is decreased) and dark urine (due to increased glomerular filtration of conjugated bilirubin). Jaundice is usually first detected in the sclera, although the bilirubin is actually deposited in the overlying conjunctival membranes. Yellow skin without scleral icterus should suggest carotenemia or the ingestion of such drugs as quinacrine.

Most patients with jaundice, excluding those in whom it is secondary to hemolysis, have nausea, anorexia and discomfort over the liver. There may be hepatomegaly, masses in the epigastrium or pancreas or a dilatated gallbladder. Signs of chronic liver disease such as spider nevi or palmar erythema are important. Pruritus may result, presumably from the deposition of bile salts (or a retained pruritogen normally excreted in bile) in the skin.

Several genetic defects in the conjugation or excretion of bilirubin may cause long-standing unconjugated or conjugated hyperbilirubinemia.

15.4 Approach to Diagnosis
Initially the most important information is whether the jaundice is due to conjugated or unconjugated hyperbilirubinemia (Figure 3). Serum bilirubin can be fractionated from "total" into conjugated and unconjugated, but the presence of bile in the urine determined by a test strip at the bedside confirms that the bilirubin rise is predominantly in the conjugated form. If the bilirubin is unconjugated, hemolysis or genetic defects are implicated. If the bilirubin is

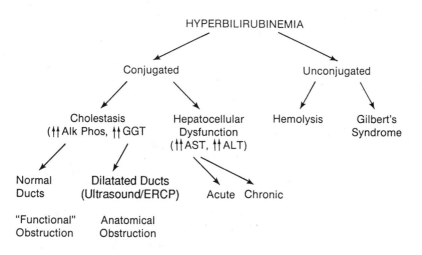

FIGURE 3.   Causes of hyperbilirubinemia.

conjugated, "liver biochemical tests" (AST, ALT, GGT and alkaline phosphatase) will help determine if the jaundice is primarily due to obstruction/cholestasis (high GGT and alkaline phosphatase) or hepatocellular damage (high AST and ALT). Cholestatic jaundice requires ultrasound as the best, first test to detect biliary tract disease. If the jaundice is cholestatic, then an ultrasound of the abdomen is required to determine if there is obstruction of the ducts or intrahepatic bile duct dilatation.

15.5 Management
The management of obstructive jaundice is directed toward the cause where possible (e.g., removal of obstructing gallstone). Jaundice secondary to hepatocellular disease, such as viral hepatitis, does not require any specific treatment. Jaundice due to alcohol, toxin or drug requires withdrawal of the offending agent.

16. ASCITES IN CHRONIC LIVER DISEASE / L.J. Scully

16.1 Definition
Ascites is the accumulation of nonsanguinous fluid in the peritoneal cavity.

16.2 Mechanisms
With significant liver disease, albumin synthesis is reduced. Low serum albu-

TABLE 3. The important causes of upper GI bleeding

Duodenal ulcer
Gastric ulcer
Gastric erosions
Ulcerative esophagitis
Esophagogastric varices
Mallory-Weiss tear
Carcinoma, lymphoma
Angiodysplasia

min results in a decrease in intravascular osmotic pressure. This causes renal blood flow changes, resulting in sodium and water retention. Increased aldosterone levels, possibly due to decreased catabolism of this hormone by the liver, also contribute. There is a generalized salt and water retention, but the fluid accumulation may be confined to the peritoneal cavity or may be associated with peripheral edema. Ascites develops because of increased portal pressure and the transudation of fluid from the capillaries in the portal system to the peritoneal cavity. Hepatic lymph production also increases and extravasates directly into the peritoneal cavity.

16.3 Signs and Symptoms
Ascites most commonly presents with increasing abdominal girth, often associated with an uncomfortable feeling of distention, and sometimes nausea and anorexia. Shortness of breath may develop, resulting from either elevation of the diaphragm or pleural effusion. Ankle edema may accompany ascites.

Clinical examination reveals flank fullness on inspection. "Shifting dullness" or a "fluid thrill" may be elicited. Smaller amounts of fluid may be detected on ultrasound when clinical signs are absent. One should look for other signs of portal hypertension, such as dilatated abdominal wall veins or an enlarged spleen.

16.4 Differential Diagnosis
Newly developed ascites must have a diagnostic aspiration to determine the albumin level, cell count and cytology. The fluid should be clear and straw-colored. Occasionally, lymph can accumulate in the peritoneal cavity, causing "chylous ascites," which requires different management. Ascitic fluid may become infected, in which case the white blood cell count will be elevated in the fluid. If the fluid is sanguinous, other causes – such as infection or malignancy – must be sought. The serum ascites albumin gradient is the best way of

TABLE 4.   The important causes of lower GI bleeding

Hemorrhoids, anal fissure
Carcinoma, adenomatous polyps
Angiodysplasia
Ulcerative colitis
Crohn's disease
Diverticular disease
Ischemic colitis
Certain bacterial infections
Amebic colitis
Meckel's diverticulum

---

confirming if the ascitic fluid is secondary to portal hypertension. In this situation the gradient is high – i.e., >11 g/L – whereas it is low if the ascites is due to peritoneal carcinomatosis. This is far more accurate than our previous assessment of transudative versus exudative ascites.

16.5 Approach to Management
Management initially includes bed rest and salt restriction. Most cases also require adding a diuretic such as spironolactone. Careful aspiration of large quantities (up to 4 L) of ascitic fluid may be necessary in some resistant cases; this can be safely performed if an intravenous infusion of albumin is given before the paracentesis.

17. GASTROINTESTINAL BLEEDING / R.R. Gillies

17.1 Description
Blood issuing from the GI tract is a cause for alarm, and justifiably so! The visible evidence is described as hematemesis, hematochezia and/or melena.

Hematemesis – vomited blood, either red (fresh) or dark brown (altered by reaction with HCl) – comes from a source proximal to the duodenojejunal junction.

Hematochezia – blood in the stool – comes from the left colon, or even above if the volume of blood is large and the transit rapid.

Melena – black, tarry, smelly stool, looser and larger with larger hemorrhages – comes from the upper GI tract, in which case bacterial action has longer to break down the blood. It may even come from the lower tract when transit is delayed. The important causes of upper gastrointestinal bleeding are shown in Table 3, and of lower gastrointestinal bleeding in Table 4.

17.2 Important Historical Points and Physical Examination Features

Vomiting blood usually signifies a major hemorrhage. In a briskly bleeding duodenal ulcer, rapid transit may result in passage of red blood and clots per rectum without vomiting. Even before being passed per rectum, a large hemorrhage into the upper tract will announce itself by hyperactive bowel sounds. It is obvious that such a large-volume blood loss will have major cardiovascular effects compared to a rectal lesion causing passage of red blood and clots.

The symptoms associated with blood loss may occur before any blood appears externally (e.g., the features of an acute anemia – weakness, faintness, sweating, pallor, thirst and collapse). While the first clues as to the site of bleeding are gathered, we need to know more about how the patient is tolerating the blood loss. A rapid, thready pulse; hypotension; cold, sweaty skin; and pallor tell us that emergency restoration of blood volume is needed to keep the patient alive. Vital signs may be normal while the patient is recumbent, but a blood pressure fall of 15 mm Hg when the patient sits up indicates a significant blood loss. Cardiovascular compensation may be perfect – for the moment! A large-diameter IV line (at least 18 gauge) must be inserted. The patient should be given first saline or plasma and then, as soon as it is available, blood as indicated by any features of hypovolemia.

Once resuscitation is under way, one can assess the site and etiology of the bleeding. First, take a detailed history, particularly noting upper and lower GI symptoms, previous episodes of bleeding, previous GI surgery, ASA or NSAID intake, ethanol abuse, and diseases or treatments that could cause clotting defects. Ulcer pain often stops as bleeding starts; ulcer pain does not precede ulcer bleeding in 20–25% of cases.

Next, do a thorough physical examination, with attention to vascular lesions of the skin and mucosa, ecchymoses, the liver, peripheral signs of cirrhosis, splenomegaly and prominent superficial abdominal veins. Inspection of the nares and oropharynx avoids the embarrassment of missing epistaxis as a source of swallowed blood. Rectal examination allows stool examination.

17.3 Approach to Diagnosis (Figure 4)

When the passage of blood from either end of the GI tract has been reported but not observed, or when hematochezia or melena without hematemesis has been observed, the passage of a nasogastric tube for a single aspiration will help determine if bleeding is proximal or distal to the pylorus. Providing the patient's response to IV volume replacement is satisfactory, one can make a decision as to the timing and type of investigation needed to identify the cause

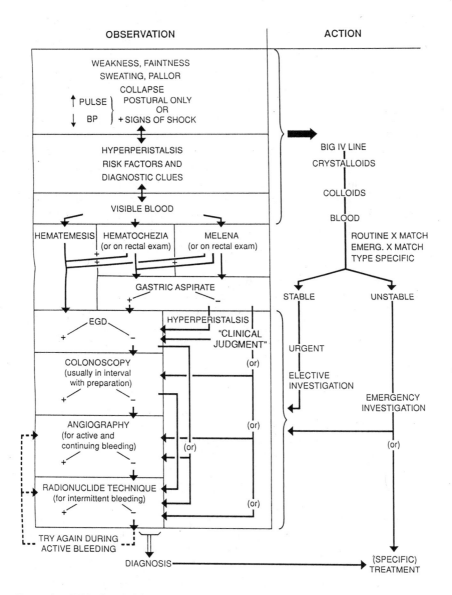

FIGURE 4.   GI bleeding decision tree.

of bleeding. Upper GI endoscopy is the most reliable technique to detect lesions proximal to the duodenojejunal junction. Sometimes perendoscopic injection, heater probe application or snare-cautery polypectomy may be employed to stop bleeding from identified lesions. Whether endoscopy is emergent, urgent or elective depends on the status of the patient. Remember that the status may rapidly deteriorate. One must be prepared to change the plan just as rapidly.

Bleeding lower GI tract lesions may be identified and treated endoscopically. Usually this is feasible only later, after proper bowel preparation removes the accumulated blood. When active bleeding continues from the small or large bowel, mesenteric angiography is the best choice to discover the bleeding site. If the bleeding is less brisk and is intermittent, radionuclide imaging may point to the site. Bleeding must occur during either test to make it useful.

When all else fails, total enteroscopy – endoscopy of the entire small bowel – should be done. Usually this is more efficient at laparotomy where the surgeon can assist by manipulating the loops of bowel over the advancing scope.

17.4 Approach to Management
Remember that the objective is a live patient. Continued, careful assessment of the patient's cardiovascular response to blood loss and replacement will guide interventions, including surgical. Specific treatment depends upon the underlying disease and will be dealt with in subsequent sections.

18. ABDOMINAL MASS / S. Gregoire

18.1 Description
When an abdominal mass is discovered on physical examination, one must define its nature. Using a systematic approach often permits the identification of the mass before the use of sophisticated tests.

18.2 Important Points in History and Physical Examination
Important clues in the history and general physical examination may help to identify the enlarged viscus. For example, the discovery of a nontender right upper quadrant mass in a jaundiced 72-year-old female who complains of pruritus, weight loss and anorexia, and who takes no medication or alcohol, suggests metastatic liver disease or cancer of the pancreas with an enlarged gallbladder. However, an abdominal mass may be discovered during physical examination of an asymptomatic individual. Certain observations made during the abdominal examination may be helpful.

18.2.1 *INSPECTION*
Where is the mass located? A practical approach is to divide the abdomen into four quadrants. Starting from the principle that an abdominal mass originates from an organ, surface anatomy may suggest which one is enlarged. A mass seen in the left lower quadrant, for example, could be of colonic or ovarian origin but, unless there is situs inversus, one would not consider an appendiceal abscess!

Does the mass move with respiration? In the upper abdomen a mobile intra-abdominal mass will move downward with inspiration with the hemidiaphragms, while a more fixed organ (e.g., aorta, pancreas) or an abdominal wall mass (e.g., hematoma of rectus muscle) will not.

18.2.2 *AUSCULTATION*
Careful auscultation for bowel sounds, bruit or rub over an abdominal mass is part of the systematic approach.

18.2.3 *DEFINING THE CONTOUR AND SURFACE OF THE MASS*
This is achieved by inspection, percussion and palpation. Is the organ air-filled (e.g., stomach) or fluid-filled? Is it a well-defined mass (e.g., liver, spleen) or are its borders difficult to define (matted loops of small bowel)? Is the surface regular? An enlarged liver due to fatty infiltration may have a smooth surface, while a cirrhotic organ is irregular and nodular. What is the consistency of the mass? Is it pulsatile? In the absence of ascites, ballottement of an organ situated in either upper quadrant more likely identifies an enlarged kidney (more posterior structure) than hepatomegaly or splenomegaly.

18.3 Differential Diagnosis
The following suggests an approach to the differential diagnosis of an abdominal mass located in each quadrant:

18.3.1 *RIGHT UPPER QUADRANT*
This location suggests liver, right kidney, gallbladder and, less commonly, a colon or gastroduodenal mass. A pancreatic mass is rarely palpable.

18.3.1.1 *Liver*
As a subdiaphragmatic organ, the liver moves downward with inspiration. This anterior organ has an easily palpable lower border, which permits assessment of its consistency. A bruit or venous hum can be heard in certain conditions.

18.3.1.2 Right kidney

The kidney may protrude anteriorly when enlarged and be difficult to differentiate from a Riedel's lobe of the liver. It may be balloted.

18.3.1.3 Gallbladder

This oval-shaped organ moves downward with inspiration and is usually smooth and regular.

18.3.1.4 Colon

Colon masses are deep and ill-defined, and do not move with respiration. High-pitched bowel sounds suggest obstruction.

18.3.2 LEFT UPPER QUADRANT

Location in the left upper quadrant suggests spleen or left kidney. Less commonly, a colonic (splenic flexure) or gastric mass can be felt. A pancreatic mass is rarely palpable.

18.3.2.1 Spleen

This anterior organ moves downward with inspiration. Since it has an oblique longitudinal axis, it extends toward the right lower quadrant when enlarged. It has a medial notch and the edge is sharp.

18.3.2.2 Left kidney

Its more posterior position and the presence of ballottement helps distinguish the left kidney from the spleen.

18.3.2.3 Colon, pancreas, stomach

It is practically impossible to differentiate masses in these by physical examination. The history helps but often one must resort to radiology or endoscopy.

18.3.3 RIGHT LOWER QUADRANT

A mass in this area has its origin either in the lower GI tract (colon, distal small bowel, appendix) or in a pelvic structure (ovary, uterus, fallopian tube).

18.3.3.1 Lower GI tract

These deeper organs are usually ill-defined, but occasionally the tubular shape of the cecum can be felt.

18.3.3.2 Pelvic organs

Bimanual palpation is the preferred method.

18.3.4 *LEFT LOWER QUADRANT*
As with a right lower quadrant mass, the differential diagnosis here is between lower GI (in this quadrant the sigmoid colon) and pelvic origin. The shape of the organ and pelvic examination should help differentiate the two.

18.4 Approach to Diagnosis
To complete the assessment of an abdominal mass, one may choose among several different investigational tools. The use of specific tests depends on availability and on the organ studied.

Generally, ultrasound is useful. This noninvasive, safe, cheap and widely available method identifies the mass and provides information on its origin and nature. Ultrasound may also be used to direct a biopsy. Other noninvasive modalities are nuclear imaging and CT scan. Hollow organs may be demonstrated radiographically through the use of contrast media (e.g., barium enema, GI series, intravenous pyelogram, endoscopic retrograde cholangiopancreatography, etc.). Sometimes, laparotomy will be necessary to make the diagnosis.

19. PROCTALGIA FUGAX / W.G. Thompson

19.1 Description
Proctalgia fugax is a sudden severe pain in the anus lasting several seconds or minutes and then disappearing completely.

19.2 Mechanism
The pathophysiology of proctalgia fugax is uncertain. Although some observations (under obviously fortuitous circumstances) suggest a rectal motility disorder, the symptom appears more likely to result from spasm of the skeletal muscle of the pelvic floor (specifically, the puborectalis).

19.3 History and Physical Examination
Proctalgia fugax occurs in about 14% of adults and is somewhat more common in females than males. The pain may be excruciating, but since it is so short-lived patients seldom report it to their physician. In 90% of instances it lasts less than five minutes and in many cases less than a minute. About one-third of patients suffer attacks following defecation. A small minority report attacks following sexual activity. There are no physical signs.

19.4 Differential Diagnosis
Perianal disease may cause pain but it usually accompanies, rather than fol-

lows, defecation. One should be particularly careful to exclude the presence of an anal fissure, which may be difficult to see on anal inspection. Pain originating from the coccyx may be accompanied by coccygeal tenderness both externally and from within the rectum.

19.5 Management
Beyond reassurance there is no treatment.

2
Nutrition in Gastrointestinal Disease

J.S. Whittaker, U.P. Steinbrecher, M. Lemoyne and H.J. Freeman

1. INTRODUCTION

FOOD ASSIMILATION is the major function of the gastrointestinal tract, and important manifestations of many gastrointestinal diseases are their nutritional effects. Digestion and absorption of nutrients are discussed elsewhere. This chapter reviews physiologic considerations that are essential for planning proper nutritional management. The focus will be on the role of the liver in regulating the supply of carbohydrate and lipid fuels as well as ensuring the availability of essential substrates to peripheral tissues. The clinical features of malnutrition and specific effects of malnutrition on the gastrointestinal tract and liver will be discussed along with diet therapy in gastrointestinal disease. Finally, an approach to clinical nutrition will be presented, including nutritional assessment and the rational use of enteral and parenteral nutritional support.

2. ESSENTIAL PHYSIOLOGIC CONCEPTS IN NUTRITION

To maintain a continuous supply of nutrients in the bloodstream in the face of intermittent dietary intake, a complex set of regulatory mechanisms have evolved. These allow the storage of nutrients during feeding, and their release from storage pools during the interdigestive period so as to maintain nutrient levels in the bloodstream within remarkably narrow limits. Short-term regulation between the fed state and the interdigestive state is mediated principally by (1) the concentration of several key substrates and (2) a set of regulatory hormones, which include insulin, glucagon, catecholamines and corticosteroids (Table 1).

TABLE 1. Hormonal regulation of nutrient metabolism

Hormone	Principal metabolic actions
Insulin	Increases glucose uptake in peripheral tissues Stimulates protein synthesis Inhibits lipolysis and glycolysis
Glucagon	Increases cyclic AMP levels in the liver and adipose tissue, with stimulation of fatty acid mobilization, glycogenolysis, glycolysis and gluconeogenesis
Catecholamines	Increase cyclic AMP levels in the liver, skeletal muscle and adipose tissue, with release of glucose, free fatty acids and lactate
Corticosteroids	Increase gluconeogenesis Increase amino acid mobilization from the periphery (chiefly skeletal muscle) Increase fatty acid release Decrease glucose utilization by peripheral tissues

The fate of glucose in the fed and the fasting states is detailed in Figure 1. Glucose is rapidly absorbed following ingestion as starch, disaccharides or monosaccharides. The glucose is transported via the portal system to the liver, which extracts a considerable fraction of portal venous glucose. The remainder enters the systemic circulation and causes pancreatic secretion of insulin. The high portal vein insulin and glucose concentrations lead to hepatic glucose uptake with conversion to glycogen and fatty acid. The peripheral rise in insulin, which occurs in association with the rise in plasma glucose concentration, causes a large peripheral uptake of glucose, first by muscle cells, and second by adipocytes. Glucose is the essential substrate for brain, renal medulla and red cell metabolism; other organs mainly use fatty acids for energy. The rise in plasma insulin also leads to amino acid uptake by muscle and has an antiproteolytic effect. These effects on muscle protein have led to the designation of insulin as an "anabolic hormone." In the postabsorptive or interdigestive state, plasma glucose is low, with low plasma insulin levels. The low plasma insulin influences the metabolism of all three macronutrients (i.e., carbohydrates, fat and protein). Glycogenolysis occurs in the liver to maintain plasma glucose levels. The low plasma insulin also allows lipolysis to take place, such that fatty acids can be utilized as the major energy substrate. Finally, the low plasma insulin leads to proteolysis, particularly of muscle protein, which leads to release of alanine and glutamine, which can be used for gluconeogenesis in the liver. This gluconeogenesis occurs in concert with glycogenolysis to assure an ongoing supply of glucose for the body.

A. Fed state

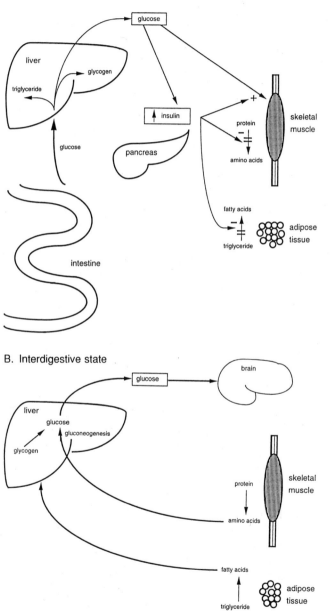

B. Interdigestive state

FIGURE 1.   Carbohydrate and protein metabolism.

Other hormones, such as glucagon, catecholamines and growth hormone, play less important roles in macronutrient metabolism, but in general have been termed the "stress hormones," since they are released during times of stress and have anti-insulin effects. In particular, if for any reason there is a low blood sugar, all these hormones are released and will promote an elevation in plasma glucose.

The flux of lipid nutrients in the fed and the interdigestive states is contrasted in Figure 2. In the fed state, fat enters the circulation from the intestine as chylomicrons, which are large droplets of triglyceride emulsified by a surface monolayer of phospholipid and apolipoproteins. Additional apolipoproteins are transferred onto the chylomicrons from HDL. The artificial fat emulsions used for parenteral nutrition are very similar to chylomicrons in that they contain a core of triglyceride with a surface monolayer of phospholipid. They initially contain no apolipoproteins, but acquire these from HDL very rapidly once they have entered the circulation. One of the apolipoproteins, apolipoprotein C-II, is particularly important in that it is an essential cofactor for the action of lipoprotein lipase. This enzyme is attached to the capillary endothelium in tissues, such as the heart and adipose tissue, that are active in utilizing fatty acids. Chylomicrons bind to the enzyme and the core triglyceride is rapidly hydrolyzed. The released fatty acids are then taken up and utilized in the peripheral tissues. As the chylomicron particle shrinks in size, the excess surface material is transferred back to HDL, and ultimately the remnant particles are cleared via a specific receptor in the liver. The process of lipolysis is extremely efficient, and the half-life of chylomicron triglyceride in the circulation is normally less than 15 minutes. The lower panel of Figure 2 depicts the postabsorptive or interdigestive state. Chylomicrons are absent, but triglyceride fuels are available in the circulation in the form of VLDL, which are secreted by the liver. The substrates for triglyceride assembly include free fatty acids released from adipose tissue through the action of a hormone-sensitive lipase, and fatty acids synthesized in the liver from acetyl-CoA. The newly secreted VLDL acquire apolipoproteins and cholesterol ester from HDL. Lipolysis of VLDL in peripheral tissues is mediated by lipoprotein lipase. As the particle decreases in size, free cholesterol transfers to HDL, where it is esterified through the action of lecithin-cholesterol acyltransferase (LCAT), and the resultant cholesterol ester is then transferred back to the lipolyzed particle, where it forms part of the core. When lipolysis is completed, what is left behind is termed an LDL particle. This is smaller and more dense than VLDL, has lost all apolipoproteins except apolipoprotein B, and has a core of cholesterol ester rather than triglyceride. LDL is cleared relatively slowly, with a half-life of several days. The uptake of LDL is mediated

A. Fed state

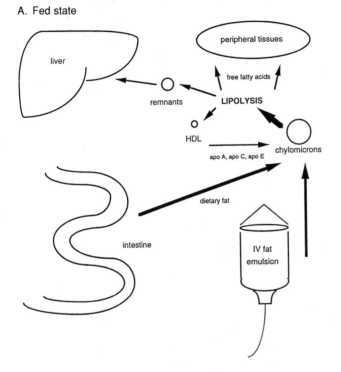

B. Postabsorptive state

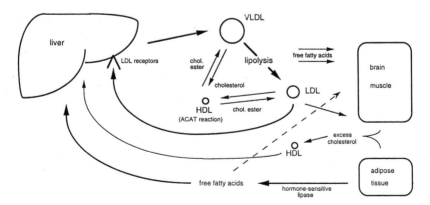

FIGURE 2. Lipoprotein metabolism.

by a specific membrane receptor, termed the LDL receptor, whose activity in turn is regulated by intracellular cholesterol levels. The most active tissues (on a weight basis) for LDL clearance are steroidogenic tissues, such as the adrenals, gonads and the liver; because of its size, the liver accounts for over half of total LDL catabolism. As peripheral tissues cannot degrade cholesterol, excess cholesterol is returned to the liver via HDL, where it is used for bile acid synthesis or excreted in the bile.

In addition to the short-term regulation mediated by substrates and hormones outlined above, additional adaptive responses occur in response to particular dietary circumstances. For example, a diet rich in carbohydrate at the expense of fat will lead to the induction of enzymes involved in glycolysis, the pentose phosphate pathway and fatty acid synthesis (e.g., glucokinase, glucose-6-phosphate dehydrogenase, 6-phosphogluconate dehydrogenase, acetyl-CoA carboxylase). A diet containing predominantly fat at the expense of carbohydrate will lead to induction of fatty acid oxidation, with increased acyl-CoA-carnitine acyltransferase, and induction of enzymes involved in gluconeogenesis, including glucose-6-phosphatase, fructose diphosphatase and transaminases. A diet rich in protein but low in carbohydrate will also lead to induction of gluconeogenic enzymes and transaminases, as well as other enzymes involved in amino acid interconversion and degradation, and induction of urea cycle enzymes to deal with the enhanced production of ammonia.

Starvation leads to a number of adaptive responses. There is a depletion of liver glycogen within 24 to 48 hours, with stimulation of gluconeogenic enzymes to allow the production of glucose from amino acids released through protein breakdown in skeletal muscle. Lipolysis in adipose tissue leads to increased fatty acid levels and activation of enzymes responsible for ß-oxidation of fatty acid in the liver (acyl-CoA-carnitine acyltransferase). In addition to acetyl-CoA, fatty acid oxidation generates ketone bodies. One important adaptive response to starvation is the induction of ß-hydroxybutyrate dehydrogenase in the brain, which allows this organ to utilize ketone bodies as a fuel. Decreased dependence on glucose reduces the need for excess gluconeogenesis and spares muscle protein. In a relatively lean 70 kg man with 12% body fat, survival without food can be expected to be about 60 days or longer.

3. CLINICAL AND LABORATORY FEATURES OF PROTEIN-ENERGY MALNUTRITION

Protein-energy malnutrition may result from a number of causes. These are shown in Table 2. Intake or assimilation may be impaired or, alternatively,

TABLE 2.   Causes of protein-energy malnutrition

Impaired intake
Insufficient quantity or quality
Impaired intake due to systemic disease (e.g., cerebrovascular accident, chronic infections)
Impaired intake due to localized gastrointestinal disease (e.g., benign or malignant esophageal
    stricture)

Impaired digestion and/or absorption
Selective enzyme defect (e.g., enterokinase deficiency, trypsinogen deficiency)
Generalized enzyme defect (e.g., pancreatic exocrine insufficiency)
Impaired small intestinal assimilation (e.g., celiac disease)

Excessive enteric protein loss
Gastric or intestinal mucosal disease (e.g., Ménétrier's disease, intestinal lymphangiectasia)
Extraintestinal disease with lymphatic blockage (e.g., pericarditis, lymphoma)

Disorders with multiple causes
Advanced malignancy
Chronic renal failure with uremia
Other chronic debilitating diseases

---

losses may be increased, as occurs with excessive enteric protein loss in
protein-losing enteropathies. In some disorders, multiple causes may be
present. Moreover, requirements may be significantly increased in some
patients as a result of growth, pregnancy, tissue injury or a superimposed disease process. In some patients with chronic debilitating diseases, multiple factors may be responsible.

Attempts have been made to classify malnutrition into a predominantly
protein-depleted (i.e., kwashiorkor) or calorie- (energy-) starved (i.e., marasmus) state. In kwashiorkor, the subject ingests a moderate number of calories,
usually as complex carbohydrate (e.g., rice), but very little protein. The carbohydrate is absorbed as glucose, causing rises in plasma glucose and insulin,
and leading to decreased lipolysis and proteolysis. The liver is therefore supplied with inadequate amino acids, with little oral intake and little peripheral
mobilization from skeletal muscle stores. Transport of triglyceride made from
ingested glucose is impaired since there is inadequate production of apoprotein, which is needed for the formation of VLDL. The liver becomes fatty and
enlarged. Furthermore, other proteins, including albumin, are inadequately
produced by the liver in kwashiorkor, and serum albumin falls, with resulting
peripheral edema. With marasmus the subject takes inadequate amounts of
protein and calories. The low caloric intake means that only small amounts of

carbohydrate are taken; plasma glucose and insulin are low. Hence, lipolysis and proteolysis occur, with adequate delivery of amino acids from muscle to the liver for protein production. Fatty liver does not occur, and serum albumin levels tend to be normal, with no peripheral edema. Often patients fall between these two extremes of nutritional states, but there are examples of kwashiorkor and marasmus in Western clinical practice. Anorexia nervosa is a classic example of marasmus. Marked muscle wasting and loss of subcutaneous tissue (adipose tissue) occur with normal-sized nonfatty livers and no peripheral edema. In contrast, the intensive care unit patient who has received intravenous dextrose (glucose) for a prolonged period will often show a fatty liver and marked hypoalbuminemia and edema.

Clinical features of protein-energy malnutrition vary depending on the severity and duration of nutrient deficiency, age at onset and the presence or absence of other contributing or conditioning factors. With minimal deficiency, abnormalities may be subtle – particularly in adults, in whom growth requirements are minimal. In these patients muscle wasting and loss of subcutaneous fat may be present. Weakness and minimal changes in psychomotor function may develop. Nontender parotid enlargement may occur, sometimes bilaterally. Patchy brown pigmentation, particularly over the malar eminences of the face, may occur. A lackluster appearance with thinning and increased shedding of hair from the sides of the head, particularly on combing or brushing, may develop. Bradycardia may occur. Variable degrees of hepatomegaly may result, sometimes with steatosis. In patients with protein-energy malnutrition following jejunoileal bypass a wide spectrum of histopathologic change has been observed, similar to findings frequently associated with alcoholic liver disease. Other changes that may occur that can affect the liver are listed in Table 3.

In adults with severe protein-energy malnutrition and in growing children, clinical features may be even more significant. Muscle wasting, subcutaneous fat loss, dependent edema and weight loss may be marked. Severe mental apathy and reduced physical activity may occur. Abnormalities in the hair, particularly of children, may be striking. Severe dyspigmentation may develop, especially distally; rarely, alternating strands of light and dark hair are observed. Hair may be removed without pain. Nails may become brittle, with horizontal grooves. An asymmetrical confluent pattern of skin hyperpigmentation may be seen, particularly over perineal and exposed areas, such as the face. Extensive desquamation may occur, leaving depigmented areas of superficial ulcers, particularly on the buttocks and backs of the thighs. Gastrointestinal symptoms are common but variable. These include marked constipation, diarrhea, anorexia or hyperphagia, nausea, vomiting and dehy-

TABLE 3.   Effects of specific nutritional disorders on the liver

Nutritional disorders	Effects on the liver
Common conditions	
Alcoholism	Steatosis, alcoholic hepatitis and cirrhosis
Obesity	Steatosis, steatohepatitis and cholelithiasis
Uncontrolled diabetes	Glycogenosis, steatosis and steatohepatitis
Protein deficiency	Pigment stones
Kwashiorkor	Steatosis and decreased protein synthesis
Fasting	Mild unconjugated hyperbilirubinemia, especially in Gilbert's syndrome
Uncommon conditions	
Jejunoileal bypass	Steatosis and steatohepatitis
Gross dietary iron excess	Bantu siderosis/hemochromatosis
Senecio alkaloids	Veno-occlusive disease
Dietary aflatoxins	Hepatocellular carcinoma (?)
Chronic arsenic ingestion	Noncirrhotic portal hypertension, angiosarcoma and hepatocellular carcinoma
Hypervitaminosis A	Hepatic fibrosis and cirrhosis

dration. Laboratory features are also variable. Serum proteins may be substantially reduced, including serum albumin and some higher-molecular-weight transfer proteins, such as transferrin, ceruloplasmin, lipoproteins, thyroxin and cortisol binding proteins. Serum amino acid analysis may show a decrease in essential amino acids (i.e., leucine, isoleucine, valine, methionine), and either normal or depressed levels of nonessentials (i.e., glycine, serine, glutamine). The urinary excretion of urea, creatinine and hydroxyproline may decrease. Severe electrolyte abnormalities develop, although serum levels may be normal.

Clinical vitamin deficiencies are listed in Table 4. Except for cheilosis and glossitis, which are seen with multiple vitamin B deficiencies, physical findings of single or isolated vitamin deficiencies are seldom observed in protein-calorie malnourished patients in developed countries. Trace elements are elements that are required in small quantities (mg amounts or less) for normal growth and/or function. Essential trace elements for humans include iron, iodine, zinc, chromium, copper, selenium and cobalt, and possibly molybdenum, manganese and vanadium. Except for iron deficiency due to blood loss and/or poor intake, deficiency states of trace elements are rare in subjects with some oral intake, since only minute amounts are required.

TABLE 4. Vitamin deficiency syndromes

Vitamin	Name of deficiency state	Clinical occurrence	Common clinical features
1. Water-soluble			
B₁ (thiamine)	Beriberi: Dry (neurologic) Wet (cardiac)	Refeeding after starvation	Neurologic: Peripheral neuropathy, Wernicke-Korsakoff
	Wernicke-Korsakoff syndrome		Cardiac: Heart failure
B₂ (riboflavin)	—	Rare	B-complex deficiency*
B₆ (pyridoxine)	—	Only with pyridoxine-antagonist drugs (isoniazid, cycloserine, penicillamine)	Neurologic: Convulsions B-complex deficiency*
B₁₂ (cyanocobalamin)	Pernicious anemia (when secondary to idiopathic gastric atrophy)	Achlorhydria Terminal ileal disease or resection Bacterial overgrowth Diphyllobothrium latum Pancreatic insufficiency	Hematologic: Pancytopenia Neurologic: Subacute combined degeneration Peripheral neuropathy Glossitis
Folic acid	—	Pregnancy Poor intake Malabsorption	Hematologic: Pancytopenia Glossitis
Niacin	Pellagra	Poor diet	Characteristic dermatitis Dementia Diarrhea
Pantothenic acid	—	Rare	—
Biotin	—	Excess egg white ingestion ? TPN	Dermatitis Depression Nausea
C (ascorbic acid)	Scurvy	Infants, the elderly and alcoholics with very poor intake	Purpura Gum disease (when teeth present)

TABLE 4. Vitamin deficiency syndromes (cont'd)

Vitamin	Name of deficiency state	Clinical occurrence	Common clinical features
2. *Fat-soluble*			
A	—	Third World children Severe low intake	Night blindness, corneal changes, xerophthalmia, xeroderma and hyperkeratosis
D	—	Inadequate sun exposure Inadequate intake Renal disease	Osteomalacia (rickets in children) Hypocalcemia
E	—	Cholestatic liver disease (especially children)	Neurologic: Posterior column degeneration, areflexia
K	—	Warfarin anticoagulant Long-term antibiotics (especially with TPN) Newborn infants	Hemorrhage with prolonged prothrombin time

*B-complex deficiency: cheilosis, angular stomatitis, glossitis.

4. EFFECTS OF MALNUTRITION ON THE GASTROINTESTINAL TRACT AND PANCREAS

Protein-energy malnutrition may produce major structural and functional changes in the gastrointestinal tract and pancreas, which, in turn, may aggravate the underlying poor nutritional condition. In severe protein-energy malnutrition, for example, acinar cell atrophy occurs and exocrine cells have decreased numbers of zymogen granules. Pancreatic secretion may be reduced following stimulation with cholecystokinin and/or secretin. With malnutrition, the activities of enzymes contained in pancreatic juice (i.e., trypsin, chymotrypsin, lipase, amylase) are reduced. With reversal of malnutrition these can return to normal levels, but this may require several weeks.

In addition to pancreatic exocrine changes, the entire wall and mucosal lining of the stomach and intestine may be reduced in thickness. This change appears to be reversible, as a more normal macroscopic appearance can follow nutritional repletion. Microscopically, marked changes may develop, including severe "flattening" of the small intestinal mucosa, similar to celiac disease. In contrast to celiac disease, however, reduced numbers of crypt mitoses are seen; the mucosa is hypoplastic rather than hyperplastic. In this setting, correction of the nutritional state per se can produce a complete reversion to normal. Nonspecific ultrastructural changes also occur, including epithelial cell lipid droplets. Changes may be present throughout the small intestine in an irregular patchy distribution, although the jejunum appears to be most severely affected. Qualitative and quantitative changes in the intestinal microflora, particularly anaerobes, also occur in protein-energy malnutrition. However, their role in altering mucosal structure and function requires definition. Some brush-border enzymes (i.e., disaccharidases) may be reduced; as a result, malabsorption of a variety of substances (e.g., lactose) may be observed. Altered uptake of glucose and D-xylose has also been reported, and steatorrhea may be present with impaired absorption of fat and some fat-soluble vitamins. In addition, loss of fecal nitrogen and serum protein into the gastrointestinal tract may be increased. Finally, specific nutrients may be deficient and cause alterations in certain tissues. For example, folic acid and vitamin B_{12} deficiencies have well-recognized effects on rapidly dividing hematopoietic precursor cells in the bone marrow; for similar reasons, as shown in Table 5, analogous changes may be anticipated in the small intestinal epithelium.

There is increasing evidence that the colonic mucosa uses short-chain fatty acids (especially butyrate) as an energy source. In patients who undergo a colostomy, the bowel that is left distally does not have a fecal stream. The

TABLE 5. Effects of depletion of specific nutrients on the intestine

Nutrient	Effects
Protein-energy malnutrition (e.g., especially, kwashiorkor)	Total or subtotal villous "atrophy" and crypt hypoplasia
Folic acid deficiency	Total or subtotal villous "atrophy" and crypt hypoplasia; macrocytic and/or "megaloblastic" enterocytes
Vitamin B_{12} deficiency	Total or subtotal villous "atrophy" and crypt hypoplasia; macrocytic and/or "megaloblastic" enterocytes
Vitamin E deficiency	(?) Small intestinal ceroidosis (i.e., "brown bowel syndrome")
Vitamin A deficiency	Reduced numbers of intestinal goblet cells

mucosa of this bowel may develop inflammation, called "diversion colitis." This condition can be corrected by administering short-chain fatty acid enemas. A major source of the short-chain fatty acids in the colon is fermented dietary fiber, and thus fiber may be considered a "nutrient."

5. DIETARY THERAPY IN GASTROINTESTINAL DISEASE

5.1 General Principles

A number of specific diets are useful in different gastrointestinal disorders. These may involve diet restriction or supplementation, or alternatively, a change in the consistency or content of specific nutrients. In patients with steatorrhea, for example, luminal fatty acids are present and involved in the pathogenesis of diarrhea. In these patients, reduction in diarrhea can be accomplished, in part, by a reduction in the oral intake of triglycerides; a low-fat diet may be beneficial. In some patients with steatorrhea, supplementation with medium-chain triglycerides may be useful because these are hydrolyzed more rapidly by pancreatic enzymes, do not require bile acid micelles for absorption, and are primarily directed to the portal rather than the lymphatic circulation. Because medium-chain triglycerides undergo ω-oxidation to metabolically nonutilizable dicarboxylic acids, the effective caloric content of medium-chain triglycerides is less than expected. Medium-chain triglycerides in a daily dose of 60 mL will provide approximately 370 calories. Low-fat dietary supplements may be provided in the form of a number of commercially available products prepared as complete nutritional supplements. Fat-soluble vitamins can be replaced using oral water-miscible formulations, if steatorrhea is present. For vitamin K, a water-soluble form is available. Fat-soluble vitamins require bile acid micelles for absorption; thus, if steatorrhea is due to bile acid depletion (as might occur in the short bowel syndrome following surgical resection for extensive Crohn's disease), increased amounts of vitamins may be required.

Bloating and cramping pain may follow ingestion of lactose-containing foods. This may be due to lactase deficiency (e.g., small bowel disease, "ethnic" lactase deficiency). Dietary lactose restriction may be indicated in patients if there is a history of lactose intolerance or a positive lactose tolerance test (i.e., rise in blood sugar less than 20 mg/dL after 50 g of lactose) accompanied by characteristic symptoms. An alternative test involves measurement of breath hydrogen; a rise of more than 20 ppm is consistent with lactose intolerance. Lactose may be found in milk, including buttermilk, even if it has been naturally fermented. Commercial yogurt should also be avoided, since this often has milk or cream added after fermentation to avoid the sour taste produced by fermenting lactose. Ice cream and sherbets have high lactose concentrations and should be avoided. Cheese or desserts made from milk or milk chocolate as well as sauces or stuffings made from milk, cream or cheese should also be avoided. Calcium supplements may be necessary with dairy product restriction, particularly in postmenopausal women. Liquid dairy products may be used to a limited extent by patients who have lactose intolerance; in these patients, a yeast enzyme preparation (i.e., lactase from Kluyveromyces lactis) added to milk at 4°C can hydrolyze up to 70% of the lactose in one day and 90% in two or three days. Nonliquid dairy products cannot be treated with enzyme preparations, although lactase tablets may be chewed prior to eating solid food.

5.2 Celiac Disease
Celiac disease, also known as gluten-sensitive enteropathy or celiac sprue, is a malabsorption disorder resulting from ingestion of proteins derived from certain cereal grains of the grass family, Gramineae: wheat, rye, barley and possibly oats. It is believed that the alcohol-soluble gliadin fraction of wheat gluten or similar alcohol-soluble proteins from the other grains (termed *prolamins*) cause the intestinal damage. Consequently, absolute restriction is required for life. Table 6 provides some dietary guidelines for celiac disease patients. Gluten, however, is a particularly ubiquitous substance and can be found in coffee, catsup, dip, frozen TV dinners, ice cream and even in the capsules of medications! Although wheat, rye, barley and possibly oats are important, corn and rice do not appear to activate celiac disease. Data on other grains are not as clear. Buckwheat is not derived from the grass family and is usually

TABLE 6.   Dietary guidelines for celiac disease patients

Foods to avoid
Wheat, rye, barley, oat products
Triticale (wheat–rye hybrid)
Millet and sorghum
Malt and hydrolyzed vegetable protein

Acceptable foods
Corn, rice, buckwheat products
Wine and distilled alcoholic beverages
Fruits and vegetables
Meat
Nuts
Dairy products (unless lactose-intolerant)

---

permitted. Millet and sorghum are often allowed, but have not been thoroughly evaluated. Triticale, a hybrid of wheat and rye, should be avoided. Rye whiskey, Scotch whiskey and other cereal-derived alcohols can be consumed, since gluten is not present in distilled spirits. Similarly, brandy and wine made from fruit pose no difficulties. Beer and ale are produced from barley; it is not entirely clear if they can activate disease and would best be avoided. Malt made from barley should be avoided, as well as hydrolyzed vegetable proteins used as flavor enhancers in processed foods, since they may be made from soy, wheat and other cereal proteins.

For both symptomatic and asymptomatic patients with celiac disease, a lifelong gluten-free diet is recommended. Multivitamin supplements are frequently required and specific vitamin, mineral and trace element deficiencies should be corrected. Iron and folate supplementation may be needed and poor absorption of oral iron may sometimes necessitate parenteral administration. Supplements of calcium and vitamin D may be required to prevent mobilization of skeletal calcium, and in some patients magnesium may be needed.

5.3 Inflammatory Bowel Disease

Malnutrition in patients with inflammatory bowel disease is a frequent problem. Weight loss may be seen in over 65% of patients and growth retardation may be observed in up to 40% of children. As shown in Table 7, there are multiple causes for malnutrition, especially in patients with Crohn's disease and small bowel involvement. The goal of nutritional management is to ensure adequate nutrient intake with modifications that reduce symptoms. Although only limited studies are available, evidence suggests that energy expenditure

TABLE 7. Malnutrition in inflammatory bowel disease

Reduced oral intake
Disease-induced (e.g., postprandial abdominal pain and diarrhea, sitophobia, anorexia, nausea and vomiting)
Iatrogenic (e.g., restrictive diets, "fad" diets)

Malabsorption
Reduced absorptive surface (e.g., shortened small intestine due to prior resection, diseased segments)
Bacterial overgrowth (e.g., associated with strictures and bypassed loops, stasis)
Bile salt deficiency after ileal resection (e.g., impaired micelle formation and steatorrhea)
Lactase deficiency (e.g., associated with small bowel disease)
Drug-induced malabsorption

Increased nutrient loss
Protein-losing enteropathy
Diarrhea losses of electrolytes, minerals and trace elements (e.g., potassium, zinc)
Gastrointestinal blood loss (e.g., iron loss)

Drug-induced malabsorption
Cholestyramine (e.g., bile acids; fat; fat-soluble vitamins, including vitamins D and K)
Sulfasalazine (e.g., folic deficiency associated with reduced absorption and increased requirement related to hemolysis)
Steroids (e.g., calcium absorption and mobilization)

Increased requirements
Chronic inflammatory disease, fever, superimposed infection

---

is no greater than one would predict for a healthy individual unless the disease is complicated by fever or sepsis. There may be increased caloric as well as nutrient requirements, however, particularly if gastrointestinal losses are substantial and malabsorption is significant. Attention should also be placed on micronutrient deficiencies in these patients, particularly if concomitant malabsorption is present. For example, patients with significant ileal disease or resection require regularly administered parenteral vitamin B_{12}.

Frequently, the diet consistency or form will require modification to permit intake of adequate amounts of various nutrients. Thus, a low-fiber or low-residue diet may be recommended if symptoms are associated with stenotic bowel segments. In some, symptoms may be improved by a diet with increased fiber. Increased amounts of pectin or guar, for example, may be helpful in patients with increased stool water content, as these fibers tend to have a significant water-retaining capacity.

Lactose intolerance may be common in patients with inflammatory bowel disease, particularly with small intestinal involvement, as well as in ethnic groups with a high frequency of primary lactase deficiency. In patients with a limited ileal resection, diarrhea may result from impaired ileal bile salt reabsorption. With more extensive ileal resection, particularly if over 100 cm, bile salt depletion may occur. As a result, micelle formation may be suboptimal, and fat malabsorption results. In addition, fecal fat and/or fatty acids may bind to calcium, magnesium, zinc and copper; increased fecal losses of these divalent cations may result. Increased fat-soluble vitamin loss may occur. Finally, patients with Crohn's disease and an ileal resection with steatorrhea are more prone to develop calcium oxalate kidney stones. This is due to increased urinary oxalate concentrations associated with enhanced absorption of dietary oxalate, largely in the colon. Steatorrhea causes enteric hyperoxaluria because calcium binds to unabsorbed fatty acids. As a result, more oxalate is available for passive colonic diffusion. In addition, fatty acids appear to increase colonic permeability to oxalate. By reducing dietary fat, oxalate absorption is also reduced.

Specific drugs may also alter nutrient absorption. For example, sulfasalazine is a competitive inhibitor of intestinal folate absorption. In addition, patients on sulfasalazine may have hemolysis secondary to red cell oxidant injury from sulfapyridine. Thus, folate requirements are increased.

6. DIETARY THERAPY IN LIVER DISEASE

Two important manifestations of chronic liver disease, ascites and portal-systemic encephalopathy, can be effectively treated with dietary modifications. The prime dietary objective in the treatment of ascites is sodium restriction. Some authorities have recommended restriction of dietary sodium intake to as little as 10–20 mmol/day for patients with symptomatic, large-volume ascites. However, it is almost impossible to design a palatable diet or provide sufficient protein to maintain nitrogen balance with such stringent restrictions, and therefore these will not be satisfactory for long-term use. Well-motivated patients can often be maintained on a 40 mmol sodium diet (equivalent to about 1 g of sodium or 2.5 g of sodium chloride).

The treatment of portal-systemic encephalopathy includes dietary protein restriction. Management will obviously need to be individualized for patients with fulminant hepatic failure or stage IV coma, but patients with chronic liver disease and mild to moderate encephalopathy should usually have dietary protein intake restricted to 0.5–0.8 g/kg body weight. Even more rigorous restriction may be necessary to control encephalopathy in the short term, but is difficult to maintain for prolonged periods because of limited patient compliance and negative nitrogen balance. It is believed that vegetable protein may be less ammoniagenic than meat, but part of this may relate to decreased efficiency of absorption of vegetable protein. Disproportionately high levels of aromatic amino acids are found in plasma of patients with decompensated cirrhosis. Hence, nutritional supplements rich in branched-chain amino acids have been advocated; however, unequivocal evidence for their efficacy is lacking.

Patients with advanced cirrhosis often have hepatic glycogen depletion. During fasting, glucagon and catecholamines will be released to maintain blood glucose levels. In the absence of hepatic glycogen stores, this requires gluconeogenesis, and the substrate is provided to a significant extent from muscle catabolism. Utilization of the amino acids for gluconeogenesis will lead to ammonia production. It is not known whether dietary manipulations designed to provide a continuous supply of glucose, and therefore to reduce gluconeogenesis, would improve the hyperammonemia in these individuals. Cholestatic liver diseases, including primary biliary cirrhosis (PBC), secondary biliary cirrhosis, sclerosing cholangitis and biliary atresia, may be accompanied by malabsorption of fat-soluble vitamins. Vitamin K deficiency can be easily confirmed with the demonstration of a prolonged prothrombin time that corrects with administration of parenteral vitamin K. Assays for vitamins D, A and E are generally available only in specialized laboratories. If confirmatory tests are not available and if there are strong clinical grounds for suspecting a deficiency state, appropriate replacement therapy should be initiated. Table 8 lists a number of hereditary liver diseases for which appropriate therapy includes specific dietary interventions.

7. NUTRITION INTERVENTION

7.1 Nitrogen Requirements
In a well-nourished adult in steady state, total nitrogen intake will equal nitrogen output in urine, stool and skin. This is termed (zero) "nitrogen balance." Nitrogen is assimilated almost exclusively as protein, and, on average, 6.25 g protein is equivalent to 1 g nitrogen. The nitrogen is excreted predominantly as urea in the urine, but stool and skin losses account for about 2–3 g daily. If a 70 kg man consumes 1 g protein/kg (= 70 g protein or 11.2 g N), then about 8–9 g of nitrogen can be expected in the urine, assuming nitrogen balance. In the steady state, ingestion of more nitrogen will merely result in excretion of more nitrogen in the urine. In growing children or in malnourished adults, the nutritional goal is a positive nitrogen balance, meaning that body tissue is being formed in excess of what is being broken down (i.e., there is net growth).

TABLE 8. Diet therapy for hereditary liver diseases

Disorder	Dietary intervention
Tyrosinemia	Low-phenylalanine diet
Hereditary fructose intolerance	Low-fructose, low-sucrose diet
Galactosemia	Galactose-free diet
Glycogen storage disease	Continuous glucose feeding
Cerebrotendinous xanthomatosis	Deoxycholic acid supplementation
Wilson's disease	Low-copper diet, zinc supplementation (together with chelating agent)
Hemochromatosis	Avoidance of excess dietary iron, selection of foods containing phytates or tannins to reduce iron absorption (together with appropriate phlebotomy treatment)
Cystic fibrosis	Low-fat diet, pancreatic enzyme supplements, fat-soluble vitamin supplements

Nitrogen balance studies have shown that well-nourished adults can maintain nitrogen balance when given as little as 0.5 g/kg protein intake, if energy requirements are met or exceeded. It is important that the protein supplied be of high quality; it should include all essential amino acids and a balanced mix of nonessential amino acids. Malnourished, septic, injured or burned patients will require more protein, in the order of 1.5–2.0 g/kg daily. Pregnant patients should also be given 1.5 g/kg protein daily. It is less clear that patients with conditions associated with protein loss, such as nephrotic syndrome and protein-losing enteropathy, benefit from extra protein intake.

7.2 Energy Requirements
Basal energy requirements in healthy subjects are accurately predicted by the Harris-Benedict equation:

MALES: Energy (kcal/d) = 66 + (13.75 × W) + (5.00 × H) − (6.78 × A)

FEMALES: Energy (kcal/d) = 655 + (9.56 × W) + (1.85 × H) − (4.68 × A) where W = weight in kg, H = height in cm and A = age in years.

Basal energy requirements, as predicted by these equations, increase in the presence of fever (13% per °C), sepsis or injury (up to 20–30%), and burns (up to 100%). Modest physical activity usually requires about 30% above basal requirements.

7.3 Types of Nutritional Intervention

The options for refeeding include oral refeeding, tube feeding and total parenteral nutrition. An assessment by a dietitian regarding current food intake and food preferences is essential. It may well be possible by determining food preferences to provide a well-balanced, nutritionally complete diet. In addition, supplements of high-calorie, high-protein foods such as milkshakes or commercially prepared liquid formula diets may allow for adequate intake. If the patient will not or cannot eat, however, nutritional intervention may be indicated. Examples of patients who will not eat include those with anorexia due to tumor or chemotherapy, and those with anorexia nervosa. Such patients generally have a normal or near-normal nonobstructed bowel, and can be fed enterally. Patients who cannot eat because of severe gastrointestinal illness include those with bowel obstruction or ileus. If nutritional intervention is required in these patients, parenteral (intravenous) nutrition will be necessary.

7.3.1 ENTERAL NUTRITION

Enteral nutrition generally refers to nutrition provided through a tube that has been inserted into the gastrointestinal tract. Usually the tube is a fine-bore (10 French [3.3 mm] or less) Silastic® or polyurethane tube placed via the nose into the stomach, duodenum or jejunum. When long-term feeding is required, it is often preferable for cosmetic and comfort reasons to perform a gastrostomy, which can now be done endoscopically or radiologically with only local anesthetic and mild sedation. If pulmonary aspiration is a potential problem, the tube should be placed into the jejunum.

A multitude of commercial enteral formulas are available for infusion. The formulas have been traditionally divided into polymeric, oligomeric and modular. Polymeric formulas (also called defined formula diets) provide nitrogen as whole protein, often casein, egg white solids or soy protein. Carbohydrate is provided as corn syrup, maltodextrins or glucose oligosaccharides, with sucrose added for sweetness in oral formulas. Fat is usually provided as soy oil, although corn oil and safflower oil may be used. Medium-chain triglycerides (MCT oil) are rarely used. Protein may be provided as milk (usually dry or skim), with lactose as a major carbohydrate. These formulas are contraindicated in patients with lactose intolerance.

Oligomeric formulas (also called elemental diets) provide nitrogen as oligopeptides from partially hydrolyzed whole protein or as crystalline amino acids. Carbohydrate tends to be provided as glucose oligosaccharides or glucose. Fat is usually present in small quantities, enough to meet the requirement for linoleic acid (an essential fatty acid), which is about 2–4% of total calories. MCT oil is added to some formulas. The oligomeric diets were formulated to require minimal digestion by the gastrointestinal tract, with little necessity for bile and pancreatic secretions, and minimal "work" by the enterocyte in terms of brush-border enzyme activity or re-esterification. Hence, these diets have been commercially promoted as ideal for patients with decreased bile output (cholestasis), pancreatic insufficiency and short bowel. However, there is little evidence that these diets are superior to polymeric diets, except with pancreatic insufficiency. Crohn's disease is another condition in which elemental diets may be superior to polymeric diets, although this too remains controversial. Furthermore, since the diet is "predigested," osmolality is high. Finally, the high cost of these diets (often 5 to 10 times that of polymeric diets) rarely justifies their use except in patients with severe pancreatic disease or possibly Crohn's disease.

Most of these formulas provide enough protein, calories, water, electrolytes, minerals, vitamins and trace elements in 2 L/day for most "nonstressed" patients. In other words, these diets are "complete." Excess requirements may exist in patients with multiple injuries, major infections or burns.

Modular formulas are those that contain or predominantly contain one kind of nutrient. There are commercially available modules for protein, fat, carbohydrates, vitamins, electrolytes and trace elements. These modules are not required for the majority of patients, and are rarely used. However, they may be used if different nitrogen-to-calorie ratios are indicated for a patient. Examples of this might include burns or protein-losing enteropathy, if more protein is to be given, or liver disease, if less protein is to be given. Modular feeding is time-consuming, since solutions must be mixed by the hospital, and are more expensive than "complete" formulas.

Finally, specialized amino acid solutions have been made for use in special circumstances – for example, liver disease, renal disease and "stress," such as trauma and sepsis. For liver disease, these solutions are composed mostly or exclusively of branched-chain amino acids, whereas for renal disease the solutions are predominantly essential amino acids. In general, these solutions are expensive and their efficacy is controversial.

Complications of enteral feeding may be divided into aspiration, mechanical, gastrointestinal and metabolic. In general, enteral feeding is well tolerated, and provided the complications are known, preventive and/or corrective measures may be undertaken to minimize patient risk.

Aspiration of the infused formula, with development of pneumonia, is a potentially lethal complication of tube feeding. Proper positioning of the tube requires radiographic verification. Risk factors for aspiration include patients on a ventilator and those with gastroesophageal reflux, poor or absent gag reflex, and impaired mentation. To minimize aspiration, it is suggested that patients, when possible, be fed with the head of the bed elevated 20–30°. Gastric contents should initially be checked by aspirating the tube every four to six hours, and if residue is present more than two hours following infusion, it should be temporarily stopped. Unfortunately, the small nasoenteric tubes in current use often collapse when aspirated, so small returns do not guarantee that the stomach is not becoming distended with fluid. Hence, examination for epigastric distention and succussion splash should be done. If there is any concern, an upright (if possible) plain film to assess gastric size may be useful. It has also been suggested that the feeding tube be placed into the small bowel well beyond the pylorus to minimize aspiration in those at risk.

Mechanical problems in patients with nasoenteric tubes include problems in the upper respiratory tract, esophagitis with development of esophageal ulceration and stenosis, tracheoesophageal fistula, and gastric outlet and small bowel obstruction. Upper respiratory problems include pharyngeal irritation, nasal erosions and necrosis, sinusitis and otitis media. These mechanical problems can be largely avoided by the use of soft, small-bore nasoenteric tubes.

Gastrointestinal problems related to nasoenteric feeding are common, occurring in 20–30% of patients. The most frequent complaints are nausea, vomiting, abdominal distention and altered bowel habit. Symptoms may be minimized by feeding at a slow rate with dilute solutions, but these symptoms may be just as common as with full-rate, full-strength solutions. Alternatively, a different enteral solution may be tried. If a lactose-containing solution is being used (generally not recommended for tube feeding), changing to a lactose-free solution is indicated. For constipation, fiber-containing solutions may be tried, although they are often unhelpful. Fiber, however, is a potential energy source for the colon, as previously discussed, and may therefore be important for maintenance of the colonic mucosa. At the present time, fiber-containing solutions are not routinely used.

Metabolic complications include overhydration, dehydration, hyperglycemia (including hyperosmolar nonketotic coma) and electrolyte disturbances.

Electrolyte problems include hyponatremia, hyper- and hypokalemia, hyper- and hypophosphatemia and hypomagnesemia. In healthy, reasonably nourished individuals with normal cardiac, liver and renal function, these problems are not common. It is recommended that appropriate blood tests be done at intervals over the first few weeks to check for these potential problems.

7.3.2 TOTAL PARENTERAL NUTRITION

Total parenteral nutrition (TPN) involves intravenous administration of all known essential nutrients. This form of therapy is as effective as oral or enteral intake in terms of growth and maintaining body nitrogen. Indications include inability to eat for a minimum of 7 to 10 days with a nonfunctional gut. Total parenteral nutrition is also used for "bowel rest," especially in Crohn's disease, intestinal fistulas and pancreatitis, even if adequate absorption is possible. Several studies suggest, however, that bowel rest is not helpful in Crohn's disease. Furthermore, other studies have shown that elemental diets can be used instead of TPN, except when bowel obstruction is present. In general, if the gut is functional, enteral feeding is preferred since it is safer, cheaper and more physiologic.

7.3.2.1 Solutions

7.3.2.1.1 *Amino acids* "Protein" is supplied as synthetic crystalline, L-amino acid solutions; these are commercially available in 7–10% concentrations. Most available amino acid mixtures are devised for patients without special requirements. Solutions with added branched-chain amino acids are available for hepatic failure, and solutions with essential amino acids are available for renal failure.

7.3.2.1.2 *Fat* There is a human requirement for linoleic acid, which is a precursor of arachidonic acid, which is in turn a precursor of prostaglandins. Linoleic acid, an essential fatty acid, cannot be produced by humans. It has been recommended that this be supplied as 4% or more of total caloric intake. Commercial fat solutions consist of soybean or safflower oil, emulsified with egg phospholipid, and made isotonic at 300 mOsmol/L with added glycerol. Commercially available fat emulsions are available at concentrations of 10% or 20%.

7.3.2.1.3 *Carbohydrate* Glucose is the preferred carbohydrate for intravenous use. Glucose is widely available in concentrations from 5–70%. The osmolality of these solutions may be markedly hyperosmolar up to about 2,500 mOsmol/L.

7.3.2.1.4 *Nonprotein energy source* Once the initial 100 g of glucose is provided for use in the brain, renal medulla and red blood cells, glucose and fat are equally effective in preserving body nitrogen after an equilibration period of four to five days. Glucose is very inexpensive as an energy source, but requires insulin for uptake into cells, and hyperglycemia can be a problem when large amounts of glucose are utilized. The high osmolality of glucose solutions means that only dilute solutions can be used in peripheral veins, and if glucose is used as a major energy source, a large central vein is necessary to prevent thrombosis. Finally, glucose has a respiratory quotient (R.Q. = CO_2 produced/O_2 consumed) of 1.0, meaning that large amounts of carbon dioxide may be produced. This may be deleterious for patients being weaned from ventilators, or with borderline respiratory function.

Lipid solutions offer the benefit of being iso-osmolar, containing linoleic acid and having a lower respiratory quotient of 0.7, with less carbon dioxide production. Drawbacks include somewhat higher cost compared to glucose, and poor tolerance in patients with hyperlipidemia.

7.3.2.2 Routes of delivery

7.3.2.2.1 *Central* The most flexible way to deliver total parenteral nutrition is through a large central vein, usually the superior vena cava, via either the internal jugular or subclavian approach. With the large flow through the superior vena cava, solution osmolality is not of great concern, and thrombosis of this vessel is rare.

7.3.2.2.2 *Peripheral* Ten percent amino acid solutions approach 1,000 mOsmol/L, and 50% dextrose solutions are over 2,500 mOsmol/L, while intravenous fat solutions are, as mentioned, iso-osmolar at about 300 mOsmol/L. Therefore, fat must become the major caloric source in a system that infuses total parenteral nutrition into a peripheral vein. There is a minimum requirement of a 1:1 ratio of amino acid/dextrose solution to the lipid solution. The typical peripheral total parenteral nutrition regimen will consist of 1 L of 5% amino acid/10% dextrose solution, Y-connected to 1.5 L of 10% lipid. This provides 50 g "protein," 350 kcal as glucose and 1,650 kcal as lipid, with the final osmolality over 600 mOsmol/L. Because of this hypertonicity, it is still necessary to rotate the catheter site every 48 hours to prevent phlebitis.

7.3.2.3 Complications
Complications of total parenteral nutrition may be divided into local and systemic. Local problems relate to the catheter site, and in the case of central

lines involve all the complications of central catheters, including inadvertent arterial catheterization with bleeding, pneumothorax, hemothorax and inadvertent infusion of solutions into the pleural cavity. The complication of pneumothorax is much more common with subclavian insertion than with internal jugular insertion, meaning that internal jugular insertion is a safer technique, overall. Air embolism may occur at the time of insertion or any time thereafter with a central line. Catheter embolization may occur, and as mentioned, thrombosis has been reported, particularly with the use of stiff catheters. For long-term use, Silastic® catheters are preferred. It is essential that catheter placement be done by persons with considerable experience to minimize these complications.

Systemic complications include sepsis, metabolic problems and bone disease. Bacteremia or fungemia occurs in 3–7% of patients given total parenteral nutrition, and this appears to arise predominantly from the hub where the catheter joins the intravenous tubing. Catheters are always inserted in a strictly aseptic manner, with personnel fully gowned and gloved. Metabolic problems include hyperglycemia, which can be treated by reducing the amount of glucose given in the solutions, hypertriglyceridemia when excess calories and/or excess lipid is given, and alterations in electrolytes. In particular, total parenteral nutrition causes anabolism with increased intracellular water, so that potassium and phosphate are driven into cells, leading to possible hypokalemia and hypophosphatemia. These complications are very uncommon if adequate amounts of these electrolytes are provided and careful monitoring is performed. Liver disease remains a frustrating complication of total parenteral nutrition and occurs in up to 90% of cases. In general, mild elevations in AST and alkaline phosphatase occur in the second week, with occasional elevations in bilirubin occurring later. Liver biopsy may show mild cholestasis. Overfeeding, particularly with glucose calories, may result in steatosis; this can be treated by reducing total calories and glucose.

3
Gastroenterology and Medical Ethics

J.J. Sidorov

BASIC MORAL PRINCIPLES and rules of medical ethics are as old as the medical profession itself. They were succinctly formulated in such codes as the Hippocratic Oath and Maimonides' Prayer, and have served for centuries as an unchanged moral base for medical practice. Major social and moral changes, particularly those of the second half of the 20th century, have challenged many of these classical values and modified others: witness the introduction of new attitudes toward sexuality and developments in transplantation of human tissues and organs, and opposing views on abortion. Promotion of the patient's autonomy and of human rights has led to the firm establishment of the right of the individual patient to be fully informed and consulted on all medical considerations and decisions related to his or her well-being, health and even death. The influence of such professionals as philosophers, ethicists, sociologists, anthropologists and lawyers has altered concepts of the patient–doctor relationship.

The change from a classical paternalistic to a modern participatory patient–doctor relationship has significantly altered the pattern of medical practice. When a patient consults a physician, a contractual arrangement takes place. The patient provides the physician with the personal, intimate information necessary for proper evaluation and rational management. Complete patient care must take into consideration the patient as a total person, including his or her personal moral values.

The rapid expansion of medical knowledge and technology has also introduced a range of expensive, complex, and often aggressive diagnostic and therapeutic procedures. The rising costs of many new, highly skilled, labor-intensive techniques have led to the rationing of our progressively diminishing

TABLE 1. Ethical principles and professional obligations

Ethical principles	Professional obligations
Beneficence	Confidentiality
Nonmaleficence	Fidelity (promise-keeping)
Respect for autonomy	Interest
Justice, fairness	Veracity (truth-telling)

health-care resources and raised difficult questions of fairness and priorities: who gets what and why, at whose expense, and under what circumstances?

Application of current biomedical ethical principles to the changing clinical and social situation has thus become an essential part of the practice of modern medicine (Table 1).

Gastroenterologists share common ethical principles with and encounter problems similar to those faced by their colleagues in other medical disciplines. Like other specialists, gastroenterologists must often apply general medical ethical principles to specific areas of their activities. One such area is diagnostic and therapeutic endoscopy. Others include the treatment of patients with new, potent drugs, the active participation of gastroenterologists in drug trial studies, and their relationship with industry.

Transplantation of the liver, intestine and pancreas also raises ethical issues, particularly related to economy of resources. The demands that organ transplantation places on society lead to political rather than purely medical decisions concerning the allocation of resources and assignment of priorities. These decisions are not only based on the principle of individual beneficence, but they also are greatly influenced by social perceptions of justice and fairness. Gastroenterologists are being exposed to escalating pressure to control costs, ration resources and act as gatekeepers for organ transplantation. In addition to purely medical decisions, assessing patient suitability involves ethical issues. Should, for example, an individual with self-induced liver disease from abusing alcohol or other drugs, or from following a particular lifestyle, be accepted for transplantation?

Commerce involving organs or parts of organs is another area of ethical concern. Organ sale elsewhere in the world has been justified in that it is the only way to meet current needs. The issue is clouded by a lack of absolute ethical standards that could be uniformly applied in all parts of the world. Although medicine is generally transcultural, ethics is often culture-specific, as it depends on historical, religious, social and cultural factors. Ethical principles applicable to contemporary Western societies do not apply to parts of the world with completely different cultural and social traditions.

The advent of fiberoptic endoscopy has had a major impact on research and clinical practice in gastroenterology. Ethical issues peculiar to gastrointestinal endoscopy are often not obvious. Gross violations of a code of ethics are easily detected and identified. The difficulty arises, however, when assessing skill, competence and quality control. It is often difficult to draw a clear line between professional competence and the safety of a procedure on one hand, and ethical behavior on the other.

A fully informed consent ensures that the patient clearly understands the necessity, benefits and risks of the proposed procedure. Failure to obtain such consent is not only a medicolegal omission, but is unethical. Equally unethical is the performance of a procedure in excess of diagnostic and therapeutic requirements.

An innovative procedure or a significant modification of a standard procedure cannot be undertaken without prior approval by the institutional review board or the hospital ethics committee, and without the fully informed consent of the patient.

Close cooperation between the pharmaceutical industry and the medical profession has greatly contributed to recent progress in research and to educational opportunities. The industry, however, is particularly concerned with the sponsorship of new products, potentially coloring this relationship.

The development of new drugs requires clinical trials. Development of a new drug from the initial invention of a chemical structure until its final approval for general use takes an average of 10 to 15 years and may cost up to $100 million before realizing any financial return. Compliance with certain study protocols may at times conflict with optimal patient care. Yet clinical studies are essential to identify the pharmacology, benefits and side effects of any therapeutic modality. The industry is quite aware that commercial objectives must not override ethical considerations and has developed the guidelines used in many countries. By subscribing to such codes, the industry has accepted responsibility for proper monitoring and supervision of sound clinical trials. For their part, those physicians involved in a clinical study must possess adequate knowledge and devote the necessary time.

It is unethical to enter a patient into a trial unless the investigator truly believes that the new drug or procedure will provide benefits beyond those already available. The investigator must be free to publish the results regardless of the outcome, unencumbered by the private interests of the sponsor. The principal investigator shares with the sponsor the responsibility for the scientific validity, ethical content and correctness of the clinical evaluation of the product undergoing trial. The investigator may be remunerated for clinical work (such as physical examination, endoscopies and other technical procedures) if charged for at standard rates. It is unethical, however, to derive personal financial benefit as a reward for participating in or conducting the study. Support by industry of continued medical education (CME) at the international, national or local level is another area of concern, because of the potential for marketing and product promotion. There are undeniable benefits derived from this support; most of these activities are of exemplary scientific standard. Nevertheless, subtle ethical issues can arise when a product-related symposium is organized by the sponsor of a drug trial while the trial is still in progress. Such an interim symposium may be viewed as a form of product promotion, particularly if industry dictates the program design and selects the invited speakers and their topics. Social aspects of these symposia (such as entertainment and personal gifts by the industry) require particularly close scrutiny. The code of practice published by the Association of the British Pharmaceutical Industry states that "entertainment or hospitality offered ... should always be secondary to the main purpose of the meeting ... [and should] not exceed that level which the recipients might normally adopt when paying for themselves." This code is similar to that adopted by Canadian industry and medical associations.

Medical research using human subjects requires careful scrutiny. A recent study by an international group of reviewers found that a significant proportion of studies involving humans, and published in some of the leading gastroenterology journals, failed to meet ethical standards as defined by the reviewers. Approximately 40% would have been rejected by reviewers had they been members of the review boards at the institutions where the work was done. Some 12% of these "rejections" involved perceived danger to participating patients; the remainder involved poor study design or problems of statistical analysis. Between 10 and 15% of medications used were subsequently discovered to be potentially toxic.

There seem to be several places where a potential deficiency may originate. Concern about personal career development and academic pressure to demonstrate research productivity might induce an investigator to disregard what might at first appear to be a trivial issue. Casual supervision and inadequate quality control by senior, experienced and established investigators could be another factor. Poorly conducted research leading to faulty conclusions based on avoidable deficiencies and errors is unethical. Just because a project has received the approval of an institutional review board, there is no guarantee that it will remain ethical throughout. Finally, the system of peer review, the traditional method of ensuring the quality of scientific investigation, is not infallible. Close supervision based on clearly defined institutional publication policies and periodic careful review of the study's progress may eliminate many of these ethical pitfalls. The ethical component must be part of the scientific review.

The complexity of current scientific, technical, philosophical and social developments and other conditions in the second half of 20th century present a plethora of ethical issues that we need to consider in our daily work – clinical practice, research or teaching. We should always consider the patient not only as a collection of symptoms, signs and pathological processes but also as an individual with emotions, problems and moral standards. Biomedical ethics is an integral part of such care. Familiarity with basic bioethical principles (Table 1) is as essential for the practice of medicine as the knowledge of pathophysiology is for the understanding of the disease process.

SUGGESTED READING LIST

Bricker BM. Industrial marketing and medical ethics. N Engl J Med 1989; 320:1690–1692.

Canada. Health Protection Branch, Health and Welfare Canada. Code of good monitoring practice for clinical investigators. 1983.

CMA guidelines for drug–company supported CME. CMAJ 1986; 135:384A.

Davies IB, Grind IM, Pottage A, Turner P. Development of new drugs in man: a review. J Roy Soc Med 1986; 79:96–99.

DeDombal PT, Holt PR, Sidorov JJ. Ethics in gastroenterology: proceedings of a workshop meeting of the World Organisation of Gastroenterology held at St. George's House, Windsor Castle, Berkshire, England, 29 April – 2 May 1986. Leeds: University of Leeds Printing Service, 1986:21–24.

Duggan JM. Resource allocation and bioethics. Lancet 1989; 1:772–773.

Engler RL, Covell JW, Friedman PJ, Kitcher PS, Peters RM. Misrepresentation and responsibility in medical research. N Engl J Med 1987; 317:1383–1389.

Gibinski K. Ethics and training in digestive endoscopy. Endoscopy 1989; 21:232–233.

Grad MR. Human experimentation and informed consent. CMAJ 1984; 131:932–935.

Leaf A. The doctor's dilemma — and society's too. N Engl J Med 1984; 310:718–720.

McGregor M. Pharmaceutical "generosity" and the medical profession. Ann RCPSC 1988; 21:289.

Omery A, Caswell D. A nursing perspective on the ethical issues surrounding liver transplantation. Heart and Lung 1988; 17:626–630.

Rawlins MD. Doctors and the drug makers. Lancet 1984; 2:276–278.

Reagan MD. Health care rationing: what does it mean? N Engl J Med 1988; 319:1149–1151.

Reagan MD. Physicians as gatekeepers: a complex challenge. N Engl J Med 1987; 317:1731–1733.

The Royal College of Physicians of London. The relationship between physicians and the pharmaceutical industry: a report of the Royal College of Physicians. J Roy Col Phy of London 1986; 20:235–241.

Sabesin SM, Williams JW, Evans LS. Ethical and economic issues. In: Maddrey WC (ed.), Transplantation of the liver. New York: Elsevier, 1988:331–343.

Sidorov JJ. Ethics in gastrointestinal research. Scand J Gastroenterol 1988; 23(Suppl. 144):100–113.

Singer PA, Siegler M, Whitington RF, et al. Ethics of liver transplantation with living donors. N Engl J Med 1989; 321:620–621.

Sircus W. Ethics of diagnostic and therapeutic endoscopic procedures. Scand J Gastroenterol 1988; 23(Suppl. 144):105–106.

Thompson WG. The ethics of physician–pharmaceutical company relationships. CMAJ 1988; 129:835–836.

Williams JR. Human organ sales. Ann RCPSC 1985; 18:401–404.

Younger SJ, Allen M, Bartlet ET, et al. Psychosocial and ethical implications of organ retrieval. N Engl J Med 1985; 313:321–323.

4
Research and Clinical Trials: The Basis for New Knowledge

A. Archambault

1. INTRODUCTION

THE SCIENTIFIC STUDY of drugs in humans represents an important aspect of the clinical research conducted in university teaching medical centers and large community hospitals. In the field of gastroenterology, pharmacological studies and clinical trials are principally developed for acid peptic disorders and inflammatory bowel diseases.

The world pharmaceutical market is divided into three approximately equal parts: (1) North America, (2) the European countries and (3) the group including Aşia, Africa and Australia. Canada represents only 3% of the market for this highly specialized and competitive activity.

The development of a new drug before it reaches market may require 10 to 15 years of investment; only one of more than 8,000 substances initially tested in animal models may stand the course from original chemical discovery to the development of a useful drug for clinical therapy in human subjects. This time-consuming and very expensive process requires the work of numerous biological and medical specialists who must combine extraordinary talent and devotion to develop each agent.

2. CLINICAL RESEARCH REGULATIONS AND SUPERVISION

In the United States, the first regulation governing unapproved new drugs and their admissibility for clinical investigational use dates as far back as 1938. Following the dramatic events involving thalidomide, important amendments were adopted, making preclinical data, informed consent and report findings mandatory after 1962. Rules establishing good clinical practices were adopted for sponsors in 1977 and for investigators in 1978. Investigational new drug (IND) regulation was established in 1987.

In Canada, the Medical Research Council of Canada (MRC) approved guidelines for research involving human subjects in 1987. The latest guidelines for good clinical research practices are stipulated in a document entitled "Conduct of Clinical Investigations," and were officially adopted by the Health Protection Branch (HPB) of the Canadian government in 1989. France, Germany, the Nordic countries, the United Kingdom and Japan adopted similar guidelines and regulations in 1989 and 1990.

The most recent and comprehensive set of guidelines for trials of medicinal products emerged in October 1990 from a meeting where the tenets of good practice were compared by scientists of the European community and North America.

Although some differences exist among countries in government policy and regulations controlling clinical research in humans, the consensus on guidelines for good clinical practices in research is becoming more uniform.

Both sponsors (pharmaceutical companies) and investigators (basic researchers or clinicians) must share the responsibility for producing very high quality data and adhering to the ethical recommendations guiding physicians who conduct biomedical research on human subjects. The Declaration of Helsinki – first adopted in Finland in 1964, and last revised by the World Medical Assembly in Hong Kong in September 1989 – is the universally accepted ethical code.

3. CLINICAL RESEARCH DEVELOPMENT

The research process includes preclinical studies and clinical trials.

3.1 Preclinical Studies

Preclinical studies are conducted in the experimental research laboratories of pharmaceutical companies and university centers.

The chemical industry, continuously in search of active substances for patent rights and formulation, selects various chemical structures for synthesis in active form on a laboratory scale and for assays on animal models.

A pharmacological expert analyzes the main effect of the compound, its duration of action and any adverse effects in various animal species. Pharmacokinetic studies determine the action and fate of each substance in the animal organism – i.e., absorption, distribution, metabolism and excretion. Toxicological studies to observe any possible mutagenic and teratogenic effects are important. Subsequent studies are completed to determine the optimal dosage and route of administration. From these studies a candidate drug is selected for further large-scale development. These goals can usually be achieved within 2 to 4 years. The submission to the government authorities for authorization to administer a new drug to humans is a well-defined and rigid procedure that may require an additional 2 to 12 months.

3.2 Clinical Trials

The U.S. Food and Drug Administration is among the most rigid and respected regulation boards in the world. The Health Protection Branch in Canada complies with a similar policy; for this reason, multicenter trials are very common between these two countries.

Medical clinical research guidelines accept four phases for clinical trials.

3.2.1 PHASE I

These are the first trials of any new active ingredient on human subjects. They are performed on 20 to 50 subjects, ordinarily healthy volunteers, to identify a safe dosage regimen and the optimal route of administration. These tolerance studies are done first with a single dose, then with multiple doses. All pharmacokinetic/dynamic profile studies in humans must be performed under close medical surveillance; some require appropriate resuscitation facilities. During Phase I, there is continuous monitoring of long-term animal studies for toxicity and potential carcinogenicity.

3.2.2 PHASE II

At this phase, therapeutic pilot studies evaluate the activity and safety of a new drug in patients suffering from a specific disease. The studies are usually short-term and placebo-controlled: they are done on a limited number of patients (100–200). Dose range/regimens and dose/response relationship must provide an optimal background for the eventual design of wider therapeutic trials.

The animal studies for toxicity and carcinogenicity are still kept under scrutiny during this phase.

3.2.3 PHASE III

These comparative studies are conducted in a large sampling of patients (500–5,000) in the setting of normal clinical practice. The circumstances of the trials are maintained as close as possible to the normal conditions of use of the drug. Fixed doses of the medication in controlled studies are usually compared with conventional therapy for short- and long-term efficacy and safety.

The results of these trials define the therapeutic profile of the drug and determine the final indications, dosage, route of administration and contraindications, as well as the reported warnings regarding side effects and possible interactions with concomitant medications.

Concurrently, the manufacturing process is developed.

The duration of Phases II and III ranges from three to five years. Even with the most satisfactory results, a submission to government authorities requesting authorization to market a new drug must be filed, and may take an additional two to three years to be approved.

During the postmarketing surveillance period, new indications, new formulations or effective combinations may be explored, and the therapeutic value of the medication may be reassessed or new strategies developed. These studies are considered part of the Phase III development of a drug.

3.2.4 PHASE IV

Clinical studies are performed on approved or marketed drugs to gather more information on possible adverse events, to compare them with alternative therapy and to detect interaction with other drugs.

4. METHODOLOGY IN CLINICAL RESEARCH

Preferably, clinical trials in Phases II and III should be controlled and double-blinded to allow valid comparison with similar groups and to avoid bias. Controlled studies involve a matched placebo (or alternative treatment) group, randomization (with access to a treatment code in the event of an emergency), various blinding techniques with proper drug matching, strict labeling and meticulous statistical analysis. Avoidance of any bias should ensure that the differences between study subjects' responses are due only to the difference between drug treatments. Uncontrolled trials are acceptable in Phase I pilot studies or in Phase IV, for the long-term evaluation of biochemical changes and drug interactions.

The knowledge of a new medication, however, grows gradually through the various phases of chemical research. It is likely never to be 100% complete. All new findings should be documented and reported even after the product has been on the market for several years.

5. GOALS AND REQUIREMENTS IN CLINICAL RESEARCH

In most countries, the efficacy and safety of a drug must be well established and demonstrated by the appropriate therapeutic trials before the agent can be approved for general clinical use in patients. Internationally acceptable standards, agreed-upon scientific principles and sound clinical practice rules are among the prerequisites for the design and conduct of these trials. They must also comply with the national laws and requirements of the various regulatory authorities supervising medical research throughout the world. The major authorities in North America are the Food and Drug Administration in the United States and the Health Protection Branch in Canada. The randomized clinical trial is considered the "gold standard" for establishing the validity of medical therapy. It must comprise sound scientific design, competent investigators, a reasonable balance between risks and benefits and an unbiased selection of subjects.

6. PLANNING OF CLINICAL TRIALS

The medical departments of pharmaceutical companies develop a study protocol for each drug to be submitted for clinical trials in humans. This procedure follows standard and rigid principles and may involve advice and expertise from scientists and clinicians interested in the nature of the drug. A steering committee for a study may be organized. It may advise that modifications be made to the protocol, or influence the selection of the investigators and study centers.

7. SELECTION OF INVESTIGATORS AND CENTERS

The selection of the principal investigators for clinical research will depend on the nature of the drug and the phase of its development. Experts in clinical pharmacology are necessary for Phase I and II studies; experts in clinical trials or medical specialties conduct Phase III and IV studies. The principal investigator in each center is responsible for carrying out the study in accordance with the protocol and for the accurate and complete reporting of the results. This person must sign a formal statement of agreement for the study and take responsibility for its commitments. Investigators must show initial and continuing personal involvement. Selection is based on several criteria, including their past record in peer-reviewed medical research, their current interest in the proposed study and the time they have available for participation. They must show evidence of appropriate clinical facilities with adequate space and equipment, safe drug storage and assistance from a research-oriented registered nurse or qualified interviewer. Access to a certified laboratory must be available. The laboratory must be able to conduct the study according to the guidelines of good laboratory practices adopted by the Food and Drug Administration in 1978. In addition, the investigators should make a predictive analysis estimating the number of study subjects required for a valid outcome, positive or negative. The investigators must agree to be audited at any time by the sponsor's representatives or by the government authorities.

8. PROTOCOL DESIGN

For Phase I–III trials, the study protocol must be approved by the Food and Drug Administration in the United States or the Health Protection Branch in Canada. Consultation with a biostatistician is desirable to select a suitable study design (open, single, double-blind, parallel or crossover, placebo or active treatment control). Within limits of the exclusion and inclusion criteria of a study, the selection of patients must be representative of the population in distribution and randomization. A brief introduction usually summarizes the source and chemical nature of the drug, and describes its pharmacology, toxicology and prior clinical investigation. The objective of the study states exactly which question is to be answered. The treatment schedule explains the drug administration, including dosage, strength, route of administration, the blinding process, packaging and labeling.

Measurement and evaluation procedures of the trial describe the following: medical parameters (inclusion and exclusion criteria, baseline, pre- and post-treatment), follow-up visit observations, clinical and laboratory investigations, relevant hazards, concomitant treatments, precautions (particularly in case of possible pregnancy), adverse events, management of overdose and treatment endpoints. The procedure to discontinue the study must be outlined in case of lack of efficacy of the drug, intolerable side effects or poor patient compliance. The statistical analysis, publication rules, institutional review committee and insurance and liability requirements are also discussed.

For the patient's protection, relevant facts in all documents used by the patient must be explained in lay language. Diary forms and informed consent papers must be absolutely clear, and must be translated into the patient's language when needed.

9. INFORMED CONSENT FORM AND ETHICAL ISSUES

The informed consent form involves a written description of the nature and purpose of the trial, the randomization uncertainties, the benefits, the foreseeable risks, the discomforts, the potential side effects and the availability of alternative treatment.

This form is an acknowledgment that specific information has been given;

it is never proof that the subject has been fully informed. It does not indicate the degree of comprehension or autonomy of the patient. Specific rules must be adopted for the unconscious or disabled patient. Even if the informed consent is for the protection of the investigator and the patient, it has no legal power in North America.

The investigator or a qualified delegate must present the consent form to the patient, preferably in the presence of an impartial witness. Sufficient time must be allowed for the patient to consider the information and to ask questions. The patient must be informed of his or her right to withdraw from the study at any time without prejudice.

10. CLINICAL MONITORING

A very important aspect of clinical research is the clinical monitoring of the trial by the sponsor's delegates. Accountability for the drug dispensed to the patients must be very accurate. This implies continuous surveillance of the expiry date, lot numbers, stability and storage conditions, and return of all unused medication.

Accuracy of drug records requires that all clinical information be registered at the time of the patient's visit. Possible deficiencies in the trial may be corrected following the visits of the clinical monitor. The patient's condition before, during and after the treatment period, the laboratory data, the concomitant therapy, the special events and side effects are all duly recorded at specific times in the trial. Source-data verification against the patient's clinical records is required by the principles of good clinical practices. The amount and extent of this verification will vary with each study.

At the completion of the study, the final evaluation of the recorded data for efficacy and safety is assured by a review of the investigation for accuracy, completeness and legibility. The results and conclusion must be signed by the investigator.

11. INSTITUTIONAL REVIEW COMMITTEE (IRC)

No patient can be enrolled in a clinical trial before an institutional review committee has accepted the protocol and the informed consent form. The scientific aspects of a trial are evaluated by clinical peer reviewers and experienced clinical researchers in each institution where the study is performed. Suggested modification requirements must be accepted by both the sponsor and investigator.

The committee should comprise at least five sufficiently qualified members. Both sexes must be represented and members should be sensitive to local racial and cultural issues. There should be at least one nonscientist member and one member who is not affiliated with the institution. No committee member should have any conflicting interests.

The Declaration of Helsinki represents the most important piece of information worldwide for those choosing to become involved in clinical research.

BIBLIOGRAPHY

Canada. Health Protection Branch, Health and Welfare Canada. Drugs Directorate guidelines.
a. Preparation of human new drug submissions (1991).
b. Conduct of clinical investigations. No. H42-2/14 (July 1989).

Canada. Medical Research Council of Canada. Guidelines on research involving human subjects. Minister of Supply and Services Canada, 1987. No. MR 21-5/1987E.

The clinical trial in Canada, USA, in Nordic and EEC countries. 2nd Symposium on drug development sponsored by the Faculty of Pharmacy of the Université de Montréal and the Health Protection Branch, Canada, May 6–7, 1990, Montréal, Québec. Montréal: Université de Montréal, 1990 (binder).

Declaration of Helsinki: Recommendations Guiding Physicians in Biomedical Research Involving Human Subjects.

France. Ministère des affaires sociales et de l'emploi. Ministre chargé de la santé et de la famille. Bulletin officiel. Direction des journaux officiels, 26, rue Desaix, 75105 Paris, France.

Good Clinical Research Practices Limited. Clinical study monitoring (binder).
Three-day course presented in Mississauga, Ontario, March 1991.
Bolaychuk WP, Ph.D.
Ball GT, C.D., Ph.D.
Kimpton DJ.
European office: Round Windows, Grayshott Road, Headly Down, Hampshire, U.K. GU 358JL.

Guidelines for research and ethical rules from FDA (U.S.A.)

Review articles. Drug Information Journal (January/June 1982):7–96.

5
The Esophagus

W.G. Paterson

1. INTRODUCTION

THE ESOPHAGUS is a hollow muscular organ whose primary function is to propel into the stomach the food or fluid bolus that it receives from the pharynx. Symptoms of esophageal disease are among the most commonly encountered in gastroenterology. Fortunately, most symptoms are due to benign disease that can be easily remedied. The physician must be on the lookout, however, for the more serious disorders, which can present with a similar spectrum of symptoms. This chapter will focus on the pathophysiology, diagnosis and management of the more common esophageal disorders. Rare diseases involving the esophagus will be dealt with only briefly.

2. ANATOMY

2.1 Muscular Anatomy

The esophagus is a hollow muscular tube closed proximally by the upper esophageal sphincter (UES) and distally by the lower esophageal sphincter (LES). The UES consists predominantly of the cricopharyngeus and the caudal fibers of the inferior pharyngeal constrictor muscles. The UES forms a transverse slit at the C5–C6 vertebral level due to surrounding bony structures and cartilage. In the proximal one-quarter to one-third of the esophagus, the muscle is striated. There is then a transition zone of variable length where there is a mixture of both smooth and striated muscle. The distal one-half to one-third of the esophageal body and LES are composed of smooth muscle. The LES is located at the junction between the esophagus and stomach, usually localized at or just below the diaphragmatic hiatus. Despite its distinct physiological function, it is not easily distinguished anatomically.

2.2 Innervation

The motor innervation of the esophagus is via the vagus nerves. The cell bodies of the vagal efferent fibers innervating the UES and the proximal striated-muscle esophagus arise in the nucleus ambiguus, whereas fibers destined for the distal smooth-muscle segment and the LES originate in the dorsal motor nucleus. The esophagus and LES also receive sympathetic nerve supply (both motor and sensory) arising from spinal segments T1–T10. Sensory innervation is also carried via the vagus and consists of bipolar nerves that have their cell bodies in the nodose ganglion and project from there to the brainstem.

2.3 Blood Supply

Arterial blood supply to the UES and cervical esophagus is via branches of the inferior thyroid artery. Most of the thoracic esophagus is supplied by paired aortic esophageal arteries or terminal branches of bronchial arteries. The LES and the most distal segment of the esophagus are supplied by the left gastric artery and by a branch of the left phrenic artery. Venous drainage is via an extensive submucosal plexus that drains into the superior vena cava from the proximal esophagus and into the azygous system from the mid-esophagus. In the distal esophagus, collaterals from the left gastric vein (a branch of the portal vein) and the azygos interconnect in the submucosa. This connection between the portal and systemic venous systems is clinically important; when there is hypertension, variceal dilatation can occur in this area. These submucosal esophageal varices can be the source of major gastrointestinal hemorrhage.

2.4 Lymphatic Drainage

In the proximal third of the esophagus, lymphatics drain into the deep cervical lymph nodes, whereas in the middle third, drainage is into the superior and posterior mediastinal nodes. The distal-third lymphatics follow the left gastric artery to the gastric and celiac lymph nodes. There is considerable interconnection among these three drainage regions.

2.5 Histology

The wall of the esophagus consists of mucosa, submucosa and muscularis propria. Unlike other areas of the gut, it does not have a distinct serosal covering, but is covered by a thin layer of loose connective tissue. The mucosa consists of stratified squamous epithelium in all regions of the esophagus except the

LES, where both squamous and columnar epithelium may coexist. Beneath the epithelium are the lamina propria and the longitudinally oriented muscularis mucosa. The submucosa contains connective tissue as well as lymphocytes, plasma cells and nerve cells (Meissner's plexus). The muscularis propria consists of an inner circular and an outer longitudinal muscle layer. The circular muscle layer provides the sequential peristaltic contraction that propels the food bolus toward the stomach. Between the circular and longitudinal muscle layers lies another nerve plexus called the myenteric or Auerbach's plexus, which mediates much of the intrinsic nervous control of esophageal motor function.

3. PHYSIOLOGY

The major function of the esophagus is to propel swallowed food or fluid into the stomach. This is carried out by sequential or "peristaltic" contraction of the esophageal body in concert with appropriately timed relaxation of the upper and lower esophageal sphincters. The esophagus also clears any refluxed gastric contents back into the stomach and takes part in such reflex activities as vomiting and belching.

3.1 Deglutition: Primary Peristalsis

The act of deglutition is a complex reflex activity. The initial phase is under voluntary control. Food is chewed, mixed with saliva and formed into an appropriately sized bolus before being thrust to the posterior pharynx by the tongue. Once the bolus reaches the posterior pharynx, receptors are activated that initiate the involuntary phase of deglutition. This involves the carefully sequenced contraction of myriad head and neck muscles. The food bolus is rapidly engulfed and pushed toward the esophagus by the pharyngeal constrictor muscles. Simultaneously there is activation of muscles that lift the palate and close off and elevate the larynx in order to prevent misdirection of the bolus. Almost immediately upon activation of this reflex, the UES opens just long enough to allow the food bolus to pass through; it then rapidly shuts to prevent retrograde passage of the bolus. The oropharyngeal phase is thus completed and the esophageal phase takes over. This involves two major phenomena: (1) the sequential contraction of the circular muscle of the esophageal body, which results in a contractile wave that migrates toward the stomach; and (2) the relaxation and opening of the LES, which allows the bolus to pass. The peristaltic sequence and associated UES and LES relaxation induced by swallowing are termed *primary peristalsis*. These can be assessed manometrically using an intraluminal tube to measure pressures. The typical sequence seen during primary peristalsis is depicted in Figure 1. *Secondary peristalsis* refers to a peristaltic sequence that occurs in response to distention of the esophagus. This is a localized peristaltic wave that usually begins just above the area of distention. It is associated with LES relaxation, but not with UES relaxation or deglutition.

3.2 Upper Esophageal Sphincter Function

The UES serves as a pressure barrier to prevent retrograde flow of esophageal contents and the entry of air into the esophagus during inspiration. This high-pressure zone is created by tonic contraction of the UES muscles, which is produced by tonic neuronal discharge of vagal lower motor neurons. With deglutition this neuronal discharge ceases temporarily and permits relaxation of the UES. UES opening will not occur with relaxation of the muscles alone; it requires elevation and anterior displacement of the larynx, which is mediated by contraction of the suprahyoid muscles. Relaxation lasts for only one second and is followed by a postrelaxation contraction (Figure 1).

3.3 Esophageal Body Peristalsis

There is a fundamental difference in the control mechanisms of peristalsis between the upper (striated-muscle) esophagus and the lower (smooth-muscle) esophagus. In the striated-muscle segment, peristalsis is produced by sequential firing of vagal lower motor neurons so that upper segments contract first and more aboral segments subsequently. In the smooth-muscle segment, the vagal preganglionic efferent fibers have some role in the aboral sequencing of contraction, but intrinsic neurons are also capable of evoking peristalsis independently of the extrinsic nervous system. Transection of vagal motor fibers to the esophagus in experimental animals will abolish primary peristalsis throughout the esophagus; however, in this setting, distention-induced or secondary peristalsis will be maintained in the smooth-muscle but not in the striated-muscle segment. Furthermore, if vagal efferent fibers are stimulated electrically (Figure 2), a simultaneous contraction will be produced in the striated-muscle esophagus that begins with the onset of the electrical stimulus, lasts throughout the stimulus, and ends abruptly when the stimulus is terminated. In the smooth-muscle esophagus, however, the response to vagal efferent nerve stimulation is quite different, in that the onset of contractions is delayed relative to the onset of the stimulus. The latency to onset of the contraction increases in the more distal segments of the esophagus (i.e., the evoked contractions are peristaltic).

This experimental observation indicates that intrinsic neuromuscular mechanisms exist and can mediate peristalsis on their own. Further evidence for

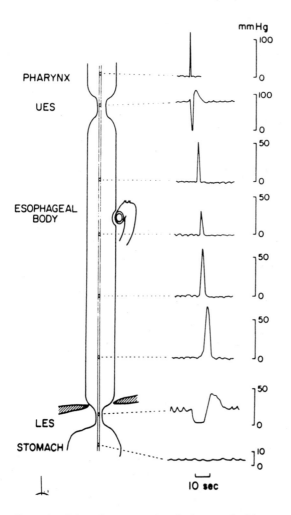

FIGURE 1.   Schematic representation of primary peristalsis as recorded by intraluminal manometry. Swallowing is marked by a rapid pharyngeal contraction coincident with abrupt relaxation of
the UES. This is followed by postrelaxation contraction of the UES and sequential contraction of
the esophageal body, which produces a pressure wave that migrates toward the stomach. A swallowed food bolus is pushed in front of this migrating contraction wave. The LES relaxes within 1
to 2 seconds of the onset of swallowing and remains relaxed until the esophageal pressure wave
has reached the distal esophagus. LES pressure then recovers and is followed by a postrelaxation
contraction, which occurs in continuity with the distal esophageal contraction.
SOURCE: Goyal RK, Paterson WG. Esophageal motility. In: Wood JD (ed.), Handbook of physiology: motility and circulation, vol. 4. Washington DC: American Physiological Society, 1989.
Used with permission.

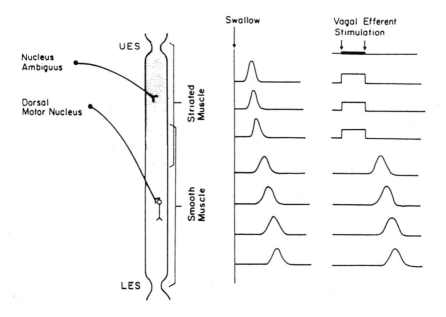

Swallow

Vagal Efferent
Stimulation

Nucleus Ambiguus

Dorsal Motor Nucleus

UES

Striated Muscle

Smooth Muscle

LES

FIGURE 2. Schematic representation of esophageal peristaltic contractions as evoked by swallowing and vagal efferent nerve stimulation. Swallowing evokes sequential esophageal contractions that pass smoothly from the striated- to the smooth-muscle segment. Electrical stimulation of the distal cut end of a vagus nerve, which simultaneously activates all vagal efferent fibers, evokes peristaltic contractions only in the smooth-muscle segment of the esophagus. In the striated-muscle esophagus, vagal stimulation causes simultaneous contractions that occur only during the period of stimulation. This demonstrates that the striated-muscle esophagus is dependent on central neuronal sequencing for its peristaltic contraction, whereas intrinsic neuronal mechanisms are capable of producing a peristaltic sequence in the smooth-muscle segment.
SOURCE: Goyal RK, Paterson WG. Esophageal motility. In: Wood JD (ed.), Handbook of physiology: motility and circulation, vol. 4. Washington DC: American Physiological Society, 1989. Used with permission.

this mechanism is found in studies where strips of esophageal circular smooth muscle are stimulated electrically in vitro. The latency to contraction after stimulation is shortest in the strips taken from the proximal smooth-muscle segment and increases progressively in the more distal strips.

This latency gradient of contraction is clearly important in the production of esophageal peristalsis. Although the exact mechanisms are unclear, initial or deglutitive inhibition is important. With primary or secondary peristalsis, a wave of neurally mediated inhibition initially spreads rapidly down the esophagus. This is caused by the release of a nonadrenergic, noncholinergic inhibitory neurotransmitter (most likely nitric oxide) that produces hyperpolarization (inhibition) of the circular smooth muscle. It is only after recovery from this initial hyperpolarization that esophageal muscle contraction (which is mediated primarily by cholinergic neurons) can occur. Thus, the duration of this initial inhibition is important with respect to the differential timing of the subsequent contraction. Derangements of the mechanisms behind this latency gradient lead to nonperistaltic contractions and dysphagia. Such derangements could result from problems with either the intrinsic neural mechanisms (enteric nervous system) or the central neuronal sequencing.

3.4 Lower Esophageal Sphincter Function

The LES is an intraluminal high-pressure zone caused by tonic contraction of a region of physiologically distinct circular smooth muscle at the junction of the esophagus and stomach. This results in a pressure barrier that separates the esophagus from the stomach and serves to prevent reflux of gastric contents up into the esophagus. In normal individuals, resting LES pressure averages between 10 and 30 mm Hg above intragastric pressure. Patients with very feeble resting LES pressure are prone to develop gastroesophageal reflux disease (GERD). Unlike that of the UES, the resting tone of the LES is primarily due to myogenic factors that result in tonic contraction of the sphincter. Extrinsic innervation as well as circulating hormones can modify the resting tone; however, the muscle fibers themselves have inherent properties that result in their being tonically contracted.

At the time of deglutition or when the esophagus is distended, the LES promptly relaxes. Swallow-induced LES relaxation is mediated by vagal efferent fibers that synapse on nonadrenergic, noncholinergic inhibitory neurons of the myenteric plexus. The inhibitory neurotransmitter released from these intrinsic neurons is probably nitric oxide. LES relaxation usually lasts about five to seven seconds, and is sufficient to abolish the gastroesophageal pressure barrier. This permits the food bolus to pass unimpeded from the esophagus to the stomach. The LES also relaxes to permit belching or vomiting. Inadequate LES relaxation is seen in achalasia and results in dysphagia.

4. SYMPTOMS AND SIGNS OF ESOPHAGEAL DISEASES

4.1 Symptoms

4.1.1 DYSPHAGIA

This sensation of food sticking during swallowing is a manifestation of impaired transit of food through the mouth, pharynx or esophagus. It is important to differentiate oropharyngeal ("transfer") dysphagia from esophageal dysphagia. If the patient has problems getting the bolus out of the mouth, then one can be certain of an oropharyngeal cause; if the food sticks retrosternally, an esophageal cause is indicated. Some patients, however, will sense food sticking at the level of the suprasternal notch when the actual obstruction is the distal esophagus. Thus, it can be difficult to determine the site of the problem when patients refer their dysphagia to the suprasternal notch or throat area. With these patients it is important to elicit any ancillary symptoms of oropharyngeal-type dysphagia, such as choking or nasal regurgitation. It may also be helpful to observe the patient swallowing in an attempt to determine the timing of the symptom; with esophageal dysphagia referred to the suprasternal notch, the sensation of dysphagia onsets several seconds after swallowing begins.

The history can also be used to help differentiate structural from functional (i.e., motility disorders) causes of dysphagia. Dysphagia that is episodic and occurs with both liquids and solids from the outset suggests a motor disorder, whereas when the dysphagia is initially for solids such as meat and bread, and then progresses with time to semisolids and liquids, one should suspect a structural cause (e.g., stricture). If such a progression is rapid and associated with significant weight loss, a malignant stricture is suspected.

Associated symptoms help determine the etiology of dysphagia. For instance, a reflux-induced stricture should be suspected if the dysphagia is associated with heartburn or regurgitation, esophageal cancer if there is associated mid-back pain and weight loss, a motor disorder such as diffuse esophageal spasm if there is angina-like chest pain, and a "scleroderma esophagus" if there is arthralgia, skin changes or Raynaud's phenomenon.

4.1.2 ODYNOPHAGIA

This refers to the sensation of pain on swallowing. Local inflammation or neoplasia in the mouth and pharynx can produce such pain. When the pain is retrosternal, one should suspect nonreflux-induced forms of esophagitis, such as infection, radiation or pill-induced (chemical) injury. Less commonly it occurs with esophageal cancer, a deep esophageal ulcer (e.g., Barrett's ulcer) or esophageal motor disorders.

4.1.3 HEARTBURN OR PYROSIS

The sensation here is one of retrosternal burning. Typically it begins in the low retrosternal area and radiates up to the throat. It may be precipitated by bending over or lying down, and usually begins shortly after consuming certain foods or beverages. It is often associated with regurgitation of acidic material into the back of the throat. "Heartburn" with these features indicates gastroesophageal reflux. This very common symptom has been experienced at one time or another by over one-third of the population and therefore does not necessarily indicate serious disease. Many patients will complain of "heartburn," but this should not be taken at face value: this term is used by some patients to describe unrelated symptomatology. It is therefore important to have patients describe exactly what they mean by the term *heartburn*.

4.1.4 *REGURGITATION*
This refers to the spontaneous appearance of food or fluid in the back of the throat or in the mouth. Some patients describe this symptom as "vomiting"; therefore it is important to determine whether there is associated nausea, retching, etc., when patients present with "vomiting." The taste and consistency of the regurgitated material is an important historical detail. Regurgitation of acidic or bile-stained fluid indicates gastroesophageal reflux. Regurgitation of undigested food or stagnant fluid devoid of an acidic taste indicates an esophageal transport problem (e.g., achalasia). (With achlorhydria, gastric contents also lack acid.) In motor disorders and mechanical obstruction of the esophagus, food may become stuck and then rather quickly will be regurgitated if it does not pass through into the stomach. Some patients regurgitate food back into their mouths after a meal only to chew and swallow it all over again. This is called *rumination* and, although a rarity in humans, it is a normal physiological event in certain animals.

4.1.5 *NONHEARTBURN CHEST PAIN*
This can also indicate esophageal disease. Chest pain, and in particular mid-dorsal pain, is seen in advanced esophageal cancer. The most common type of nonheartburn esophageal chest pain, however, is a pain that is qualitatively similar to the pain of ischemic heart disease. This pain can be squeezing or crushing and can radiate into the jaw or arms. Unlike ischemic heart pain, angina-like chest pain of esophageal origin is not predictably elicited by exertion and often occurs spontaneously, in relationship to meals or in the middle of the night. It is associated with other esophageal symptoms. Clearly, patients with this type of pain need to have ischemic heart disease excluded. Once this is done, many will be found to have some form of esophageal motor disorder. In addition, this angina-like pain can be precipitated by gastroesophageal reflux.

4.1.6 *WATERBRASH*
This sudden appearance of copious amounts of saliva in the mouth must be differentiated from regurgitation of fluid. With waterbrash, acid reflux into the esophagus stimulates hypersalivation via a (cholinergic) neural reflex.

4.1.7 *BLEEDING*
This may be a symptom of certain esophageal diseases. Esophageal varices can cause massive hematemesis and melena. Deep esophageal ulcers may also bleed massively, but this is uncommon. Usually the bleeding from ulcerative lesions of the esophagus is occult. When the patient does present with hematemesis or melena from esophagitis, the rate of bleeding is usually slow; therefore, significant hemodynamic compromise is uncommon.

4.1.8 *RESPIRATORY SYMPTOMS*
These may be a manifestation of esophageal disease or oropharyngeal swallowing disorders. Aspiration at the time of swallowing will cause coughing, choking and eventual hoarseness. In addition, patients with motor disorders or GERD may regurgitate esophageal or gastric contents up into the larynx and subsequently aspirate. These patients may present with pneumonia, chronic cough, wheezing or hoarseness. Gastroesophageal reflux may also trigger coughing and wheezing via a vasovagal reflex.

4.2 Signs
It is uncommon for esophageal disease to be associated with specific physical findings. Signs of weight loss and malnutrition can be found if the esophageal problem is so severe that adequate caloric intake is not maintained. There may be signs of metastatic disease (e.g., hepatomegaly, supraclavicular lymphadenopathy) in esophageal cancer. Patients with GERD rarely have respiratory tract signs such as wheezing, hoarseness or lung consolidation. It is important to look for signs of connective tissue disease (especially scleroderma) in patients with reflux symptoms or dysphagia.

The physical examination is more often helpful in patients with oropharyngeal dysphagia. Careful examination of the head and neck for structural and neurologic abnormalities is mandatory. It is also important to look for more generalized neurologic or connective tissue abnormalities. Observing the patient swallow is also useful when oropharyngeal dysphagia is present.

5. INVESTIGATIONS USED IN THE DIAGNOSIS OF ESOPHAGEAL DISEASE

5.1 Barium X-ray
This most commonly used method of investigating the esophagus evaluates both structural lesions and motor disorders. It is the single most important test in evaluating patients with dysphagia. Proper communication between physician and radiologist is vital. Videotaping the barium swallow allows for play-

back and slow-motion review. This is very helpful in assessing the rapid events of the oropharyngeal phase of swallowing. Use of marshmallows, barium-coated cookies and different consistencies of barium further assesses swallowing disorders, as delays in transport may not be apparent with simple liquid barium. The disadvantage of barium x-rays is that they are relatively insensitive in detecting mucosal disease, even if air contrast technique is added.

5.2 Endoscopy with Mucosal Biopsy and Brush Cytology

Fiberoptic endoscopy directly visualizes the esophageal mucosa as well as other areas of the upper gastrointestinal tract. Its direct view is superior to barium x-rays for assessing mucosal disease of the esophagus, and the esophagoscope permits assessment of structural lesions that are identified. Furthermore, pinch biopsies and/or brush cytology of specific lesions are easily obtained through the endoscope. Microscopic evidence of esophagitis may be found even when the mucosa looks grossly normal. Endoscopy is the single most useful test in the evaluation of patients with reflux symptoms, as it permits one to establish the presence or absence of esophagitis or Barrett's esophagus (Section 7.3). Endoscopy gives little reliable information regarding esophageal function.

5.3 Bernstein (Acid Perfusion) Test

This tests the sensitivity of the patient's esophagus to acid perfusion. A tube is placed into the distal esophagus and saline, acid and then antacid are infused sequentially, with the patient kept unaware as to what is being administered. The patient is questioned periodically about the presence or absence of symptoms and their quality. This test is useful in determining whether a patient's atypical chest or epigastric pain is secondary to acid reflux. The test is positive if the patient's presenting pain is reproduced during acid perfusion and relieved by antacid perfusion.

5.4 Esophageal Manometry

This involves recording intraluminal pressures at multiple sites along the esophagus (Figure 1). The most commonly used method involves a perfused multilumen catheter bundle with side holes at 5 cm intervals. Each catheter is connected to a pressure transducer, which in turn is attached to a physiograph. LES pressure and swallow-induced LES relaxation are measured, as are pressure responses to swallowing at several esophageal sites. Pharyngeal peristalsis and UES function can also be measured. Esophageal manometry is the "gold standard" in the assessment of esophageal motor disorders. Motor dysfunction, however, may be intermittent and therefore not detected at the time of the study. Manometry is now commonly combined with provocative tests (acid perfusion, balloon distention and/or pharmacological stimulation of the esophagus with bethanechol or edrophonium) in an attempt to evoke abnormal contractions and reproduce the patient's chest pain (Section 11).

5.5 pH Reflux Studies

These are performed using a pH electrode passed via the nose or mouth into the distal esophagus. The traditional short-duration study measures acid reflux events (pH drop to < 4) after various postural maneuvers. This has now been largely replaced by a miniature system that with computer assistance allows 24-hour ambulatory studies. The results of this test are compared to a healthy control population to determine whether an abnormal degree of gastroesophageal reflux is present. They also can be correlated to any spontaneous symptoms that occur with acid reflux events. Despite initial enthusiasm for this test in determining the presence or absence of GERD, recent reports have found a high false-negative rate.

5.6 Radionuclide Studies

These assess either gastroesophageal reflux or esophageal transit. In the latter instance, food or fluid labeled with a radioisotope is swallowed and gamma camera scanning is performed over the chest. Computer programs measure transit time in the upper, middle and lower thirds of the esophagus. This has been reported to be a sensitive way of detecting motor dysfunction in patients with dysphagia. It may therefore be a useful screening test, but fails to give information concerning the type of motor disorder present. Gastroesophageal reflux can be quantitated by having the patient ingest the radioisotope and then scanning over the chest and upper abdomen. Binders are placed over the abdomen to increase intra-abdominal pressure; reflux is present if the isotope is seen to travel back up into the esophagus. The role of this test in the assessment of patients with reflux disease remains to be defined, as its sensitivity and specificity are rather poor.

6. ANATOMIC VARIANTS

6.1 Congenital Anomalies

Embryologically the gastrointestinal and respiratory tracts start out as a single tube; however, by the second month of gestation they have completely divided. Problems with this process lead to various congenital anomalies, the most common being tracheoesophageal fistula with esophageal atresia. In 85–

90% of cases, the proximal esophagus ends in a blind pouch while the distal esophagus consists of a blind pouch in continuity with the stomach. Neonates with this abnormality develop immediate aspiration with feeding. There is no air in the bowel on x-ray films of the abdomen, contrary to what is observed in those with fistulas involving the distal esophagus. In 1–2% of cases there is an "H-type" fistula with atresia. The patient presents with repeated pulmonary infections and abdominal distention. The latter is caused by air getting into the gastrointestinal tract via the fistula when the infant cries. Because the H-type fistula may be very small, the condition may go unnoticed until adulthood, when it is detected during the investigation of recurrent pulmonary infections. Some of these fistulas may close spontaneously but produce paraesophageal inflammation and ultimately localized esophageal stricture formation.

Treatment of esophageal fistulas (with or without atresia) is surgical. The prognosis is now quite good and mortality is usually related to coexistent congenital malformations. It is important to remember that many of these patients will have gastroesophageal reflux as well as abnormal esophageal peristalsis following surgery, which may cause significant long-term problems.

Congenital esophageal stenosis is a rare anomaly that is also probably related to abnormal differentiation of the gastrointestinal and respiratory tracts, as resected specimens have been found to have pulmonary epithelium and/or bronchial remnants. Sequestered pulmonary remnants with connections to the esophagus but not associated with stenosis have also been described.

6.2 Hiatus Hernia

The majority of hiatus hernias are acquired. Rarely, a hiatus hernia can be caused by a congenitally short esophagus. Hiatus hernias can be divided into two types: (1) sliding and (2) paraesophageal (Figures 3 and 4, respectively). A *sliding hiatus hernia* refers to the condition where a circumferential cuff of cardia and proximal stomach migrates up through the diaphragmatic hiatus and into the thorax. This may reduce and reform spontaneously. These hernias are very common and increase in incidence with advancing age. Generally they are of no clinical significance, despite the fact that many patients and physicians persist in attributing a wide variety of symptoms to them. Large hiatus hernias may be associated with iron deficiency anemia that is presumably caused by recurrent superficial ulcerations at the site where the diaphragm exerts pressure on the herniated stomach. If no other source of GI blood loss is discovered after thorough investigation, and patients continue to be iron-deficient despite supplementation and antiulcer treatment, surgical correction of the hernia should be performed.

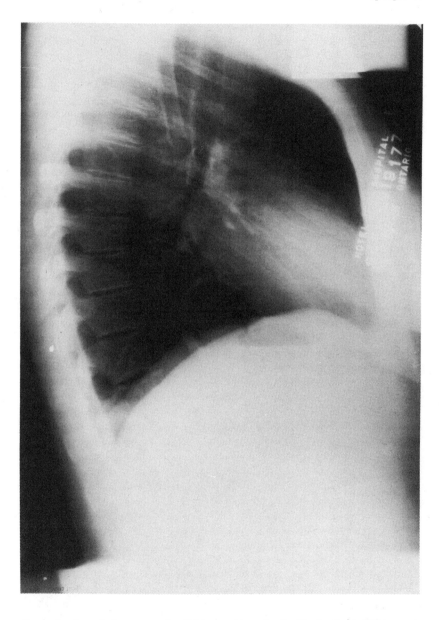

FIGURE 3. Lateral chest x-ray of a sliding-type hiatus hernia. The fundic air bubble can be clearly seen in the chest, posterior to the cardiac silhouette, indicating that the gastroesophageal junction and upper stomach have slid up through the diaphragmatic hiatus.

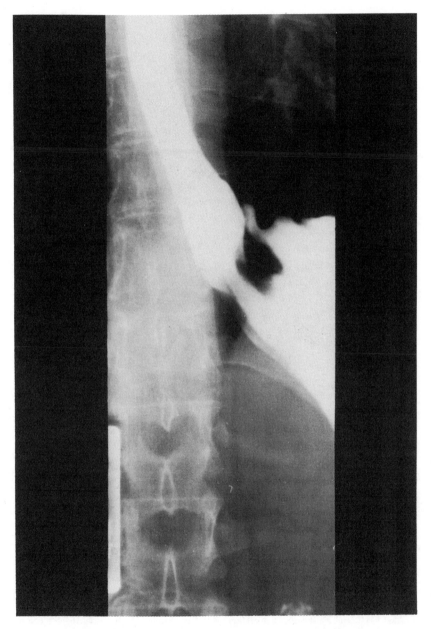

FIGURE 4.   Barium contrast study of a paraesophageal-type hiatus hernia. Note that the gastro-esophageal junction has maintained its normal position at the hiatus, but a small portion of the gastric fundus has migrated up through the hiatus alongside the esophagus.

The etiology of the sliding hiatus hernia is obscure. Certainly there is laxity and dilatation of the diaphragmatic hiatus and associated laxity of the phreno-esophageal ligament; however, these may well be secondary and not primary pathophysiologic factors. In some cases, persistent gastroesophageal reflux may result in inflammation and consequent esophageal shortening, which in turn leads to the development of a hiatus hernia.

A sliding hiatus hernia is often seen in association with GERD; the precise role of the hernia in the pathogenesis of the reflux remains obscure. Certainly the majority of people with hiatus hernias do not have significant reflux disease, and occasionally patients with severe reflux esophagitis will not have a hiatus hernia. It appears that a hiatus hernia may contribute somewhat to gastroesophageal reflux, but it is most unlikely that this is the prime etiologic factor. A hiatus hernia may contribute to GERD by providing a reservoir of gastric acid that has ready access to the distal esophagus whenever the LES relaxes.

Paraesophageal hiatus hernias are uncommon. These consist of the fundus of the stomach migrating through the hiatus alongside the esophagus without any displacement of the gastroesophageal junction. Although these hernias are often asymptomatic, most physicians believe that they should be treated surgically when the diagnosis is made because the herniated portion may become strangulated and infarcted.

7. GASTROESOPHAGEAL REFLUX DISEASE (GERD)

GERD is the most common condition to affect the esophagus. The disease spectrum ranges from patients with heartburn and other reflux symptoms without morphologic evidence of esophagitis (the so-called acid-sensitive esophagus) to patients with deep ulcer, stricture or Barrett's epithelium. Everyone has some degree of gastroesophageal reflux; it becomes pathological only when associated with troublesome symptoms or complications. Fortunately, the vast majority of patients suffering from GERD have an easily controlled disorder. At the other end of the spectrum, there are patients who develop severe damage to the esophagus. Some will develop Barrett's metaplasia as a consequence of gastroesophageal reflux, which in turn predisposes them to adenocarcinoma.

7.1 Pathophysiology

GERD results from the reflux of gastric contents into the esophageal lumen. Early pathogenesis concepts focused on anatomic factors: reflux was considered a mechanical problem, related to the development of a hiatus hernia. We now know, however, that a hiatus hernia can occur without GERD, and conversely, GERD can occur without a hiatus hernia. Many factors are involved in the pathogenesis of GERD.

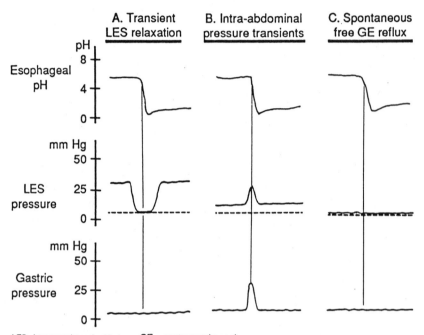

LES= lower esophageal sphincter   GE = gastroesophageal

FIGURE 5.   Schematic representation of three different mechanisms of gastroesophageal (GE) reflux.

A. Transient LES relaxation refers to the sudden occurrence of LES relaxation that causes obliteration of the gastroesophageal pressure barrier and permits gastric contents to reflux up into the esophagus. The reflux event is marked by the sudden drop in esophageal pH. These transient LES relaxations are sometimes related to incomplete or failed peristalsis but may also occur in isolation.

B. Intra-abdominal pressure transients are sudden increases in intragastric pressure caused by coughing, sneezing or deep inspiration. The increased intragastric pressure overcomes the LES pressure and results in reflux.

C. Spontaneous free reflux occurs when there is very low or nonexistent LES pressure, which permits spontaneous reflux across the gastroesophageal junction. In healthy volunteers without GERD, virtually all reflux episodes are due to transient LES relaxation. In patients with reflux esophagitis, approximately two-thirds of the reflux episodes are due to transient LES relaxation. The remaining one-third are caused by either intra-abdominal pressure transients or spontaneous free gastroesophageal reflux.

SOURCE: Dodds WJ, Dent J, Hogan WJ, et al. Mechanisms of gastroesophageal reflux in patients with reflux esophagitis. N Engl J M 1982; 307:1547–1552. Used with permission.

7.1.1 *BARRIERS TO GASTROESOPHAGEAL REFLUX*

By far the most important barrier to gastroesophageal reflux is the LES. Factors such as the intra-abdominal location of the sphincter, extrinsic compression exerted by the diaphragmatic crura and the angle of His (which forms a "mucosal flap valve") may augment this barrier but play a minor role relative to the LES itself. Some patients developing reflux esophagitis have feeble LES tone, but in most, resting LES pressure is nearly normal. Gastroesophageal reflux occurs by three major mechanisms, as outlined in Figure 5.

7.1.2 *ESOPHAGEAL CLEARANCE*

Once reflux occurs, the duration of insult to the esophageal mucosa depends on the rapidity with which the esophagus clears this material. Once the initial (primary) peristaltic wave has passed, the bolus (a portion of which frequently remains) is cleared by one or two secondary peristaltic waves. The remaining small adherent acidic residue is then neutralized by saliva, which is carried down by successive swallows. Disorders of salivation or esophageal motor function will impair this clearance mechanism and predispose to the development of GERD.

Patients with severe GERD may have frequent prolonged nighttime reflux episodes because during sleep, peristalsis seldom occurs and salivary flow virtually ceases. Hence the contact time of refluxed material with the esophagus is markedly increased.

7.1.3 *GASTRODUODENAL FACTORS*

In some patients delayed gastric emptying further predisposes to the development of GERD. Bile salts and pancreatic enzymes, if refluxed back into the stomach, can in turn reflux into the esophagus and may inflict worse damage than when gastric juice is refluxed alone. Such reflux into the stomach and then the esophagus may occur after gastric surgery, when the pylorus is destroyed. Whenever there is increased gastric pressure or an increase in gastric contents, there is greater likelihood that reflux will occur when the sphincter barrier becomes deficient.

7.1.4 *MUCOSAL RESISTANCE*

The degree of damage to esophageal mucosa depends not only on the composition of the refluxed material and the amount and duration of reflux, but also on defensive factors within the mucosa itself. Certain patients are more susceptible to the development of actual mucosal damage, for reasons that are not clear.

TABLE 1. Diagnostic tests in GERD

Tests to determine the presence of reflux
Barium meal
Radionuclide scintigraphy
pH reflux study (short-duration or 24-hour ambulatory)

Tests to determine whether symptoms are due to reflux
Bernstein (acid perfusion) test
24-hour pH recording

Tests to determine the presence of mucosal damage
Barium meal
Endoscopy
Mucosal biopsy

7.2 Clinical Features

Most patients present with heartburn and acid regurgitation that onset after eating certain foods or following various postural maneuvers (e.g., bending over, lying flat). Frequency varies from once a week or less to daily episodes with disruption of sleep. Other presenting symptoms include waterbrash, angina-like chest pain, dysphagia and various respiratory symptoms (hoarseness, cough, wheezing). The dysphagia may be due to the development of a reflux-induced stricture or to abnormal motility induced by the refluxed acid. Odynophagia is rarely a symptom of GERD and should alert the physician to another diagnosis such as infectious esophagitis.

Reflux symptoms are common during pregnancy because of increased intra-abdominal pressures and the LES-relaxant effect of progesterone.

Physical examination in patients with GERD rarely reveals associated physical signs. In severe cases with stricture formation there may be weight loss secondary to decreased caloric intake, or findings of consolidation or bronchospasm on respiratory examination in patients who have GE reflux with aspiration.

7.3 Diagnosis

In the vast majority of patients, GERD can be diagnosed from the history alone and treated without further investigation. Several tests are useful in the assessment of suspected GERD, depending on the information sought: Is there an abnormal degree of reflux? Are symptoms in fact due to reflux? Is there mucosal damage or other complications (Table 1)? Some specialists believe that all patients with symptomatic gastroesophageal reflux should undergo endoscopy. The argument in favor of this approach is that Barrett's esophagus will be found in up to 10–15% of these patients. This identifies those at increased risk for the development of adenocarcinoma (Section 7.5.2). Most physicians, however, feel that in young patients with typical symptoms that are infrequent and relatively mild, empiric therapy should be instituted first without further investigation. In patients with frequent or more severe symptoms but without symptoms that suggest complications, endoscopy is necessary to rule out other diseases and to document the presence or absence of mucosal damage or Barrett's metaplasia. Endoscopic biopsy will also detect microscopic esophagitis, which may appear normal otherwise.

Many patients will have normal endoscopy and biopsy even though significant GERD is present. In these patients or in patients with atypical or multiple symptoms, it is worthwhile to do a Bernstein test and/or a 24-hour pH reflux study to establish that the symptom(s) are in fact due to acid reflux. It is important to first rule out ischemic heart disease if the presenting symptom is angina-like chest pain.

All patients who present with symptoms of complicated GERD (i.e., dysphagia, bleeding or respiratory symptoms) need to be fully investigated. If dysphagia is present, a barium x-ray study should be performed, followed by endoscopy. Further investigations will depend on the results of the initial tests. Esophageal manometry has little role to play in the routine assessment of patients with GERD. It is useful in the assessment of patients with atypical symptoms, and can be combined with an acid perfusion (Bernstein) test as well as with other provocative tests. It is important to perform manometry prior to surgical intervention, because patients with significant underlying primary motor disorders of the esophagus (e.g., scleroderma) often develop severe dysphagia following an antireflux procedure.

7.4 Treatment

7.4.1 MEDICAL TREATMENT

The treatment of GERD is directed toward the abnormal pathophysiology (Table 2). In patients with mild or infrequent symptoms, lifestyle modifications, dietary advice, elevation of the head of the bed and p.r.n. antacids are usually all that is required. If possible, the patient should avoid ingestion of various agents that are known to inhibit LES tone and promote reflux (Table 3). In patients with more severe symptoms or who do not respond to these simple measures, addition of an H_2-receptor antagonist is indicated. Prokinetic agents such as cisapride may also be used alone or in combination with other agents in the treatment of GERD, but are probably best suited for the subgroup of patients who have gastroparesis or coexistent functional, nonulcer

TABLE 2. Medical therapy of gastroesophageal reflux disease: a pathophysiologic approach

---

Decrease frequency of reflux episodes
Improve LES function (prokinetic drugs; avoid certain drugs and foods)
Elevate head of bed 4–6 inches on blocks
Weight loss

Augment clearing mechanisms; decrease duration of reflux episodes
Bethanechol (?also metoclopramide, domperidone, cisapride)
Other agents to stimulate salivation
Gravity (elevate head of bed, avoid bending over)

Decrease irritant quality and volume of gastric juice
Antacids, alginic acid
H_2-receptor antagonists (cimetidine, ranitidine, famotidine, nizatidine)
M_1 antagonists (pirenzepine)
Proton pump inhibitors (omeprazole)
Prokinetic agents (bethanechol, metoclopramide, domperidone, cisapride)

Augment esophageal mucosal defenses
Sucralfate
?Misoprostol

---

subgroup of patients who have gastroparesis or coexistent functional, nonulcer dyspepsia (gas-bloat syndrome). The most efficacious therapy for GERD currently available is the proton pump inhibitor omeprazole. This should be used in patients with complicated GERD (e.g., frank erosive esophagitis, peptic stricture or Barrett's ulcer) or in patients who have not responded to H_2-receptor antagonists.

GERD is a chronic relapsing condition that usually requires long-term treatment. As a general rule the physician should use the simplest, least expensive and least potent therapeutic regime that will keep the patient's symptoms in check.

7.4.2 SURGICAL TREATMENT
Antireflux surgery should be considered in patients with reflux esophagitis whose symptoms are not controlled with the aforementioned medical regimen. Some patients who develop the complications of GERD (Section 7.5) are also best managed surgically. Several different operative techniques are used for this condition. The most popular are the Nissen fundoplication, the Belsey Mark IV repair and the Hill posterior gastropexy. At some centers antireflux surgery is being performed via the laparoscopic route. All procedures adhere to the same basic principles: restoration of the LES to an intra-abdominal

TABLE 3.   Agents known to decrease LES tone

Theophylline
Caffeine
Fatty meal
Chocolate
Peppermint
Smoking
Ethanol
Calcium channel blockers
Morphine
Meperidine
Benzodiazepines
β-adrenergic agonists
Nitrates
Anticholinergics (including tricyclic antidepressants)

position, extrinsic bolstering of the LES pressure and repair of the patulous hiatus. Use of a ring-like prosthesis (Angelchik prosthesis) simplifies the surgery but produces significant long-term complications; it probably should not be used.

The results of antireflux surgery depend more on the expertise and experience of the surgeon than on the specific operative procedure. In expert hands, surgery will produce a good-to-excellent result in 85–95% of patients; however, in up to 50% of these patients, objective evidence of recurrent pathological reflux will be present five years after surgery, even though symptomatic benefit is maintained. Overall operative mortality for first-time operations is in the order of 0.5%. Between 10 and 20% of patients develop significant problems with dysphagia and/or gas-bloat symptoms after surgery. In most cases these problems resolve with time.

7.5 Complicated GERD

7.5.1 PEPTIC STRICTURE
Chronic GERD may lead to peptic stricture formation. This is a fibrous stricture related to collagen deposition that occurs in the course of repair of esophagitis. Patients are usually asymptomatic until the luminal narrowing has reached 12–14 mm. At this point dysphagia to solids occurs. As the stricture progresses, the dysphagia gradually progresses to semisolids and then liquids. Treatment of peptic strictures involves peroral dilation, using either mercury-filled rubber bougies or dilators passed over guidewires. In close to 50% of

patients one or two dilation sessions prove adequate, and no further dilations are required because ongoing medical treatment of the reflux is successful. In others, the stricture recurs and periodic dilations are required to maintain luminal patency. In patients who are otherwise healthy, consideration should be given to antireflux surgery if frequent dilations are required to maintain luminal patency. The success rate of antireflux surgery is lower in such patients with peptic stricture. Strictures are less likely to recur following dilation if the patient is treated with omeprazole. For this reason, long-term treatment with this agent seems appropriate for patients with peptic stricture.

7.5.2 BARRETT'S ESOPHAGUS

This develops in up to 10% of patients with chronic GERD. In this condition the squamous epithelium of the distal esophagus is replaced by metaplastic columnar epithelium. Deep ulcers as well as strictures at the new squamocolumnar junction may also develop. Severe hemorrhage may complicate the deep ulcers.

Barrett's epithelium is a premalignant condition. At the time of initial presentation, about 10% of patients found to have Barrett's esophagus will have coexistent adenocarcinoma arising in the Barrett's epithelium. This number gives an exaggerated impression of the magnitude of risk, because Barrett's esophagus patients with cancer are more likely to seek medical attention. The true incidence of adenocarcinoma developing in Barrett's epithelium is only about 1 case for every 200 patient-years of follow-up. This nevertheless represents about a 30- to 40-fold increase over the risk faced by the general population. For this reason patients with Barrett's esophagus should be followed periodically with endoscopy and mucosal biopsy in order to detect early cancer. Most patients will develop severe dysplasia before frank invasive carcinoma occurs. Thus, if patients are found to have severe dysplasia or early mucosal carcinoma, esophageal resection should be considered in order to prevent the development of invasive carcinoma. Although there have been case reports of Barrett's esophagus regressing after successful antireflux surgery, it is unlikely that such surgery decreases the risk of cancer in the majority of patients. For this reason, Barrett's esophagus per se should not be an indication for antireflux surgery. Surgery should be performed if the patient has symptoms or complications not readily managed by medical therapy.

7.5.3 RESPIRATORY COMPLICATIONS

In some patients the refluxed gastric contents may get past the UES and into the larynx and lungs. This produces recurrent chest infections, chronic cough and laryngitis. In addition, gastroesophageal reflux may trigger bronchospasm or cough via a neural reflex. GERD with aspiration is more commonly seen in the pediatric age group; when present, antireflux surgery should be performed unless there is a well-documented response to medical therapy.

8. NONREFLUX-INDUCED ESOPHAGITIS

8.1 Infectious Esophagitis
Bacteria rarely cause primary esophageal infection, although the esophagus can be involved secondarily by direct extension from the lung. The two most common forms of infectious esophagitis are caused by Candida and herpes. Other viruses and fungi also cause esophagitis; however, this is uncommon and almost invariably associated with immunosuppression.

8.1.1 *CANDIDA ESOPHAGITIS*
This is by far the most common form of infectious esophagitis. Usually there is a predisposing cause, such as diabetes mellitus, antibiotic therapy or some form of immunocompromise. The patient may be asymptomatic. Not all patients will have associated oral thrush. More commonly, however, patients present with odynophagia, retrosternal chest pain and/or dysphagia. Severe cases can be complicated by bleeding, a stricture and sinus tract formation with secondary lung abscess. Barium x-rays reveal an irregular granular or even cobblestone appearance to the esophageal mucosa. Approximately 25% of patients will have a normal barium esophagogram; for this reason, endoscopy with biopsy and brushing are required to make the diagnosis. The typical endoscopic appearance is the presence of small raised whitish plaques. When the plaques are removed the underlying mucosa is seen to be erythematous and friable. Specimens obtained by biopsy or brush cytology should be cultured and examined microscopically for the presence of typical Candida yeast with pseudohyphae formation. Most patients can be treated with oral nystatin; however, in immunocompromised patients ketoconazole should be initial therapy. Amphotericin B is required if there is evidence of systemic spread.

8.1.2 *HERPES SIMPLEX ESOPHAGITIS*
Next to Candida, this is the most common form of infectious esophagitis. The clinical presentation is much the same as with Candida esophagitis. There may also be constitutional symptoms of a viral upper respiratory tract infection preceding the esophageal symptoms. Herpetic mouth or skin lesions may also develop. This infection occurs most frequently in immunosuppressed patients, but also develops sporadically in healthy young adults. Endoscopy

with biopsy and brush cytology is required to confirm the diagnosis. The pathognomonic finding is the eosinophilic "Cowdry's Type A" intranuclear inclusion body. Herpetic esophagitis is self-limiting in immunocompetent individuals; specific treatment is not indicated. Symptoms of odynophagia often respond to a combination of antacids mixed with viscous Xylocaine®. In severely immunocompromised patients, intravenous acyclovir treatment should be instituted.

8.2 Esophagitis Associated with Immune-Mediated Disease

Rarely, esophagitis can occur in association with Crohn's disease or Behçet's syndrome. The typical lesion is scattered aphthous-type ulcerations, although severe transmural involvement with stricture formation can occur. The esophagus can also be severely involved in pemphigoid, in pemphigus and in epidermolysis bullosa.

Esophagitis occurs in as many as one-third of patients who develop chronic graft-versus-host disease after bone marrow transplantation. The typical lesion is a generalized epithelial desquamation of the upper and middle esophagus. There may be associated ring-like narrowings or strictures due to submucosal fibrosis. A nonspecific esophageal motor disorder may also develop and result in superimposed reflux esophagitis because of poor esophageal clearing. Sarcoidosis and eosinophilic gastroenteritis are two other immune-mediated diseases that (rarely) cause esophageal inflammation.

8.3 Chemical-Induced Esophagitis

8.3.1 CAUSTIC CHEMICAL INGESTION

Strong acids or alkalis ingested accidentally or as a suicidal gesture cause marked esophagitis. Alkali tends to be more injurious to the esophageal mucosa than acid and produces liquefaction necrosis as well as thermal burns (due to heat release when the alkali is hydrated by gut secretions). Acids tend to produce superficial coagulation necrosis and eschar formation. Typically the patient develops immediate chest pain and odynophagia. Oral burns also may produce local pain and drooling. There may be respiratory symptoms such as stridor, dyspnea and hoarseness if the airway is contaminated. Symptoms alone do not permit accurate prediction of the presence or absence of esophageal injury; therefore early diagnostic endoscopy should be carried out in most patients. Clearly, endoscopy should not be performed if there is evidence of esophageal perforation. In the management of these patients, it is imperative to maintain an adequate airway. Oral intake must be stopped and intravenous fluids administered. Empiric treatment classically has involved antibiotics and corticosteroids, but there is no good evidence documenting the efficacy of this approach. Patients who survive the acute phase of the injury are at risk of developing strictures because of the intense collagen deposition associated with healing. This often requires repeated esophageal dilation to maintain luminal patency.

Lye-induced injury increases the risk of developing squamous cell carcinoma of the esophagus. Typically there is a 30- to 50-year lag time before the development of cancer. For this reason any patient with previous lye injury and new esophageal symptoms should be promptly investigated. The extent of the risk is such that periodic endoscopic surveillance is not indicated.

8.3.2 *PILL-INDUCED ESOPHAGITIS*

A large number of oral agents can cause localized esophageal injury. The antibiotic doxycycline and the anticholinergic emepronium bromide are two of the most common culprits. Patients with this type of injury typically take their medication with a small amount of water and then immediately lie down to go to bed. They may then wake up several hours later with severe retrosternal chest pain and odynophagia. Capsules and tablets are notorious for being transported through the esophagus quite poorly unless adequate amounts of fluid are ingested at the same time. This is an important point to remember in counseling all patients who take medicines at bedtime. Rarely, the medication becomes lodged and causes a deep esophageal ulcer with perforation. More commonly the ulceration is superficial and heals in a few weeks. Late stricture formation may occur. Patients with esophageal motility disorders are particularly prone to this complication.

8.4 **Radiation-Induced Esophagitis**

When included in the field of irradiation the esophagus becomes inflamed in up to 80% of patients receiving therapeutic radiation for cancer. The risk of esophagitis is greater if there is concomitant chemotherapy. The patients typically develop chest pain, dysphagia and odynophagia shortly after the initiation of therapy. This can be a serious problem in such patients, who are already often severely malnourished. Late stricture formation is a well-recognized complication.

9. **DISORDERS OF THE OROPHARYNGEAL PHASE OF DEGLUTITION**

A variety of structural and functional disorders can disrupt the oropharyngeal phase of deglutition and result in oropharyngeal or "transfer"-type dysphagia

TABLE 4.   Classification of disorders causing oropharyngeal dysphagia

---

Central nervous system disease
Cerebrovascular accident (brainstem, pseudobulbar palsy)
Wilson's disease
Multiple sclerosis
Amyotrophic lateral sclerosis
Brainstem neoplasm
Tabes dorsalis

Peripheral nervous system disease
Bulbar poliomyelitis
Miscellaneous peripheral neuropathies
Head and neck neoplasms
Post–radical neck surgery

Muscle disease
Muscular dystrophy
Polymyositis and dermatomyositis
Metabolic myopathy (e.g., hypo- and hyperthyroidism)
Amyloidosis
Systemic lupus erythematosus
Myasthenia gravis

Local disorders
Oropharyngeal inflammation
Oropharyngeal neoplasms
Zenker's diverticulum

Idiopathic
Cricopharyngeal achalasia
Idiopathic oropharyngeal incoordination

(Table 4). In the assessment of these patients it is important to exclude disorders for which specific treatment is available.

The most important investigation is a carefully performed video fluoroscopic study of the swallowing mechanism. In addition to the usual barium studies, it is helpful to observe deglutition when the patient swallows barium-soaked cookies or bread. Not only will this examination identify and characterize disorders of oropharyngeal coordination, it will also help exclude structural lesions. If an inflammatory, neoplastic or other structural lesion is suspected, direct or indirect laryngoscopy is indicated. At present manometric studies of the pharynx and UES add little to what can be learned from radiologic studies. This is partly because of limitations in recording methods, but also because complex motor events occurring during deglutition (e.g., closure of the nasopharynx, elevation and closure of the larynx – see Section 3, "Physiology") are not amenable to manometric study.

Ideally, treatment of oropharyngeal motor disorders should be directed at the underlying disease. Frequently this is not possible, and nonspecific treatment must be instituted. In some cases reassurance and education are all that is required. Many patients will be able to control their symptoms simply by eating slowly and carefully in a relaxed atmosphere. In patients in whom aspiration develops because of inadequate clearing of the hypopharynx after the initial swallow, it is beneficial to have the patient immediately follow a "bolus" swallow with a second, "dry" swallow. Correcting denture problems and avoiding foods of certain consistency may also help. Most speech pathologists have special expertise as swallowing therapists and can be extremely helpful in the management of these patients.

For patients in whom these simple measures are not helpful and whose symptoms are such that respiratory and nutritional complications are developing, cricopharyngeal myotomy is often performed. This helps patients with true cricopharyngeal achalasia or Zenker's diverticulum (Section 13). Unfortunately, the response to myotomy is inconsistent in most other patients with oropharyngeal dysphagia, because inadequate opening of the UES is rarely due to dysfunction of the cricopharyngeal muscle alone. More often there is associated weakness of the suprahyoid muscles, which actually open the sphincter, and/or associated problems with pharyngeal peristalsis. Cricopharyngeal myotomy does little to improve such altered physiology. Once cricopharyngeal myotomy has been performed, the patient has lost an important defense mechanism against the aspiration of refluxed material. The patient should therefore be instructed to elevate the head of his or her bed on blocks in order to minimize this risk. For this same reason patients with gross GERD should not undergo cricopharyngeal myotomy unless the reflux can be controlled.

When all other measures fail and nutritional and respiratory complications develop, percutaneous endoscopic gastrostomy should be performed. If the problem is so severe that the patient cannot handle salivary secretions, it is sometimes necessary to also perform laryngeal exclusion and tracheotomy.

10. MOTOR DISORDERS OF THE ESOPHAGUS AND LOWER ESOPHAGEAL SPHINCTER

Esophageal motor disorders can be classified as either primary or secondary. Primary disorders refer to those that usually affect the esophagus alone and

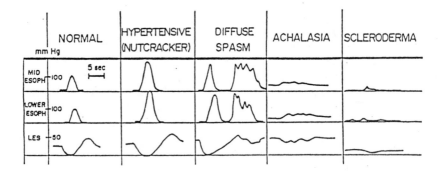

FIGURE 6. Manometric features of the major esophageal motor disorders. A *normal* tracing is on the left and depicts sequential "peristaltic" contractions in the esophageal body with full LES relaxation. *Hypertensive peristalsis* or *"nutcracker" esophagus* is characterized by normal peristalsis and LES relaxation, but the amplitude of contraction in the distal esophagus is abnormally high (> 180 mm Hg). In *diffuse esophageal spasm*, normal peristaltic waves are interspersed with high-pressure, nonpropulsive (simultaneous) contraction waves that are often repetitive. The resting LES pressure may be abnormally high, but swallow-induced LES relaxation is normal. In *achalasia* there is complete absence of normal peristalsis in the smooth-muscle segment of the esophageal body. The LES is usually hypertensive, and swallow-induced LES relaxation is either absent or incomplete. Note also that resting intraesophageal pressures are elevated. *Scleroderma* is characterized by the presence of weak, nonperistaltic esophageal conditions and a markedly hypotensive LES that relaxes normally with swallowing.

have no known etiology. Secondary disorders are motility derangements caused by some other systemic or local condition. Examples of secondary disorders include acid-reflux–induced dysmotility, dysmotility related to the neuropathy associated with diabetes or alcoholism, and motor dysfunction secondary to esophageal involvement in scleroderma or other connective tissue disorders. The well-defined primary motor disorders include the hypertensive peristaltic or "nutcracker" esophagus, diffuse esophageal spasm and achalasia (Figure 6). Many cases of primary motility disorders are actually "nonspecific," having a variety of abnormalities that do not fulfill criteria established for the well-defined motor disorders of the esophagus.

Patients with primary motor disorders typically present with dysphagia and/ or chest pain. The pain is often qualitatively similar to angina pectoris and is attributed to smooth-muscle spasm. Some patients with motor disorders will have secondary GERD because of poor clearing or poor LES function. Here, heartburn and regurgitation may be prominent symptoms.

The diagnosis of a motor disorder can be made on the basis of history and barium swallow x-ray. If there is dysphagia referred to the retrosternal area and no evidence of a structural lesion on x-ray, then by exclusion the patient's dysphagia is related to a motor disorder. As mentioned previously, the quality of the dysphagia (e.g., sporadic, unpredictable dysphagia to both liquids and solids) is also helpful in differentiating motor disorders from structural causes of dysphagia. During fluoroscopy, the radiologist is usually able to detect abnormalities of motor function as the barium is swallowed. Endoscopy primarily rules out secondary causes of the disorder (i.e., ulcerative esophagitis and neoplasm). In order to define specifically the type of motor disorder present, however, esophageal motility studies are required. The manometric features of the important esophageal motor disorders are depicted schematically in Figure 6.

10.1 "Nutcracker" Esophagus
This motility disorder is characterized by normally propagated but high-amplitude peristaltic waves in the distal esophagus. The duration of the contraction wave is also often prolonged. LES relaxation is normal, although in many patients the resting LES pressure is elevated. Patients often present with angina-like chest pain and usually do not complain of dysphagia. Nutcracker esophagus is the most frequent abnormal manometric finding in patients referred for evaluation of noncardiac angina-like chest pain. The etiology is unknown. Rarely, this disorder progresses to diffuse esophageal spasm or even vigorous achalasia. Reassurance that the pain is not cardiac but is secondary to a benign esophageal condition is the most important part of treatment. Nitrates and calcium channel blockers (to relax smooth muscle) have been used extensively, but have no proven benefit. In some patients with nutcracker esophagus, pain is actually triggered by acid reflux; these patients often respond dramatically to appropriate antireflux therapy.

10.2 Diffuse Esophageal Spasm
This is characterized by normal peristalsis interspersed with frequent high-pressure nonpropagated or "tertiary" waves and multipeaked waves. Patients often present with dysphagia and chest pain. In advanced diffuse esophageal spasm, the x-ray will show a corkscrew pattern as different segments of the esophagus vigorously and simultaneously contract. The etiology is obscure, but may relate to degenerative changes in the intrinsic and extrinsic esophageal nerves. Management involves reassurance and the use of nitrates or calcium channel blocking agents. Patients with severe disease unresponsive to medical measures may benefit from a long esophageal myotomy.

10.3 Achalasia
This uncommon primary motility disorder is characterized by aperistalsis in

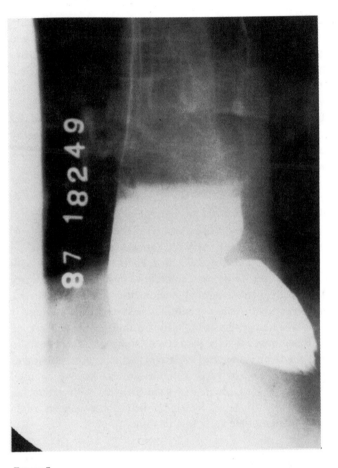

FIGURE 7.
A. Typical barium x-ray in a patient with achalasia. Note that the esophagus is dilatated and an air-barium level is present, indicating stasis. There is also tortuosity of the distal esophagus, which is often referred to as a "sigmoid" esophagus. At the gastroesophageal junction (lower right) there is a beak-like narrowing, which is caused by the nonrelaxing LES. The mucosal contour at this narrow area appears normal.
B. Barium x-ray of a patient with advanced scleroderma esophagus. The esophagus is dilatated, with evidence of retained food debris. Note that the narrowing at the gastroesophageal junction is somewhat irregular on one wall. This is due to an area of structuring caused by gastroesophageal reflux. This x-ray appearance can be confused with that of achalasia (Figure 7A) and points out the need to confirm a diagnosis of achalasia or scleroderma by performing endoscopy and esophageal manometry.

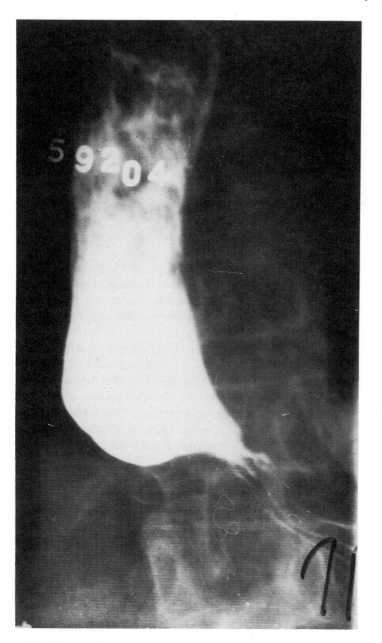

the body of the esophagus, an elevated LES pressure and absent or incomplete LES relaxation in response to swallowing. Failure of LES relaxation leads to progressive proximal dilatation of the esophagus with consequent elevated resting intraesophageal pressures. On x-ray the esophagus is dilatated, and retained food and fluid may be present. The distal esophagus narrows in a beak-like fashion (Figure 7A). This "beak" represents the hypertonic, nonrelaxing LES. In some patients there are associated vigorous nonperistaltic contractions in the esophageal body, a condition called *vigorous achalasia*. Achalasia is caused by degeneration of inhibitory neurons within the esophageal and LES myenteric plexus. Nerve damage also occurs in the vagal nerve trunks and the dorsal motor nuclei. The parasite Trypanosoma cruzi, which is endemic in Brazil, can cause achalasia by destroying myenteric neurons (Chagas' disease). Neoplastic disease can also interfere with esophageal and LES nerve function and cause "secondary" achalasia. The cause of the degeneration is unknown in most cases, however.

The cardinal symptom of achalasia is dysphagia, although chest pain and even heartburn may be present. The heartburn is not due to gastroesophageal reflux. It may be caused by lactic acid formed by fermentation of stagnant esophageal contents. Another common symptom of achalasia is regurgitation of esophageal contents.

In mild cases treatment can begin with the use of calcium channel blockers or long-acting nitrates, which have been shown to decrease LES pressure. This is rarely successful in the long term, however. The treatment then required is pneumatic balloon dilation of the LES. This consists of passing a balloon across the sphincter and inflating it rapidly so that the sphincter is forcefully dilated. Pneumatic dilation is successful in alleviating the dysphagia and improving esophageal transport in approximately 70–75% of patients. Patients who do not respond to pneumatic dilation should be treated with Heller myotomy. This consists of a longitudinal incision through the muscle of the LES. (Laparoscopic techniques are being developed.) Following either pneumatic dilation or Heller myotomy, the patient can develop severe GERD, because the pressure barrier preventing reflux has been destroyed. This tends to be worse after Heller myotomy and has led some surgeons to perform a modified antireflux procedure at the time of myotomy. Because of this problem all patients having successful myotomy or pneumatic dilation should be instructed regarding lifelong antireflux therapy. Usually dietary and posture-type treatment are all that is needed, but in some patients drug therapy is required. Achalasia patients have an increased risk of developing esophageal cancer and need to be thoroughly investigated if new esophageal symptoms develop.

10.4 Scleroderma Esophagus

Patients with scleroderma frequently have esophageal involvement. This may occur even in the absence of obvious skin and joint involvement. The initial event is damage to small blood vessels, which in turn leads to intramural neuronal dysfunction. With time, actual muscle damage and fibrosis occur. This results in a very hypotensive LES, as well as weak nonpropulsive esophageal contractions. Scleroderma may also involve the stomach and cause delayed gastric emptying. As a result, patients develop gross GERD. They present with heartburn and regurgitation, as well as dysphagia. The dysphagia can be due to poor esophageal propulsion and/or reflux-induced stricture (Figure 7B). These patients need very aggressive treatment for GERD. Because they have very poor peristaltic function, increasing the barrier at the LES with antireflux surgery may markedly worsen the dysphagia.

11. THE ESOPHAGUS AS A CAUSE OF ANGINA-LIKE CHEST PAIN

At least one-third of the patients referred to a cardiologist or admitted to a coronary care unit because of angina-like chest pain will have cardiac causes excluded. In most, an alternative etiology is not apparent. Lack of a specific diagnosis may lead to ongoing anxiety, changes in lifestyle and frequent medical consultations if the patient continues to worry that serious heart disease may be present. Such patients should be evaluated for esophageal disease, although the cost-effectiveness of this approach is not known.

Initial investigations include a barium esophagogram and/or upper GI endoscopy to screen for gross esophageal dysmotility and esophagitis. These studies, however, are frequently negative. For this reason, esophageal motility studies with provocative testing (acid perfusion, drug provocation with edrophonium or bethanechol, intraesophageal balloon distention) are usually required to establish an esophageal cause for the pain (Figure 8). In many of these patients, abnormalities of esophageal motility can be documented, suggesting that esophageal dysfunction may be responsible for the pain. Of more diagnostic importance, however, is the demonstration that "provoking" the esophagus with acid perfusion, balloon distention or cholinergic stimulation reproduces the patient's pain.

The pathophysiology of this angina-like chest pain of esophageal origin is poorly understood. In some patients acid reflux is the cause: these patients experience angina-like chest pain under circumstances in which most people would experience heartburn. In others, the pain is caused by abnormal "spastic" contractions of the esophagus that either occur spontaneously or are sec-

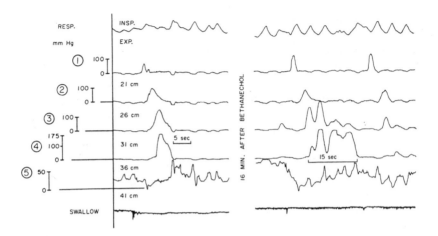

FIGURE 8.   Esophageal motility study in a patient with hypertensive esophageal contractions (nutcracker esophagus) and angina-like chest pain. Calibration (mm Hg) for each "lead" is shown on the left of the record. Zero is set at atmospheric pressure. The uppermost tracing shows respiratory excursion as measured with a belt pneumograph. The lowest tracing is an electromyograph of the neck muscles and indicates the onset of pharyngeal swallowing movement. The lowermost recording lead is positioned in the LES, 41 cm from the incisors. The other leads are recording pressures in the esophageal body 36, 31, 26 and 21 cm from the incisors. The tracing on the left depicts a normal peristaltic sequence; however, the pressures recorded in the distal esophagus are high. The right-hand panel depicts the tracing 16 minutes after the subcutaneous injection of the muscarinic agonist bethanechol. Note that at this time the tracing has become disorganized, with many high-pressure, prolonged and repetitive waves being recorded. During this time the patient experienced reproduction of angina-like chest pain.
SOURCE: Beck IT. Chest pain and the esophagus. Ann RCPSC 1984; 17:13–22. Used with permission.

ondary to acid reflux. In most cases there is a poor correlation between spastic esophageal contractions and the occurrence of pain. Many of these patients appear to have an abnormal esophageal pain threshold; pain episodes may be triggered by multiple different stimuli that in normal subjects would not be perceived as painful.

Both pH and esophageal pressure can be monitored over 24 hours. This method is probably more sensitive and specific than conventional tests, but the equipment is expensive and the test is of limited value in patients with infrequent pain attacks.

Management of angina-like chest pain of esophageal origin should be directed at the specific pathophysiological process. If the pain is triggered by gastroesophageal reflux, then antireflux treatment may be quite helpful. If the pain is due to esophageal spasm, smooth-muscle relaxants such as nitrates, calcium channel blockers, hydralazine and anticholinergics should help, although few controlled clinical trials have demonstrated any significant benefit. Tricyclic antidepressants in relatively low dosage have been shown to be beneficial and should be tried in patients with incapacitating symptoms when other forms of treatment have failed. These are most likely to be useful in patients with abnormal visceral nociception, or the so-called irritable esophagus. Many of these patients will have a significant functional overlay with many other somatic complaints. Simple reassurance is probably the most important part of treatment. Symptoms usually improve once the patient is given a positive diagnosis and no longer fears that underlying heart disease is the cause.

12. ESOPHAGEAL NEOPLASMS

A large number of different tumors can involve the esophagus (Table 5). The vast majority are extremely rare and often do not produce clinical disease. Unfortunately, the most common esophageal neoplasm is squamous cell carcinoma, which has a five-year survival rate (< 10%) that is among the lowest for any neoplastic disease.

12.1 Benign Tumors

Leiomyoma is the most common benign esophageal tumor. Esophageal leiomyomas may produce dysphagia and retrosternal chest pain, but in most cases are asymptomatic. Unlike gastric leiomyomas, they rarely hemorrhage. On barium x-ray a characteristic smooth, round luminal defect is seen projecting from one wall. Its endoscopic appearance is a clearly demarcated projection into the lumen; the overlying mucosa is normal. Endoscopic biopsy is not helpful, as the lesion is submucosal and cannot be reached with biopsy forceps. If leiomyomas are symptomatic, surgical enucleation is indicated.

Squamous cell papillomas consist of frond-like projections of the lamina propria that are covered by squamous epithelium and develop at several sites simultaneously. They rarely grow large enough to produce dysphagia. They occur in association with acanthosis nigricans and tylosis. Except when associated with tylosis, these lesions are not considered to be precursors of squamous cell carcinoma.

Fibrovascular polyps consist of a core of loose fibrous connective tissue, fat and blood vessels covered by a thick layer of squamous epithelium. Such a polyp may become quite large, with a very long stalk that permits the lesions to flop back and forth in the esophageal lumen. Patients with this lesion have

TABLE 5.   Classification of esophageal tumors

Benign tumors
Epithelial origin
  Squamous cell papilloma
Non-epithelial origin
  Leiomyoma
  Granular cell tumor
  Hemangioma
  Lymphangioma

Malignant tumors
Epithelial origin
  Squamous cell carcinoma
  Adenocarcinoma
  Adenoid cystic carcinoma
  Mucoepidermoid carcinoma
  Adenosquamous carcinoma
  Undifferentiated carcinoma; small-cell carcinoma
Non-epithelial origin
  Leiomyosarcoma
  Carcinosarcoma
  Malignant melanoma
Secondary tumors
  Malignant melanoma
  Breast carcinoma

Tumor-like lesions
  Fibrovascular polyp
  Heterotopia
  Congenital cyst
  Glycogen acanthosis

presented with regurgitation of the free end of the polyp into the mouth; in other instances, the regurgitated polyp has caused sudden death by obstructing the larynx.

Granular cell tumors are submucosal lesions with intact mucosal covering that are usually picked up incidentally at endoscopy. They may originate from neural elements. They rarely cause symptoms, although there have been occasional reports of dysphagia due to large granular cell tumors. There have also been rare reports of malignant granular cell tumors in the esophagus. Symptomatic tumors need to be removed surgically.

12.2 Malignant Tumors

Carcinoma of the esophagus is a relatively uncommon malignancy in Canada, with only 3 to 4 new cases per 100,000 population per year in males and just over 1 new case per 100,000 population per year in females. Nevertheless, because of its poor prognosis, esophageal cancer ranks among the 10 leading causes of cancer death in Canadian men 45 years of age and older.

Although several different types of primary and secondary malignancies can involve the esophagus (Table 5), squamous cell carcinoma and adenocarcinoma are by far the most common esophageal malignancies.

12.2.1 ADENOCARCINOMA

Adenocarcinoma makes up close to 10% of all esophageal cancers. Rarely, primary esophageal adenocarcinomas arise from embryonic remnants of columnar epithelium or from superficial or deep glandular epithelium. In most instances, adenocarcinoma arises from metaplastic Barrett's epithelium in the distal esophagus. Adenocarcinoma of the cardia of the stomach may also involve the distal esophagus and give the appearance that the cancer arises from the esophagus.

The prevalence of adenocarcinoma in patients with Barrett's esophagus is approximately 10%. Incidence data are incomplete, but suggest that patients with Barrett's esophagus will develop adenocarcinoma at a rate of about 0.5% per year. This is a significant problem given the large number of reflux patients with Barrett's metaplasia (estimated at 10% of all patients with chronic GERD). Because dysplasia develops prior to frank carcinoma in Barrett's epithelium, most experts suggest that these patients should undergo yearly surveillance endoscopy with multiple biopsies to identify those who are likely to progress to cancer (Section 7).

The clinical presentation and diagnostic evaluation of patients with adenocarcinoma of the esophagus are similar to squamous cell carcinoma (Section 12.2.2). These lesions are not radiosensitive and their response to various chemotherapeutic agents is not very satisfactory. Surgical resection or palliation with laser, peroral dilation and/or stent placement are the preferred treatments. The prognosis is similar to that for gastric adenocarcinoma – i.e., an overall five-year survival rate of < 10%.

12.2.2 SQUAMOUS CELL CARCINOMA

The occurrence of squamous cell carcinoma of the esophagus shows striking geographic variability, with high frequencies in certain regions of Iran, Africa, China and the former USSR. This has led to several theories concerning cer-

TABLE 6.   Esophageal squamous cell carcinoma: possible etiological factors

---

Alcohol
Tobacco
Nutritional exposures
  Nitrosamines; "bush teas" containing tannin and/or diterpene phorbol esters
Nutritional deficiencies (riboflavin, niacin, iron)
Chronic esophagitis
Achalasia
Previous lye-induced injury
Tylosis

---

tain environmental agents that may be important etiologically (Table 6). In North America, squamous cell carcinoma is associated with alcohol ingestion, tobacco use and lower socioeconomic status. It is also significantly more common in blacks and in males.

Characteristically these cancers extend microscopically in the submucosa for substantial distances above and below the area of the gross involvement. They also have a propensity to extend through the esophageal wall and to regional lymphatics quite early. Furthermore, they usually produce symptoms only when they have become locally quite advanced. For these reasons approximately 95% of these cancers are diagnosed at a time when surgical cure is impossible.

In most studies, the mid-esophagus is the most common site of origin; however, others have reported distal cancers to be most common. The lungs and liver are the most common sites of distant metastases.

Most patients present with progressive, predictable dysphagia and weight loss. Other symptoms include odynophagia, chest pain (which may radiate to the mid-scapular region), hoarseness (due to recurrent laryngeal nerve involvement) and blood loss. Pulmonary complications due to either direct aspiration or esophagorespiratory fistulas are also quite common during the course of the disease. Physical examination is usually negative aside from signs of weight loss. Hepatomegaly or enlarged cervical or supraclavicular lymph nodes may be detected in cases of disseminated metastases.

Barium swallow is usually diagnostic, although small cancers can be missed in up to 30% of cases. Endoscopy with multiple directed biopsies combined with brush cytology is required to confirm the diagnosis. This should be followed by careful attempts to stage the disease prior to deciding on therapeutic intervention. In addition to a careful physical examination, chest x-ray and blood tests for transaminases, alkaline phosphatase and bilirubin, an ultrasound of the abdomen should be performed to look for liver metastasis. If this is negative, one should proceed to a CT scan of the thorax in order to define the extent of local spread. Unfortunately the CT scan lacks sensitivity in this regard. Endoscopic ultrasound appears promising in accurately assessing depth of tumor involvement and presence or absence of enlarged mediastinal lymph nodes. If the above investigations are negative, some experts recommend bronchoscopy, mediastinoscopy and scalene node biopsy prior to attempting surgical resection.

Treatment results of squamous cell carcinoma of the esophagus are discouraging. Although it is traditionally taught that surgical resection is the only chance for a cure, there is no convincing evidence that "curative" surgery is better than "curative" radiotherapy. These tumors are quite radiosensitive; however, most centers give radiotherapy to patients who have advanced unresectable tumors or other health problems that make them poor surgical candidates. This understandably leads to very poor overall survival following radiotherapy. In the few reports where radiotherapy is used as the primary mode of therapy in patients who might otherwise be considered surgical candidates, the five-year survival rate is as high as 17%, which compares quite favorably to surgical results. Both forms of treatment have significant morbidity, and the mortality following esophageal resection is at least 10%. Controlled trials are needed, but in only a small proportion of the total population of esophageal cancer patients is cure a realistic goal. In the majority the disease is too far advanced. New regimens that combine radiotherapy and chemotherapy, with or without surgery, are currently being evaluated.

The goal of treatment has to be palliation in most patients. Both radiotherapy and modified surgery can be used in this setting; however, other modalities are often necessary. The dysphagia can be relieved with peroral dilation, but in many patients this becomes exceedingly difficult as the disease progresses. If this is the case, a prosthetic device can sometimes be placed across the tumor to maintain luminal patency. These stents can work quite well, although tube blockage, tube migration and erosion through the esophageal wall are important complications. These prosthetic devices are the best treatment for an esophagorespiratory fistula. Endoscopic Nd-YAG laser therapy has been used to destroy tumors that obstruct the esophageal lumen. This appears to be a very useful form of palliation, but it is expensive and has not as yet been documented to be superior to dilation and stent placement. The caring physician must also provide emotional support, nutritional support and adequate pain therapy for these unfortunate patients.

13. MISCELLANEOUS DISORDERS OF THE ESOPHAGUS

13.1 Webs and Rings

Webs are thin, membrane-like structures that project into the esophageal lumen. They are covered on both sides with squamous epithelium and are most commonly found in the cervical esophagus. Webs are usually detected incidentally during barium x-rays and rarely occlude enough of the esophageal lumen to cause dysphagia. The etiology of these webs is unclear. Most are probably congenital in origin. In some instances postcricoid esophageal webs are associated with iron deficiency and dysphagia – the so-called *Plummer-Vinson* or *Paterson-Kelly syndrome*. This syndrome is associated with increased risk of hypopharyngeal cancer and should be managed with bougienage, iron replacement and careful follow-up. Esophageal webs may also form after esophageal injury, such as that induced by pills or lye ingestion, and have also been reported in association with graft-versus-host disease.

The lower esophageal or *Schatzki's ring* is also a membrane-like structure, but unlike webs is lined by squamous epithelium on its superior aspect and columnar epithelium inferiorly. Such a ring is quite common, being detected in up to 10% of all upper GI barium x-rays. Few produce sufficient luminal obstruction to cause dysphagia (yet a lower esophageal ring is a common cause of dysphagia). When the lumen is narrowed to a diameter of 13 mm or less, the patient will experience intermittent solid-food dysphagia or even episodic food-bolus obstruction. Treatment of a symptomatic Schatzki's ring involves shattering the ring with a large-diameter bougie or a balloon dilator.

13.2 Diverticula

Pharyngoesophageal diverticula are outpouchings of one or more layers of the pharyngeal or esophageal wall and are classified according to their location.

13.2.1 *ZENKER'S DIVERTICULUM* (Figure 9)

This diverticulum arises posteriorly in the midline between the oblique and transverse (cricopharyngeal) fibers of the inferior pharyngeal constrictor muscles. As this diverticulum enlarges, it usually shifts to the left of the midline. Zenker's diverticulum forms because of decreased compliance of the cricopharyngeal muscle, which results in abnormally high pressures in the hypopharynx during deglutition. If large, the diverticulum may cause dysphagia secondary to external compression of the cervical esophagus. In addition to oropharyngeal-type dysphagia, Zenker's diverticulum may be associated with effortless regurgitation of stagnant, foul-tasting food, as well as aspiration. A very large diverticulum can produce a neck mass, usually on the left side.

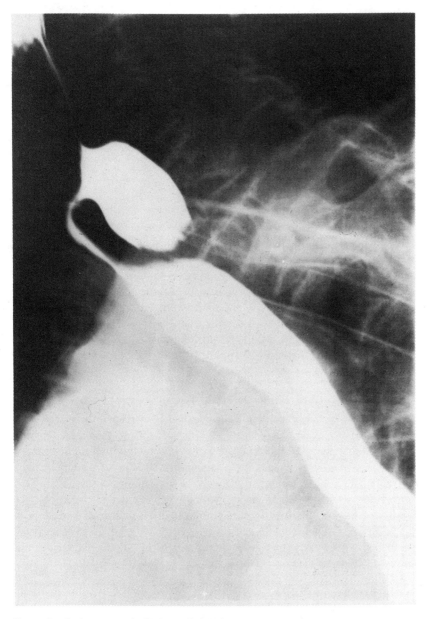

FIGURE 9.   Barium x-ray of a Zenker's diverticulum. Note that barium has filled the diverticulum, which originates posteriorly, just above the cricopharyngeal muscle. Most of these diverticula shift to the left of the midline as they enlarge.

Treatment of a symptomatic Zenker's diverticulum is surgical. Most surgeons will either resect the diverticulum or suspend it (diverticulopexy) so that it cannot fill. This is combined with cricopharyngeal myotomy. In many cases cricopharyngeal myotomy alone will alleviate symptoms. Once the cricopharyngeal myotomy has been performed, the patient has lost an important defense mechanism to prevent the aspiration of refluxed material. The patient should therefore be instructed to elevate the head of the bed in order to minimize this risk. For the same reason patients with gross GERD should not undergo cricopharyngeal myotomy unless the reflux can be controlled either medically or surgically.

13.2.2 MIDESOPHAGEAL DIVERTICULA
Traditionally, midesophageal diverticula have been called "traction" diverticula because of their supposed etiology. They were believed to arise secondary to old mediastinal inflammation, such as tuberculosis, that caused adherence of mediastinal structures to the outer esophageal wall so that outward traction occurred during peristalsis. It now appears likely that very few midesophageal diverticula arise this way. In most there is an associated motility disorder and it is likely that this is actually a "pulsion" diverticulum formed when a peristaltic wave deteriorates into a simultaneous or spastic contraction in the smooth-muscle esophagus. Midesophageal diverticula rarely require specific therapy. Rather, only the associated motor disorder requires treatment if symptomatic.

13.2.3 LOWER ESOPHAGEAL OR EPIPHRENIC DIVERTICULA
These "pulsion" diverticula form just above the LES and are invariably associated with an esophageal motor disorder – usually diffuse esophageal spasm, with or without abnormal relaxation of the LES. Patients with these diverticula usually present with dysphagia and/or angina-like chest pain. In addition, they may complain of nocturnal regurgitation of large quantities of stagnant fluid.

If symptoms are present, treatment with nitrates or calcium channel blockers may be helpful. If this is not successful, surgery is indicated. Any surgical attack on these diverticula should involve a myotomy of the spastic distal esophagus and/or LES. Resection of the diverticula alone seldom affords long-term benefit.

13.2.4 INTRAMURAL DIVERTICULOSIS
This disorder has a characteristic radiologic appearance consisting of numerous tiny, flask-shaped outpouchings from the esophageal lumen. There is usually an associated smooth stricture in the proximal esophagus. Patients

typically present with dysphagia that responds to peroral dilation. The out-pouchings are actually dilatated ducts coming from submucosal glands and thus are not true diverticula. The etiology is obscure. Some cases are associated with esophageal candidiasis, but this organism does not appear to be of etiological importance.

13.3 Esophageal Trauma

Blunt or penetrating trauma to the chest can cause esophageal injury. In addition, esophageal instrumentation such as that used in bougienage or endoscopy may cause perforation or mucosal laceration. Severe retching or vomiting can also cause esophageal perforation *(Boerhaave's syndrome)* or mucosal laceration *(Mallory-Weiss syndrome)*. Boerhaave's syndrome is a life-threatening condition that requires immediate surgery to drain the mediastinum and repair the defect in the esophageal wall. Patients, typically alcoholics, present with sudden epigastric and/or chest pain following a bout of vomiting and usually have fever and signs of hypovolemia or shock.

The mucosal laceration of Mallory-Weiss syndrome is probably better classified as a disorder of the stomach, because in most cases the laceration starts at the EG junction and extends down into the stomach. These patients present with hematemesis or melena following a bout of retching or vomiting. The bleeding usually stops spontaneously and only supportive therapy is required. If bleeding persists, endoscopically applied hemostasis or surgical intervention may be necessary.

13.4 Food-Bolus Obstruction and Foreign Bodies

A surprising variety of foreign bodies can lodge in the esophagus after being swallowed either inadvertently or deliberately. The three most common sites where foreign bodies become stuck are the piriform sinuses, at the aortic arch and just above the LES. The patient can usually localize the site of the obstruction quite accurately, and this can be confirmed using routine x-rays if the object is radiopaque. Otherwise, x-rays using small amounts of water-soluble contrast media may be necessary. Most foreign bodies can be removed by an expert endoscopist. Surgery is rarely required, except when perforation has occurred.

A more common clinical problem is esophageal food-bolus obstruction. This typically occurs when a patient with a motility disorder, stricture or Schatzki's (lower esophageal) ring swallows a large solid-food bolus. The patient notices immediate chest pain, usually well localized to the site of obstruction. Attempts to swallow anything further are unsuccessful and usually lead to prompt regurgitation.

Many physicians will initially treat these patients with smooth-muscle relaxants such as intravenous glucagon, sublingual nitroglycerin or nifedipine; however, there is little evidence that this approach is efficacious. If the food bolus does not pass on spontaneously within a few hours, endoscopy should be performed, at which time the bolus can either be removed per os or pushed through into the stomach. These patients should not be left too long, as the bolus is capable of causing significant maceration to the esophageal mucosa. Giving the patient meat tenderizer, in an attempt to dissolve the bolus, is probably of no value and may be very harmful; papain can digest the esophageal mucosa and has been reported to cause severe hemorrhagic pulmonary edema when aspirated.

ACKNOWLEDGMENT

I would like to acknowledge Dr. I.T. Beck's valuable input, including his contribution of several of the figures for the chapter and valuable editorial advice.

OBJECTIVES

Anatomy and Physiology
1. Know the anatomy and physiology of the normal esophagus and esophago-gastric junction.
2. Describe the process of deglutition and esophageal peristalsis.
3. Understand the different physiological control mechanisms between the upper striated-muscle esophagus and distal smooth-muscle esophagus.

Congenital and Anatomic Abnormalities
1. Define esophageal atresia and tracheoesophageal fistula, and describe how they present.
2. Define hiatus hernia with regard to anatomic type (sliding versus para-esophageal).

Gastroesophageal Reflux Disease (GERD)
1. Outline the clinical symptoms of GERD.
2. Describe the anatomic and physiological factors predisposing to GERD.
3. Discuss the procedures used in the diagnosis of GERD.
4. Discuss medical management of GERD.
5. List the indications for operative management of GERD and discuss the physiological basis for the antireflux procedures.
6. List the complications of gastroesophageal reflux disease.

Nonreflux-Induced Esophagitis
1. List the major infectious causes of esophagitis (Candida, herpetic) and describe how they present.
2. List other causes of esophagitis.

Disorders of the Oropharyngeal Phase of Deglutition
1. Categorize the major causes of oropharyngeal deglutition.
2. Describe how oropharyngeal dysphagia can be differentiated from esophageal dysphagia based on history.
3. Describe the investigations required in the assessment of oropharyngeal dysphagia.
4. What are the complications of oropharyngeal dysphagia?

Motor Disorders of the Esophagus
1. List the major primary and secondary esophageal motor disorders.
2. Describe the clinical symptoms typically associated with different esophageal motor disorders.

Esophageal Tumors
1. List the symptoms suggestive of an esophageal malignancy.
2. Outline a diagnostic plan for evaluating a patient with suspected esophageal tumor.
3. Describe the natural history of malignant esophageal neoplasms.
4. Describe the treatment options for esophageal malignancy.
5. List the common types of benign esophageal tumors.

Miscellaneous Esophageal Disorders
1. Be able to describe the presenting symptomatology and typical x-ray findings of esophageal webs, and Zenker's and esophageal diverticula.
2. Outline the clinical presentation and management of patients presenting with (a) Boerhaave's syndrome and (b) esophageal foreign body or food-bolus obstruction.

Skills
1. Demonstrate the ability to read a barium swallow in patients with sliding and paraesophageal hiatus hernia, esophageal cancer, Zenker's diverticulum, esophageal diverticulum and achalasia.
2. Describe the motility abnormalities in achalasia, diffuse esophageal spasm, "nutcracker" esophagus and scleroderma esophagus.
3. Develop an approach for diagnostic evaluation of a patient with dysphagia.

6
The Stomach and Duodenum

B.J. Salena and R.H. Hunt

1. INTRODUCTION

DISEASES OF THE GI tract are common, accounting for one out of seven complaints, and disorders of the stomach and duodenum make up a large part of these.

It has been known for many centuries that the gastric juice is acid in nature, but it was not until 1824 that William Prout established that the acid in the stomach is hydrochloric acid. Since then physicians have been fascinated by the ability of the healthy stomach and duodenum to withstand hydrochloric acid and pepsin. In particular they have studied extensively the mechanisms controlling gastric secretion in the hope of finding a satisfactory way of explaining and treating peptic ulcer disease. Recent attention has turned to the role of mucus, bicarbonate and prostaglandins in maintenance and defense of the gastric mucosa against acid injury. This chapter will review the anatomy, physiology and related common disorders of the stomach and duodenum.

2. ANATOMY

2.1 General Anatomy

The stomach is the most capacious part of the GI tract and lies between the distal esophagus and the duodenum. It is situated entirely within the abdomen below the diaphragm (Figure 1). The body of the stomach lies slightly to the left of the midline, the antrum across the spinal vertebrae at the level of T10–L1 and the pylorus to the right of the vertebral column. The duodenum is predominantly retroperitoneal and comprises the cap, descending and distal portions.

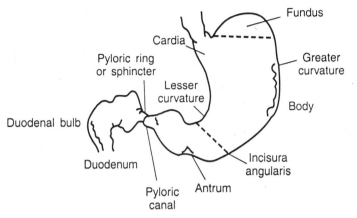

FIGURE 1.   Anatomic divisions of the stomach.

The greater curvature is some three or four times the length of the lesser curvature. A point known as the angulus or incisura may be defined on the lesser curvature. This point is relatively constant and marks a change from the prominent rugal folds of the body of the stomach to the smoother, less prominent folds of the antrum.

The stomach and duodenum lie in close proximity to a number of important anatomic structures. Anterosuperiorly are the left diaphragm and left lobe of the liver, while the body and tail of the pancreas lie posteriorly. Laterally to the left are the hilum of the left kidney, the left adrenal gland and, above that, the spleen. These organs form the stomach bed and are separated from it by the lesser omentum and the lesser sac. The duodenum, apart from the cap, lies retroperitoneally. The second and distal parts surround the head of the pancreas while the cap, which is attached to the lesser omentum, lies anterior to the head of the pancreas.

2.2 Blood Supply

The main arterial blood supply (Figure 2) arises from the celiac axis. The common hepatic artery gives rise to the gastroduodenal artery and the right gastric artery, which then anastomoses with the left gastric artery. The splenic artery gives rise to the short gastric arteries that supply the body along the greater curvature of the stomach. The right and left gastroepiploic arteries also form an anastomosis along the greater curvature.

Venous drainage essentially follows the arterial supply but passes to the portal venous system and its tributaries, the splenic vein and the superior mesenteric vein. Veins from the fundus communicate with veins draining the

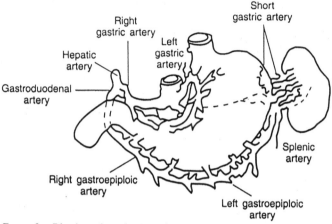

FIGURE 2. Blood supply to the stomach.

lower third of the esophagus and form a connection between the systemic and portal venous systems. This connection assumes clinical importance if portal venous pressure rises, when venous flow is reversed through the esophageal veins, leading to esophageal or fundal varices.

Lymphatic drainage is to the pancreaticosplenic nodes, the left gastric nodes and the pyloric nodes, and then via the celiac group to the preaortic lymph nodes and the cisterna chyli.

2.3 Nerve Supply

The nerve supply is both sympathetic and parasympathetic. The vagal supply arises via the anterior and posterior trunks, which pass through the diaphragm on either side of the esophagus before giving rise to the hepatic and celiac branches. The hepatic branch supplies further branches to the anterior surface of the body of the stomach and to the pyloric region, while the celiac branch passes to the celiac plexus and the posterior aspect of the body of the stomach. The vagal fibers anastomose with ganglion cells of the stomach within the muscle layers, forming Auerbach's plexus or, in the submucosa, forming Meissner's plexus.

The sympathetic nerve supply arises from the spinal cord between T6 and T10 and passes to the sympathetic ganglia. The parasympathetic supply contracts the stomach, relaxes the pylorus and stimulates acid, pepsin and mucus secretion, whereas sympathetic stimulation constricts the blood supply and reduces gastric motor activity and secretion while the pylorus is contracted.

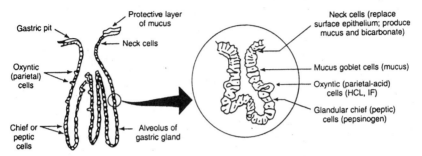

FIGURE 3. Microscopic appearances of gastric pit and glands.

2.4 Structure of the Stomach and Duodenum

The stomach and duodenum comprise an outer serosal coat, a muscular layer, submucosa and mucus membrane. The mucosal surface is ridged by the rugal folds created by contractions of the muscularis mucosa, especially prominent in the body of the stomach and less obvious in the antrum. The glands of the stomach are of two main types – gastric and pyloric – both of which are closely packed in the columnar epithelium. The gastric glands (known as oxyntic glands) make up 70–80% of the total and are responsible for secreting mucus, pepsinogen, hydrochloric acid and intrinsic factor (Figure 3). The pyloric glands, which secrete mucus and gastrin, make up only about 15%. A line of demarcation can usually be seen between the gastric and pyloric glands in the region of the incisura.

The gastric glands differ in cell type: the chief or peptic cells secrete pepsinogen, while the parietal or oxyntic cells secrete hydrochloric acid and intrinsic factor. The endocrine cells of the antrum secrete gastrin and 5-hydroxytryptamine. In the duodenum the first 4–5 cm of mucosa are smooth, but in the descending duodenum the mucosa is thrown into crescentic folds. The mucosa is lined with columnar, goblet, Paneth's and endocrine cells. The columnar cells line the villi and crypts, which increase in size in the second and third parts of the duodenum. A characteristic feature in the duodenal submucosa is the presence of Brunner's glands, which are similar to pyloric glands.

3. PHYSIOLOGY

The stomach has three major functions: motor, secretory and endocrine (Table 1). The motor functions include temporary storage of food and fluid, mixing of ingested materials with gastric juice and regulated emptying of gastric contents. The most important substances secreted into the lumen of the stomach

TABLE 1.   Functions of the stomach

Motor
Vagus-mediated and gastrin-induced receptive relaxation
Mixing and emptying

Secretory
Acid, pepsin, intrinsic factor, volume, water, electrolytes

Endocrine
Gastrin, serotonin, somatostatin

---

include hydrochloric acid, pepsin, mucus, bicarbonate, intrinsic factor and water. The stomach releases two hormones into the blood: gastrin and somatostatin. Serotonin-staining (ECL) cells are also present in the gastric fundus and antrum. Gastrin stimulates acid secretion by the stomach, and somatostatin inhibits the release of gastrin.

3.1 Gastric Motility

The motor functions of the stomach include serving as a reservoir, mixing its contents, kneading and churning solid food, and regulating the emptying of its contents into the duodenum. The reservoir function involves temporary storage of ingested and secreted substances. Above a certain threshold volume, the stomach is "full" (whether the volume is large or small); i.e., the intragastric pressure increases very little with the addition of more food and fluid because the walls of the stomach relax to accommodate the load. The stomach also mixes ingested substances with gastric juice to dissolve and dilute food, kneads solid materials to a particle size of less than 1 mm diameter, and finally, empties its contents into the duodenum slowly and in small volumes.

Gastric motility is controlled centrally and by local neurohormonal control of muscle. The muscle layers include the outer longitudinal, middle circular and inner oblique fibers. Neuronal control involves the intrinsic myenteric plexus, the extrinsic postganglionic sympathetic fibers of the celiac plexus, and the preganglionic parasympathetic fibers of the vagus nerve. The vagal afferents are both relaxatory and excitatory. These vagal fibers are neither cholinergic nor adrenergic.

Factors that influence gastric motility may be classified as myogenic, neural and chemical. The resting potential difference of the gastric smooth muscle is 5–15 mV and there is a rhythmic depolarization, with this basic electrical rhythm being set by the gastric pacemaker, which gives rise to slow-wave activity. The action potential produces peristalsis and is influenced by gastrin.

The force of the contraction is increased with vagal activity, gastrin and motilin, and is decreased with gastric secretion.

Gastric distention by food or liquid stimulates both intrinsic nerves and vagal afferents. There is increased spike burst activity, more forceful peristaltic contractions and increased gastric emptying. Pyloric sphincter relaxation occurs so that the antral lumen is not occluded by peristaltic waves. Gastric contents are propelled both forward and backward toward the body of the stomach and are thoroughly mixed. Gastrin delays gastric emptying by decreasing gastric motility and at the same time increasing duodenal motility and pyloric tone (events that are mediated by fat, protein or acid in the duodenum). This increase in duodenal motility and pyloric tone is effected by stimulation of duodenal osmoreceptors and by the release of secretin, cholecystokinin (CCK) and gastric inhibitory polypeptide (GIP).

Gastric motility is inhibited for the stomach to accommodate food. Vagal relaxatory fibers are stimulated by swallowing, esophageal or gastric distention, and neurogenic stimulation. Sympathetic and adrenergic fibers influence these cholinergic neurons.

The emptying of the stomach is influenced by the substance, volume, osmolality and composition of the ingested meal. Liquids empty more rapidly than solids. The rate of gastric emptying is related to the square root of the volume, so that a constant proportion of the gastric contents empties per unit time. Stimulation of duodenal osmoreceptors with triglycerides, fatty acids or hydrochloric acid slows gastric emptying.

The gastric body serves as a reservoir, whereas the antrum has the function of mixing, churning and emptying. A high-pressure gradient exists at the gastroduodenal junction, with the pyloric sphincter playing an important role in the coordinated activity of emptying the antral contents into the duodenum.

When the volume of the stomach increases with relaxation, the intragastric pressure does not increase, because of receptive relaxation mediated by way of a vagal reflex and the splanchnic nerves. Receptive relaxation occurs primarily in the gastric fundus and body. Vagotomy, fundoplication and extensive involvement of the stomach by adenocarcinoma result in a loss of this capacity, leading to early satiety. Gastric fundal contractions are infrequent, and of large amplitude and long duration (45 seconds). These contractions propel contents to the body and antrum for mixing to occur.

The distal two-thirds of the stomach is under intrinsic myogenic control. Electrical slow-wave activity can be detected on the greater curvature, with aboral contractions passing from the greater to the lesser curvature at a rate of about 3 per minute. Although antral contractions occur only in response to neural stimulation, the muscle will contract only when a slow wave occurs.

The gastric pacemaker controls the frequency and direction of propagated contractions. This control can be altered by the insertion of an electrical pacemaker, potentially changing the frequency of contraction and reversing its direction. It is possible that some clinical disorders of gastric emptying may give rise to chronic nausea, vomiting, fullness and distention.

As antral contractions pass distally, velocity increases, with near simultaneous contractions of distal antrum and pylorus. A small amount of gastric chyme may enter the duodenum, but most passes back into the stomach, where further mixing and churning takes place.

The pyloric sphincter is recognized macroscopically by thickening of the distal circular antral muscle, forming a muscular ring. However, it is difficult to accept this as a true physiologic sphincter, since in its resting phase it is open, and the rapid closure with antral peristalsis serves more to retard than to facilitate the aboral passage of gastric chyme. The pylorus acts to limit duodenogastric reflux. Duodenal acidification or infusion of secretin results in an increase in pyloric sphincter pressure. Patients with gastric ulcer or bile gastritis experience increased reflux of duodenal contents (including bile and pancreatic enzymes) into the stomach, apparently secondary to a pyloric defect. If the sphincter is ablated by pyloroplasty for duodenal ulcer disease, bile reflux is inevitable.

3.2 Gastric Secretion

Gastric juice contains many substances. The six most important of these are hydrogen ion, pepsin, mucus, bicarbonate, intrinsic factor and water. Hydrochloric acid and the enzyme pepsin participate in the digestion of proteins. Mucus lubricates ingested solids. Mucus and bicarbonate probably protect the mucosal lining against digestion by acid and pepsin. The intrinsic factor is required for normal absorption of ingested cobalamin (vitamin B_{12}). Each day the stomach secretes about 2 L of water in an adult.

3.2.1 GASTRIC ACID SECRETION

It is generally accepted that acid secretion is activated by three separate pathways: the neural, hormonal and paracrinal (local) pathways. The major chemical transmitter substances are acetylcholine, gastrin and histamine.

The vagus and branches from the celiac plexus and ganglia traveling along the celiac artery are the major extrinsic nervous supply to the acid-secreting portion of the stomach. The postganglionic neurons of the vagi that terminate in the oxyntic gland near the oxyntic cells are predominantly cholinergic. These cholinergic fibers are rarely seen in contact with the oxyntic cells, and therefore acetylcholine released by these nerve endings must diffuse a relatively long distance to the cells. There are two types of muscarinic binding sites on oxyntic cells: M_1 and M_2 receptors. The cholinergic binding results in a dose-dependent acid secretory response. Additionally, there may be muscarinic receptors on histamine-containing cells resulting in indirect stimulation by histamine release on paracrine cells.

Histamine has a direct stimulatory action on oxyntic cells via an H_2 receptor. The stimulatory action of histamine on oxyntic cells is competitively antagonized by a group of histamine analogues (such as cimetidine, ranitidine, famotidine, nizatidine and others) that specifically interact with the H_2 receptor. The histamine antagonists binding to the H_1 receptor can decrease gastric histamine, but at much higher doses.

Gastrin, the other major secretagogue, also interacts with oxyntic cells via a gastrin receptor. The weak stimulatory effect of gastrin on acid production can be competitively inhibited by proglumide, a glutamic acid derivative known to antagonize CCK. Since CCK binds with the same affinity and produces a similar weak secretory response, the question has been raised whether the receptor may be a CCK receptor instead of a gastrin receptor, or whether the receptor may be related to the well-known trophic effect of gastrin rather than the acid-secreting effects.

The binding of secretagogues to the oxyntic cell receptors is coupled to at least two possible intracellular messengers, Ca^{++} and cyclic AMP. Cholinergic action controls the influx of extracellular Ca^{++} into the oxyntic cell, with subsequent activation of undefined intracellular events resulting in acid secretion. The weak stimulatory effect of gastrin is also Ca^{++} dependent. Histamine does not require extracellular Ca^{++} for stimulation of acid secretion. Cyclic AMP is the intracellular messenger coupling the effect of histamine to hydrogen ion production and secretion.

After the oxyntic cells have been stimulated, intracellular endoplasmic tubular structures known as tubulovesicles disappear from the cytoplasm, while the microvilli in the secretory canaliculi increase in length to enlarge the secretory surface. The tubulovesicle membranes contain H^+/K^+ ATPase, the enzyme responsible for driving the H^+ pump, exchanging K^+ for H^+. These membranes have a low permeability to K^+ and, at rest, prevent sufficient K^+ from entering the lumen of the tubulovesicles, thus preventing H^+ transport. Stimulatory activity occurs only with a cellular signal from secretagogues.

It is evident that the overall process of acid secretion is controlled by a complex interaction of a number of pathways that will be further elucidated in the future.

3.2.2 PEPSINOGEN SECRETION
Pepsinogens are present in the mucus cells of cardiac glands, in the chief and

mucus neck cells of oxyntic glands, in the mucus cells of pyloric glands and in the mucus cells of duodenal Brunner's glands. These proenzymes are secreted and activated by acids to the active form, pepsin. Furthermore, pepsin can activate additional pepsinogen autocatalytically.

The mucosal lining of the stomach contains four types of immunologically distinct pepsinogens with the ability to digest proteins at acid pH. Pepsinogens and hydrochloric acid secretion respond to much the same stimulants. Cephalic-vagal stimulation strongly stimulates pepsinogen secretion. Anticholinergics, histamine H_2-receptor antagonists and vagotomy decrease pepsinogen secretion. Elevated serum type 1 pepsinogen has been associated with duodenal ulcer and gastrinoma, while atrophic gastritis (with or without pernicious anemia) has been associated with low levels of type 1 pepsinogen.

3.2.3 INTRINSIC FACTOR SECRETION

Intrinsic factor (IF) is a glycoprotein secreted by oxyntic cells. It is important in vitamin B_{12} absorption. B_{12} is released from dietary protein by gastric acid and pepsin; it binds to IF and to R protein, which is secreted into saliva. B_{12} binds more efficiently to the R proteins at low pH, so most of the B_{12} is initially complexed with the R proteins. In the upper small bowel, pancreatic enzymes cleave the complexes and the free B_{12} binds to IF, which eventually binds to a specific ileal receptor and is subsequently absorbed and transported to the tissues by another B_{12}-binding protein, transcobalamin II.

Stimulants of acid secretion also stimulate IF secretion. Patients with low or absent acid secretion often have reduced IF secretion. Continued IF secretion is low but the amounts may be adequate to prevent vitamin B_{12} deficiency and pernicious anemia. Rarely, IF secretion can be absent with normal acid secretion. Circulating antibodies to IF and oxyntic cells are found in many patients with atrophic gastritis, achlorhydria or hypochlorhydria, and pernicious anemia.

3.3 Gastric Mucosal Barrier

Healthy gastric mucosa has the ability to resist high intraluminal concentrations of hydrochloric acid and peptic activity. The physiologic basis of this barrier involves several factors.

The tight junctions between the surface epithelial cells seal off the paracellular route for transport between cells. Transport can also occur across the bilipid layer membrane at the apical surface of the mucosal epithelial cells. The fluidity of this membrane can vary and influence permeability to various macromolecules. While there is active and passive transport of H^+, Na^+ and K^+ ions, an electric potential difference exists across the mucosa. With disruption of this barrier, a fall in potential difference occurs.

In the presence of luminal acid, the gastroduodenal pH approaches pH 2, while the immediately adjacent epithelium may be near neutral (pH 7). This pH gradient, which plays some role in protection from acid-peptic digestion, is probably dependent on the combined secretion of mucus and bicarbonate. How the gastric mucosa secretes acid while maintaining a near-neutral pH adjacent to the surface epithelium requires elucidation.

Gastric mucus consists of about 95% water and 5% glycoprotein. It provides lubrication for food particles and its gel-like nature retains water and bicarbonate close to the surface epithelium. Mucus is secreted by exocytosis, apical expulsion and exfoliation, and formed with bicarbonate in the surface epithelial cells, in the epithelial cells of the gastric gland neck and by the Brunner's glands of the duodenum. The mucus layer varies in thickness but averages about 100 μm. The role of mucus in protection against acid-peptic activity is unclear. It does provide a relatively thick unstirred layer adjacent to the mucosa, allowing a rate of diffusion of H^+ ions four times slower than through a similar thickness of unstirred water. This contributes to the maintenance of a hydrogen ion gradient between the gastric lumen and the surface epithelium. That is, when the pH in the gastric lumen is 2, the pH at the gastric membrane will be 6.8 to 7. ASA and nonsteroidal anti-inflammatory agents inhibit mucus synthesis and release, while prostaglandins increase mucus synthesis. Mucus synthesis is decreased after stress and may play a role in stress ulceration. Mucus limits the diffusion of pepsin and other large molecules, thus preventing further injury.

Bicarbonate secretion is an active process dependent on the metabolic integrity of a healthy epithelium. Secretion is stimulated by acetylcholine, prostaglandins, glucagon and cyclic GMP, and inhibited by α-adrenergic agonists and GIP. Luminal acid also appears to stimulate gastric and duodenal bicarbonate secretion. Low concentrations of bile salts in the stomach inhibit gastric bicarbonate secretion.

Prostaglandins probably play an important role in mucosal defense. These saturated, oxygenated fatty acids are derived from arachidonic acid. They may protect the mucosa by maintaining or increasing gastric mucosal blood flow and hence stimulating mucus production and bicarbonate secretion, and increasing protein synthesis (which is necessary for the maintenance and regeneration of cells). It is not known whether prostaglandins play a role in the maintenance of normal membrane function and tight junctions, but they probably maintain sulfhydryl groups, which act as oxidative scavengers.

The development of gastritis and gastric ulcer is thought to arise as a result of defective defense mechanisms. There may be increased degradation of mucus by pepsinogen 1, bile or pancreatic secretions; by infection with Helicobacter pylori; or through mechanical factors. A quantitatively or qualitatively defective secretion of mucus is also possible. Bicarbonate secretion may be reduced or mucosal blood flow and/or mucosal metabolism compromised, as occurs in stress ulceration.

3.4 Gastric Endocrine Secretion

The stomach produces regulatory peptides, such as gastrin and somatostatin. Each agent is a polypeptide; gastrin is known to exist in multiple forms in the body. These peptides are produced by enterochromaffin cells of the gastric mucosa. The cell that produces gastrin is called the "G cell" and is found in high concentrations in the antral mucosa.

Gastrin is the most important peptide in the regulation of gastric acid secretion. Under physiologic conditions gastrin is released continually, with increased amounts appearing in the blood at mealtimes. Gastrin is a hormone that increases the rate of oxyntic cell secretion of H^+ and peptic cell secretion of pepsinogen. Gastrin increases contraction of antral smooth muscle and increases mucosal blood flow.

Extragastric actions of gastrin include contraction of the lower esophageal sphincter, stimulation of pancreatic enzyme secretion, gallbladder contraction, increased small intestine motility, and the regulation of glucose-stimulated insulin release. Gastrin is a trophic hormone that stimulates protein synthesis and growth of certain gastrointestinal tissues, such as the mucosal lining of the stomach and gut, and the parenchyma of the pancreas.

Somatostatin inhibits the release of gastrin from the G cells, probably acting as a paracrine substance. In addition, the nerves of the gastric mucosa contain vasoactive intestinal peptide (VIP) and gastrin-releasing peptide (GRP or bombesin). VIP is probably responsible for mediating the relaxation of gastric smooth muscle. Bombesin mediates the release of gastrin in response to vagal stimulation.

3.5 Assessment of Gastric Acid Secretion

Basal acid output (BAO) refers to the quantity of hydrochloric acid (HCl) secreted per hour by the stomach in the unstimulated basal state, expressed in milliequivalents of HCl per hour. The normal range is 1–5 mEq of HCl per hour. The acid output is the product of the volume of gastric juices (in liters) multiplied by the concentration of hydrogen ion (in milliequivalents per liter).

Maximal acid output refers to the total acid output during the hour after stimulation with pentagastrin (6 µg/kg IM or SC) or histamine (40 µg/kg SC). This value is determined by adding the results of either four 15-minute or six

10-minute sample collections after stimulation. The normal range is 25–55 mEq HCl per hour.

Peak acid output reflects the two highest consecutive 15-minute periods of stimulated output, multiplied by a factor of 2 to yield a value for a one-hour output.

Gastric secretory studies may be useful in patients with suspected gastric hypersecretion and in the evaluation of the efficacy of medical and surgical therapy in the reduction of gastric acid output. In suspected Zollinger-Ellison syndrome, elevated basal hypersecretion may point to the diagnosis, but usually gastric acid secretory studies are more useful in establishing the therapeutic response to acid-suppressive pharmacotherapy.

4. PATHOPHYSIOLOGY OF PEPTIC ULCER DISEASE

4.1 Gastric Ulcer Disease

Acute ulcers may occur in the patient with burns (Curling's ulcer), midbrain disease (Cushing's ulcer) and chronic debilitating disease. ASA-containing analgesics and nonsteroidal anti-inflammatory drugs may also induce acute ulcer bleeding, though the risk of this complication has probably been overstated. There is epidemiologic evidence suggesting that the incidence and behavior of chronic peptic ulcers vary according to the site at which they occur. Therefore, gastric and duodenal ulcers will be considered separately, although the basic defects that cause either type relate to an imbalance of aggressive and protective factors.

Numerous pathophysiologic defects have been identified in gastric ulcer disease (Table 2A). Not all of these factors are present in each patient. These defects include decreased acid secretion, decreased parietal cell mass and back-diffusion of acid. Many patients with chronic gastric ulcers have associated gastritis. There may be increased concentration of bile acids and pancreatic juice in the stomach as a result of duodenogastric reflux. Delayed gastric emptying has also been identified in some patients with gastric ulcers, and this may accentuate the release of gastrin and the secretion of hydrochloric acid. It has yet to be determined whether delayed gastric emptying is the cause or secondary effect of gastric ulcer disease. However, as a result of back-diffusion of acid, the actual concentration of acid in the gastric lumen may be underestimated. Hypergastrinemia and hyperchloremia are not commonly thought to be associated with gastric ulcers. The pressure of the pyloric sphincter may be inappropriately decreased under basal conditions and may fail to respond normally to acid or fat in the duodenum, thereby predisposing to duodenogastric reflux.

TABLE 2.   Pathophysiologic defects in some patients with:

A. *Peptic ulcer disease/gastric ulcer disease*
Decreased acid secretion, decreased parietal cell mass (PCM), back-diffusion of acid
Chronic superficial and atrophic gastritis
Increased concentration of bile acids and pancreatic juice in stomach (duodenogastric reflux)
Delayed gastric emptying
Inappropriately decreased pyloric sphincter pressure under basal conditions and in response to
   acid (secretin) or fat (cholecystokinin) in the duodenum

B. *Duodenal ulcer disease*
Increased parietal cell mass
Increased sensitivity of parietal cells to gastrin and secretagogues
Increased secretory drive
Decreased acid-induced inhibition of meal-stimulated gastrin release
Increased gastric emptying
Increased duodenal acid/pepsin loads

4.2 Duodenal Ulcer Disease

A number of pathophysiologic defects have also been identified in some patients with duodenal ulcer disease (Table 2B). These include increased parietal cell mass (leading to increased maximal and peak acid output); increased sensitivity of the parietal cells to gastrin and other secretagogues; increased secretory drive; decreased acid-induced inhibition of meal-stimulated gastrin release; and increased gastric emptying (leading to increased duodenal acid and pepsin loads).

Apart from an increased parietal cell population (and possibly G-cell hyperplasia), the gastric mucosa is histologically normal in duodenal ulcer. By contrast, in gastric ulcer the nonparietal mucosal area is usually increased, especially on the lesser curvature, and there is often some degree of histologically demonstrable gastritis. Biliary reflux through the pylorus is also a common finding in patients with gastric ulcers, and it has been suggested that the combination of bile and acid may be particularly damaging to the mucosa, probably by causing back-diffusion of hydrogen ions into it and thus disrupting intracellular organelles.

4.3 Hereditary Factors

Hereditary factors are important in the pathogenesis of peptic ulcer disease, as suggested by a higher prevalence of peptic ulcer disease in certain genetic syndromes. A number of familial aggregations have been noted in patients with peptic ulcer disease. These include hyperpepsinogenemia 1, normal pepsinogenemia 1, antral G-cell hyperfunction, rapid gastric emptying, childhood duodenal ulcer and immunologic forms of peptic ulcer disease. Heredity also plays a role in the development of ulceration and is associated with the syndrome of multiple endocrine adenomatosis 1 (adenomas of the pancreas, pituitary and parathyroid). Parents, siblings and children of ulcer patients are more likely to have peptic ulcer disease than control individuals. There is greater concordance for ulcer disease in identical than in fraternal twins. Hyperpepsinogenemia 1 appears to be an autosomal dominant trait. Families have been described in which a number of physiologic abnormalities associated with the development of ulcer disease have been noted, including increased meal-stimulated gastrin release and altered gastric emptying.

4.4 Interplay of Acid, Pepsin and Other Factors
Peptic ulcer disease is thought to occur as a result of an interplay between acid and pepsin. Peptic ulcers occur more commonly in the duodenum and less commonly in the stomach and esophagus. They usually occur near mucosal junctions. Rarely, peptic ulcers occur in the jejunum; this should raise the possibility of the Zollinger-Ellison syndrome. When gastric mucosa is present in a Meckel's diverticulum in the ileum, peptic ulceration and bleeding can occur.

4.5 The Patient and the Environment
When considering the pathogenesis of any disease, we need to examine environmental factors, hereditary associations and pathophysiologic abnormalities. Environmental factors (Table 3) that have been examined include drugs, smoking, alcohol, caffeine-containing beverages and stress. Nonsteroidal anti-inflammatory agents such as ASA are thought to cause ulceration, mostly as a result of damage to the protected mucosal barrier. Smoking is associated with a higher prevalence of peptic ulcer disease and may be associated with impaired healing of duodenal and gastric ulcer disease. Also, death rates from peptic ulcer disease are higher in individuals who smoke. Alcohol and caffeine-containing beverages may affect acid secretion, and have been considered in the pathogenesis of peptic ulcer disease. However, it is fair to say that the role of coffee, alcohol, nonsteroidal anti-inflammatory agents and corticosteroids in the pathogenesis of peptic ulcer disease remains unclear.

Both patients and physicians often express the concern that "stress" is important in the initiation or perpetuation of peptic ulcer disease. Some patients with duodenal ulcer disease may have an exaggerated sense of self-sufficiency and demonstrate overambitiousness and aggressiveness. Some psychiatric views suggest that these attitudes represent a defense against an awareness of dependency. It is possible but unproven that patients exposed to excess stress may

TABLE 3.   Environmental factors in pathogenesis of peptic ulcer disease (PUD)

Drugs
NSAIDs

Smoking
Prevalence of PUD
Healing of duodenal ulcer (DU) and gastric ulcer (GU)
Death rates from PUD

Alcohol and caffeine-containing beverages
Acid secretion

Stress
Exaggerated self-sufficiency
Ambition
Aggression
Defense against awareness of dependency
More frequent and more sensitive symptoms
Perforation

have more frequent ulceration, may be more sensitive to the symptoms of peptic ulcer disease, and may be more likely to develop perforations.

Recent studies from Israel and the United States have identified a number of predictors of duodenal ulcer disease in men. These are psychosocial and biological. The important psychosocial factors include anxiety – stress, brooding (i.e., difficulty coping and difficulty expressing emotions) and inadequate caring, particularly lack of family support. Biological factors include age, lower blood pressure, use of cigarettes and leanness.

4.6 The Molecular Level

At a molecular level, the pathogenesis of ulcer disease is believed to reflect an imbalance between increased aggressive factors and decreased protective factors. In considering the possible aggressive factors, we need to briefly review the normal mechanism of acid secretion. Acid secretion is divided into the cephalic, gastric and intestinal phases. As a result of vagal stimulation arising from the sight, smell, taste or thought of food, acetylcholine is released and acts on the parietal cells to produce acid. In addition, vagal afferents stimulate the antral G cells to release gastrin. Food in the stomach gives rise to antral distention, and this along with peptide breakdown products stimulates the antral G cells to produce gastrin. The gastrin and acetylcholine act directly on the parietal cells or the mast cells. The mast cells in turn release histamine, which stimulates gastric acid secretion.

Once acid secretion has been initiated, how is further acid secretion limited? Clearly, there will be loss of vagal stimulation, loss of antral distention and loss of stimulated release of gastrin as food is virtually digested and emptied from the stomach into the duodenum. Also, the acid released from the parietal cells acidifies the antrum and thereby inhibits the further release of gastrin. The presence of food in the intestine further stimulates the release of a number of gastrointestinal hormones (including secretin, somatostatin, GIP and VIP) that inhibit the secretion of acid by parietal cells.

In health, a basal acid output obtained under unstimulated conditions is 5–10 mmol/hr. Following the administration of 6 mg/kg of pentagastrin, the parietal cell mass will be stimulated to produce hydrochloric acid. The maximal acid output will be less than 35 mmol/hr, and the peak acid output will be less than 60 mmol/hr. In health, the ratio of basal to maximum acid output or basal to peak acid output will be less than 0.25. The peak or maximum acid output reflects the parietal cell mass, whereas the ratio of BAO/PAO reflects the parietal cell function under basal conditions.

In disease, acid secretion may change. With gastric atrophy, both the basal and stimulated acid outputs are reduced. Peak acid output is increased in approximately one-half of patients with duodenal ulcer disease, whereas in patients with the Zollinger-Ellison syndrome, the major change is in the increased basal acid output. In patients with gastric ulcers, basal and peak acid output are usually normal or reduced. It must be stressed that this represents the acid measured in the gastric lumen and does not necessarily reflect the acid-secreting ability of the parietal cells in patients with gastric ulcer disease. That is, as a result of associated gastritis and back-diffusion of acid, these patients may secrete normal amounts of acid, which then diffuse back into the parietal cell. Therefore, the amount of acid measured in the gastric lumen would be normal or reduced.

Gastrin, histamine, acetylcholine and unspecified inhibitors influence the gastric secretory drive. Gastrin concentrations may be increased physiologically following food intake, with an increase of less than 100% above basal or fasting values. Secretory drive may be increased in the Zollinger-Ellison syndrome, G-cell hyperplasia or retained antrum. In the short bowel syndrome, temporary gastric hypersecretion may occur. The pathogenesis of this abnormality is unknown, and may relate to the loss of gastrin inhibitory factor in the small bowel. Gastrin levels are commonly increased in renal failure and pernicious anemia, and more rarely in diabetes mellitus and rheumatoid arthritis. In the latter two conditions, it is presumed that the gastrin levels are increased as a result of hypochlorhydria.

Once the stimulants of acid secretion (gastrin and acetylcholine) have been released, parietal cells are stimulated to secrete acid. The receptor for acetylcholine and gastrin may be on the mast cells, which are then stimulated to release histamine, which acts directly on the parietal cells to produce acid. Alternatively, there may be three separate receptors on the parietal cell: those for gastrin, acetylcholine and histamine. The histamine acts on adenylate cyclase in the parietal cell membrane to increase the production of cyclic AMP. In the presence of calcium, a protein kinase is stimulated, which then acts on the H^+/K^+ ATPase to secrete hydrochloric acid. This H^+/K^+ ATPase is known as the "proton pump." It represents the final common pathway for hydrogen ion secretion. Acetylcholine may act on the mast cells to release histamine, but may also act on the parietal cells to increase the influx of calcium ions, which then stimulate the protein kinase. The intracellular mechanism of gastric-mediated acid secretion is not known, although gastrin may stimulate the mast cells to release histamine, which further stimulates acid secretion.

This discussion of the mechanism of acid secretion provides the basis for understanding the pathogenesis of peptic ulcer disease. The parietal cell mass may be increased, and this may be reflected by an increase in the peak acid output or in serum pepsinogen 1. Secretory drive may be increased, and this is reflected by an increase in the ratio of BAO/PAO. Stimulated secretion is abnormal, as reflected by an increased parietal cell sensitivity to gastrin and possibly to histamine. Finally, the acid load in the duodenum is increased (as a result of increased acid secretion, as well as an increased rate of gastric emptying) in duodenal ulcer disease.

4.7 Diagnosis

Radiology for the diagnosis of peptic ulcer disease is being increasingly replaced by upper gastrointestinal endoscopy (esophagogastroduodenoscopy, or EGD). A chronic lesser-curve ulcer is usually seen as a distinct niche or pocket of barium projecting out from the line of the barium-filled stomach. The crater has a clean, smooth outline, and often its upper part contains a fluid level between the barium below and gastric' juice or gas above. A posterior-wall gastric ulcer is often best seen *en face* as a barium-filled niche after a small amount of the barium suspension has been drunk, and when the abdomen has been compressed. A spastic notch on the greater curvature opposite the ulcer is a common feature of chronic gastric ulcer. Occasionally, a gross horizontal fibrous contracture in association with long-standing ulceration can cause a permanent hourglass constriction, or the lesser curvature can shorten longitudinally. Antral or prepyloric ulcers present special diagnostic difficulties to the radiologist, because the associated spasm or inflammatory swelling cannot always be distinguished from the appearance of gastric cancer. Greater-curvature ulceration is uncommon, and is seldom malignant. Lesser-curvature ulcers above the angulus can usually confidently be separated from malignant disease by their regularity and relative absence of mucosal distortion within the line of the barium-filled viscus (except by the classical appearances of fibrous contracture). The size of a gastric ulcer is not a guide to the presence of malignancy or to the severity of symptoms; furthermore, large gastric ulcers often respond better to medical treatment than small ones (Figure 4A, 4B).

The radiologic diagnosis of duodenal ulcer is complicated by the problem of distinguishing simple deformity (scarring) in the duodenal bulb (due to previous and now healed ulceration) from deformity with active ulceration. Ulceration in an undeformed cap is relatively uncommon. It may be seen either as a niche in profile on one border of the bulb (Figure 5A, 5B) or *en face* through the bulb when the bulb contains a small quantity of barium suspension and is compressed or examined in air contrast films (e.g., in a posterior view with the patient lying slightly on the left side). Scarring of the bulb can induce a number of deformities, such as trefoil deformity following ulceration at the base of the bulb, and pseudodiverticulum formation. A minority of ulcers occur in the immediate postbulbar region of the duodenum. Close attention to this region is needed if they are to be found.

4.8 Endoscopy
Modern fiberoptic instruments used in endoscopic examination have greatly increased its safety and diagnostic range, and the patient's comfort. The available instruments are either end- or side-viewing. The former are good general-purpose instruments that allow an adequate view of the esophagus, stomach and upper duodenum. Side-viewing instruments are more specialized and are used in the duodenal loop.

4.9 Therapy of Peptic Ulcer Disease
Medications used in the treatment of peptic ulcer disease can be classified into those that inhibit or neutralize acid secretion and those that are cytoprotective (Figure 6). Acid that has already been secreted can be neutralized with antacids, or the synthesis of acid can be inhibited by the use of H_2 blockers (such as ranitidine and cimetidine), anticholinergics (such as pirenzepine) or antigastrin agents (such as proglumide). The cytoprotective agents include licorice extracts, sucralfate and prostaglandins. Recent attention has turned to combin-

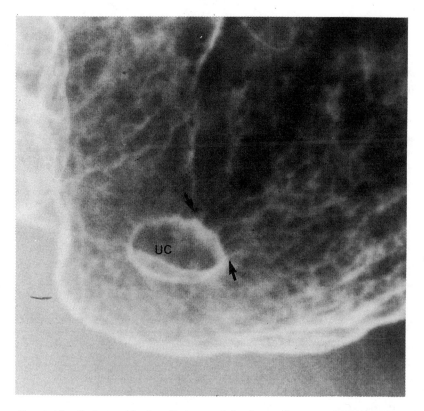

FIGURE 4A.   Benign gastric ulcer. Barium meal showing an ulcer crater (UC) situated on the greater curvature of the stomach, in the gastric antrum. The ulcer is visualized *en face* with a slightly oblique projection. Smooth mucosal folds radiating from the edge of the crater (arrows) in a regular fashion are a pathognomonic sign of a benign gastric ulcer. (Courtesy of Dr. J. Rawlinson).

ing various therapeutic agents with antibiotic therapy to treat both the peptic ulcer and the Helicobacter pylori–associated gastritis in an attempt to prevent ulcer recurrence (see Section 8.2.3 for a further discussion).

The medications that inhibit acid secretion act either on the three receptors on the parietal cell or on the acid pump. These include H_2-receptor antagonists (cimetidine and ranitidine), muscarinic-receptor antagonists (pirenzepine, propantheline), gastrin-receptor antagonists (proglumide) and H^+/K^+-ATPase inhibitors (omeprazole).

Cimetidine is structurally similar to histamine, with an imidazole ring. The

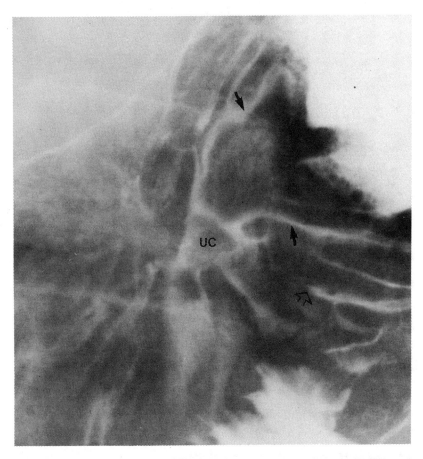

FIGURE 4B. Malignant gastric ulcer. Barium meal demonstrating an ulcer crater (UC) on the lesser curvature of the stomach, also visualized *en face*. In this case the radiating mucosal folds are irregularly thickened (e.g., between closed arrows) and do not extend to the edge of the crater (open arrow) – features indicating a local infiltrative, malignant process. (Courtesy of Dr. J. Rawlinson.)

side structure of ranitidine is vaguely similar to that of cimetidine, but there is a furan rather than an imidazole ring. This difference in ring structure may account for the differences in side effects of these two H_2-receptor antagonists. Many side effects have been ascribed to H_2 blockers (Table 4). It must be stressed, however, that these side effects are rare with cimetidine. Cimetidine is metabolized by the cytochrome P-450 system, as are a number of cardiovascular, anoretic, CNS, analgesic and anesthetic medications.

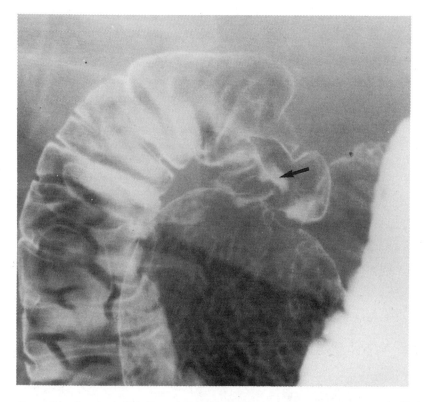

FIGURE 5A.   Duodenal ulcer. Situated at the base of the duodenal cap, the ulcer crater is filled with barium (arrow). The surrounding inflammatory process has considerably distorted the normal bulbar configuration of the proximal duodenum. (Courtesy of Dr. J. Rawlinson.)

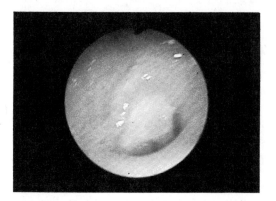

FIGURE 5B.   Duodenal ulcer. Endoscopic view of the duodenal cap ulcer.

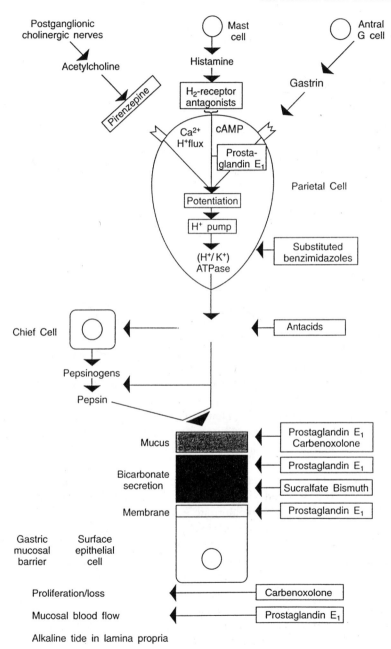

FIGURE 6.   Therapeutic intervention in a pathophysiologic scheme.

TABLE 4. Side effects of H_2 blockers

CNS	Confusion, dizziness
CVS	Bradycardia
Endocrine	Gynecomastia
	Antiandrogenic
	Prolactinemia
Blood	Neutropenia
	Immune system
Liver	Blood flow
	Increased serum transaminases
	Cytochrome P-450 (cimetidine)
Kidney	Increased plasma creatinine
	(1–2% of patients)
Intestine	Diarrhea
Skin	Rash
Muscle	Pain

Those in common use include diazepam, warfarin, theophylline, propranolol, phenytoin and lidocaine. As a result of this interaction, patients receiving cimetidine must have a reduction in the dose of any medication that is also metabolized by the cytochrome P-450 system. Ranitidine is not metabolized to the same degree by this hepatic oxidative system; therefore no adjustment in the dosage of other medications is necessary in patients on this H_2-receptor antagonist. Furthermore, antiandrogenic effects, particularly gynecomastia, are exceedingly rare in patients taking ranitidine.

The basic aluminum salt of the sulfated disaccharide sucralfate enhances mucosal defense, possibly by providing a protective barrier at the ulcer base, inhibiting the action of pepsin and bile, and blocking the back-diffusion of acid.

What is the practical approach to the management of patients with ulcer disease? Based on the history and physical examination, peptic ulcer disease may be suspected. If the patient's symptoms are mild and of short duration, then the use of antacids and avoidance of obviously irritating agents should be undertaken. If the antacids are ineffective or if the symptoms are severe or prolonged, then either an upper gastrointestinal series or an endoscopy should be performed. Because of the approximately 20% false-positive and false-negative rate of an upper GI series, many family physicians prefer to refer a patient for endoscopy. In this way the diagnosis is confirmed, and if a gastric ulcer is demonstrated, then biopsies and cytology can be performed to exclude gastric malignancy. Although the new potent antacids have a high neutralizing effect, they must be taken in large volumes frequently throughout the day, are generally unpalatable, and cause side effects (e.g., diarrhea). Therapy of gastric and duodenal ulcer disease is now recommended to begin with an H_2-receptor antagonist. If the patient is elderly or on multiple-drug therapy, the agent of choice is ranitidine 150 mg b.i.d. or 300 mg h.s. Alternatively, in the majority of patients cimetidine may be given as an 800 mg h.s. dose. If the ulcer does not heal after six weeks of therapy with one of these agents, and if the diagnosis is certain, then the H_2-receptor antagonist can be stopped and the patient switched to sucralfate 2 g b.i.d. As long as there is no evidence of gastric outlet obstruction, metoclopramide 10 mg q.i.d. one-half hour before meals and at night can be used in a patient with mild nausea and bloating. If the patient's ulcer still has not healed, then a fasting gastrin concentration must be obtained to exclude hypergastrinemia, endoscopy must be performed or repeated to exclude malignancy, and every effort must be taken to ensure that the patient is not taking nonsteroidal anti-inflammatory agents. Patients over the age of 40 years complaining of dyspepsia should be investigated with endoscopy.

4.10 Other Agents

A number of tricyclic agents are available to reduce acid secretion. The tricyclic antidepressants have been shown to be modestly useful in the treatment of acid-peptic disorders. The non-antidepressant tricyclic agent pirenzepine is efficacious in the healing of duodenal ulcer disease when given in a dose of 50 mg b.i.d., but this dose is associated with prevalent side effects (including bradycardia, dry mouth and difficulty in focusing the eyes). Because of its anticholinergic effects, this medication is contraindicated in patients with glaucoma or with GI or genitourinary obstruction. The tricyclic agents are generally not considered to be the first line of therapy.

Omeprazole is the first agent of a class of substituted benzimidazoles that are able to specifically block the H^+/K^+-ATPase enzyme that is unique to the secretory canaliculus for the parietal cell. Inhibition of this final common pathway of gastric acid secretion is able to abolish the secretory response to all known secretagogues. Omeprazole is a weak base absorbed from the proximal small intestine at the highly acidic compartment of the secretory canaliculus, leading to activation of a sulfoxide metabolite, which is either rapidly inactivated or binds to the H^+/K^+-ATPase enzyme. Binding to the H^+/K^+ ATPase inactivates the enzyme and profoundly inhibits gastric acid secretion. Omeprazole will act in the stimulated parietal cell only when the drug can be trapped and converted to its active form in the highly acidic compartment. Peak absorption occurs 3 to 4 hours after oral administration, and the plasma levels are undetectable by about 11 hours after a single dose of the drug. The bioavailability of omeprazole increases with repeated doses up to about four days, probably as a result of increasing drug absorption as intragastric acidity decreases. Gastric acid inhibition approaches 98% following omeprazole 30 mg daily for one week.

The powerful antisecretory effects of omeprazole result in an elevation of serum gastrin concentrations, which in humans appear to be related to the degree of acid suppression. However, toxicologic studies in the rat in which massive doses of omeprazole have been used have shown markedly elevated gastrin levels associated with ECL-cell hyperplasia and gastric carcinoid tumors, which have been found after long-term treatment. Omeprazole at present is approved for short-term clinical use. It is an effective agent in the treatment of peptic ulcer disease and reflux esophagitis. Omeprazole inhibits the hepatic microsomal P-450 mono-oxygenase system, and the plasma half-life of drugs metabolized by this route may be extended.

Another therapeutic approach to the patient with peptic ulcer disease, based on different pathophysiologic mechanisms, includes the use of drugs that enhance mucosal defense. Colloidal bismuth compounds (e.g., tripotassium dicitrato bismuthate [De Nol®]) are used in the United Kingdom to treat peptic ulcer disease. Licorice extracts have been used for many years for the treatment of peptic ulcer disease, but the active agent, carbenoxolone, is unfortunately associated with significant aldosterone-like side effects and this compound has not gained wide acceptance. We have already considered the potential application of prostaglandins for the treatment of gastric and duodenal ulcer disease; current clinical studies have shown that methylated prostaglandins E_2 given by mouth may be as effective as H_2-receptor antagonists in the rapid healing of peptic ulcers.

It is likely that in the future, prostaglandins will become the drug of choice for the treatment of gastritis and gastric ulcer. Since the side effects from these medications are few, prostaglandins may in time replace H_2-receptor antagonists or sucralfate in the treatment of peptic ulcer disease. Because of their frequent side effects, anticholinergics are generally avoided except in the patient with nighttime pain despite maximal doses of H_2-receptor antagonists. Depression, both overt and masked, occurs in patients with peptic ulcer disease. These individuals may improve with an antidepressant; trimipramine has been shown to accelerate the healing of duodenal ulcer disease.

4.11 General Recommendations

What therapeutic recommendations can be made? The proportion of patients whose ulcers heal after six weeks of cimetidine, ranitidine, sucralfate or prostaglandin is comparable. Recommendations must therefore be made on other factors, including convenience, side effects, cost and maintenance of healing. Liquid antacids are inconvenient to take, and patient compliance is poor. Side effects from the anticholinergics are frequent, and cimetidine should be avoided in the older patient or in the individual taking multiple drugs. A therapeutic dose of each of these agents – that is, a dose necessary to obtain ulcer healing – is comparable and expensive (about $60 to heal an ulcer).

Peptic ulcer disease has a natural history of recurrence. Once an ulcer has healed, there is a 75% chance that the ulcer will recur in 12 months; 50% will be symptomatic, whereas 25% will be asymptomatic. If patients are maintained on low-dose H_2-receptor antagonists, then only 25% of the patients will have an ulcer recurrence in 12 months. There is no widely accepted practice advised for maintenance therapy. The general rule of thumb would be to advise maintenance therapy for the patient with severe aggressive recurrent ulcer disease.

More recently, attention has turned to the role of Helicobacter pylori in ulcer recurrence. In particular, Helicobacter pylori is associated with an antral gastritis seen in 95% of duodenal ulcer patients. Eradication of Helicobacter pylori infection associated with duodenal ulcer disease through antibiotic therapy may eliminate ulcer recurrence (see Section 8.2.3).

4.12 Failure of Medical Therapy

If the ulcer fails to heal with medical therapy, the patient may have taken inadequate doses of medication for an inadequate duration, or the medication may have been taken improperly. For example, an antacid must be taken one and three hours after meals; sucralfate must be taken one hour before meals and concurrent antisecretory therapy and antacid use must be avoided; and H_2-receptor antagonists must be taken with meals. The possibility of malabsorption of the medication must be considered. An ulcer complicated by penetration or pancreatitis may be associated with continued symptoms. The continuation of the environmental factors responsible for the initial development of the ulcer may be responsible for lack of healing. The adequacy of the diagnosis must be questioned, and it is for this reason that endoscopy is generally recommended for the proper diagnosis of peptic ulcer disease. Finally, concurrent infection of the stomach or duodenum with Helicobacter pylori may be a factor in a resistant ulcer (see Section 8.2.3).

An additional cause of failure of medical therapy and failure of ulcer healing is the presence of a hypersecretory state, possibly due to hypergastrinemia. It is disputed whether G-cell hyperplasia occurs in patients with duodenal ulcer disease. Clearly, however, a small proportion of patients with ulcer disease would have a hypersecretory state due to the presence of a gastrinoma (which will lead to basal and/or stimulated hypergastrinemia). Other conditions leading to basal hypergastrinemia include retained antrum, pyloric obstruction, pernicious anemia, hypercalcemia, renal failure, massive small bowel resection and portacaval anastomoses. Peptic ulcer disease does not occur in patients with pernicious anemia, because they lack parietal cells. However, these other conditions associated with basal hypergastrinemia may also be associated with hyperchlorhydria and associated peptic ulcer disease. It is unclear whether hypergastrinemia also occurs in patients with diabetes mellitus or rheumatoid arthritis.

For the complications of hemorrhage, obstruction, perforation or intractability, surgery will be necessary. There is no consensus regarding the procedure of choice, but generally some form of vagotomy (e.g., truncal, selective or parietal cell) with a drainage procedure (pyloroplasty or antrectomy) is advised.

In general, a vagotomy is performed with a gastric draining procedure (pyloroplasty/gastroenterostomy) and/or a gastric resection to avoid gastric stasis (Figure 7). Three forms of vagotomy are in vogue: truncal, selective and parietal cell. A Billroth I or Billroth II anastomosis may also be performed, particularly when the antrum or portions of the body of the stomach are resected. A drainage procedure is needed to avoid the gastric atony resulting from the vagotomy and associated delayed gastric emptying.

4.13 Gastrinoma

The Zollinger-Ellison (ZE) syndrome is characterized by autonomous gastrin production by an adenoma or adenocarcinoma of the pancreas or duodenum. Patients may present either with severe acute ulcer disease or recurrent ulcer disease; the ulcers will often occur in unusual sites and be associated with diarrhea. The Zollinger-Ellison syndrome is distinguished from peptic ulcer disease by the demonstration of fasting hypergastrinemia. There are many causes of fasting hypergastrinemia (gastritis, vagotomy and pyloroplasty, the short bowel syndrome, rheumatoid arthritis, retained antrum, G-cell hyperplasia), but only two conditions – atrophic gastritis and renal failure – are associated with gastrin levels increased several times above the upper limit of the normal range. However, in a patient with peptic ulcer disease and hypergastrinemia, it is important to exclude the Zollinger-Ellison syndrome. Gastric analysis may be helpful: the finding of a dramatically increased basal output relative to a modestly increased maximal acid output (i.e., BAO/MAO greater than 0.6) is suggestive of this syndrome. Ingestion of a protein-containing meal normally produces a doubling of the gastrin concentration (a.c. versus p.c.), but an exaggerated response is seen in G-cell hyperplasia rather than in

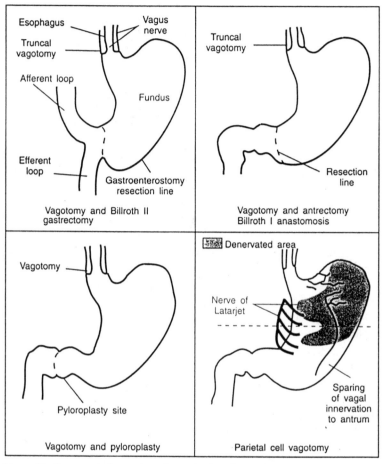

FIGURE 7.   Some surgical procedures for peptic ulcer disease.

gastrinoma syndrome. Infusion of calcium intravenously results in an increase in gastrin concentration in normal individuals and an exaggeration of this response in patients with the Zollinger-Ellison syndrome. However, the most useful diagnostic test is the secretin infusion. In normal individuals or those with G-cell hyperplasia, injection of secretin results in a rapid decline in plasma gastrin concentrations, whereas in patients with the Zollinger-Ellison syndrome, the gastrin concentration will increase in response to secretin.

The Zollinger-Ellison syndrome arises from a gastrinoma, a tumor in the pancreas. This may be a localized or diffuse tumor. The presence of hypergastrinemia leads to hypersecretion; while the maximal acid output may be increased, the major defect is basal hypergastrinemia and a marked increase in the basal acid output. The patient will have aggressive peptic ulcer disease with ulceration in unusual sites, or multiple ulcers that fail to heal on medical therapy. Hypertrophic gastric folds and diarrhea may be prominent features. The presence of a gastrinoma should be suspected from the history, and confirmed with provocative tests. A protein meal will increase the serum gastrin concentration in patients with G-cell hyperplasia; a calcium infusion will markedly increase the gastrin concentration in patients with gastrinoma, and have a lesser effect in normal patients and patients with G-cell hyperplasia. The best test to diagnose a gastrinoma is a secretin test in which the basal gastrin concentration increases dramatically, in contrast to the reduction in gastrin concentration that occurs following secretin infusion in patients with G-cell hyperplasia or a normal stomach. A CT scan or an angiogram may be useful in identifying the gastrinoma, although these tumors are often small and difficult to identify. A laparotomy will be necessary to determine whether there is a localized tumor. Since one-half of these tumors are malignant, it is worthwhile to undertake surgery in the hope that resection of the tumor will produce a cure.

If the high dose of H_2-receptor antagonists does not sufficiently relieve the patient's pain, then nighttime anticholinergics can be used. A trial of parietal cell vagotomy is under way, but this is not yet accepted therapy.

5. POSTGASTRECTOMY PROBLEMS

Numerous problems follow peptic ulcer surgery. These postgastrectomy problems may occur early after surgery or many months later. The early problems relate to the surgery itself. There are many late postgastrectomy syndromes (Table 5); these may be more disabling than the dyspeptic symptoms that led to the surgery in the first place.

5.1 Esophageal Symptoms
The incidence of gastroesophageal reflux after vagotomy or partial gastric resection is unknown, although it is a common symptom even in unoperated patients. The effect of vagotomy on lower esophageal sphincter pressure is uncertain, but operations involving mobilization and manipulation of the proximal stomach can damage the sphincter. Operations that involve the antrum and pylorus may allow duodenal juice to reflux into the stomach. From there it may enter and damage the esophagus, an additional factor that may contribute to therapeutic problems. Assessment of patients with symp-

TABLE 5.   Complications of gastric surgery

Esophagus
Gastroesophageal reflux
Dysphagia

Stomach
Delayed gastric emptying
Bezoars
Outlet obstruction
Stomatitis
Recurrent ulcers
Stump carcinoma
Afferent loop syndrome

Small intestine
Diarrhea
  Dumping syndrome
  Bacterial contamination syndrome
  Unmasked celiac disease, unmasked pancreatic
    insufficiency or unmasked lactase deficiency
Weight loss and malabsorption
  Iron
  Folate
  Vitamin B_{12}
  Calcium
  Fats
Anemia

Gallbladder
Cholelithiasis

---

toms of gastroesophageal reflux should include a barium swallow and endoscopy. If the patient's acid output is low, then the esophagitis may be due to the reflux of bile and pancreatic juice from the duodenum into the stomach and esophagus. If the bile-induced esophagitis does not respond to bile acid binding agents (cholestyramine, sucralfate, aluminum hydroxide antacid), then surgical revision with a Roux-en-Y anastomosis may be necessary.

One of the more troublesome postgastrectomy syndromes is that of dysphagia. This usually occurs in the early postoperative period. Although spontaneous improvement is the rule, occasionally esophagitis and stricture may occur. This dysphagia may result from trauma to the esophagus at the time of surgery, the development of a periesophageal hematoma, or a vagotomy.

5.2 Delayed Gastric Emptying

Delayed gastric emptying may result from recurrent ulceration, stomal edema, fibrosis or decreased gastric tone and motility, and may lead to bezoar formation. The patient may suffer early satiety or postprandial fullness. Gastric bezoars are secretions of food or foreign material in the stomach. Vegetable bezoars are called phytobezoars; those composed of hair are called trichobezoars. These develop following antrectomy and vagotomy, and probably relate to inadequate chewing, hypochlorhydria, and a high-fiber diet. Bezoars may be suspected on plain film of the abdomen or upper GI series and may be confirmed at endoscopy. It is occasionally possible at endoscopy to fragment the bezoar, but therapy with papain (an enzyme that digests protein, and thus helps dissolve either type of bezoar) is usually necessary.

If stomal fibrosis is present, surgery is usually indicated. Intravenous therapy may be required if the obstruction is severe, but if the outlet is patent, metoclopramide or domperidone may improve gastric emptying. Alternatively it may be necessary to revise the surgical anastomosis.

5.3 Recurrent Ulcers

Ulcers that recur following gastric surgery bear many names (e.g., stomal ulceration, recurrent ulcers, postgastrectomy ulcers). These recurrent ulcers may be due to incomplete vagotomy, incomplete resection of G cells or acid-producing cells, retained antrum, delayed gastric emptying, duodenogastric reflux, ulcerogenic drugs or gastrinoma. Naturally, these benign conditions must be excluded from a stump ulcer. Recurrent ulceration with edema and partial obstruction may benefit from a trial of an H_2-receptor antagonist.

5.4 Carcinoma

Carcinoma of the gastric stump may develop 20 or more years following gastric surgery for benign peptic ulcer disease. Stump carcinoma appears to be more common following a Billroth II anastomosis. The carcinoma develops at the anastomosis, or in the gastric body or fundus. The pathogenesis is thought to be related to the development of chronic atrophic gastritis. Initially, there may be metaplasia of the Paneth's and goblet cells, and then subsequent dysplasia. These morphologic changes seem to relate to chronic bile and alkaline reflux.

5.5 Afferent Loop Syndrome

In patients with a gastrojejunostomy or a Billroth II anastomosis, obstruction of the afferent loop may occur. Symptoms may be acute or chronic and due to the presence of an internal hernia, kinking, the formation of adhesions or stenosis of the stoma. The acute afferent loop syndrome occurs in the early postoperative period. There may be partial or complete obstruction of the afferent loop, giving rise to pain, nausea, vomiting of nonbilious material, the palpation of an abdominal mass, and occasionally elevation in the serum amylase and liver function tests. The chronic afferent loop syndrome is due to partial obstruction of the afferent loop. The patient will complain of postprandial bilious vomiting without food. This vomiting will be intermittent, severe and painful.

5.6 Diarrhea

Diarrhea commonly occurs immediately after truncal vagotomy; various mechanisms have been suggested, including the dumping syndrome, the bacterial overgrowth syndrome, use of excessive amounts of magnesium-containing antacids, the Zollinger-Ellison syndrome, unmasked celiac disease, unmasked lactose intolerance and unmasked pancreatic insufficiency. Other causes of diarrhea seen in patients without previous gastric surgery or vagotomy also need to be considered.

Most cases of postvagotomy diarrhea improve with time. Antidiarrheal agents such as loperamide and diphenoxylate may improve symptoms; in those patients who do not respond, cholestyramine or antibiotics are sometimes helpful. More persistent diarrhea should be fully investigated to rule out infection, malabsorption or gastrin-secreting tumors. In extreme cases, surgical intervention may be necessary.

"Early dumping" occurs 10 to 20 minutes after meals and has three components: gastrointestinal, vasomotor and cardiovascular. The patient may develop pain, nausea, vomiting, fullness and diarrhea. Vasomotor symptoms include weakness, dizziness, faintness, pallor and sweating; cardiovascular symptoms include palpitations and tachycardia. The early dumping syndrome is caused by rapid emptying of gastric contents with osmotic fluid shifts, abdominal distention and release of vasoactive substances. The intestinal distention produces the pain, nausea and vomiting, whereas the vasomotor and cardiovascular symptoms are due to the release of serotonin and bradykinin.

The "late dumping" syndrome occurs 1 to 3 hours after meals, particularly meals containing large amounts of carbohydrate. The late dumping syndrome is characterized by evidence of sympathetic discharge due to hypoglycemia. These symptoms include weakness, sweating, hunger and confusion. The pathophysiologic basis for this dumping syndrome is straightforward: rapid gastric emptying, rapid absorption of glucose, release of large amounts of insulin, rapid decline in blood sugar levels due to the rapid cessation of glucose absorption, and excessively high insulin levels.

The dumping syndrome may be treated with dietary therapy: six small meals per day containing high-protein, low-carbohydrate foods, and the ingestion of liquids between rather than with meals. This is effective for most patients, but in some individuals anticholinergics will be necessary before meals, or the serotonin antagonist cyproheptadine may be prescribed. Tolbutamide or pectin may be useful in some individuals. When all else fails, a Billroth II anastomosis will need to be converted into a Billroth I. If the patient already has a Billroth I, then in rare cases an antiperistaltic loop of small bowel will need to be inserted.

5.7 Weight Loss and Malabsorption
Weight loss occurs after surgery in 30–60% of patients; it is less common with vagotomy alone than with vagotomy and antrectomy. The most common cause is decreased caloric intake because of early satiety, but in patients with severe malnutrition or persistent diarrhea, an investigation of malabsorption should be undertaken.

5.8 Anemia
Anemia is common following gastric surgery. Iron deficiency may be due to a preoperative iron deficiency, surgical blood loss inadequately replaced during or following surgery, postoperative GI or GU losses, or malabsorption of iron resulting from reduction in gastric acid (necessary for the absorption of food iron) or bypassing of the duodenum (the optimal site for the absorption of all forms of iron). In some patients, an associated malabsorption syndrome unmasked by the gastric surgery will result in folate deficiency from inadequate intake or malabsorption of folate. B_{12} deficiency may occur if a sufficient number of intrinsic-factor–producing cells have been resected. B_{12} deficiency may also occur if there is associated bacterial overgrowth syndrome, and rarely if there is pancreatic insufficiency. In patients with pernicious anemia, the urinary excretion of vitamin B_{12} (Schilling test) will increase to normal when the intrinsic factor is given together with a low dose of vitamin.

5.9 Cholelithiasis
Cholelithiasis occurs more frequently following a truncal than other types of vagotomy. The mechanism is thought to be decreased bile flow and gallbladder contraction, associated with increased gallbladder size and the development of lithogenic bile.

TABLE 6.   Classification of gastritis

Autoimmune	Congenital pernicious anemia
Granulomatous	Tuberculosis, Crohn's disease
Infectious	Helicobacter pylori
Hypertrophic	Ménétrier's disease
Eosinophilic	Eosinophilic gastroenteritis
Chemical	NSAIDs, alcohol, bile reflux
Miscellaneous	Senility, iron deficiency, radiation

6. GASTRITIS

6.1 Acute Gastritis

Acute gastritis is an acute self-limiting syndrome caused by irritation of the gastric mucosa by alcohol, corrosive poisons, and the various bacterial and oral causes of food poisoning. It is characterized by anorexia, nausea and vomiting. In some patients, the same causal agents produce acute ulcers that may bleed or perforate. The role of analgesics is not clear.

6.2 Chronic Gastritis

Three main types of gastritis are recognized by histological examination: superficial gastritis, atrophic gastritis and gastric atrophy. Chronic gastritis is characterized by mononuclear and polymorphonuclear cell infiltration of mucosa, glandular atrophy and intestinal metaplasia. In superficial gastritis inflammation is marked and glandular atrophy is minimal, whereas in gastric atrophy inflammatory cells are few and glandular atrophy is extensive. These represent different degrees of gastritis, though not necessarily all cases that progress to atrophy must be preceded by the two lesser lesions.

With progressive degeneration of the mucosa, gastric secretion progressively fails. Hydrochloric acid secretion fails first, followed by pepsinogen secretion and finally by the secretion of intrinsic factor. As intrinsic factor secretion fails, the body becomes depleted of vitamin B_{12} and pernicious anemia develops. Antibodies to parietal cells and intrinsic factor appear in the serum. The presence of these antibodies together with a partial response to steroids suggests that autoimmunity may play an etiologic role.

The cause of chronic gastritis is unknown, but it is probably due to a combination of genetic and acquired factors (Table 6). Among the latter may be included repeated minor trauma due to alcohol and analgesics, reflux of duodenal contents and gastric irradiation. Deficiencies of vitamin B_{12}, folic acid and iron interfere with the regenerative and functional capacity of the gastric mucosa.

Predisposition to gastric cancer is probably due to an unknown biochemical lesion within the cell that leads to secretory failure, cellular degeneration and in some cases gastric carcinoma. While most of the causes of hypochlorhydria are associated with gastritis, it remains disputed whether gastritis is necessarily associated with an increased risk of gastric cancer. Gastric cancer is 5 to 10 times as common as expected in those with chronic atrophic gastritis; the same increased incidence is also found in first-degree relatives of patients with gastric cancer and pernicious anemia.

It is uncertain whether chronic gastritis causes symptoms. Chronic gastritis can be diagnosed only by gastric biopsy of body or fundic mucosa. Marked gastric hyposecretion or anacidity is present if the lesion is diffuse

6.2.1 COMPLETE GASTRIC ATROPHY AND PERNICIOUS ANEMIA

There are many causes of hypochlorhydria (Table 7). The ability to produce acid, pepsin and intrinsic factor is lost altogether in patients with complete gastric atrophy. However, vitamin B_{12} deficiency – which leads to pernicious anemia or (much more rarely) to subacute combined degeneration of the spinal cord – takes several years to supervene because of the large liver stores of the vitamin. In the complete atrophy of pernicious anemia, gastric glandular and all parietal cells are lost, and the mucosa is infiltrated by large numbers of plasma cells and lymphocytes. Pentagastrin stimulation will demonstrate that the patient is achlorhydric. Studies will demonstrate antibodies to intrinsic factor and to parietal cells in serum, gastric secretions and mucosa in most patients. Though the presence of such antibodies is a useful marker, it is not diagnostic: intrinsic factor antibodies can be demonstrated occasionally (and parietal cell antibodies frequently) in patients with simple atrophic gastritis or chronic superficial gastritis without vitamin B_{12} malabsorption.

Hydroxocobalamin has replaced cyanocobalamin for the treatment of pernicious anemia, because it is better retained in the body. A dose of 200 μg by injection every month is more than sufficient to maintain body stores after loading treatment with 200 μg on three alternate days.

6.2.2 CONGENITAL PERNICIOUS ANEMIA

Congenital pernicious anemia is a rare condition, inherited as a Mendelian recessive, and is due to an inherited inability to secrete intrinsic factor in adequate amounts. It presents as megaloblastic anemia in infancy and is associated with normal acid secretory potential. The specific failure of intrinsic factor synthesis in this condition must be distinguished from congenital ileal receptor deficiency for the vitamin B_{12}-intrinsic factor complex (the Imers-

TABLE 7.   Causes of hypochlorhydria

Chronic gastritis (Table 6)
Gastric ulcer or cancer or polyposis
Resection

---

lund-Graesbeck syndrome) and from vitamin B_{12} deficiency due to gastric failure in the hypoparathyroidism-candidiasis syndrome.

The cause of pernicious anemia is unknown. The presence of auto-antibodies, mucosal infiltration by plasma cells and reversibility of the gastric lesion by corticosteroids suggest an autoimmune process. There is also a small but definite genetic predisposition; like gastric cancer, the disease is slightly more common in individuals of group A than in those of the remaining ABO groups. Exogenous factors that predispose to gastric cancer also seem likely to predispose to pernicious anemia. It is unclear why most patients present with pernicious anemia while a few develop the neurological condition of subacute degeneration of the spinal cord without anemia.

6.3 Chronic Superficial Gastritis
In this form of gastritis, inflammatory cells, mainly polymorphonuclear, infiltrate the superficial mucosa but gastric glands are well preserved. It has been found with increased frequency in those who smoke excessively or who consume large amounts of alcohol or hot beverages. No specific symptom pattern has been correlated with it, and it does not seem necessarily to predispose to gastric atrophy. Chronic superficial gastritis is commonly found in patients with chronic gastric ulcer, but is not a universal concomitant.

6.4 Chronic Atrophic Gastritis
With chronic atrophic gastritis, in addition to cellular infiltration, predominantly lymphocytic and plasma cell in pattern, there is a loss of gastric glands, and acid and pepsin secretory capacity is reduced in parallel. It does not cause symptoms, but in a minority of patients there is progression to the complete atrophy of pernicious anemia. Patients with atrophic gastritis probably develop eventual gastric cancer approximately as often as those with pernicious anemia.

6.5 Giant Mucosal Rugal Hypertrophy
Giant mucosal rugal hypertrophy is a histologic change occurring in association with the Zollinger-Ellison syndrome and rarely as an isolated entity.

Ménétrier's disease (giant hypertrophic gastritis), a rare condition associated with mucosal hypertrophy, involves reduced acid secretion. Hypertrophic-hypersecretory gastropathy, another associated condition, involves increased acid secretion. In giant mucosal rugal hypertrophy, as a result of protein loss into the gastric lumen, the serum albumin concentration will be reduced. The condition usually occurs in males between the ages of 30 and 50, and the patient will present with pain, nausea, vomiting, weight loss, bleeding, or edema as a result of hypoalbuminemia. The condition is suspected from the presence of large rugal folds identified on upper GI series or at endoscopy. A biopsy will demonstrate hyperplasia of the parietal, chief and mucus cells. There may be cystic structures in the mucosa and submucosa as well. The condition must be distinguished from giant hypertrophic gastritis, the Zollinger-Ellison syndrome, gastric carcinoma, lymphoma and amyloidosis. The protein loss may be reduced with anticholinergics. If gastric hyper-secretion occurs, as in the case of hypertrophic-hypersecretory gastropathy, H_2 blockers will prove useful. If pain, bleeding and protein loss persist, then a vagotomy and pyloroplasty or subtotal gastrectomy is necessary.

6.6 Granulomatous Gastritis
Chronic inflammatory changes in the gastric mucosa may occur in Crohn's disease, tuberculosis, syphilis and sarcoidosis, and granulomas may be present. These diseases are all uncommon.

6.7 Eosinophilic Gastritis
The cause of eosinophilic gastritis is unknown. There is extensive infiltration of the gastric and often the small intestinal mucosa by eosinophils, in association with peripheral eosinophilia. The disease produces nonspecific dyspeptic symptoms, and antral distortion is radiographically visible. Spontaneous cure is common, but some patients require steroid therapy and in a few the disease is progressive.

6.8 Bile Gastritis
The common occurrence of gastritis following gastric surgery is thought to be due to the effect of bile and alkaline duodenal secretion damaging the gastric mucosal barrier and giving rise to an inflammatory reaction. Some patients will respond to medical treatment with cholestyramine, aluminum hydroxide or sucralfate. Cholestyramine and aluminum hydroxide act by binding bile acids and pepsin, and providing a protective surface to the gastric mucosa. When the condition persists and is associated with pain or bleeding, a surgical procedure (Roux-en-Y) will be necessary.

6.9 Miscellaneous

There are two forms of gastritis that fall outside the classifications listed above. One is intestinal metaplasia, where a large number of cells with the histochemical properties of intestinal mucosal cells are found in the stomach. This is commonly associated with chronic gastritis. The second is Ménétrier's disease or giant hypertrophic gastritis, where the giant mucosal folds may be confused with neoplastic disease; excess protein loss from the folds may cause a syndrome of protein depletion (protein-losing enteropathy). Erosive gastritis and hyperplastic atrophic gastritis are less well defined entities.

7. PREMALIGNANT CONDITIONS OF THE STOMACH AND GASTRIC CANCER

7.1 Premalignant Conditions

Possible premalignant gastric conditions include pernicious anemia, atrophic gastritis, polyps and previous gastric surgery. People with a family history that is positive for gastric cancer also have an increased risk of developing this disease. Benign gastric ulcer is not a premalignant condition, but can appear so because of the long natural history of some ulcerating cancers. At present, regular endoscopy is not necessary for most patients with conditions predisposing to gastric ulcer. A high index of suspicion for cancer, however, must be maintained. If endoscopy and biopsy have been performed and distinct dysplastic changes are found in the epithelium, regular follow-up endoscopy and biopsy are advised.

7.1.1 *PERNICIOUS ANEMIA*

Patients with pernicious anemia have long been considered at risk for gastric cancer, but the risk is likely to be low and does not justify intensive endoscopic screening. Pernicious anemia is invariably associated with fundal gland atrophy, usually with intestinal metaplasia and sometimes with polyps. When cancer develops, it tends to occur in the body or fundus of the stomach.

7.1.2 *ATROPHIC GASTRITIS*

There are two main types of atrophic gastritis: fundal gland (type A), and pyloric (antral) gland (type B). These occur in older people. Antral gastritis increasingly involves the fundal gland area with advanced age. Both types A and B are associated with intestinal metaplasia and a predisposition to gastric cancer. Type A gastritis is less common and its distribution in the stomach resembles that of pernicious anemia. Type B gastritis is predominant in those areas of the body where gastric cancer is common and appears to be a risk factor mainly for the intestinal type of gastric cancer. Helicobacter pylori, which is the cause of type B gastritis, has been implicated as a risk factor for gastric cancer.

7.1.3 GASTRIC POLYPS

There are two main types of gastric polyps: hyperplastic and adenomatous. Hyperplastic polyps are small and do not become malignant. Hyperplastic polyps should be removed endoscopically but, when multiple, they need not all be removed. Adenomatous polyps are uncommon and are usually larger than 2 cm in diameter. They are premalignant, and a substantial minority show areas of cancer at the time of detection. Endoscopic or surgical excision is recommended.

7.1.4 PREVIOUS GASTRIC SURGERY

Patients who have had a partial gastrectomy for peptic ulcer disease may have an increased probability of developing gastric cancer some 15 to 20 years after the operation. Endoscopic surveillance of these patients does not appear to be justified in North America, since the risk is low.

7.2 Other Conditions

Individuals with a parent or sibling with gastric cancer are three times as likely to develop gastric cancer as the general population. People born in a country where gastric cancer is common (e.g., Japan or Eastern Europe) are also at increased risk, even if they have lived in North America for many years. Although regular screening is not warranted in either case, minor symptoms should be promptly and thoroughly investigated.

Barrett's epithelium (columnar cell lining of the lower esophagus) is a proven precursor of esophageal adenocarcinoma, and there is increasing suspicion that lesser degrees of Barrett's epithelium may predispose to the much more common adenocarcinoma of the gastric cardia.

7.3 Gastric Cancer

Adenocarcinoma is the most common gastric cancer, but lymphoma and leiomyosarcoma also occur. The frequency of gastric cancer has decreased considerably over the past 50 years in North America, but it still ranks as the second most common GI malignancy (after colon cancer). Most patients are over 60 years of age. Men are affected about twice as often as women. The cancer usually involves the antrum, body or cardia with about equal frequency. The three main macroscopic types are polypoid, ulcerative and infiltrative. The two main microscopic types are intestinal and diffuse. The intestinal type is often associated with atrophic gastritis and intestinal metaplasia; the diffuse type is often manifest as a linitis plastica.

Most patients have advanced incurable disease by the time they have significant complaints, but some patients with early gastric cancer may have mild epigastric discomfort or ulcer-like symptoms. Physical examination is usually normal but may reveal a mass or a succussion splash in a minority of patients. There may be evidence of metastases, such as a supraclavicular node, hepatomegaly, ascites, a "shelf" on a rectal examination, an ovarian mass or an umbilical node. Iron deficiency anemia is found in about 50% of patients and occult blood is present in the stool in about 75% of cases. Occasionally, the neurological signs of subacute combined degeneration of the spinal cord from associated pernicious anemia will be found. Measurement of gastric acid secretion or carcinoembryonic antigen (CEA) is not helpful. Barium radiograph is usually the first diagnostic procedure. Experienced radiologists can show some abnormality in up to 90% of patients, particularly if double contrast techniques are used. While there are distinguishing clinical and radiological features, every patient with a presumed benign gastric ulcer should have biopsies obtained to exclude a malignant ulcer. Endoscopy and biopsy, with or without brush cytology, are required to establish the diagnosis.

The diffuse type of gastric cancer often manifests itself as a linitis plastica. It is harder to diagnose than the intestinal type, particularly in the earlier stages. Thus, although diagnostic techniques have improved, some gastric cancers are still missed on the initial investigation. Although routine endoscopic screening is not feasible in North America, minor symptoms should be thoroughly investigated in people with predisposing conditions. It is also important to ensure that only benign gastric ulcers are treated medically; if a gastric ulcer fails to heal after three months of intensive medical therapy, surgery is generally recommended.

Early surgery offers the only hope for cure, but is not performed if there is evidence of metastatic disease, unless the patient suffers from gastric outlet obstruction. Cancers of the distal and mid-stomach are treated by subtotal gastrectomy. In order to remove the regional lymph nodes, the lesser and greater omenta are resected and, if necessary, the spleen is removed. Cancers of the proximal stomach are usually treated by esophagogastrectomy. With the increased proportion of diffusely infiltrating cancer, total gastrectomy with biliary diversion is being performed more often. Palliative resection, bypass, surgery or laser photoablation is justified in those patients with gastric outlet obstruction. Palliative esophagogastrectomy or total gastrectomy is not recommended. The prognosis after surgical treatment is related to the depth of the tumor's penetration. Overall, about 10–15% of patients survive five years. Occasionally, patients have a long course without treatment or with only palliative surgery.

Therapy includes chemotherapy with 5-fluorouracil, doxorubicin and mitomycin (FAM). This approach achieves a response rate of up to 40% but gives a disappointing median survival of less than one year. Occasionally, good responses are obtained, and a trial is recommended for patients in good condition and with advanced disease. Adjuvant chemotherapy or radiotherapy remains of unproven value, but palliative radiotherapy is useful to control bleeding, to alleviate pain from bone metastases and to relieve dysphagia. Esophageal dilation and endoscopically placed plastic tubes can also help dysphagia caused by persistent spread of a cardia tumor.

General supportive care is important, including dietary advice, replacement of iron and vitamin B_{12}, judicious use of analgesics, antiemetics, and antacid support. Emotional support is particularly important and increasingly includes guidance in interpreting the common, overoptimistic "breakthroughs" reported in the press.

8. OTHER GASTRIC DISEASES

8.1 Acute

Partial (antral) or total gastric volvulus is a rare cause of acute upper abdominal pain and vomiting. These obstructions can arise by themselves, or as torsion within a hiatus hernia. Volvulus within a hernia is not uncommon in the elderly, when there may be no symptoms. The belief that twisting obstruction poses an important risk to the blood supply is probably unjustified. Gastric aspiration is followed by surgical relief of the volvulus in those who present with obstruction.

Sudden gross gastric distention and acute dilatation of the stomach can arise after any form of upper abdominal surgery, including cholecystectomy, and especially after vagotomy, after childbirth and in diabetic coma. The causes are uncertain. Vomiting of relatively clear gastric contents is succeeded by the production of dirty brown or feculent material and the development of abdominal distention. Prompt decompression with a large-bore stomach tube and intravenous fluid replacement are required. After a variable interval the condition should then resolve spontaneously.

8.1.1 *GASTRIC RUPTURE*

Acute, nontraumatic, spontaneous rupture of the stomach is a rare, catastrophic and poorly understood event. The majority of ruptures occur on the lesser curvature. They have also been reported to occur during upper gastrointestinal radiography using barium, sodium bicarbonate ingestion, nasal oxygen therapy, cardiopulmonary resuscitation and labor, and during the postpartum period.

8.2 Chronic

Hypertrophic pyloric stenosis is an idiopathic condition that may occur in infants or adults. The muscle of the pyloric canal is unduly hypertrophied. Infantile hypertrophic pyloric stenosis is more common in boys than in girls (the sex ratio is approximately 10:1), is a frequent anomaly (its incidence is about 3 per 1,000 live births) and is thought to be due to a combination of genetic predisposition and some abnormality of fetal or early postnatal development. Symptoms usually develop in the first few weeks after birth and characteristically consist of copious projectile vomiting of the gastric contents after feeding. On examination there is usually visible gastric peristalsis; a lump can be felt abdominally in the region of the pylorus. Barium-meal examination is not usually necessary but will confirm the presence of a narrow segment, 1–2 cm long, at the pylorus. The condition must be distinguished clinically from esophageal atresia (which involves onset at birth of difficulties with swallowing) and duodenal obstruction/atresia (which involves bile-stained vomitus). A minor proportion of all cases settle in the first two to three months with conservative management with anticholinergic drugs, but most patients will require early surgery with Ramstedt's procedure (pyloromyotomy).

Occasionally, adult patients present with obstructive symptoms resulting from pyloric stenosis associated with muscular hypertrophy. This is rarely if ever caused by recurrence of infantile pyloric stenosis; it is usually associated with juxtapyloric peptic ulceration, but sometimes the problem seems to be due to primary hypertrophic stenosis arising in adult life. The differential also includes pyloric mucosal diaphragm and annular pancreas. Pyloric obstruction requires pyloroplasty together with a procedure such as vagotomy if there is an associated ulcer.

8.2.1 GASTRIC DIVERTICULA

Gastric diverticula occur most commonly near the cardia on the lesser curve, but occasionally are found in the prepyloric region. They seldom cause symptoms. Their principal importance lies in the likelihood of confusion with gastric ulceration.

8.2.2 PSEUDOLYMPHOMA

Localized lymphoid hyperplasia of the stomach is also known as pseudolymphoma. The lesions are raised, flat or nodular folds, and are often associated with gastric ulceration. The etiology of this condition remains unclear, but Helicobacter pylori infection has been implicated. It is difficult to exclude lymphoma using radiology or endoscopic biopsy; thus, a resected specimen is required for diagnosis.

8.2.3 GASTRIC INFECTIONS AND INFESTATIONS

Gastric acid provides a bactericidal barrier against infection. Acid-suppressive pharmacotherapy, hypochlorhydria or gastric surgery may increase the risk of bacterial infection. Recent attention has been turned to Helicobacter pylori, a spiral bacillus found in the upper gastrointestinal tract, particularly the gastric antrum. H. pylori has been associated with chronic gastritis in addition to peptic ulcer disease.

Viral infections such as cytomegalovirus (CMV) and herpes simplex virus are very often found in immunocompromised hosts. They are associated with gastric erosions, although CMV has been found in intact mucosa. Cultures or endoscopic biopsies and smears demonstrating intranuclear inclusions are helpful in establishing a diagnosis. Candida albicans is commonly found in the gastric ulcers or erosions of immunocompromised hosts. Candidal infection should be a consideration in an ulcer that fails to heal. In the immunocompromised host, parasites such as Strongyloides stercoralis may become overwhelmingly disseminated. Histoplasmosis and mucomycosis involving the stomach are rare causes of gastric ulceration and bleeding.

8.2.3.1 Helicobacter pylori gastritis

Helicobacter pylori (H. pylori) is a small (3×0.5 μm) gram-negative, microaerophilic urease-producing rod-shaped bacillus, which has been closely linked to both acute and chronic active type B gastritis, especially of the antrum. H. pylori is an important pathogenic factor in peptic ulcer disease.

H. pylori is present in almost all cases of chronic active gastritis, which most commonly involves antral inflammation but may spread to the whole stomach over time. H. pylori does not colonize areas of intestinal metaplasia, but has been seen in the distal esophagus of some patients with Barrett's esophagus.

The source of H. pylori is unknown, although person-to-person spread is probably demonstrated by intrafamilial clustering and a high prevalence of seropositivity in institutionalized persons, those of low economic status, and populations in less developed countries. The prevalence of H. pylori infection increases with age; in Western countries it is uncommon before the third decade but thereafter increases with seropositivity at the rate of approximately 1% per year of age.

Most people with H. pylori–associated gastritis are asymptomatic and have normal-appearing gastric mucosa at endoscopy. The histologic spectrum of H. pylori–associated gastritis ranges from minimal to severe inflammation, but the organisms noted in the mucous layer are associated with severe depletion of mucus and an intense inflammation, which most often is chronic, although neutrophils can be noted in some instances. Eradication of H. pylori with antibiotics has resulted in a marked lessening in the severity of the gastritis.

8.2.3.1.1 *Diagnosis* The organism can be identified on histology with conventional hematoxylin- and eosin-stained sections at high-power magnification, but is more easily seen with the Warthin-Starry or the modified Giemsa stains. The enzyme-linked immunosorbent assay (ELISA) is the most widely employed serologic method; its sensitivity and specificity are greater than 90%. Rapid urease tests can be performed on tissue biopsies in the endoscopy unit since H. pylori produces large amounts of urease, which can convert urea into ammonia and carbon dioxide. Rapid urease tests involve urease and pH indicator gel, into which the biopsy is placed. The presence of H. pylori results in an alkaline pH of the medium and a color change when the pH rises. Approximately 75% of the positive tests occur between 20 minutes and 1 hour, and 90% are positive between 6 and 24 hours. Carbon-urea breath tests using carbon ^{13}C and ^{14}C employ carbon-labeled urea that is fed to the patient and is subsequently hydolyzed by the H. pylori urease, resulting in the formation of ammonia and carbon dioxide. This labeled carbon dioxide in the breath is then measured.

8.2.3.1.2 *H. pylori association with peptic ulcer disease* Numerous studies have established the close association of antral H. pylori and peptic ulcer disease. Over 90% of patients with duodenal ulcer have H. pylori identified in gastric antral biopsies. The association for gastric ulcer and H. pylori is up to 85%. Although ulcers can be healed with a variety of agents that do not eradicate H. pylori, in these cases relapse is common. However, when the H. pylori organism is eradicated the impact on the subsequent course of duodenal ulcer is dramatic. The recurrence rate in patients in whom H. pylori is eradicated ranges from 0–4% per year. This is in marked contrast to those who remain H. pylori–positive, whose recurrence rates vary from 40–80% per year. Unfortunately the current treatment of H. pylori is complex, with poor compliance and problems of antibiotic resistance. A triple drug regimen using bismuth sub-salicylate, metronidazole and tetracycline or amoxicillin can be expected to eradicate H. pylori in 75–90% cases. A more attractive alternative is the use of a proton pump inhibitor plus amoxicillin, with an efficacy in excess of 80% eradication.

Antral H. pylori infection may be a significant factor in acid hypersecretion and duodenal ulcer. The ulcer diathesis may be caused either by direct epithelial damage or by the inflammation secondary to the damage promoted by the organism and the subsequent weakening of mucosal defenses. The G cells are gastrin-producing cells that reside in the gastric antrum and are regulated by somatostatin and the presence of hydrochloric acid. The mechanism is disrupted in H. pylori infection and inflammation, resulting in an increased gastrin release and acid secretory response. The ulcer diathesis may reflect more damaging strains of the organisms, greater density of the infecting organisms or an exaggerated host inflammatory response.

8.2.3.1.3 *Nonulcer dyspepsia and H. pylori*   The role of H. pylori infection in nonulcer dyspepsia remains an important question. There may be a subset of patients with nonulcer dyspepsia whose symptoms are due to H. pylori infection. However, many patients harboring H. pylori are symptom-free. Acute infection with H. pylori is associated with belching, pyrosis and malaise, and may be associated with decreased gastric acid secretion. At present, there is no evidence to suggest that the presence of H. pylori is associated with any particular symptom cluster related to functional dyspepsia.

7
The Small Intestine

A.B.R. Thomson, P. Paré and R.N. Fedorak

1. GROSS ANATOMY OF THE SMALL INTESTINE

1.1 Duodenum

THE TERM *duodenum* (a Latin derivation from the Greek *dodekadaktulon*, "12 fingers") is applied to the most proximal segment of the small intestine because of its length – 12 fingers' breadth. The duodenum is subdivided into four portions: the first portion, which corresponds to the radiologic designation of duodenal bulb or cap; the second (descending) portion; the third (transverse) portion; and the fourth (ascending) portion.

Situated immediately above the first portion of the duodenum are the quadrate lobe of the liver and the gallbladder. The gallbladder normally can impinge on the lesser curve of the duodenal cap to produce the smooth concavity seen in radiographs. Behind the first portion of the duodenum is the head of the pancreas. Because of this relationship, the pancreas is the commonest site of penetration by a duodenal ulcer.

The second portion of the duodenum is concave; it hugs the head of the pancreas. A carcinoma or inflammatory mass in the head of the pancreas can occasionally affect the mucosal pattern along the medial aspect of the second portion of the duodenum. Congenital duodenal diverticula are commonly seen extending from the medial aspect of the second portion.

The third portion of the duodenum lies horizontally at the level of the third lumbar vertebra. The superior mesenteric artery, vein and nerve run anterior to its middle segment. In a thin individual or a person with recent massive weight loss, the superior mesenteric vessel sheath may impinge on the third portion of the duodenum, which is associated with chronic, intermittent obstruction of the duodenum.

The fourth portion of the duodenum as it ascends to the level of the second lumbar vertebra is in intimate contact with the aorta. This intimacy of duodenum and aorta can lead to fatal complications of aortic grafting when the graft erodes the duodenal wall, resulting in massive hemorrhage.

The mucosal pattern of the first portion (the duodenal cap or bulb) can be distinguished radiologically and endoscopically from the remaining duodenum. In the cap, shallow folds run longitudinally and are obliterated as the cap is distended. Beginning at the junction between the first and second portions of the duodenum, permanent transverse conniventes, characteristic of the small intestine, begin.

1.2 Jejunum and Ileum

The length of the small intestine is approximately 6 m. The proximal 40% of the small intestine is referred to as the *jejunum* (from the Latin, meaning "empty"), and the distal 60% is designated as the *ileum* (from the Greek *eilein*, "to roll or twist"). The wall of the jejunum is thicker and its lumen wider than the ileum's. There is also a gradual diminution in the caliber of the lumen from duodenum to ileum. Because of its narrower lumen, the ileum is prone to obstruction. There is a characteristic difference in the mesentery between jejunum and ileum. The fat is thicker in the ileal mesentery and extends fully to the intestinal attachment. In Crohn's disease, the thickened mesenteric fat encroaches further beneath the serosa of the small intestine. On x-ray, the mucosa in the proximal and ileal segments of the small intestine also differs. In the jejunum, the valvulae conniventes are thick, tall and numerous, giving a feathery mucosal pattern on x-ray. This contrasts with the sausage-shaped ileal loops, where the valvulae conniventes are progressively fewer and less prominent but are more clearly seen as transverse folds on x-ray.

2. SMALL INTESTINAL MOTILITY

The main function of the small intestine is digestion and absorption of nutrients. In this process, the role of small bowel motility is to mix food products with the digestive enzymes, to promote contact of chyme with the absorptive cells over a sufficient length of bowel and finally to propel remnants into the colon. Well-organized motility patterns occur in the small intestine to accomplish these goals in the fed as well as the fasting state. During fasting, a migrating motor complex (MMC) exists. This complex is characterized by a front of intense spiking activity (phase III activity) that migrates down the entire small intestine; as the front reaches the terminal ileum, another front develops in the gastroduodenal area and progresses down the intestine. The purpose of this phase III myoelectric and contractile activity is to sweep remnants of the previous meal into the colon and prevent starvation and bacterial overgrowth. The MMC often starts in the lower esophagus. Sweeping through the stomach, it removes debris and residual material not emptied with the last meal. Absence of phase III activity is associated with bacterial overgrowth and diarrhea. Thus, the small bowel is active even during fasting.

During meals, this cycle is interrupted and the motility pattern in the small bowel becomes an irregular spiking activity called the fed pattern. This fed pattern of motility does not seem to move intestinal contents forward to any great extent but does mix these contents with digestive juices, spreading them again and again over the absorptive surface of the brush border. Diarrhea can thus occur when this normal fed pattern is replaced by aggressive propulsive contractions.

3. PRINCIPLES OF ABSORPTION

Understanding the pathophysiology of diarrhea and malabsorption is based on understanding the normal steps in the digestion and absorption of food. The normal gastrointestinal tract is a finely integrated system geared to carry out the assimilation of ingested foodstuffs. Assimilation (the process by which ingested foods reach body fluids and cells) consists of two stages: (1) digestion (the breakdown of large molecules in the lumen of the intestine into their component small molecules) and (2) absorption (the transport across the intestinal mucosa to systemic body fluids).

Many disease processes directly or indirectly alter gastrointestinal physiology in such a manner that normal absorptive mechanisms are compromised, resulting in maldigestion or malabsorption of one or more dietary constituents. Too simplistic an approach to these diseases may be confusing because of the large number of illnesses involved and because of the plethora of diagnostic tests. This chapter will (1) present a classification of malabsorption and (2) outline the usefulness and potential pitfalls of common tests of intestinal function.

4. ABSORPTION OF VITAMINS AND MINERALS

4.1 Folic Acid (Pteroylglutamic Acid, $PteGlu_1$)

4.1.1 *FOOD SOURCES*
Dietary folates (folacins) are synthesized by bacteria and plants. They occur

mostly as polyglutamates, which are not absorbed intact. All folacins, or poly-pteroylglutamates (PteGlu$_n$), are hydrolyzed to folic acid, or pteroylglutamic acid (PteGlu$_1$), during absorption. Pteroylglutamic acid (PteGlu$_1$) is absorbed at a faster rate than larger polymers (PteGlu$_n$). Only 25–50% of dietary folacin is nutritionally available; boiling destroys much of folate activity. Therefore, uncooked foods with a large portion of the monoglutamate form (PteGlu$_1$) – e.g., bananas, lima beans, liver and yeast – contain the highest availability of folacin. Average Canadian diets contain 242 μg of folate a day. The daily requirement for folate is approximately 100 μg, although the recommended dietary allowance is 400 μg. Tissue stores of folate are only about 3 mg; therefore, malabsorption can totally deplete the body of folate within one month.

4.1.2 HYDROLYSIS AND ABSORPTION OF POLYGLUTAMATE FOLATES

Polyglutamate forms of folate (PteGlu$_n$) hydrolyze sequentially down to the monoglutamate form (PteGlu$_1$). This hydrolysis takes place at the brush border by the enzyme folate conjugase (Figure 1). Folic acid (PteGlu$_1$) is absorbed from the intestinal lumen by a sodium-dependent carrier. Once in the intestinal epithelial cell, folic acid is methylated and reduced to the tetrahydro form (CH$_3$H$_4$PteGlu$_1$).

Interference with folic acid absorption at the brush-border carrier site occurs with phenytoin and sulfasalazine. In addition, folic acid deficiency itself can impair folic acid absorption by producing "megaloblastic" changes in columnar epithelial cells of the gut – an abnormal epithelium.

4.2 Cobalamin (Vitamin B$_{12}$)

4.2.1 FOOD SOURCES

Cobalamin refers to cobalt-containing compounds with a corrin ring: these have biological activity for humans. Vitamin B$_{12}$ is the generic term for all of these compounds with bioactivity in any species. Cobalamin is therefore the preferred term to distinguish those compounds that are active in humans from the many analogues produced by bacteria. Cobalamin enters animal tissues when the animal ingests bacteria-containing foods or from production in the animal's rumen. Microorganisms in the human colon synthesize cobalamin, but it is not absorbed. Thus, strict vegetarians who do not eat cobalamin-containing meats will develop cobalamin deficiency. The average Western diet contains 10–20 μg per day. The daily requirement for cobalamin is 1 μg. The human liver is the repository of approximately 5 mg of cobalamin. These large hepatic stores account for the delay of several years in the clinical appearance of deficiency after cobalamin malabsorption begins.

INTESTINAL
LUMEN

INTESTINAL
EPITHELIUM

MESENTERIC
CIRCULATION

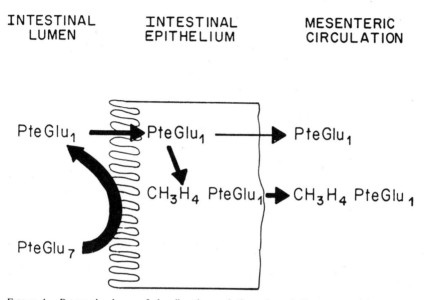

FIGURE 1. Proposed scheme of the digestion and absorption of dietary pteroylglutamates. Hydrolysis of polypteroylglutamates (shown here as $PteGlu_7$) probably occurs outside the intestinal epithelial cell. The overall rate of absorption into the mesenteric circulation is governed by the rate of transport of the monoglutamyl product ($PteGlu_1$). At physiologic doses, a substantial amount of $PteGlu_1$ is reduced and then methylated to $CH_3H_4PteGlu_1$ in the intestinal cell before release to the circulation.

SOURCE: Rosenberg IH. Folate absorption and malabsorption. N Engl J Med 1975; 293:1303.

4.2.2 ROLE OF THE STOMACH, PANCREAS AND ILEUM

Once cobalamin is liberated from food, it is bound at acid pH to R proteins (so called because of their rapid movement during electrophoresis). R proteins are glycoproteins present in many body secretions, including serum, bile, saliva and gastric and pancreatic juices. Most of the gastric R protein is from swallowed saliva. The R proteins cannot mediate the absorption of cobalamin alone, and their physiologic function is incompletely understood. Rare cases of complete R-protein deficiency have occurred without obvious clinical effect on the patient.

The cobalamin/R-protein complex leaves the stomach along with free intrinsic factor (Figure 2). In the duodenum, pancreatic proteases in the presence of bicarbonate (i.e., neutral pH) hydrolyze the R protein, thereby liberating free cobalamin. The cobalamin now combines with intrinsic factor. A conformational change takes place, allowing the cobalamin/intrinsic-factor

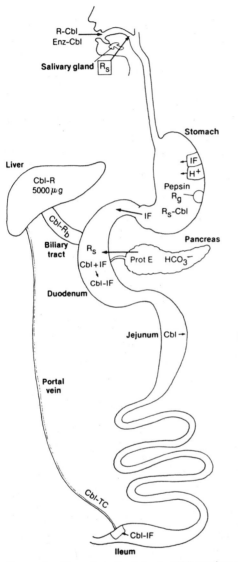

FIGURE 2.   Absorption of cobalamin (Cbl) requires proteolysis and intrinsic factor (IF). The intrinsic factor secreted is far in excess of that needed for binding the available cobalamin. R protein derived from saliva is also present in great abundance. Note that Cbl binds initially to R protein in the stomach at acid pH. Only after R protein is degraded by protease does Cbl bind to IF. After Cbl is absorbed in the ileum, it is bound to transcobalamin II.

SOURCE: Kalser MH. Absorption of cobalamin (vitamin B_{12}), folate, and other water-soluble vitamins. In: Berk JE (ed.), Bockus gastroenterology, vol. 3. 4th ed. Philadelphia: WB Saunders, 1985:1556.

TABLE 1. Abnormalities of cobalamin absorption that produce deficiency

Physiologic step	Disorder
Impaired food digestion	Gastrectomy, achlorhydria
Decreased IF secretion	Pernicious anemia, gastrectomy
Impaired transfer to IF (acidic pH)	Pancreatic insufficiency
Competition for uptake	Bacterial overgrowth
Impaired attachment to ileal receptor	Ileal disease or resection
Impaired passage through the ileal cell wall	Familial cobalamin malabsorption
Impaired uptake into blood	Transcobalamin II deficiency

complex to be resistant to proteolytic digestion. This resistance allows the complex to safely traverse the small intestine and reach the ileum, its site of active absorption.

Since transfer of cobalamin from R protein to intrinsic factor depends upon pH, pancreatic insufficiency (with deficient bicarbonate production) or the Zollinger-Ellison syndrome (with excess hydrogen ion production) interferes with this process and may result in cobalamin deficiency.

In the ileum, the cobalamin/intrinsic-factor complex binds to a specific receptor located on the brush border. Free cobalamin does not bind to the ileal receptor. After passage across the enterocytes, cobalamin is transported in blood bound to circulating proteins known as transcobalamins.

Understanding the normal absorptive processes allows a classification of cobalamin malabsorption and deficiency (Table 1).

4.3 Iron

4.3.1 FOOD SOURCES

Iron is available for absorption from vegetables (nonheme iron) and from meats (heme iron). Heme iron is better absorbed (10–20%) and is unaffected by intraluminal factors or its dietary composition. Nonheme iron is poorly absorbed, with an efficiency of 1–6%, and absorption is largely controlled by luminal events. The average dietary intake of iron is 10–20 mg/day. Men absorb 1–2 mg/day, while menstruating women and iron-deficient patients absorb 3–4 mg/day. In acute blood loss, increased absorption of iron does not occur until three days later. Nonheme iron (in the ferric, Fe^{+++} state), when ingested into a stomach unable to produce acid, forms insoluble iron complexes, which are not available for absorption (Figure 3). In the presence of gastric acid and such agents as ascorbic acid, however, ferrous iron (Fe^{++}) forms. The ferrous iron complexes bind to a mucopolysaccharide of about

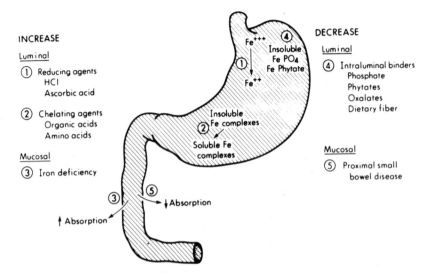

FIGURE 3. Factors that affect iron absorption. Nonheme iron absorption is affected both by intraluminal factors (1, 2 and 4) and by the total iron body content (3) as well as by small bowel disease (5). Heme iron absorption is altered only by those factors that affect the mucosa itself (3 and 5).

SOURCE: Alpers DH. Absorption of water-soluble vitamins, folate, minerals, and vitamin D. In: Sleisenger MH, Fordtran JS (eds.), Gastrointestinal disease: pathophysiology, diagnosis, management. 3d ed. Philadelphia: WB Saunders, 1983:835.

200,000 MW_r and are transported as an insoluble complex into the duodenum and proximal jejunum. Here, with the assistance of ascorbic acid, glucose and cysteine, the iron is absorbed. Dietary factors such as phosphate, phytate and phosphoproteins can render the iron insoluble and so inhibit nonheme iron absorption.

Heme iron (ferrous, Fe^{++}) is ingested as myoglobin and hemoglobin. In the presence of gastric acid, the globin molecule is split off, and ferrous iron is liberated and transported with its phosphorin ring from the stomach into the duodenum and jejunum for absorption.

Both heme and nonheme iron are absorbed most rapidly in the duodenum. Some of the iron taken up is deposited as ferritin within the enterocyte, and the remainder is transferred to the plasma-bound transferrin. When the enterocyte defoliates, iron deposited as ferritin is lost into the intestinal lumen. This mechanism for loss is probably overwhelmed by the large amounts of iron ingested. The amount of iron entering the body depends largely upon two factors: (1) total body iron content and (2) the rate of erythropoiesis.

5. ABSORPTION OF WATER AND ELECTROLYTES

5.1 Passive Permeability to Ions and Water

The epithelium of the small intestine exhibits a high passive permeability to salt and water that is a consequence of the leakiness of the junctions between epithelial cells. Osmotic equilibration between plasma and lumen is fairly rapid; therefore, large differences in ion concentration do not develop. These intercellular junctions are more permeable to cations than anions, so that lumen-to-blood concentration differences for Na^+ and K^+ are generally smaller than those for Cl^- and HCO_3. The colonic epithelium displays lower passive permeability. This permeability diminishes from cecum to rectum. It also decreases from duodenum to ileum. One consequence of this lower passive ionic permeability (higher electrical resistance) is that electric potential differences across the epithelium are an order of magnitude greater than those in the small intestine (remember Ohm's law, $E = IR$, where E is electrical potential, I is electrical current, and R is electrical resistance). Active Na^+ absorption, which is the main transport activity of the distal colon, generates a serosa-positive charge or potential difference (PD). Under the influence of aldosterone (i.e., salt depletion), this PD can be 60 mV or even higher. A 60 mV PD will thus sustain a 10-fold concentration difference for a monovalent ion such as K^+. Most of the high K^+ concentration in the rectum is accounted for, therefore, by the PD. Despite the high fecal K^+ level, little K^+ is lost in the stool, since stool volume (about 200–300 mL per day) is normally so low. In contrast, during high-volume (several liters per day) diarrhea of small bowel origin, the stool K^+ concentration is considerably lower (10–30 mM) but stool K^+ loss is nonetheless great because of the large volumes involved. In such states, the stool K^+ concentration is low (and the Na^+ concentration relatively high) because diarrheal fluid passes through the colon too rapidly to equilibrate across the colonic epithelium.

5.2 Active Electrolyte Absorption along the Intestine

The intestine, especially the small intestine, has the largest capacity for secreting water and electrolytes of any organ system in the body. In both the small bowel and the colon, secretion appears to arise predominantly, if not exclusively, in crypts; the more superficial villus tip epithelium is absorptive. Disease processes that result in damage to the villus or to superficial portions of the intestinal epithelium (e.g., viral enteritis) inevitably shift the overall balance between absorption and secretion toward secretion. This is especially important in celiac disease, where there is not only villous atrophy but also crypt hypertrophy.

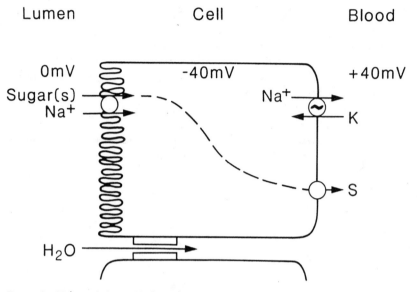

FIGURE 4. Na^+-coupled sugar(s) absorption.

In the small intestine, active electrolyte and fluid absorption can be conceived of as either *nutrient-dependent* or *nutrient-independent*.

5.2.1 NUTRIENT-DEPENDENT TRANSPORT

The absorptive processes for the nutrients glucose and neutral amino acids are Na^+-dependent – i.e., one Na^+ molecule is translocated across the brush border with each glucose or amino acid molecule (Figure 4). The sodium pump (Na^+/K^+-ATPase), which is located exclusively in the basolateral membrane, extrudes Na^+ that has entered the cell from the lumen, thereby maintaining a low intracellular Na^+, a high intracellular K^+ and a negative intracellular electric potential. This Na^+/K^+ pump provides the potential energy for uphill sugar and amino acid absorption. Glucose is cotransported with sodium. Patients in intestinal secretory states such as cholera can absorb glucose normally. Na^+ (and thus water) are also absorbed, accompanying the transport of glucose. As a consequence, the fluid losses incurred by these patients can be replaced by oral glucose-electrolyte solutions[1] and do not require intravenous fluids unless the patient is comatose or too nauseated to drink the necessary

---

[1] The WHO oral rehydration solution contains in mmol/L: glucose, 111; Na^+, 90; K^+, 20; Cl^-, 80; HCO_3^-, 30.

Lumen   Cell   Blood

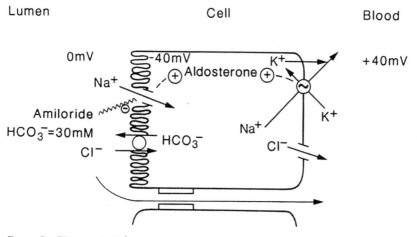

FIGURE 5.   Electrogenic Na$^+$ absorption and Cl$^-$/HCO$_3^-$ exchange.

large volumes of fluid. Application of this knowledge has had a major impact on world health, since the parts of the world where cholera-like diarrheas are prevalent generally have very limited hospital facilities and insufficient supplies of sterile electrolyte solutions.

5.2.2 NUTRIENT-INDEPENDENT TRANSPORT

Nutrient-independent active absorption of electrolytes and water by intestinal epithelial cells occurs through three or four specific mechanisms, located at different levels of the mammalian intestinal tract (Figures 5 and 6). All of these mechanisms have in common an Na$^+$/K$^+$-ATPase pump, located on the basolateral membrane and also a requirement for luminal Na$^+$.

In the distal colon (Figure 5), the luminal membrane contains Na$^+$ channels, which can be blocked by low concentrations of the pyrazine diuretic amiloride. The Na$^+$ entering through these channels in the luminal membrane is then extruded across the basolateral membrane by the Na$^+$/K$^+$-ATPase pump. Aldosterone increases the number of these channels and also, more slowly, increases the number of Na$^+$/K$^+$-ATPase pumps. Aldosterone therefore enhances active Na$^+$ absorption in the distal colon. To a more limited extent, aldosterone also causes the appearance of Na$^+$ channels more proximally in the colon and even in the distal ileum. Cl$^-$ is absorbed along with Na$^+$ and traverses the epithelium by both cellular and paracellular routes. Its transcellular route involves a Cl$^-$/HCO$_3^-$ exchanger in the luminal membrane and Cl$^-$ channels in the basolateral membrane. Intracellular mediators such as cyclic AMP (cAMP) do not appear to affect these Na$^+$ channels; thus, patients with

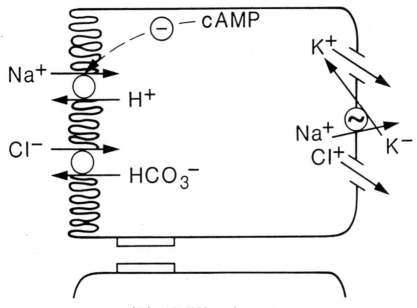

FIGURE 6.   Electroneutral Na^+/H^+ and Cl^-/HCO_3^- exchanges.

secretory diarrheas, especially those who are salt-depleted and therefore have elevated blood levels of aldosterone, are able to reabsorb some of the secreted fluid in their distal colon. Spironolactone, which inhibits the action of aldosterone, can increase the severity of diarrhea in such patients.

In the more proximal colon and in the ileum, the luminal membrane contains Na^+/H^+ exchangers that permit net Na^+ entry (Figure 6). The colon and the ileum (but not the jejunum) also appear to have Cl^-/HCO_3^- exchangers in their luminal borders. Cell pH adjusts the relative rates of these two exchangers. Thus H^+ extrusion by Na^+/H^+ exchange can cause cell alkalinization, which then stimulates Cl^- entry and HCO_3^- extrusion by this Cl^-/HCO_3^- exchange. The latter exchanger increases cell H^+, thereby sustaining Na^+/H^+ exchange. Increases in cell concentrations of cAMP and free Ca^{2+} inhibit the Na^+/H^+ exchange. Cyclic AMP and its agonists thereby cause cell acidification – which, in turn, inhibits Cl^-/HCO_3^- exchange. Therefore, electrolyte absorption in small and large intestinal segments (except the distal colon) can be down-regulated by hormones, neurotransmitters and certain luminal substances (bacterial enterotoxins, bile salts, hydroxylated fatty acids) that increase cell concentrations of cAMP or free Ca^{2+}. For this reason, body fluid secreted in response to these stimuli cannot be effectively reabsorbed in the

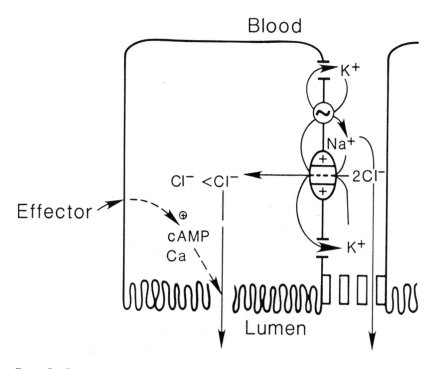

FIGURE 7. Secretory cell.

absence of amino acids and sugars, except in the distal colon. In the jejunum, where Cl^-/HCO_3^- exchange does not appear to be present, Na^+/H^+ exchange can be well sustained by anaerobic glycolysis, which generates H^+ as well as some ATP.

There is also some evidence for a direct cotransport of Na^+ and Cl^-, although this is difficult to separate experimentally from dual exchangers. This entry mechanism may exist in the ileum and proximal colon.

5.3 Active Electrolyte Secretion along the Intestine

In the secretory cell, the entry of Cl^- from the contraluminal bathing medium (blood or serosal side) is coupled to that of Na^+ and probably also K^+ by a triple cotransporter with a stoichiometry of 1 Na^+, 1 K^+ and 2 Cl^-. Na^+ entering in this fashion is then recycled to the contraluminal solution by the Na^+/K^+ exchange pump (Figure 7). K^+, entering via the pump and also the triple cotransporter, diffuses back to the contraluminal side through K^+ channels. Owing to the Na^+ gradient, Cl^- accumulates above electrochemical equilib-

TABLE 2. Hormones and neurotransmitters that stimulate intestinal secretion

	Intracellular mediator	
cAMP	Ca^{2+}	Unknown
Vasoactive intestinal peptide	Bradykinin	Bombesin
Prostaglandins	Acetylcholine	Lipoxygenase products
Bradykinin	Substance P	Thyrocalcitonin
	Neurotensin	Histamine
	Serotonin	Vasopressin

Only agents found effective in vitro have been listed. Several other hormones have been found to stimulate secretion in vivo, but it is unclear whether they act directly on the intestinal mucosa. The latter include glucagon and pentagastrin.

rium and can either (1) recycle back to the contraluminal solution through the Na$^+$/K$^+$/2 Cl$^-$ cotransporter or through basolateral membrane Cl$^-$ channels, or (2) be secreted into the lumen through luminal membrane Cl$^-$ channels. When Cl$^-$ is secreted into the lumen it generates a serosa-positive electric potential difference, which provides the driving force for Na$^+$ secretion through the paracellular pathway between cells. In the resting secretory cell, the luminal Cl$^-$ channels are closed. When secretion is stimulated by a hormone or neurotransmitter, these channels open. Secretion is initiated, therefore, by opening the Cl$^-$ "gate" in the luminal membrane of the secretory cell.

The known intracellular mediators of secretion are cAMP, cGMP and Ca^{2+} (Table 2). These can arise from the blood; nerve endings; endocrine cells in the epithelium (APUD cells); mesenchymal elements such as lymphocytes, plasma cells and mast cells; or the enterocytes themselves. Except for the cAMP agonists, lipoxygenase products and calcitonin, the actions of the other agonists are short-lived; desensitization rapidly develops. They operate to fine-tune electrolyte transport rather than invoke persistent secretion.

Predictably, since there are hormones and neurotransmitters that stimulate active electrolyte secretion in the gut, there are also agonists that inhibit secretion and/or stimulate absorption. These include adrenocorticosteroids, norepinephrine, somatostatin, enkephalins and dopamine. Glucocorticoids enhance electrolyte absorption throughout the intestinal tract, but the mechanisms involved are less well understood than for aldosterone. They may act in part by inhibiting phospholipase A$_2$ and therefore the arachidonic acid cascade. The adrenergic receptors on enterocytes are almost exclusively α$_2$ in type. The sympathetic nervous system in the intestinal mucosa releases norepinephrine (an α$_2$ antagonist) and so inhibits electrolyte secretion and stimulates absorption. Sympathectomy, whether chemical or surgical, leads to diarrhea, at least transiently. Chronic diabetics with autonomic neuropathy sometimes develop persistent diarrhea that is associated with degeneration of adrenergic nerve fibers to the gut. Somatostatin and endogenous enkephalins are also antisecretory. A physiological role for dopamine is not likely.

6. ABSORPTION OF FAT

The overall process of fat digestion and absorption consists of four distinct phases, related to the respective functions of the pancreas, liver, intestinal mucosa and lymphatics (Figure 8). Physiologically, these involve (1) lipolysis of dietary triglyceride (TG) to fatty acid (FA) and ß-monoglyceride (MG); (2) micellar solubilization with bile acid; (3) uptake into the mucosal cell, with re-esterification of the MG with FA to form TG, and chylomicron formation in the presence of cholesterol, cholesterol esters, phospholipids and protein; and (4) delivery of chylomicrons in lymphatics to the body for utilization of fat.

The average North American diet contains 60–100 g of fat each day, mostly in the form of neutral fat or triglycerides. In the proximal intestine, TG comes under hydrolytic attack by lipases, producing glycerol, FA and MG. These products of lipolysis first form an emulsion and later a micellar solution.

Following the entry of food and particularly fat into the duodenum, cholecystokinin (CCK) is released from mucosal cells, causing gallbladder contraction. Bile acids, along with other biliary constituents, thus exit into the proximal small intestine. Bile acids chemically resemble detergent molecules in that a portion of the molecule is polar and water-soluble, while another portion of the molecule is nonpolar and fat-soluble. When the bile acids are present in sufficient amounts, known as the critical micellar concentration (CMC), they form negatively charged spheres, called simple micelles. Incorporation of FA and MG forms a larger, polymolecular aggregate, a mixed micelle. All this is necessary to solubilize fat and disperse it in small packets more effectively, setting the stage for further digestion by pancreatic lipase. This enzyme acts only at oil–water interfaces and requires a large surface area.

Adequate concentrations of bile acid must be present within the jejunal lumen for effective micellar solubilization and lipolysis by pancreatic lipase, a preliminary to uptake and esterification. Such adequate concentrations are maintained by the constant reutilization of a relatively small pool of bile acid. In the liver, about 0.6 g of new bile acid is produced daily from cholesterol. This is added to the total bile acid pool of 3.0 g, which cycles 6 to 10 times daily from passive absorption in the jejunum and active absorption in the ileum. Approximately 96% of the bile acid is absorbed through these mecha-

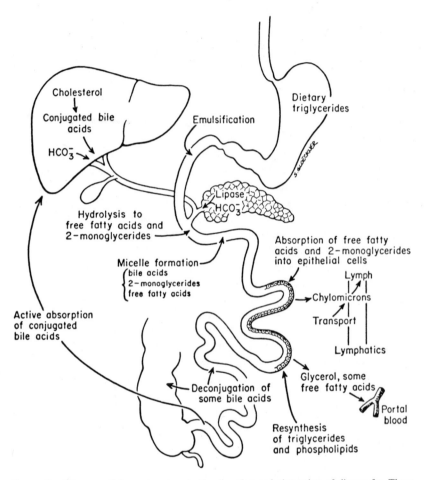

FIGURE 8. Diagram of the major steps in the digestion and absorption of dietary fat. These include (1) the lipolysis of dietary triglyceride (TG) by pancreatic enzymes; (2) micellar solubilization of the resulting long-chain fatty acids (FA) and ß-monoglycerides (ßMG; shown in figure as 2-monoglycerides) by bile acids secreted into the intestinal lumen by the liver; (3) absorption of the fatty acids and ß-monoglycerides into the mucosal cell with subsequent re-esterification and formation of chylomicrons; and, finally, (4) movement of the chylomicrons from the mucosal cell into the intestinal lymphatic system. During the process of chylomicron formation, small amounts of cholesterol (C), cholesterol ester (CE), and phospholipid (PL) as well as triglyceride are incorporated into this specific lipoprotein fraction.

SOURCE: Wilson FA, Dietschy JM. Differential diagnostic approach to clinical problems of malabsorption. Gastroenterology 1971; 61:912.

nisms with each cycle; the remainder is lost in the stool. Bile acids return to the liver via the portal vein and are excreted once more. This recirculation of bile acid between the intestine and the liver is called the enterohepatic circulation.

The principal role of the bile salt micelle is to facilitate lipid absorption by maintaining the lipid in a water-soluble form, overcoming the resistance of the unstirred water layer and maintaining a high concentration of a local source of fatty acid and cholesterol, which leave the micelle and enter the mucosal cell.

The lipid-containing bile acid micelle is now ready for mucosal uptake. Two important events occur within the mucosal cell: re-esterification and chylomicron formation. The fatty acids are first reattached to the mono-glycerides through re-esterification, and the resultant triglyceride is then combined with small amounts of cholesterol and coated with phospholipids and proteins to form a specific class of lipoproteins known as chylomicrons. The chylomicrons are then released from the basal portion of the columnar epithelial cell and find their way into the central lacteal of the intestinal villus. From there, chylomicrons travel in lymph up the thoracic duct and eventually reach the general circulation. Chylomicrons are then transported in the blood to the sites of disposal and utilization in the periphery (e.g., liver, muscle and adipose tissue).

From these physiological considerations, malabsorption of fat due to impaired lipolysis or micellar solubilization would be expected to occur in the following circumstances: (1) rapid gastric emptying and improper mixing – e.g., following vagotomy or postgastrectomy; (2) altered duodenal pH – e.g., the Zollinger-Ellison syndrome; (3) pancreatic insufficiency; (4) cholestasis – e.g., biliary obstruction, liver disease; and (5) an interrupted enterohepatic circulation – e.g., ileal disease or loss.

Fat malabsorption due to impaired mucosal uptake, assembly or delivery would be expected to occur following (1) generalized impaired enterocyte function – e.g., celiac disease, Whipple's disease; (2) failure of the packaging process – e.g., abetalipoproteinemia, which represents a genetic defect of betaprotein B synthesis with consequent impairment of chylomicron formation; (3) disorders of lymphatics – e.g., intestinal lymphangiectasia, retroperitoneal fibrosis or lymphoma; and (4) loss of mucosal surface area – e.g., the short bowel syndrome.

7. ABSORPTION OF CARBOHYDRATES

Starch, sucrose and lactose constitute the main carbohydrates in the human diet. All are inexpensive sources of food. Together they constitute the major source of calories when considered worldwide. People in the Western world

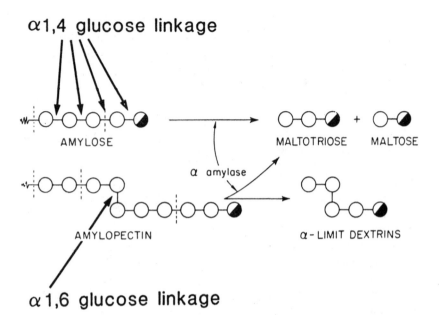

FIGURE 9. The action of pancreatic a-amylase on linear (amylose) and branched (amylopectin) starch. Circles indicate glucose residues and the reducing glucose unit.
SOURCE: Gray GM. Mechanisms of digestion and absorption of food. In: Sleisenger MH, Fordtran JS (eds.), Gastrointestinal disease: pathophysiology, diagnosis, management. 3d ed. Philadelphia: WB Saunders, 1983:851.

consume about 400 g of carbohydrates daily: 60% as starch, 30% as sucrose and 10% as lactose (milk contains 48 g of lactose per liter).

Starch in wheat, rice and corn is a polysaccharide whose molecular weight ranges from 100,000 to greater than 1,000,000. The straight chain of glucose molecules in starch is bridged by an oxygen molecule between the first carbon (C_1) of one glucose unit and the fourth carbon (C_4) of its neighbor (a1,4 glucose link). This type of starch is called amylose and makes up as much as 20% of the starch in the diet. The glucose-to-glucose bridge is of the alpha type – in contrast to the beta type, which connects glucose units in cellulose, an indigestible saccharide. The remaining 80% of the starch that humans ingest has a branch point every 25 molecules along the straight a1,4 glucose chain. This starch is called amylopectin. These branches occur via an oxygen bridge between C_6 of the glucose on the straight chain and C_1 in the branched chain (a1,6 branch points), which then continues as another a1,4 glucose-linked straight chain (Figure 9).

Salivary and pancreatic a-amylases act on interior a1,4 glucose–glucose

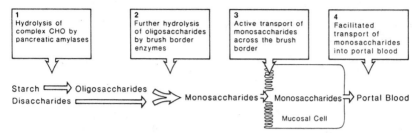

FIGURE 10.   Major steps in the digestion and absorption of dietary carbohydrate.

links of starch but cannot attack α1,4 linkages close to a 1,6 branch point. The products of amylase digestion are therefore maltose and maltotriose. Since α-amylase cannot hydrolyze the 1,6 branching links and has relatively little specificity for 1,4 links adjacent to these branch points, large oligosaccharides containing five to nine glucose units and consisting of one or more 1,6 branching links are also produced by α-amylase action. These are called α-limit dextrins, and represent about 30% of amylopectin breakdown.

The responsibility for digesting the oligosaccharides, including α-limit dextrins, and the amylose and amylopectin rests with the hydrolytic enzymes on intestinal epithelial cells (Figures 10 and 11). These hydrolytic enzymes are called disaccharidases, but most are in fact oligosaccharidases: they hydrolyze sugars containing three or more hexose units. They are present in highest concentration at the villus tips in the jejunum and persist throughout most of the ileum, but not in the colon. Lactase breaks down lactose into glucose and galactose. Glucoamylase (maltase) differs from pancreatic α-amylase since it sequentially removes a single glucose from the nonreducing end of a linear α1,4 glucose chain, breaking down maltose into glucose. Sucrase is a hybrid molecule consisting of two enzymes – one hydrolyzing sucrose and the other, the α1,6 branch points of the α-limit dextrins. This enzyme is commonly called sucrase-isomaltase, because the isomaltase moiety hydrolyzes isomaltose, the α1,6 glucosyl disaccharide. However, the only products containing α1,6 linkages after amylase action on starch are the α-limit dextrins. Thus no free isomaltose is presented to the intestinal surface and the term "isomaltase" is a misnomer. The sucrase moiety thus breaks down sucrose into glucose and fructose.

Humans normally are born with a full complement of brush-border-membrane disaccharidases. Intake of large amounts of sucrose results in an increase in sucrase activity, probably as the substrate stabilizes the enzyme and reduces its rate of breakdown. In contrast, there is no evidence that dietary manipulation can regulate human lactase or maltase.

Disaccharides ⟶ Monosaccharides

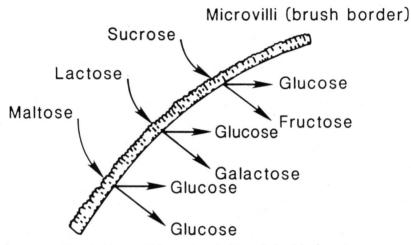

FIGURE 11. Disaccharides are split into monosaccharides at the brush border.

Once the disaccharides are broken down, how are the monosaccharides absorbed? Sodium facilitates glucose uptake by binding to the carrier along with glucose. Since intracellular Na^+ concentration is low, the Na^+ ion moves down its concentration gradient into the cell, to be pumped out subsequently at the basolateral membrane by Na^+/K^+-ATPase, an active process that utilizes energy derived from the hydrolysis of ATP. The electrochemical gradient thus developed by Na^+ provides the driving force for glucose entry. Glucose accompanies Na^+ on the brush-border carrier and is released inside the cell, where its concentrations may exceed those in the intestinal lumen. Glucose then exits from the basolateral membrane of the cell into the portal system by a non–Na^+-dependent carrier.

Fructose, released from the hydrolysis of sucrose, is transported by facilitated diffusion, a carrier-mediated process that is independent both of Na^+ and of the glucose transport mechanism.

From these physiological considerations, carbohydrate malabsorption can occur in the following circumstances: (1) severe pancreatic insufficiency; (2) selective deficiencies of brush-border disaccharidases – e.g., lactase deficiency; (3) generalized impairment of brush-border and enterocyte function –

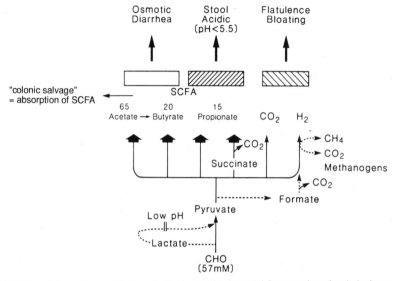

FIGURE 12.   Intermediate and end products of anaerobic bacterial fermentation of carbohydrates. Minor pathways are depicted by dashed lines.
SOURCE: Soergel KH. The role of the colon in case of inhibition of carbohydrate absorption. In: Creutzfeldt W, Fölsch UR (eds.), Delaying absorption as a therapeutic principle in metabolic diseases. Stuttgart and New York: Thieme Verlag, 1983:854.

e.g., celiac disease, tropical sprue, gastroenteritis; and (4) loss of mucosal surface area – e.g., the short bowel syndrome.

Although infants often have a deficiency of amylase, starch is not usually fed for the first few months of life. In the adult, there is a great excess of pancreatic amylase secreted into the intestinal lumen, so that even in patients with severe fat malabsorption due to pancreatic exocrine insufficiency, residual salivary and pancreatic amylase output appears to be sufficient to completely hydrolyze starch to the final oligosaccharides by the time a meal reaches the mid-jejunum. Hence, maldigestion of starch rarely, if ever, occurs in humans.

Secondary deficiency of disaccharidases results from anatomic injury of the small intestine, as in celiac disease, tropical sprue and gastroenteritis. When disaccharidase levels are sufficiently low, the particular oligosaccharide or disaccharide remains unhydrolyzed within the intestinal lumen and augments intraluminal fluid accumulation by virtue of its osmotic effect. Bacterial fermentation of disaccharides that reach the colon produces fatty acids (butyric, formic, acetic and propionic acids), alcohols and gases (H_2 and CO_2) (Figure 12). The benefits of this bacterial fermentation to the host are twofold. First,

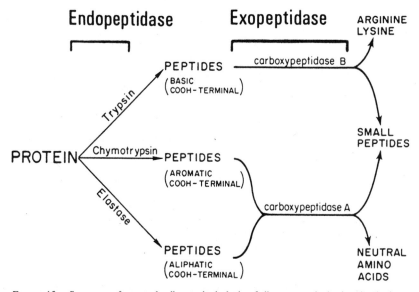

FIGURE 13.   Sequence of events leading to hydrolysis of dietary protein by intraluminal proteases.

SOURCE: Gray GM. Mechanisms of digestion and absorption of food. In: Sleisenger MH, Fordtran JS (eds.), Gastrointestinal disease: pathophysiology, diagnosis, management. 3d ed. Philadelphia: WB Saunders, 1983:854.

the bulk of the caloric value present in carbohydrates remains in the fermentative products. Reabsorption of fatty acids and alcohols in the colon "salvages" calories from malabsorbed carbohydrates. Second, this colonic "salvage" reduces the number of osmoles in the lumen and hence lessens the water lost in feces. During the fermentation of carbohydrates to organic acids, colonic bacteria liberate H_2 and CO_2 gas. In general, the passage of large quantities of rectal gas suggests that excessive carbohydrates are reaching the colon. (Remember your beer-drinking days!)

Primary (congenital) deficiencies of disaccharidases are unusual. Such entities can be differentiated from a secondary defect, since general tests of absorption and mucosal histology are normal; however, assay of an intestinal biopsy reveals the absence of hydrolytic activity for a single disaccharide. Lactase deficiency (even when secondary) is very common.

8. ABSORPTION OF PROTEIN

8.1 Intraluminal Digestion

Digestion of protein begins in the stomach under the influence of pepsin. This lasts for only one to two hours, while the pH is acidic following meal-stimulated acid secretion. Most dietary protein, however, is hydrolyzed by pancreatic proteases secreted into the proximal duodenum in inactive form. Activation of each protease is initially catalyzed by the duodenal mucosal surface enzyme enterokinase and by activated trypsin (Figure 13). Activation is virtually instantaneous in the first and second portions of the duodenal lumen. Intraluminal digestion of dietary protein occurs in the duodenum by sequential action of pancreatic endopeptidases and exopeptidases. The endopeptidases trypsin, chymotrypsin, elastase, DNAase and RNAase act on the peptide at the interior of the protein molecule. These peptides are then acted upon by the exopeptidases carboxypeptidase A and B, which remove a single amino acid from the carboxyl terminal end of the peptide, yielding basic and neutral amino acids (AAs) as well as other small peptides.

8.2 Cellular Digestion

Peptidases in the brush border then hydrolyze the residual di-, tri- and tetrapeptides that contain neutral AAs. Peptides consisting primarily of glycine, proline, hydroxyproline or dicarboxylic AA appear to be hydrolyzed inside the cell. AA and dipeptides are then transported into the mucosal cell interior. The transport system for neutral AA absorbs aromatic (phenylalanine, tyrosine, tryptophan) and aliphatic (valine, leucine, isoleucine, methionine) AAs. The basic AAs (arginine, lysine) are absorbed by a separate mechanism. There is a third mechanism for glycine, proline and hydroxyproline, and a fourth for dicarboxylic AAs (aspartic and glutamic AA).

From these physiological considerations, protein malabsorption would be expected in diseases causing (1) pancreatic insufficiency; (2) generalized impaired enterocyte function – e.g., celiac disease; and (3) loss of mucosal surface – e.g., the short bowel syndrome.

9. MALDIGESTION AND MALABSORPTION: THE MALASSIMILATION SYNDROMES

Normal digestion and absorption of foods is essential for life and well-being. Given the length of the gastrointestinal tract, the number of organs involved in digestion, and the large number of nutrients that must be taken into our bodies, it is not surprising to find a large number of disease states that impair the processes of food digestion and absorption. Clinical malassimilation occurs in only one of two ways: (1) through intraluminal disorders (maldigestion of food) and (2) through intramural disorders (malabsorption of food).

9.1 Clinical Manifestations

The list of diseases that can cause malassimilation is long (Table 3), necessitating logical history-taking.

TABLE 3.   Classification of malassimilation syndromes

Defective intraluminal digestion

Mixing disorders
  Postgastrectomy

Pancreatic insufficiency
  Primary
    Cystic fibrosis
  Secondary
    Chronic pancreatitis
    Pancreatic carcinoma
    Pancreatic resection

Reduced intestinal bile salt concentration
  Liver disease
    Hepatocellular disease
    Cholestasis (intrahepatic or extrahepatic)
  Abnormal bacterial proliferation in the small bowel
    Afferent loop stasis
    Strictures
    Fistulas
    Blind loops
    Multiple diverticula of the small bowel
    Hypomotility states (diabetes, scleroderma, intestinal pseudo-obstruction)
  Interrupted enterohepatic circulation of bile salts
    Ileal resection
    Ileal inflammatory disease (regional ileitis)
  Drugs (by sequestration or precipitation of bile salts)
    Neomycin
    Calcium carbonate
    Cholestyramine

(cont'd)

Clinical suspicion, as always, comes from the patient's history and physical examination. A patient with malassimilation may have symptoms and signs of specific nutrient deficiencies or those of the underlying disease process itself (e.g., Crohn's disease). Furthermore, considering that malassimilation usually involves multiple nutrients, the symptoms and signs of a malassimilation state can vary from a straightforward presentation to myriad symptom complexes (Tables 4 and 5).

The patient who gives a history of progressive weight loss, polyphagia, excessive flatus, diarrhea, bulky and foul-smelling stools, food particles or fat in the stool, abdominal distention, muscle wasting, bone pain, bleeding, weakness, tetany, paresthesia, glossitis, cheilosis or dermatitis is giving you the "classical" history of severe intestinal malassimilation. Rarely will you hear

TABLE 3.   Classification of malassimilation syndromes (cont'd)

Defective intramural absorption

Inadequate absorptive surface
  Intestinal resection or bypass
    Mesenteric vascular disease with massive intestinal resection
    Regional enteritis with multiple bowel resections
    Jejunoileal bypass

Mucosal absorptive defects
  Biochemical or genetic abnormalities
    Celiac disease
    Disaccharidase deficiency
    Hypogammaglobulinemia
    Abetalipoproteinemia
    Hartnup disease
    Cystinuria
    Monosaccharide malabsorption
  Inflammatory or infiltrative disorders
    Regional enteritis
    Amyloidosis
    Scleroderma
    Lymphoma
    Radiation enteritis
    Eosinophilic enteritis
    Tropical sprue
    Infectious enteritis (e.g., salmonellosis)
    Collagenous sprue
    Nonspecific ulcerative jejunitis
    Mastocytosis
    Dermatologic disorders (e.g., dermatitis herpetiformis)
  Lymphatic obstruction
    Intestinal lymphangiectasia
    Whipple's disease
    Lymphoma

---

such a history from a patient in North America. It is far more common to see patients who will have vague symptoms for which there is some abnormality in their blood chemistry that alerts you to the presence of disease.

Early symptoms of the disease may easily be overlooked, and a severely malnourished state may come to exist. Often a patient will have noticed "early" symptoms, which will become apparent only when questioned directly. Hence, the physician must inquire about minor changes in bowel habits occurring before the onset of weight loss, hyperphagia, pain, anorexia or gross changes in bowel habits. Subtle changes in stool volume or bulk

TABLE 4. Clinical signs and symptoms of malassimilation

	Clinical sign or symptom	Deficient nutrient
General	Weight loss	Calorie
	Loss of appetite, amenorrhea, decreased libido	Protein energy
Skin	Psoriasiform rash, eczematous scaling	Zinc
	Pallor	Folate, iron, vitamin B_{12}
	Follicular hyperkeratosis	Vitamin A
	Perifollicular petechiae	Vitamin C
	Flaking dermatitis	Protein energy, niacin, riboflavin, zinc
	Bruising	Vitamin K
	Pigmentation changes	Niacin, protein energy
	Scrotal dermatosis	Riboflavin
	Thickening and dryness of skin	Linoleic acid
Head	Temporal muscle wasting	Protein energy
Hair	Sparse and thin, dyspigmentation Easy to pull out	Protein
Eyes	History of night blindness	Vitamin A
	Photophobia, blurring, conjunctival inflammation	Riboflavin, vitamin A
	Corneal vascularization	Riboflavin
	Xerosis, Bitot's spots, keratomalacia	Vitamin A
Mouth	Glossitis	Riboflavin, niacin, folic acid
	Bleeding gums	Vitamin C, riboflavin
	Cheilosis	Riboflavin
	Angular stomatitis	Riboflavin, iron
	Hypogeusia	Zinc
	Tongue fissuring	Niacin
	Tongue atrophy	Riboflavin, niacin, iron
	Scarlet and raw tongue	Niacin
	Nasolabial seborrhea	Pyridoxine
Neck	Goiter	Iodine
	Parotid enlargement	Protein
Thorax	Thoracic "rosary"	Vitamin D

(cont'd)

TABLE 4. Clinical signs and symptoms of malassimilation (cont'd)

	Clinical sign or symptom	Deficient nutrient
Abdomen	Diarrhea	Niacin, folate, vitamin B_{12}
	Distention	Protein energy
	Hepatomegaly	Protein energy
Extremities	Edema	Protein, thiamine
	Softening of bone	Vitamin D, calcium, phosphorus
	Bone tenderness	Vitamin D
	Bone ache, joint pain	Vitamin C
	Muscle wasting and weakness	Protein, calories
	Muscle tenderness, muscle pain	Thiamine
	Hyporeflexia	Thiamine
Nails	Flattening, brittleness, luster loss, spooning	Iron
	Transverse lines	Protein
Neurologic	Tetany	Calcium, magnesium
	Paresthesias	Thiamine, vitamin B_{12}
	Loss of reflexes, wrist drop, foot drop	Thiamine
	Loss of vibratory and position sense, ataxia	Vitamin B_{12}
	Dementia, disorientation	Niacin
Blood	Anemia	Iron, vitamin B_{12}, folate
	Hemolysis	Phosphorus

(manifested by a slight increase in the number of bowel movements per day), consistency or odor are early manifestations of malassimilation. A slight increase in the frequency of stools occurring at a time when the patient is mildly anorexic occurs a long time before disease becomes clinically apparent. An early increase in bulk of the stool is caused by increased water and gas content and leads to an inability to flush the stool easily. It is not uncommon for the patient to think the toilet is malfunctioning because several flushings are needed to remove the stool. A greasy character and truly rancid odor are indicative of increased stool fat, but are often absent until late. These complaints are often readily passed over by the busy physician. At such time, physical findings are usually absent, but hyperactive bowel sounds may be noted, especially in small intestinal disease. If symptoms are intermittent or if they progress slowly over many years, patients may exhibit vague, seemingly

TABLE 5. Specific vitamin and mineral deficiencies

Vitamin/mineral		Clinical manifestation
Vitamin A	Eyes	Night blindness
		Xerosis (dry bulbar conjunctiva)
		Bitot's spots (conjunctiva plaques)
		Keratomalacia (corneal ulceration)
	Skin	Hyperkeratosis
Vitamin B$_{12}$	Hematologic,	Anemia
	neurologic systems	Nonreversible loss of vibratory and position sense
		Paresthesia
	GI	Diarrhea
Vitamin C	Skin	Perifollicular papules (brittle hair)
		Perifollicular hemorrhages
		Gum bleeding
		Skin purpura, ecchymosis
Vitamin D	Bone	Bone pain and softening
		Joint pain
		Rickets
Vitamin K		Bruising
		Bleeding
Vitamin B$_6$	Skin	Seborrheic dermatitis
(Pyridoxine)		Cheilosis
		Glossitis
Niacin		Dermatitis
		Diarrhea
		Dementia
Thiamine	CVS	Congestive heart failure
	CNS	Wernicke's encephalopathy
		Wernicke-Korsakoff syndrome
Zinc	Skin	Acrodermatitis enteropathica
		Alopecia
	Taste	Hypogeusia
Folate	Hematologic,	Anemia
	neurologic systems	Reversible loss of position and vibratory sense

unrelated symptoms such as chronic fatigue and depression, long before the physician considers the possibility of serious organic disease.

9.2 Manifestations of Carbohydrate Malassimilation

Carbohydrate malassimilation will result in both specific and generalized symptoms. Specific to the maldigestion and malabsorption of carbohydrates are diarrhea and excess flatus. (Unfortunately, everyone has flatus, and a definition or measure of excessive wind is lacking.) Malabsorbed carbohydrates that enter the colon are fermented by colonic bacteria to gases (CO_2, H_2 and CH_4) and organic acids (Figure 12). These organic acids produce diarrhea by acting directly on colonic epithelium to stimulate fluid secretion and by their osmotic effect, which further draws water into the lumen. The presence of organic acids in the stool reduces the pH below 6 and suggests carbohydrate malassimilation. The gas produces flatulence, with associated borborygmi and abdominal distention. The presence of intraluminal H_2 gas, eventually absorbed into the circulation and exhaled, forms the basis of the hydrogen breath test to detect carbohydrate malabsorption. Physical examination often reveals a distended tympanitic abdomen with hyperactive bowel sounds. Stools seem to float on the water because of their increased gas content (not because of their fat content).

Generally, lack of carbohydrate as an energy source will result in decreased insulin levels, increased plasma glucagon and cortisol levels and decreased peripheral T_4-to-T_3 conversion. Given sufficient time, the body will enter a state of oxidative metabolism: fat and muscle will be catabolized. Physical examination may reveal signs of weight loss from both fat stores and lean body mass. The patient will be weak and will fatigue easily. Fat loss will generally be noted as sunken cheeks and flat buttocks, with wrinkled or loose skin indicative of loss of subcutaneous fat stores. The loss of muscle mass is easily noted as thenar mass reduction and sunken soft tissues between the extensor tendons on the dorsum of the hands. There may be direct evidence of a reduced metabolic rate secondary to decreased T_3 conversion. The patient will often be mentally slowed.

9.3 Manifestations of Fat Malassimilation

Failure to digest or absorb fats results in a variety of clinical symptoms and laboratory abnormalities. These manifestations are the result of both fat malassimilation per se and a deficiency of the fat-soluble vitamins. In general, loss of fat in the stool deprives the body of calories and contributes to weight loss and malnutrition. More specific is the action of unabsorbed long-chain fatty acids, which act on the colonic mucosa to cause diarrhea by an irritant effect on the colon. In addition, fatty acids bind calcium, which would normally be available to bind oxalate. In fat malabsorption, oxalate is not bound to calcium and remains free (undissociated) within the colonic lumen, where it is readily absorbed. This results in oxaluria and calcium oxalate kidney stones. This occurs in Crohn's disease more readily than in other cases of fat malabsorption (steatorrhea).

Failure to absorb the fat-soluble vitamins A, D, E and K also results in a variety of symptoms. Vitamin K deficiency presents as subcutaneous, urinary, nasal, vaginal and gastrointestinal bleeding. Deficiencies in factors II, VII, IX and X produce defective coagulation. Vitamin A deficiency results in follicular hyperkeratosis. Vitamin E deficiency leads to a progressive demyelination of the central nervous system. Malabsorption of vitamin D causes rickets and osteopenia, as discussed later.

9.4 Manifestations of Protein Malassimilation

Severe loss of body protein may occur before the development of laboratory abnormalities. Impaired protein synthesis from liver diseases and excessive protein loss in renal disease can further aggravate protein deficiencies. Clinically, protein deficiency results in edema and diminished muscle mass. Since the immune system is dependent upon adequate proteins, protein deficiency can manifest as recurrent or severe infections. Protein deficiency in children results in growth retardation, mental apathy and irritability, weakness and muscle atrophy, edema, hair loss, deformity of skeletal bone, anorexia, vomiting and diarrhea (marasmus).

9.5 Manifestations of Iron Deficiency

Hypochromic microcytic anemia characterizes iron deficiency. Since malassimilation may result in folate or B_{12} deficiency (producing megaloblastic red cells), the microcytosis of iron deficiency may be obscured with automated cell counters; a dimorphic picture is present. Accompanying the development of anemia may be symptoms of pica and dysphagia. Pica originally referred to the eating of clay or soil; however, the commonest "pica" in North America is the eating of ice. Dysphagia may be due to the Plummer-Vinson (Paterson-Kelly) syndrome (with atrophic papillae of the tongue and postcricoid esophageal webs), and/or cheilosis (reddened lips with angular fissures). Weakness, fatigue, dyspnea and edema also can occur. Physical examination often reveals pallor, an atrophic tongue and koilonychia (brittle, flat or spoon-shaped fingernails).

The clinical picture of vitamin B_{12} and folic acid deficiency includes the nonspecific manifestations of megaloblastic anemia and its sequelae – i.e., anemia, glossitis, megaloblastosis, and elevated serum lactate dehydrogenase (LDH). In addition, deficiency of B_{12} may induce neurologic abnormalities consisting of symmetrical paresthesias in the feet and fingers, with associated disturbances of vibration sense and proprioception, progressing to ataxia with subacute combined degeneration of the spinal cord. Neurologic manifestations are not part of folic acid deficiency alone.

9.6 Manifestations of Calcium, Vitamin D and Magnesium Malabsorption

Impaired absorption of calcium, magnesium and vitamin D may lead to bone pain, fractures, paresthesias, tetany, Chvostek's sign and Trousseau's sign. Low levels of serum calcium will stimulate parathyroid activity. Increased parathormone raises the level of blood calcium by both a direct effect on bone and a renal mechanism. These processes lead to osteitis fibrosa and osteomalacia. Osteomalacia principally affects the spine, rib cage and long bones with or without fractures (Milkman's fractures), and may cause extreme pain, particularly in the spine, pelvis and leg bones. A child with calcium or vitamin D malabsorption will present with classical rickets. Hypomagnesemia may cause seizures and symptoms identical to those of hypocalcemia. In addition, hypomagnesemia may reduce the responsiveness of the parathyroids to calcium and impair parathyroid regulation of calcium homeostasis.

9.7 Investigation of Maldigestion and Malabsorption

To avoid embarking on the shotgun approach to investigation, there are several questions one must ask. First, does malassimilation exist? And second, if so, is it due to a disorder of intraluminal digestion or a disorder of intramural absorption? Physicians should attempt to restrict the use of laboratory tests to those that establish the presence of malassimilation and the cause of the malassimilation (Figure 14).

To determine if malassimilation exists, one begins, as always, with the simplest, least invasive tests. A complete blood count (CBC) and differential might reveal a macrocytic or microcytic anemia. A peripheral smear may demonstrate megaloblastosis, microcytosis and/or lymphopenia. Serum calcium, phosphorus and alkaline phosphatase will detect the presence of osteomalacia. Serum albumin can assess protein stores. Serum cholesterol, carotene and prothrombin time (vitamin K) indirectly assess fat assimilation. Iron stores from serum iron, total iron binding capacity (TIBC) and ferritin assess proximal intestinal integrity. Serum B_{12} is an index of ileal integrity. Red cell folate measures folate stores.

If their results are abnormal, the above tests suggest the presence of malassimilation and may indicate the deficient nutrient(s). Steatorrhea is the most

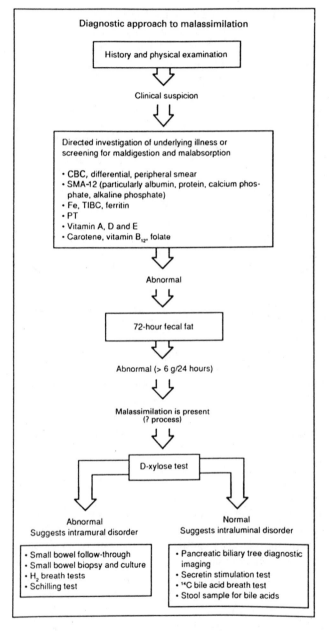

FIGURE 14.   Diagnostic approach to malassimilation.
SOURCE: Fedorak RN. Maldigestion and malabsorption. Medicine North America 1988; 3:3400.

important feature in the diagnosis of generalized malassimilation. Accurate measurement of fecal fat is extremely important. Qualitative Sudan stain for fat globules on suspension of stool will give an indication of significant steatorrhea. The test is simple, relatively sensitive and effective for screening. However, it cannot substitute for a quantitative fecal fat determination for a definitive diagnosis.

Quantitative fecal fat determination is the most reliable measure of steatorrhea. In the normal individual, the amount of fat appearing in the stool is relatively constant despite small changes in the quantity of dietary fat. Even when the daily fat intake is zero, the fecal fat output equals about 2.9 g/day. Presumably this is the amount of fat that is derived from endogenous sources, such as sloughed mucosal cells, excreted bile lipids (cholesterol and bile acids) and bacterial lipids. As the dietary intake of fat is increased, the fecal fat will increase to about 5 g/day on a 100 g fat diet. Fecal fat (FF) bears some relation to dietary fat: normally, the fecal fat loss is usually less than 5% of dietary intake. A defect at one of the four steps in the overall process of fat assimilation dramatically increases this fat loss. In disease the absolute value of the quantitative fecal fat output may depend on the dietary load, which must be carefully assessed prior to adequate evaluation of the test. Thus a number of conditions should be met in order to obtain a reliable quantitative stool fat output. The patient should be on a steady dietary intake of a known 60–100 g fat, there must be a regular pattern of stooling, and all stool must be collected for 72 hours.

There are numerous possible artifacts for this test. Poor food intake, interrupted food intake, constipation or incomplete stool collection all give rise to a spuriously low value for the 24-hour fecal fat output. An artifactually high value will be seen when castor oil or nut oils have been consumed, but not petroleum mineral oils. The Van de Kamer method is the most commonly used procedure to chemically determine fecal fat output. This method, however, may lead to incomplete extraction and quantitation of medium-chain triglycerides (MCT) and thus may underestimate (by 10%) the quantity of fecal fats in patients whose diet has been supplemented with MCT. Steatorrhea does not indicate into which category of malassimilation the patient falls. An elevated fecal fat may be due to intraluminal maldigestion or intramural malabsorption. Therefore, further investigations are required to fully characterize the problem (Figure 15).

9.8 Intraluminal Maldigestion
Intraluminal maldigestion will occur with (1) inadequate mixing; (2) pancreatic insufficiency; and (3) reduced bile salt concentration. If the D-xylose

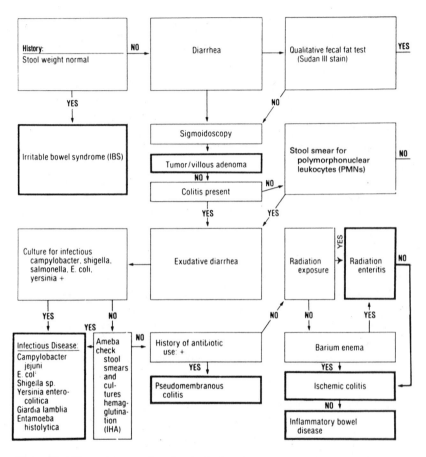

FIGURE 15.   Diagnostic approach to chronic diarrhea.
SOURCE: Knapp AB, Farkas PS. Diagnostic diagrams: gastroenterology. Baltimore: Williams and Wilkins, 1985:54–55.

absorption test and small bowel x-rays are normal, then it is likely but not absolutely certain that malassimilation is due to an intraluminal disorder. Pancreatic function is assessed by the secretin stimulation test used to measure secretory capacity of the exocrine pancreas. A tube placed in the duodenum adjacent to the ampullae of Vater collects pancreatic juice to measure volume, bicarbonate and enzyme (amylase) output. Maximal secretion should reach 2 mL/min at 90 minutes after injection of 2 units of secretin/kg of body weight, and bicarbonate concentration is normally 90 mEq/L. Both enzyme and bicarbonate secretion are diminished in chronic pancreatitis. Partial duct obstruc-

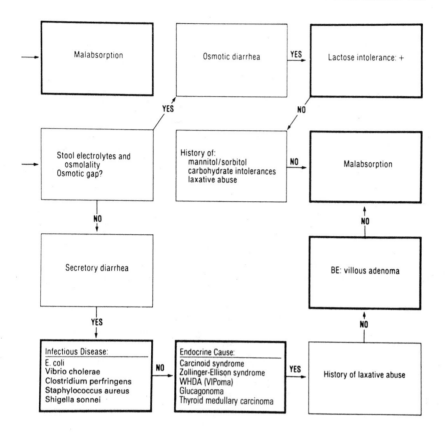

tion resulting from pancreatic cancer often reduces the volume of secretion without reducing bicarbonate concentration. The test is cumbersome and not very sensitive.

Assessment of biliary disease includes liver biochemistry, ultrasound and, where indicated, transhepatic or endoscopic cholangiography to ensure patency of the ductal system. In the bacterial overgrowth syndrome, bile acids are deconjugated and rapidly absorbed in the small intestine, and are not available or active for micellar solubilization. With bacterial overgrowth, the Schilling test for vitamin B_{12} is abnormal, even with the addition of intrinsic factor. Bile salt concentration may be diminished as a result of failure of reabsorption in a diseased ileum, adding to the malabsorption from gut loss. A ^{14}C-labeled bile acid breath test detects bile acid deconjugation in the bacterial overgrowth syndrome; an isotope scan with a radiolabeled bile acid analogue measures bile acid absorption.

The bile acid breath test is used if one suspects bile acid malabsorption due to ileal dysfunction (decreased absorption) or bacterial overgrowth (deconjugation and thus diminished absorption). The basis of the test is that the amino acid (glycine) part of the bile salt is labeled with ^{14}C-glycine. Bacteria deconjugate the glycine and metabolize this amide to $^{14}CO_2$, which is then expired. With ileal dysfunction, an excess of bile salts reaches the colon, where colonic bacteria split off the glycine, producing $^{14}CO_2$. With bacterial overgrowth, the excess coliform bacteria in the jejunum metabolize these bile salts to $^{14}CO_2$.

Disordered mixing of ingested food with endogenous enzymes results from the rapid transit in postgastrectomy syndromes. Small bowel x-rays with transit times sometimes help in the diagnosis.

9.9 Intramural Malabsorption

Malabsorption from an intramural defect occurs as a result of (1) inadequate absorptive surface – e.g., the short gut syndrome; (2) mucosal absorptive defects – e.g., celiac disease; or (3) lymphatic obstruction. Since the pentose sugar D-xylose does not require intraluminal digestion, D-xylose absorption tests serve to separate patients with intramural malabsorption from those with intraluminal maldigestion. An abnormal result points toward intramural malabsorption, while a normal result points toward intraluminal maldigestion. Remember that patients with renal impairment (who cannot excrete the sugar), delayed gastric emptying, bacterial overgrowth (who metabolize the sugar in the lumen) and advanced age may have spuriously low measurements of D-xylose absorption. Clinicians therefore may elect to omit this step and advance to specific intramural or intraluminal investigations (Figure 14).

Following an abnormal D-xylose test, the next evaluation should be barium contrast x-rays of the small intestine. They may demonstrate structurally abnormal bowel patterns, dilatation of bowel lumen, segmentation of barium or a dilution of barium because of increased intraluminal fluid. Although segmentation and flocculation of barium have been used as indications of malassimilation in the past, the use of nondispersible barium sulfate in recent years rarely allows us to observe such signs. Additionally, x-ray films may demonstrate diverticula as sites of bacterial overgrowth or thickening of folds resulting from infiltration or edema.

Following the x-ray, endoscopic or suction biopsy of the small intestine will identify evidence of specific mucosal disease. Once the position and/or etiology of the intramural disease is known, further tests can be carried out to

TABLE 6. Therapy for malassimilation syndromes

Site of defect	Therapy
Pancreas	Enzyme supplements; insulin; dietary counseling; surgery for pancreatic duct obstruction or cancer
Hepatobiliary	Surgery for obstruction of biliary tree
Mucosa	Diet, such as gluten withdrawal or milk-free diet; nutrient supplements; steroids for Crohn's disease; antibiotics for bacterial overgrowth or Whipple's disease
Lymphatics	Low-fat diet; medium-chain triglycerides (MCTs)

determine the extent of functional derangement. Tests can help define unabsorbed carbohydrate as a result of disaccharidase deficiency, generalized mucosal damage, inadequate surface area or bacterial overgrowth. Unabsorbed carbohydrate produces stool with an acid pH, easily tested on pH paper strip. The hydrogen breath test will detect an increase in expired hydrogen, which might result when an ingested carbohydrate is not absorbed. This test is used to diagnose suspected disaccharidase deficiencies or bacterial overgrowth. The basis of the test is that bacteria ferment sugars to fatty acids and H_2, which is expired. Normally, sugars are absorbed as monosaccharides in the small intestine and no H_2 is expired. In lactase deficiency, expired H_2 is elevated after ingestion of the test sugar lactose, since the unabsorbed sugar reaches colonic bacteria and is catabolized. In bacterial overgrowth, bacteria in the jejunum ferment the sugar before it can be absorbed and H_2 is expired. The hydrogen breath test is reliable, noninvasive and helpful in establishing the diagnosis of carbohydrate malabsorption and/or the bacterial overgrowth syndrome.

Vitamin B_{12} absorption is tested by the Schilling test. Radiolabeled vitamin B_{12} with intrinsic factor (labeled with [58]Co) and without intrinsic factor (labeled with [57]Co) are simultaneously administered orally. The excretion of both compounds is then measured in the urine over a 24-hour period. Excretion of both radiolabeled compounds is normal. Failure to excrete [57]Co-labeled vitamin B_{12} indicates absent gastric intrinsic factor – e.g., pernicious anemia or gastrectomy, while failure to excrete [58]Co- and [57]Co-labeled vitamin B_{12} indicates ileal disease or loss, or absent ileal B_{12} receptors.

9.10 Treatment
The specific treatments for malabsorption or maldigestion are given in Table 6. The nutritional therapies necessary for any associated deficiencies are given in Table 7.

TABLE 7. Representative doses for agents used in replacement therapy in patients with malassimilation syndromes

---

Minerals

Calcium	PO:	requires 1,200 mg elemental calcium daily as: (a) Calcium gluconate (93 mg Ca^{2+}/500 mg tablet), 5 g tid (b) Calcium carbonate (200 mg Ca^{2+}/500 mg tablet), 2 g daily
	IV:	Calcium gluconate, 10 mL (9.3 mg Ca^{2+}/mL) of 10% soln over 5 min
Magnesium	PO:	Magnesium gluconate (29 mg Mg^{2+}/500 mg tablet), 2–6 g/day
	IV:	Magnesium sulfate (50% soln, 1 mL contains 2.03 mmol Mg^{2+}) 2 mL bid
Iron	PO:	Ferrous fumarate (65 mg elemental Fe/200 mg tablet), 200 mg tid Ferrous gluconate (35 mg elemental Fe/300 mg tablet), 600 mg tid Ferrous sulfate (60 mg elemental Fe/300 mg tablet), 300 mg tid
	IM:	Iron dextran 1 mL once daily (calculated from existing Hb)*
	IV:	Iron dextran approx. 30 mL (calculated from existing Hb)* in 500 cc 5% D/W over 4 hrs, beginning with slow observed infusion
		*NOTE: IM/IV Fe for deficit replacement only
Zinc	PO:	Zinc sulfate (89 mg elemental zinc/220 mg capsule), 220 mg tid

Vitamins

Vitamin A	Water-miscible vitamin A (25,000 IU/capsule), 25,000 IU daily
Vitamin B_{12}	100 µg/IM monthly
Vitamin D_2	(Ergocalciferol) (50,000 IU/capsule), 50,000 IU 3 times per week
Vitamin E	Water-miscible vitamin E (100 IU/capsule), 400 IU daily
Vitamin K_1	(Phytonadione) has caused fatal reactions, thus should be avoided
Vitamin K_3	(Menadione) water-soluble PO: 5–10 mg/day IV: 5–10 mg/day
Folic acid	PO: 1 mg/day

Other
water-soluble   Multiple vitamin 1/day

(cont'd)

TABLE 7. Representative doses for agents used in replacement therapy in patients with malassimilation syndromes (cont'd)

Pancreatic supplements

Preparation	Type	Enzyme activity (IU/unit)			
		Lipase	*Trypsin*	*Proteolytic*	*Amylase*
Ku-Zyme HP®	Capsule	2,330	3,082	6,090	594,048
Festal®	Enteric-coated	2,073	488	1,800	219,200
Cotazym®	Capsule	2,014	2,797	5,840	499,200
Viokase®	Tablet	1,636	1,828	440	277,333
Pancrease®	Micro-encapsulated	>4,000	>25,000		

4–18 g/day at meals, with antacid or cimetidine (to prevent HCl inactivation of the supplement)

Bile salt binding agents
Cholestyramine 4 g (1 scoop), 3–6 times daily, according to response
Psyllium and aluminum hydroxide gel may also be effective

(cont'd)

10. ACUTE DIARRHEA

With a complaint of "diarrhea," the physician must establish if this represents a change in the patient's bowel habit and if the complaint arises from a perception of increased frequency of stool, increased volume or both.

If the diarrhea is acute (i.e., lasting less than two weeks), the malabsorption of fluid and electrolytes probably has an infectious or toxic cause (Table 8). When diarrhea lasts for a longer period of time, other explanations need to be considered. In the absence of prior gastric surgery, the four most common causes of chronic diarrhea are (1) the irritable bowel syndrome; (2) inflammatory bowel disease; (3) malabsorption; and (4) carcinoma of the colon. The physician also must consider altered bowel function due to drug or alcohol abuse (see Section 11). Associated tenesmus, urgency or a sense of incomplete evacuation suggests involvement of the rectum or sigmoid colon. The passage of blood, pus and mucus suggests bowel inflammation, ischemic bowel disease or cancer. Malassimilation syndromes (discussed in the previous section) are suspect if there is passage of food and oil droplets, or if the patient develops symptoms suggestive of nutrient deficiency, particularly weight loss.

In Western societies, stool weight is approximately 200 g/day. Since stools are 70–90% water, regardless of their consistency, excess fecal water must accompany diarrheal diseases with elevated stool weight. This concept leads

TABLE 7. Representative doses for agents used in replacement therapy in patients with malassimilation syndromes (cont'd)

Caloric supplements
Medium-chain triglyceride oil: (8 cal/mL), 60 mL/day po, 480 cal/day
Portagen®: medium-chain triglyceride + other oils: (1 cal/mL), 1 L/day
Enteral supplements:

Product	Kcal*/ 1,000 mL	Grams of protein/ 1,000 mL	Na mg/L	K mg/L	Osmolality mOsm/kg Water
Ensure®	1,060	37	740	1,270	450
Isocal®	1,040	34	530	1,320	300
Osmolite®	1,060	37	540	1,060	300
Precision Isotonic Diet®	960	29	800	960	300
Precision LR Diet®	1,110	26	700	810	525
Travasorb STD® (unflavored)	1,000	45	920	1,170	450
Standard Vivonex® (unflavored)	1,000	21	470	1,170	550
High-Nitrogen Vivonex® (unflavored)	1,000	44	530	1,170	810
Meritene Powder® In milk	1,065	69	1,000	3,000	690
Compleat B®	1,000	40	1,200	1,300	390
Formula 2®	1,000	38	600	1,760	435–510

*When prepared in standard dilution
Parenteral supplements: Intralipid® 1 L/day IV (10 mL/kg/day)
Travasol® 2 L/day IV (mix as per patient's protein requirements)

directly to consideration of the mechanisms responsible for the malabsorption or stimulated secretion of water.

Two caveats need to be remembered. First, fecal bulk varies with the diet, being influenced most notably by the content of indigestible carbohydrates (dietary fiber). Stools are smaller in developed countries than they are among societies whose members regularly ingest large amounts of dietary fiber. Second, disease of the distal colon or rectum can lead to the frequent, often painful passage of small stools (due to limited capacity as a reservoir), yet there may be little fecal water and no increase in stool weight. Proctitis characteristically produces diarrhea even though the actual weight of feces may not be increased; indeed, "constipation" may occur!

TABLE 8.   Common causes of acute diarrhea

Drugs	*Bacteria (toxin-mediated, cytotoxic)*
Laxatives	Clostridium difficile
Antacids	Staphylococcus aureus
Antibiotics	Shigella dysenteriae
Cholinergic drugs	Campylobacter jejuni
Lactose	Yersinia enterocolitica
Guanethidine	
Quinidine	*Bacteria (invasive)*
Digitalis	Salmonella
Colchicine	Enteroinvasive Escherichia coli
Potassium supplements	
Lactulose	*Bacteria (unknown mechanism)*
	Enteropathogenic Escherichia coli
	Enteroadherent Escherichia coli
	Viruses
Bacteria (toxin-mediated, cytotonic)	Parvovirus (Norwalk agent)
Enterotoxigenic Escherichia coli	Reovirus (rotavirus)
(both heat-labile and heat-	
stable toxins)	*Protozoa*
Vibrio cholerae	Cryptosporidia
Vibrio parahaemolyticus	Giardia lamblia
Clostridium perfringens	Entamoeba histolytica
Bacillus cereus	
	Parasites
	Stronglyoides
	Trichuris

Acute diarrhea is thus defined as stool weight > 200 g/day for less than 14 days' duration. It always will represent a change in bowel habit for the individual and will often be associated with an increased frequency of bowel movements.

10.1 Bacterial Diarrhea

Most enteric infections are self-limiting and resolve in less than two weeks. Acute bacterial diarrheas can be classified into *toxigenic types*, in which an enterotoxin is the major pathogenic mechanism, and *invasive types*, in which the organism penetrates the enterocyte as a primary event, although an enterotoxin may be produced as well. Enterotoxins are either *cytotonic* (producing intestinal fluid secretion by activation of intracellular enzymes, without damage to the epithelial surface) or *cytotoxic* (causing injury to the enterocyte as well as inducing fluid secretion). Three major clinical syndromes caused by bacterial infections are (1) food poisoning, (2) infectious gastroenteritis and (3) traveler's diarrhea.

10.1.1 *FOOD POISONING*

The food poisoning syndrome characteristically features the development of a brief but explosive diarrheal illness in subjects following exposure to a common food source contaminated with bacteria or bacterial toxins. Staphylococcus aureus, Salmonella, Clostridium perfringens and Bacillus cereus are responsible for 90% of these outbreaks.

Staphylococcus aureus produces a heat-stable, odorless and tasteless enterotoxin that is generated in poorly refrigerated desserts and seafoods. Ingestion of the preformed enterotoxin causes nausea, vomiting and profuse diarrhea within 4 to 8 hours. Spontaneous resolution occurs within 24 hours. No specific therapy is available or necessary.

Salmonella food poisoning has been attributed to an enterotoxin similar to that of Staphylococcus aureus, but none has been clearly identified. Within 12 to 36 hours after ingestion of contaminated foods (usually poultry products), there is a sudden onset of headaches, chills and abdominal pain, with nausea, vomiting and diarrhea. These symptoms may persist for one to four days before subsiding.

Antibiotic therapy of nontyphoidal Salmonella gastroenteritis fails to alter the rate of clinical recovery. In fact, antibiotic therapy will increase the duration of intestinal carriage of the Salmonella and is thus contraindicated.

Clostridium perfringens produces a preformed toxin from spores that germinate in contaminated meats cooked to less than 50°C. Symptoms are diarrhea and crampy abdominal pain without vomiting, beginning 8 to 24 hours after the meal. The illness lasts less than 24 hours. No specific therapy is indicated.

Bacillus cereus produces either a diarrheal syndrome or a vomiting syndrome, depending upon the enterotoxin. The vomiting syndrome is always associated with ingestion of rice and is caused by a preformed toxin that is elaborated when rice is left to cool unrefrigerated. Flash-frying later does not generate enough heat to destroy the toxin. The diarrheal syndrome occurs after ingestion of the organism itself. Both illnesses are short-lived and require no specific therapy.

The diagnosis of food poisoning is usually made by history. Except in special circumstances (e.g., botulism), isolation of the toxin is not cost-effective.

10.1.2 *GASTROENTERITIS*

The organisms responsible for bacterial gastroenteritis exert their predominant

TABLE 9. Types of Escherichia coli intestinal pathogens

Name	Toxin	Mechanism
Enteropathogenic (EPEC)	Shiga-like toxin	Adherence
Enterotoxigenic (ETEC)	Labile toxin (LT)	Activates adenylate cyclase
	Stable toxin (ST)	Activates guanylate cyclase
Enteroinvasive (EIEC)	Shiga-like toxin	Penetrates epithelium
Enteroadherent (EAEC)	—	Adherence
Enterohemorrhagic (EHEC)	Shiga-like toxin (verotoxin)	Unknown

effects by invading and destroying the intestinal epithelium or by producing various enterotoxins.

10.1.2.1 Toxin-mediated, cytotonic bacterial gastroenteritis

Vibrio cholerae is the prototypic cause of toxigenic diarrhea. The Vibrio cholerae organisms elaborate a toxin that attaches to the inner cell membrane and activates adenylate cyclase (formerly "adenyl cyclase"). The presence of adenylate cyclase then elevates cyclic AMP (cAMP) levels. Cyclic AMP then stimulates the enterocyte to secrete fluid and electrolytes while at the same time impairing their absorption. Stool output can exceed 1 L/hour. Treatment is based on restoring fluid and electrolyte balance and maintaining intravascular volume. Even though fluid and electrolyte transport is impaired, glucose transport is intact. Since glucose absorption carries Na^+ (and thus water with it), an oral rehydration solution containing glucose, sodium and water will enhance water absorption during the profound dehydration stage of cholera.

Several types of Escherichia coli (E. coli) are intestinal pathogens. Each exerts its effects through different mechanisms (Table 9).

Enterotoxigenic E. coli (ETEC) colonizes the upper small intestine after passing through the acid barrier of the stomach. The organisms colonize the surface without penetrating the mucus layer. Like cholera, ETEC causes no mucosal damage and no bacteremia. Two types of enterotoxins are produced by ETEC: the heat-labile toxin (also called "labile toxin" or LT) and the heat-stable toxin (also called "stable toxin" or ST). ETEC can elaborate LT only, ST only, or both toxins. ST produces diarrhea by stimulating intestinal secretion through guanylate cyclase and subsequently cyclic GMP. LT produces diarrhea by a similar mechanism, except that it acts through adenylate cyclase and cyclic AMP. After a 24- to 48-hour incubation period, the disease begins with upper abdominal distress followed by watery diarrhea. The infection can be mild (with only a few loose movements) or severe (mimicking cholera). Treatment is symptomatic. Antibiotic therapy is ineffective and favors the emergence of resistant ETEC strains.

Vibrio parahaemolyticus causes acute diarrheal disease after consumption of seafood: raw fish or shellfish. The common factor in most outbreaks appears to be storage of the food for several hours without proper refrigeration. Explosive, watery diarrhea is the cardinal manifestation, along with abdominal cramps, nausea and vomiting. Fever and chills occur in 25% of cases. The duration of illness is short, with a median of three days. Treatment is symptomatic; there is no role for antimicrobial therapy.

10.1.2.2 Toxin-mediated, cytotoxic bacterial gastroenteritis

After ingestion, Shigella dysenteriae organisms attack the colon, sparing the stomach and small bowel. Shigella organisms adhere to the mucosal surface, penetrate the mucosal surface, and then multiply within epithelial cells, moving laterally through the cytoplasm to adjacent cells by filopodium-like protrusions. Shigella organisms rarely penetrate below the intestinal mucosa and almost never invade the bloodstream. Both attached and intracellular organisms elaborate toxic products.

Even a small inoculum of 200 organisms (as contrasted with Salmonella, which requires greater than 10^7 organisms) will lead to crampy abdominal pain, rectal burning and fever associated with multiple small-volume bloody mucoid bowel movements. Intestinal complications include perforation and severe protein loss. Extraintestinal complications include respiratory symptoms, meningismus, seizures, the hemolytic uremic syndrome, arthritis and rashes. Ampicillin 500 mg q.i.d. or co-trimoxazole 2 tablets b.i.d. for 5 days is the treatment of choice. Amoxicillin, interestingly, is not effective therapy for shigellosis.

Campylobacter jejuni–induced diarrhea is more common than diarrhea from either Salmonella or Shigella. Infection is from consumption of improperly cooked or contaminated foodstuffs. Campylobacter attaches to the mucosa and releases an enterotoxin that destroys the surrounding epithelia. Clinically, there is often a prodrome of constitutional symptoms along with headache and generalized malaise. A prolonged diarrheal illness follows – often with a biphasic character, with initial bloody diarrhea, slight improvement, then increasing severity. The illness usually lasts less than one week, although symptoms can persist for a longer period, and relapses occur in as many as 25% of patients. Erythromycin 500 mg q.i.d. for 7 days is optimal therapy.

Yersinia enterocolitica is often transmitted to humans from pets or food sources. The organism invades epithelial cells and produces an enterotoxin. Clinically, the spectrum of illness ranges from simple gastroenteritis to invasive ileitis and colitis. This organism causes diarrheal illness most frequently in children less than 5 years of age. Children over 5 years of age develop mesenteric adenitis and associated ileitis, which mimic acute appendicitis. Yersinia is less likely to cause disease in adults; if it does, the illness is an acute diarrheal episode that may be followed two to three weeks later by joint symptoms and a rash (erythema nodosum). Treatment is symptomatic. There is no evidence that antibiotics alter the course of the gastrointestinal infection.

Clostridium difficile causes antibiotic-associated colitis (Section 10.4).

10.1.2.3 Invasive bacterial gastroenteritis

Certain strains of E. coli are invasive, producing an illness indistinguishable from shigellosis. Isolates of E. coli 0157:H7 have been identified in the stools of patients with a diarrheal illness clinically designated as "hemorrhagic colitis." Infection has been traced to contaminated hamburger meat obtained from a variety of sources, including large national restaurant chains.

Ingestion of this organism results in severe crampy abdominal pain and fever, followed within 24 hours by bloody diarrhea that lasts five to seven days. Since the organism is shed in the stool for only a short period of time, early stool collections are critical for the diagnosis. Treatment is symptomatic, as antibiotics do not appear to alter the disease course. In severe cases with possible toxic megacolon, systemic antibiotics may be in order.

Approximately 1,700 serotypes and variants of Salmonella are potential pathogens for humans. A dose of approximately 10^7–10^9 organisms is required to produce a clinical illness. Salmonella organisms invade the mucosa of the small intestine and (particularly) the colon. This form of gastroenteritis produces nausea and vomiting followed by abdominal cramps and diarrhea that lasts three to four days and then gradually subsides. In 10% of the cases bacteremia of the Salmonella organism occurs, and in approximately 5% there are disseminated infections to bones, joints and meninges. Certain conditions increase the risk of salmonellosis: hemolytic anemia, malignancy, immunosuppression, achlorhydria and ulcerative colitis. With uncomplicated Salmonella gastroenteritis, treatment is symptomatic. In fact, antibiotic therapy increases the duration of intestinal carriage of these organisms. Patients

TABLE 10. Traveler's diarrhea: recommendations for treatment

General
Avoid ice cubes, raw vegetables and fruits, raw fish and shellfish, unrefrigerated food.
Drink canned pop and beer, boiled water.
Drink oral replacement solutions for acute attacks.
Avoid over-the-counter preparations sold locally for acute attacks.

Specific
To provide symptomatic relief of acute attack:
   Diphenoxylate 1 tab, 2.5 mg, after each bowel movement to max 9 tab/day
   Loperamide 1 cap, 2.0 mg, after each bowel movement to max 8 cap/day
   Pepto-Bismol® 30 mL q 30 min × 8 doses

To decrease severity of acute attack:
   Co-trimoxazole 1 tab bid po × 3 days
   Doxycycline 100 mg bid po × 3 days

Prophylaxis:
Not recommended except for persons who are immunosuppressed or suffer chronic illness. If indicated, then:
   Co-trimoxazole 1 tab bid po × 3 days
   Doxycycline 100 mg bid po × 3 days

---

with complicated Salmonella gastroenteritis (e.g., those with predisposing conditions or sepsis, or who are very young or very old) should be treated with ampicillin or co-trimoxazole.

10.1.2.4 *Bacterial gastroenteritis of unknown mechanism*

Enterohemorrhagic E. coli–induced diarrhea tends to occur in neonates and young children. Only occasionally does it affect older children and adults. The pathogenic mechanism of this diarrhea is unclear; adherence of the organism to the intestinal epithelial cell seems to cause intestinal damage. There is no indication for specific treatment except for neonates in a nursery epidemic. In this case, oral nonabsorbable aminoglycosides should be used.

10.1.3 *TRAVELER'S DIARRHEA*

Traveler's diarrhea is a syndrome characterized by an increase in frequency of unformed bowel movements, typically four to five loose stools per day. Associated symptoms include abdominal cramps, nausea, bloating, urgency, fever and malaise. Traveler's diarrhea usually begins abruptly, during travel or soon after returning home, and is generally self-limiting, lasting three to four days. Ten percent of cases persist longer than one week, approximately 2% longer than one month and very few beyond three months. Enterotoxigenic E.

coli (ETEC) is the most common causative agent of traveler's diarrhea. These organisms adhere to the small intestine, where they multiply and produce an enterotoxin that causes fluid secretion and hence diarrhea. Salmonella gastroenteritis, Shigella dysentery, and viral enteric pathogens (rotavirus and Norwalk-like virus) are less common causes of traveler's diarrhea.

Since traveler's diarrhea is usually mild and self-limiting, with complete recovery even in the absence of therapy, therapy should be considered optional (Table 10). The value of prophylaxis for travelers is unclear. Bismuth preparations are helpful, but their use is limited by the large volumes necessary and by their taste. Antibiotic prophylaxis can reduce the likelihood of developing diarrhea, but carries its own risks.

10.2 Viral Gastroenteritis

At least two groups of viruses are capable of producing an acute diarrheal illness.

10.2.1 NORWALK VIRUS

The Norwalk virus causes a self-limiting syndrome that affects children and adults, mainly in winter. An incubation period of 24 to 48 hours is followed by a variable combination of fever, anorexia, nausea, vomiting, myalgia, abdominal pain and diarrhea. Spontaneous recovery occurs two to three days later. Immune electron microscopy of fecal filtrates demonstrates a characteristic 27 nm viral particle (the Norwalk agent). No specific treatment is available. The vomiting represents delayed gastric emptying; there are no morphologic features of gastritis.

10.2.2 ROTAVIRUSES

Rotaviruses are the most common causes of acute nonbacterial gastroenteritis in infancy and childhood. Rotaviruses invade mucosal epithelial cells. The resulting illness is more severe than that caused by the Norwalk virus. Rotavirus infection commonly requires hospital admission and intravenous fluids. Infection occurs mainly in children from 6 to 24 months old, and almost always in winter. Virus excretion is maximum three to four days after the onset of symptoms and disappears after a further three to four days. The stability of the virus and the large number of viral particles excreted make environmental contamination inevitable, with a high risk of secondary infection in susceptible contacts. For example, 20% of the rotavirus infections diagnosed in pediatric hospitals are acquired in the hospital. Most older children and adults have antibodies to rotaviruses, so any subsequent infection is generally mild.

10.3 Parasitic Enteritis

The parasites that infect the intestine may be divided into three broad groups. These include protozoa, roundworms and flatworms. The flatworms may be further divided into cestodes (tapeworms) and trematodes (flukes). This chapter will focus upon only a few relevant protozoa.

10.3.1 *GIARDIA LAMBLIA*

Giardia lamblia is endemic in many areas of the world, including Canada. Some patients with giardiasis present with an abrupt, self-limiting illness that develops one to three weeks after infection and lasts three to four days. Others may develop chronic and episodic diarrhea associated with bloating and, at times, steatorrhea and a malabsorption syndrome clinically like celiac disease. Diagnosis is made by recovery of the organism; it is found in the stool of approximately 50% of patients and in 90% of histologically examined smear preparations obtained from small bowel biopsy specimens. The treatment of choice in both asymptomatic and symptomatic patients is metronidazole 250 mg t.i.d. for 7 days. Repeat therapy will occasionally be needed to totally eradicate the organism. Quinacrine 100 mg t.i.d. for 7 days also is effective.

10.3.2 *AMEBIASIS*

This is an acute and chronic disease caused by the organism Entamoeba histolytica. Although there are numerous species of ameba that inhabit the human intestinal tract, E. histolytica seems to be the only variety that is pathogenic for humans. Its manifestations vary from the asymptomatic carrier state to a severe fulminating illness with mucosal inflammation and ulceration. Asymptomatic patients harbor only cysts in their stools and have no evidence of tissue invasion. Since the cysts are resistant to the outside environment, the disease can be transmitted by individuals unaware of their infective potential. This is in contrast to patients with acute or chronic invasive disease, who harbor a trophozoite that cannot survive outside the host.

The acute illness is characterized by diarrhea with the passage of blood and mucus, and by variable degrees of abdominal pain. In its most severe form it may mimic fulminating ulcerative colitis and may progress to a toxic dilatation (toxic megacolon) and perforation of the colon. During the acute illness, trophozoites may be recovered in the stool, from biopsies of shallow ulcers in the rectum, or from smears of rectal mucus.

Chronic infectious features may develop many years after the patient has left an endemic area. Patients present with nonspecific bowel complaints and may show radiologic changes in the distal small bowel and colon that mimic Crohn's disease, cancer or tuberculosis. Diagnosis necessitates recovering trophozoites from the stool. As an adjunct, the indirect hemagglutination test can help detect patients with invasive disease.

Intestinal complications of amebiasis include massive intestinal hemorrhage, which is rare; ameboma formation in any part of the colon, which may lead to obstruction or intussusception; permanent stricture formation during the healing stage; and postdysenteric colitis, which usually resolves over several weeks or months without specific therapy.

Systemic dissemination of the ameba may involve other organs, such as the brain, lung, pericardium and liver. Liver abscess is the most common extraintestinal infection by the ameba.

Therapeutic agents used for the treatment of amebiasis act at selected sites: intraluminally, intramurally or systemically. Treatment must therefore be individualized to the location of the disease. Asymptomatic carriers are treated with iodoquinol 650 mg t.i.d. for 20 days; this effective agent acts against amebas located intraluminally. Acute or chronic intestinal disease is treated with metronidazole 750 mg t.i.d. for 10 days. However, because metronidazole is less effective against organisms within the bowel lumen, iodoquinol (650 mg t.i.d. for 20 days) must be added.

10.3.3 *CRYPTOSPORIDIA*
Cryptosporidia are a genus of protozoa classified within the subclass Coccidia. Cryptosporidia infection has been recognized as a diarrheal disease in humans only since 1979. In immunocompetent persons it presents as a transient, self-limiting diarrheal state lasting from one to seven days. Adults are less commonly affected than young children. In most, the illness is mild and medical help is not sought. With immunological incompetence (e.g., AIDS, neoplasia, hypogammaglobulinemia or concurrent viral infection), a persistent chronic watery diarrhea may occur. Diagnosis is made by demonstrating Cryptosporidia oocysts in the stool or, better still, by mucosal biopsy and examination of the microvillus border for embedded Cryptosporidia oocysts.

A successful treatment for Cryptosporidia has not yet been found.

10.4 **Drug-Related Diarrhea**
Since almost every drug can cause diarrhea, the first question to ask a patient is "What medications, both prescribed and over-the-counter, are you currently taking?" Discontinuing the drug is often the only therapeutic move required in nonantibiotic diarrhea; even in patients with antibiotic-induced diarrhea, with or without colitis, this may be the only step necessary. Although many drugs can cause diarrhea, little is understood about the ways in which they do so. The common causes of drug-induced diarrhea with pathogenic mechanisms follow.

10.4.1 *ANTIBIOTIC-ASSOCIATED DIARRHEA AND PSEUDO-MEMBRANOUS COLITIS*

Antibiotics are the most common cause of drug-induced diarrhea. In many cases, the condition is self-limiting. The development of pseudomembranous colitis in association with antibiotics may be a serious and sometimes life-threatening condition.

Pseudomembranous colitis secondary to antibiotics was first recognized during the 1950s. Initially, it was thought to be caused by overgrowth with Staphylococcus aureus, but later research revealed that the colitis was usually caused by an enterotoxin produced by Clostridium difficile.

Pseudomembranous colitis can follow virtually any antibiotic use. The frequency of diarrhea or colitis does not appear to be related to dose or route of administration. Symptoms can occur while the patient is on the antibiotic or within six weeks following its discontinuation. Only increasing age is clearly identifiable as a risk factor. The diarrhea is usually loose with a blood-streaked mucus. Frank bleeding is uncommon. The diarrhea can be devastating, with up to 30 bowel movements in a 24-hour period. The diarrhea may be associated with varying degrees of abdominal pain and low-grade fever. Depending on the severity of the diarrhea and the amount of fluid loss, hypotension, shock and even death have been reported. In many patients the problem is self-limiting and resolves spontaneously with discontinuation of the antibiotic. Further investigation is required in those patients who have severe diarrhea associated with systemic symptoms and those whose diarrhea persists despite discontinuing the implicated antibiotic.

An accurate history is usually sufficient to suggest the diagnosis, and a sigmoidoscopy may be all that is required for confirmation. The presence of copious amounts of mucus and typical raised white pseudomembrane plaques are characteristic features on sigmoidoscopy. Biopsies help confirm the diagnosis. The distal colon is involved in most cases so that sigmoidoscopy is usually adequate. Lesions may be restricted to the right colon, necessitating colonoscopy.

Isolation of C. difficile plus toxin in the stools provides the diagnosis. If it is certain that there can be no other cause for the diarrhea, treatment can be undertaken while awaiting assay results. Treatment depends upon the condition of the patient. If symptoms are resolving with discontinuance of the antibiotic, no further therapy may be indicated. In mild cases, metronidazole 250 mg p.o. t.i.d. for 14 days is effective. In severe hospitalized cases the drug of choice is vancomycin 125 mg p.o. q.i.d. for 14 days. Vancomycin is poorly absorbed and CNS and renal toxic effects are uncommon. The high cost of this medication limits its use, even though the eradication rate is quite high; recurrence is possible with the cheaper therapeutic choice, metronidazole. If oral therapy cannot be used, as with severe ileus or recent surgery, parenteral metronidazole is preferred. Some 10–20% of treated patients will have a recurrence, usually within 4 to 21 days of stopping treatment. In this case, another course of vancomycin or metronidazole should be given. Cholestyramine (Questran®) binds the toxin and can provide symptomatic relief even though it will not eliminate the microorganism.

10.4.2 MAGNESIUM-CONTAINING ANTACIDS
Usually, the osmotic diarrhea produced by Mg^{++} is mild; it may even be welcomed by previously constipated patients. A change to a magnesium-free aluminum-containing antacid is all that is required to control the situation in some. (Magnesium can be used to induce diarrhea by the rare patient with the Münchausen syndrome seeking medical attention.)

10.4.3 ANTIARRHYTHMIC DRUGS
The antiarrhythmic drugs most commonly associated with diarrhea include quinidine, procainamide and disopyramide. The mechanism involved is unknown. Changing the antiarrhythmic drug may halt the diarrhea.

10.4.4 OTHER MEDICATIONS
Colchicine, often administered for acute gout, produces diarrhea as a common side effect. It resolves with discontinuance of the medication. The mechanism of the diarrhea is unknown, but may relate to an intestinal cytotoxic effect of colchicine. Antimetabolites (e.g., methotrexate) often cause diarrhea as a result of damage to the small or large bowel mucosa. This type of diarrhea can be devastating and difficult to control. Except for rehydration and stopping the drug, little can be done.

11. CHRONIC DIARRHEA

11.1 Pathogenesis
The four basic mechanisms that cause chronic diarrhea are osmotic, secretory and exudative factors, and abnormal intestinal transit (Table 11).

If the diarrhea ceases when fasting, or if there is a significant osmotic gap in the stool water, then an osmotic diarrhea is suspect. Examples include diarrhea after ingesting milk (a result of lactase deficiency) or drugs such as laxatives and antacids, or the excessive use of artificial sweeteners, such as sorbitol and mannitol, that contain polycyclic alcohols.

If the patient's diarrhea persists when fasting, a secretory diarrhea is likely.

TABLE 11. Pathophysiologic mechanisms of chronic diarrhea

Major disturbance	Probable mechanisms	Examples/Associated conditions
Osmotic	Ingestion	Antacids, laxatives
	Maldigestion	Pancreatic insufficiency, disaccharidase deficiency
	Malabsorption	Carbohydrate malabsorption, congenital chloridorrhea
Disorders of intestinal transit	Slow transit ("blind loop syndrome") – excessive contact time	Fistulas, strictures, diabetic neuropathy
	Rapid transit – insufficient contact time	Intestinal resection, hyperthyroidism, irritable bowel
Secretory	Bacterial enterotoxins	Vibrio cholerae, enterotoxigenic E. coli
	Secretagogues	Bile acids, fatty acids, ethanol, prostaglandins, phenolphthalein, dioctyl sodium sulfosuccinate, VIP, gastrin, calcitonin
Exudative	Increased passage of body fluids into lumen	Ulcerative colitis, Crohn's disease

Secretory diarrhea usually arises from infection or inflammation associated with toxigenic and invasive bacteria. Secretory diarrhea may also result from the spillage of excess bile acids into the colon (choleretic enteropathy) or from the cathartic effect of hydroxy fatty acids arising from the colonic bacterial action on malabsorbed fat. Very rarely, secretory diarrhea can arise from a tumor producing an intestinal secretagogue (e.g., pancreatic islet cell tumor producing vasoactive intestinal peptide).

Exudative diarrhea results from mucosal damage to the small or large bowel, which interferes with absorption of salt and water, and may be associated with the exudation of serum proteins, blood, and mucus and sloughed cells. This mechanism is seen in infectious, inflammatory and neoplastic disorders.

Disorders of intestinal transit may give rise to diarrhea secondary to abnormal intestinal motility in hyperthyroidism or diabetic neuropathy. Scleroderma leads to bacterial overgrowth and steatorrhea (as can the rapid transit in hyperthyroidism). The mechanism of diarrhea in these conditions relates to a

TABLE 12.   Causes of osmotic diarrhea

Carbohydrates
Specific disaccharidase deficiencies
Glucose–galactose malassimilation
Fructose malassimilation
Mannitol, sorbitol ingestion ("chewing gum diarrhea")
Lactulose therapy

Divalent ions
Magnesium sulfate (Epsom salts)
Sodium sulfate
Sodium phosphate
Sodium citrate
Magnesium-containing antacids

combination of bacterial overgrowth, bile salt wastage and disorders of motility (slow or rapid intestinal transit).

11.1.1 OSMOTIC DIARRHEA

Retention of solute molecules within the bowel lumen generates osmotic forces that retard the normal absorption of water (Table 12). Practical examples include poorly absorbed carbohydrates or a divalent ion. Poorly absorbed divalent ions (e.g., phosphate, sulfate and magnesium) are the laxative constituents of several common antacids and saline purges. Since the "pores" through which ions are absorbed are highly charged, these polyvalent ions tend to be absorbed slowly. Thus, they accumulate within the intestinal lumen, raise the osmolality, and so retard the normal absorption of water or even act to draw water from the circulation into the intestinal lumen.

Carbohydrates constitute the other major group of osmotic agents. Some are poorly absorbed by everybody; lactulose, for example, was developed to be a nonhydrolyzable, nonabsorbable disaccharide that would act as a cathartic. The action of lactulose mimics the effects of *primary lactase deficiency*. This condition normally develops after weaning in the majority of blacks and orientals, and occurs in 30–50% of southern Europeans. The unabsorbed lactose acts osmotically to retain water in the small intestine. In fact, any disease that interferes with carbohydrate absorption (e.g., impaired intraluminal digestion due to pancreatic disease, primary disaccharidase deficiencies, and secondary disaccharidase deficiencies due to small bowel disease) will lead to osmotic diarrhea. Since carbohydrates are not inert in the colon, their metabolism leads to further osmotic forces. Once carbohydrate reaches the fecal flora, anaerobic fermentation occurs (Figure 12). Intermediary products are ethanol and formic, succinic and lactic acids. These products are further consumed to varying degrees. CO_2 and H_2 are rapidly absorbed, and CO_2 rises in exhaled air. (Expired CO_2 is the basis for the hydrogen breath test described earlier.) Excess gas production causes borborygmi and flatus rich in H_2. Short-chain fatty acids (SCFAs) are also produced (acetic acid, propionic acid and butyric acid) and account for the acidic stool pH noted in diarrhea of carbohydrate malabsorption. The caloric loss due to carbohydrate malabsorption is diminished to the extent that short-chain fatty acids can be absorbed from the colon, thus "salvaging" some of the malabsorbed carbohydrates that enter the colon.

The consequences of malabsorption are as follows: With minor impairment of sugar absorption, colonic fermentation is complete and only small amounts of excess solute are present in stool water. Stool volume and stool pH do not initially change much, and up to three-quarters of the glucose energy is returned to the body in the form of short-chain fatty acids (colonic "salvage"). As the extent of carbohydrate malabsorption increases, more short-chain fatty acids are formed than can be reabsorbed. This results in diarrhea due to the presence of osmotically active short-chain fatty acids. The stool pH consequently begins to fall, which further decreases colonic salvage.

Clinically, osmotic diarrhea should stop when the patient stops ingesting the poorly absorbed solute. Stool analysis should not reveal fat, RBC or WBC. There should be a positive osmotic gap – that is, stool osmolality minus stool Na^+ plus stool K^+ times 2 (multiplied by 2 to account for anions) is greater than 50, the size of the osmotic gap being approximately equivalent to the concentration of poorly absorbed solutes in fecal water.

11.1.2 INTESTINAL TRANSIT AND DIARRHEA

The basal electrical rhythm of the small intestine alters the excitability of the muscle cells. The motility patterns of the small intestine consist of three essential patterns: (1) migrating motor complex (MMC), periodic bursts of contractile activity lasting at least 5 minutes that are succeeded by periods of quiescence and appear to migrate down the small intestine at a slow rate of less than 5 cm/min; (2) minute rhythm, regular groups of between 3 and 10 contractions that occur at intervals of 1 to 2 minutes, separated by periods of quiescence, and appear to migrate down the small intestine at a rapid rate of 60–120 cm/min; (3) migrating action potential complex, a single ring contraction or single burst of spike potentials that migrates down the intestine at a rate exceeding 90 cm/min.

These forms of small intestinal motility control the rate at which material travels along the intestine and hence arrives at the anus. Gastrointestinal motor activity also determines the time and hence the degree of contact between gut contents, the digestive enzymes and the absorptive epithelium. Accelerated transit of material through the gut produces diarrhea by limiting digestion and absorption.

Understanding of motility-associated diarrhea remains limited, and only rudimentary measures of intestinal myoelectrical activity exist for humans. The oral–anal transit times of radiolabeled markers, radiopaque tubing, or nonabsorbable carbohydrate markers provide the only clinical assessments. Even small intestinal motility, unlike esophageal motility, remains a research tool.

The ileocecal valve is important to gut function. The ileocecal sphincter extends over a 4 cm length of distal small intestine and produces a high-pressure zone of 20 mm Hg. Distention of the ileum results in a decrease in the ileocecal sphincter pressure, whereas distention of the colon results in an increased pressure in this area. By this mechanism the ileocecal valve is important in regulating intestinal transit. Removal of the ileocecal valve during surgery will result in marked intestinal hurry as well as the potential for bacterial overgrowth from fecal "backwash." Disorders that impair peristalsis in the small gut allow bacterial overgrowth, resulting in diarrhea. Lastly, premature evacuation of the colon because of an abnormality of its contents or because of intrinsic colonic "irritability" or inflammation results in a reduced contact between luminal contents and colonic mucosa and, therefore, in more frequent, liquid stools.

11.1.3 SECRETORY DIARRHEA

The small intestine normally secretes as well as absorbs fluid and electrolytes; the secretion rate is lower than the absorption rate. Therefore, the net effect of small bowel transport is absorption of fluid. This is an important concept, because it means that a pathophysiologic event may reduce the absorption rate in either of two ways: by stimulating secretion or inhibiting absorption. Either or both can result in what is clinically recognized as secretory diarrhea. It is usually difficult, if not impossible, to ascertain which of the two events is predominant. For clinical purposes, it seems best to consider inhibition of ion absorption and stimulation of ion secretion together.

The prototype of secretory diarrhea is Vibrio cholerae; its clinical description first aroused interest in the secretory process as a mechanism for diarrhea (Table 13).

Bacterial secretagogues fall into two major classes. The first class comprises large (MW 84,000), heat-labile proteins, of which cholera enterotoxin is

TABLE 13.   Causes of secretory diarrhea

Pathophysiologic mechanisms
Enterotoxins
Circulating secretagogues (VIP, calcitonin, prostaglandins, serotonin)
Increased hydrostatic pressure and tissue pressure
Gastric hypersecretion (Zollinger-Ellison syndrome)
Pancreatic hypersecretion
Laxatives (ricinoleic acid, bisacodyl, phenolphthalein, oxyphenisatin, dioctyl sodium sulfo-
   succinate, aloe, senna, danthron)
Bile salts
Fatty acids

Clinical syndromes
Acute secretory diarrhea
Chronic secretory diarrhea
   Surreptitious laxative ingestion
   Pancreatic cholera syndrome (VIP)
   Medullary carcinoma of the thyroid (calcitonin)
   Ganglioneuroma, ganglioneuroblastoma, neurofibroma
   Zollinger-Ellison syndrome (gastrin)
   Malignant carcinoid syndrome (serotonin)
   Idiopathic secretory diarrhea
   Congenital chloridorrhea (some cases)
   Secreting villous adenoma
   Total villous atrophy of small bowel mucosa
   Niacin deficiency
   Intestinal lymphoma
Miscellaneous
   Intestinal obstruction
   Intestinal distention/ileus

the prototype. These toxins appear to stimulate secretion by activating mucosal adenylate cyclase and thus increasing cyclic AMP levels in the mucosa. The intracellular "messenger" for secretion is less well defined; cyclic AMP is considered important, though there are additional steps that might also involve intracellular levels of Ca^{++} and the calcium regulatory protein, calmodulin. A second class of secretagogues comprises smaller proteins that are heat-stable. The best studied is the ST (heat-stable toxin) of E. coli, which stimulates secretion by activating mucosal guanylate cyclase, leading to higher levels of cyclic GMP in the mucosa.

Bacterial toxins, however, are only part of the story. Secretion is also stimulated experimentally by hormones, peptides acting locally (paracrine hormones), luminal factors (e.g., dihydroxy bile acids and fatty acids), neurotransmitters, prostaglandins and physical factors (e.g., distention). Bile acids and fatty acids not absorbed in the small intestine evoke secretion of electrolytes and water by the colon. The exact mechanism(s) for this are uncertain. Both groups have multiple effects on the bowel, including stimulation of secretion, increased intestinal permeability and transient alterations in morphology.

One or more humoral stimuli can elicit a massive secretion of water and electrolytes from the small bowel. The colon is usually not involved directly, but it may be unable to adequately reabsorb the fluid load imposed on it. A key question, difficult to answer, is "What is the responsible hormone?" Putative secretagogues include vasoactive intestinal peptides in the pancreatic cholera syndrome, calcitonin in medullary carcinoma of the thyroid, gastrin in the Zollinger-Ellison syndrome, serotonin in the malignant carcinoid syndrome, and glucagon in glucagonomas. Prostaglandins are also potent stimulators of intestinal secretion. Although no hormone-producing prostaglandin has yet been identified, prostaglandins are used therapeutically to treat gastric ulcers. Diarrhea secondary to prostaglandin-stimulated intestinal secretion is a common side effect.

The intestinal distention that occurs with obstruction or ileus also produces a local secretory state proximal to the obstruction. The mechanism is not entirely clear and may be related to changes in permeability (as tight junctions are stretched and broken) as well as to direct, perhaps neural, stimulation of secretory mechanisms.

Secretory diarrhea is recognized clinically by four features: (1) the stools are large-volume, watery and often >1 L/day; (2) the diarrhea persists during fasting; (3) measured stool osmolality is less than 10 mOsm; and (4) patients with secretory diarrhea do not have excessive fat, blood or pus in their stools.

Therapeutically, the offending agent must be removed. A variety of empirical therapies that influence the secretory process (e.g., somatostatin, prostaglandin inhibitors, phenothiazines, calcium channel blockers, α_2-adrenergic agonists and lithium) may be effective but should be reserved for use in a research center. Oral glucose-saline replacement therapy is useful for maintenance of hydration. For bile acid–induced diarrhea, cholestyramine works well.

11.1.4 EXUDATIVE DIARRHEA

Exudation is a far simpler concept. Structural disruption of the intestinal wall by diffuse ulceration, inflammation, infiltrations and tumors will add cellular debris, mucus, serum proteins and blood to the lumen. The effects on stool volume will be most pronounced when the lesions also involve the colon,

TABLE 14.   Anatomic approach to the causes of chronic diarrhea

---

Gastric
Excessive use of antacids
Hypergastrinemia/Zollinger-Ellison syndrome
Postoperative unmasked celiac disease, lactase deficiency or pancreatic
   insufficiency
Postoperative dumping syndrome*

Small intestine
Crohn's disease*
Celiac disease
Lymphoma
Whipple's disease
Bacterial, viral or parasitic infection*
Abnormal intestinal integrity: scleroderma, amyloidosis, diabetes

Large bowel
Colon neoplasia*
Irritable bowel syndrome*
Inflammatory bowel disease: ulcerative colitis, Crohn's disease*

Drugs
Antacids
Antibiotics*
Alcohol*
Antimetabolites
Laxatives
Digitalis
Colchicine

Metabolic
Hyperthyroidism
Hypoparathyroidism
Addison's disease
Diabetes
Carcinoid syndrome
VIPoma syndrome

---

*Common

since there will be little opportunity for normal mechanisms of colonic fluid
and electrolyte absorption to compensate for the increased volume of chyme.

11.1.5 *SELF-INDUCED DIARRHEA*

The possibility that the diarrhea is self-induced must be considered when a patient complains of chronic diarrhea. In general, abusing laxatives, diuretics and sometimes thyroid hormones will induce diarrhea. Often the diarrhea is sufficiently severe to cause electrolyte disturbances, acid-based problems and dehydration. The diagnosis can be extremely difficult since the history is often misleading or not obtained. The usual investigations (including sigmoidoscopy and radiographs) will be negative, unless the patient is taking a drug that can cause melanosis coli (brown-black pigmentation of the colonic mucosa). Finding packages of laxatives and other drugs in room searches is often the only method that permits the diagnosis; this approach has been criticized because of ethical considerations, but may be the only way to uncover the problem. Stool analysis for Mg^{++}, sennas or phenolphthalein may reveal the culprit.

11.2 Investigation of the Patient with Chronic Diarrhea

For a patient with chronic diarrhea, a careful history and physical examination can help define the site in the intestinal tract responsible (Table 14). This may avoid the expense and frustration of the unproductive "shotgun" approach. One possible diagnostic approach appears in Figure 15.

12. DISACCHARIDASE DEFICIENCIES

Disaccharide intolerance is a characteristic symptom complex resulting from the ingestion of ordinary dietary quantities of disaccharides, which produces a symptomatic diarrhea. The cause is a deficiency of one or more disaccharidases, but not all people with such a deficiency will experience symptoms.

Dietary carbohydrates are presented to the surface of the jejunal mucosa in the form of isomaltose, maltotriose and three major disaccharides – maltose, sucrose and lactose. Trehalose, a disaccharide contained in young mushrooms and in certain insects, is a minor component of modern Western diets. Deficiencies of disaccharidases may be *primary* (hereditary) or *secondary* (acquired) deficiencies. Characteristically in primary deficiencies, which are rare, only one enzyme is involved; the deficiency is present at birth (with the exception of the adult-onset form of lactase deficiency), not associated with intestinal disease, and irreversible. Secondary deficiencies usually involve all the disaccharidases, may occur at any age, are associated with a disorder of the small intestinal mucosa, and may be reversed if the intestinal disorder (e.g., celiac disease, stasis syndromes or acute enteritis) heals.

The clinical manifestations of enzyme deficiency result from the osmotic diarrhea following ingestion of the disaccharide. The affected individual develops crampy, abdominal distress and distention, relieved by the expulsion of liquid stool and flatus. The severity of the diarrhea varies with the disaccharide load, the degree of deficiency of enzyme activity and any associated/ causal intestinal disease. The clinical diagnosis can be confirmed by direct enzyme assay of jejunal mucosal biopsies or by indirect methods for detecting disaccharide malabsorption (e.g., the breath hydrogen test). Treatment of hereditary deficiencies is usually by elimination diets. For children and adolescents (who have high nutritional requirements) and for adults who enjoy milk, low-lactose milk is available in some localities. It can also be prepared by adding yeast lactase (available in commercial form) to milk and refrigerating it for 24 hours; 80% lactose hydrolysis can be obtained with this method.

Delayed-onset (adult-onset) hereditary lactase deficiency is extremely common and probably "normal" for humans. Beginning as early as age 2 years in some racial groups, and as late as adolescence in others, the activities of lactase in the majority of the world's populations drop sharply. This is the result of the genetically controlled "switching off" of lactase synthesis by intestinal cells. Individuals of northern European ancestry and certain groups in Africa and India, however, maintain lactase activity throughout adulthood.

13. GLUTEN-INDUCED ENTEROPATHY (CELIAC DISEASE)

In celiac disease the mucosa of the small intestine is damaged by gluten-containing foods (i.e., those containing wheat, rye, barley and possibly oats). This causes a characteristic though nonspecific lesion and subsequent malabsorption of most nutrients. The precise mechanism of gluten toxicity is unknown. Fractionation of cereal proteins reveals that the component that is toxic to the intestinal mucosa is a portion of the gluten molecule called gliadin. Although gliadin can be inactivated in a test tube by enzymatic degradation, digestion to smaller peptides by pepsin and trypsin does not alter its toxicity in humans. In susceptible people, symptoms and pathologic changes occur within 12 hours of gluten intake. The immune system is also involved. The small intestine in patients with untreated celiac disease shows an increase in lamina propria lymphocytes, plasma cells and intraepithelial lymphocytes. Immunocytochemical studies indicate that cells producing IgA, IgG and particularly IgM are increased. Increased levels of serum IgA and decreased levels of serum IgM have also been reported and appear to revert toward normal with treatment.

Genetic studies indicate that 10% of the patient's first-order relatives have asymptomatic disease. HLA-B8 and HLA-DW3, generally associated through linkage disequilibrium, are present in 80% of patients (compared to 20% of the general population). In addition, a specific antigen is present on the surface of B lymphocytes in approximately 80% of celiac disease patients (compared to

TABLE 15. Symptoms of celiac disease

Manifestations	Probable causes or deficiencies
Common	
Anemia	Iron, folate, B_{12}, pyridoxine
Glossitis	Iron, folate
Weight loss/weakness	Malassimilation – Negative nitrogen balance
Diarrhea/flatulence	Fat and carbohydrate malassimilation
Abdominal pain	Increased intestinal gas production secondary to carbohydrate malassimilation
Occasional	
Follicular hyperkeratosis and dermatitis	Vitamin A, folate
Pigmentation	Associated adrenal insufficiency
Edema	Hypoproteinemia
Tetany	Vitamin D, calcium, magnesium
Osteomalacia	Vitamin D, calcium
Purpura	Hypoprothrombinemia (vitamin K)
Rare	
Spinal cord degeneration	B_{12}
Peripheral neuritis	B_{12}, vitamin E, thiamine, pyridoxine
Psychosis	B_{12}
Malignancy (usually small bowel lymphoma)	Unknown

10–15% of controls). It is found in all parents of affected individuals, which suggests that this antigen is inherited by an autosomal recessive method.

13.1 Clinical Features

13.1.1 *CHILDHOOD PRESENTATION*
In children, onset is gradual with failure to thrive after the introduction of cereals in the diet (Table 15). The affected infant is anorexic, pale and wasted. Physical examination discloses generalized hypotonia and abdominal distention. The stools are soft, bulky, clay-colored and offensive. In the slightly older child, abdominal pain may be the presenting complaint. It may be sufficiently severe to simulate an intestinal obstruction. Older children may also present with anemia, rickets and failure to grow normally. Quite often, adolescents have a clinical quiescence of the disease. Even if relatively asymptomatic in childhood, affected people often do not attain their normal growth potential, being shorter than their sibs.

13.1.2 ADULT PRESENTATION

Celiac disease can present at any age, even after 70 years, but in adults it usually occurs between 20 and 60 years. In adult and adolescent patients, presentations with classical features of diarrhea, weight loss and malnutrition, or bone pain (osteomalacia) have become much less common. Mild and subclinical forms are frequent, occurring in more than 50% of patients. The sole presentation may be an otherwise unexplained hematologic abnormality (iron deficiency with or without anemia, folate deficiency, macrocytosis), constitutional symptoms or fatigue with minimal weight loss and no intestinal symptoms, or mild abdominal or digestive complaints. The entity is most common in those of Irish and Scottish background or those who have a family history.

Diarrhea is common but many patients experience normal bowel habits, alternating diarrhea and constipation, and even constipation. The diarrhea is usually mild, with fewer than three bowel movements per day in most. Floating stools, also common in healthy subjects excreting high amounts of stool gas, are often not reported. Indeed, stools suggesting steatorrhea (i.e., unformed, bulky and hard to flush, greasy, sticky, pale and foul-smelling) are quite uncommon. Flatulence, abdominal distention, abdominal cramps and borborygmus are common complaints. Fatigue is the most frequent symptom at presentation. Weight loss is usually moderate (averaging 10 kg) and may be absent in mild cases. Clinically overt metabolic (tetany) and bone (osteomalacia) diseases have become uncommon with our generous Western diets, but these situations are hallmarks of celiac disease.

Patients with dermatitis herpetiformis have gluten enteropathy but often without clinical impact. Overall, mucosal involvement in celiac disease progresses from duodenum to jejunoileum and is most severe proximally; the length of bowel involved determines to a great extent the clinical picture of the disease.

13.2 Laboratory Findings

Laboratory findings, as clinical signs and symptoms, vary widely. The definitive diagnosis of celiac disease requires the demonstration of small bowel mucosal villous atrophy that improves upon gluten withdrawal. In practice, several tests can be used to strengthen the suspicion of celiac disease and/or evaluate the possible biochemical consequences.

13.2.1 STOOL EXAMINATION

Steatorrhea can be confirmed by a 72-hour fecal fat study. It is usually mild

(10–20 g/24 hours) and may be absent in some patients. Its severity correlates with the extent of the intestinal lesion, so that patients whose disease is limited to the proximal small intestine often have normal stool fat excretion.

13.2.2 HEMATOLOGIC TESTS
Anemia is present in less than 50% of adult patients and may be secondary to iron, folate or (very rarely) vitamin B_{12} deficiency. Since celiac disease involves the proximal small bowel (i.e., the duodenum, where iron absorption occurs) most severely, iron deficiency is the most common laboratory abnormality. Folate deficiency also occurs, providing two laboratory screening tests for celiac disease. Decreased absorption of B_{12} and malabsorption of vitamin K (with prolonged prothrombin time) are uncommon.

13.2.3 BLOOD CHEMISTRY TEST
Depletion of minerals (zinc, magnesium) and ions (potassium) occurs only with severe disease. Plasma proteins are often within normal limits but this protein-losing enteropathy (leakage of serum protein into gut lumen) and possible malnutrition may result in decreased serum albumin. A low serum carotene (and sometimes cholesterol) level may be a clue to the presence of the disease.

13.2.4 CARBOHYDRATE TOLERANCE TEST
Approximately two-thirds of patients with celiac disease exhibit an abnormal D-xylose test. D-xylose is an aldopentose that is absorbed in the upper small intestine and is excreted in the urine almost completely within the first five hours after ingestion. Abnormal D-xylose absorption is best evaluated by the serum concentration after ingestion and points specifically to small bowel disease or luminal bacterial overgrowth. Similarly, the absorptive cell lesion also results in secondary lactase deficiency; thus, the H_2-lactose breath test may be abnormal in celiac disease.

13.2.5 RADIOGRAPHIC STUDIES
Barium studies of the small bowel generally show dilatation of the bowel and slight thickening of the mucosal folds. Intraluminal signs of malabsorption with flocculation, segmentation and clumping of the barium (features due to excess amount of fluid present within the lumen) are variable and not common. (The new barium suspensions now used have made this a rare finding.) Radiographic findings in celiac disease are not specific for this syndrome of malabsorption.

13.2.6 SMALL BOWEL BIOPSY

Small intestinal biopsies can be obtained endoscopically from the distal duodenum (at least four forceps biopsies). When diagnostic uncertainty persists, a larger mucosal specimen may be needed and obtained from the duodenojejunal area using the peroral Rubin tube.

A flat mucosal biopsy from a white adult in the Western world is almost certain to indicate celiac disease, although other disorders can be associated with similar changes (e.g., tropical sprue, diffuse lymphoma of small bowel, immunoglobulin deficiency syndromes and the Zollinger-Ellison syndrome with gastric hypersecretion). In infants, soy protein intolerance, cow's milk protein intolerance and viral gastroenteritis produce a similar appearance. Therefore, to establish unequivocally the diagnosis of celiac disease, clinical improvement with a gluten-free diet is needed. Mucosal small bowel atrophy improves similarly, although reversion of histology toward normal requires months or even years of gluten withdrawal and often is not complete in the duodenum.

Microscopically the characteristic "flat" lesion of celiac disease will demonstrate absent villus with an abnormal cuboidal surface epithelium, markedly lengthened crypts and increased numbers of plasma cells and lymphocytes in the lamina propria. The proximal small bowel is most severely involved, while the lesion decreases in severity toward the distal small intestine. Celiac disease will not spare the proximal small intestine while involving the distal small intestine, however.

13.3 Treatment

The mainstay of therapy for celiac disease is the gluten-free diet, which requires avoiding wheat, rye, barley and oats but allows widely diversified foods. Expert dietetic counseling is a major determinant of successful treatment. Supplements of iron and folic acid are often needed. If milk products cause diarrhea, commercially available lactase enzymes may be used for the first few months. Usually, clinical symptoms improve within weeks, but drastic changes may be seen in sicker patients after a few days.

13.4 Complications and Prognosis

A primary failure to respond to treatment is usually due to incomplete (often involuntary) exclusion of gluten from the diet. Revision of the diet is necessary. Motivation for continuing with the gluten-free diet is provided by contacts with the physician and dietitian. Other causes of primary failure include diagnostic error (tropical sprue, lymphoma, etc.), dysgammaglobulinemia syndromes, "functional" associated pancreatic insufficiency and refractory sprue. Deterioration after a period of clinical improvement suggests dietary indiscretions, malignancies (there is increased risk of lymphoma) or rare instances of refractory sprue, collagenous sprue and nongranulomatous ulcerative jejunoileitis.

13.4.1 *REFRACTORY SPRUE*

Refractory sprue is a disease in which malabsorptive symptoms and mucosal small bowel atrophy persist or recur on a strict gluten-free diet. Corticosteroids, total parenteral nutrition and cyclosporine therapy have been used in treatment, but their value is not clear. The prognosis is serious.

13.4.2 *NONGRANULOMATOUS ULCERATIVE JEJUNOILEITIS*

This very rare complication presents with abdominal pain, intestinal bleeding and diarrhea. Ulcers may lead to small bowel perforations or strictures. The mortality rate for this condition is very high.

13.4.3 *COLLAGENOUS SPRUE*

This rare disorder is generally associated with severe and profound malabsorption. In addition to the characteristic small intestinal biopsy of untreated celiac disease, a striking trichrome-positive band of collagen is seen beneath the surface epithelium. Changes may be patchy, necessitating multiple biopsies from different sites to confirm the diagnosis. There is no effective therapy.

13.4.4 *MALIGNANCIES*

Incidence of malignancies is increased in patients with celiac disease. Most of these are small bowel lymphomas and carcinomas of the esophagus and colon. Recent data suggest that a strict gluten-free diet might decrease this risk – another reason to reinforce a lifetime commitment to gluten avoidance. Overall, the vast majority of patients with celiac disease have a normal life expectancy.

14. **SHORT BOWEL SYNDROME**

The severity of symptoms following resections of large segments of the small bowel relates to the extent of the resection and to the specific level of the resected small bowel. The level of resection is important because absorption of nutrients is most effective in the proximal small bowel (iron, folate, calcium, bile salts, vitamin B_{12}). Resection of up to 40% of the intestine is usually tolerated provided the duodenum and proximal jejunum and distal half of the ileum and ileocecal valve are spared. In contrast, resection of the distal two-thirds of the ileum and ileocecal valve alone may induce severe diarrhea and significant malabsorption even though only 25% of the total small intestine has been resected. Resection of 50% of the small intestine results in significant malabsorption, and resection of 70% or more of the small intestine will result in severe malnutrition sufficient to cause death.

The most common cause for resection of large amounts of small intestine is diseases that compromise the blood supply of the small intestine. These include thrombosis, embolism, low-flow ischemia of the superior mesenteric artery and thrombosis of the superior mesenteric vein. Less commonly, volvulus, strangulated hernias, Crohn's disease, neoplasm and trauma necessitate massive resection.

Two major types of diarrhea can develop after massive ileal resection. One is induced primarily by malabsorbed bile acids, and the other by malabsorbed fat. When the ileal resection is small (less than 100 cm), hepatic synthesis of bile acids is sufficient to compensate for increased fecal losses. The luminal concentrations of bile acids are maintained within the micellar range, and significant steatorrhea does not occur. However, without an ileum for reabsorption, bile acids enter the colon, impairing electrolyte and water absorption. Thus the term "bile acid diarrhea" is applied to this circumstance.

When the ileal resection is extensive (greater than 100 cm), hepatic compensation for wastage of bile acids is incomplete and the concentration of bile acids in the lumen is too low for adequate micellar solubilization of fat. Steatorrhea results. Here the malabsorbed fat is primarily responsible for the diarrhea. With excessive amounts of fatty acids now in the colon, electrolyte and water absorption are further impaired.

Consistent with these proposed pathogenic mechanisms are the therapeutic observations that a reduction in the dietary intake of long-chain fats will reduce the severity of diarrhea in the second instance (extensive resection and steatorrhea), whereas a sequestrant of bile acids such as cholestyramine or aluminum hydroxide is needed for effective therapy of bile acid diarrhea.

Additional metabolic complications arise from the short bowel syndrome. These include hyperoxaluria and subsequent nephrolithiasis. Normally dietary oxalate is excreted in the feces, bound to calcium as an insoluble complex. However, in a patient with steatorrhea, fatty acids in the intestine preferentially bind to calcium, leaving the oxalate soluble and available for absorption in the colon. The short bowel syndrome may also give rise to cholelithiasis. If bile acid malabsorption is extensive, a lithogenic bile will be produced, predisposing to gallstone formation.

15. POSTGASTRECTOMY MALABSORPTION

Postgastrectomy malabsorption frequently follows gastric surgery. The small size of the gastric remnant causes inadequate mixing of food with digestive juices, particularly after a gastroenterostomy. With the loss of the pylorus, there may be rapid gastric emptying, poor mixing of bile and pancreatic secretions, and rapid transit down the small intestine. Incoordinated secretion and poor mixing of bile and pancreatic juice leads to fat maldigestion. Bacterial contamination in a blind loop (with gastroenterostomy) results in maldigestion of fat, carbohydrate, protein, vitamins and minerals. Gastric surgery that allows food to enter into the upper small intestine without dilution and with minimal digestion may "unmask" mild and subclinical celiac disease, lactase deficiency or pancreatic insufficiency.

16. NORMAL SMALL INTESTINAL FLORA

The concentration and population of microorganisms that constitute the normal intestinal flora vary with the location along the intestine. Flora in the stomach, duodenum, jejunum and proximal ileum are sparse, usually less than 10^5/mL. The distal ileum represents a transitional zone between the sparse flora of the proximal small intestine and the luxuriant flora of the lower bowel, where microorganism concentrations reach 10^{11}/mL. The predominant species are strict anaerobes, including bacteroides, anaerobic streptococci, bifidobacteria and Clostridium. The commonest aerobic organisms are E. coli; however, their concentration (10^8/mL) is only 1/1,000 of the usual concentration of anaerobes in the colon.

Normally, bacterial flora are present in the intestinal lumen and in the mucus layer overlying the epithelium, and attached to the mucosal cells themselves. There is a specific tissue or cell type to which each microbial species attaches. For example, Streptococcus mutans, the oral organism that causes tooth decay, attaches only to the enamel surface of teeth; removal of the teeth leads to the disappearance of S. mutans from the oral microflora. This phenomenon of adherence may play an important role in the establishment and maintenance of a normal flora.

What are the mechanisms controlling normal small intestinal flora? First, in the stomach, acid suppresses the growth of most organisms that enter from the oropharynx. Bile added in the duodenum has additional antibacterial properties. Second, small intestinal motility mechanically sweeps bacteria downstream, helping to maintain a low concentration of organisms in the proximal small intestine. Third, the ileocecal valve plays an important role in preventing reflux of large amounts of colonic organisms. Additionally, mucus secreted by goblet cells and immunoglobulins has antibacterial properties.

Whereas the small intestine regulates the number of organisms present, in the colon the microorganisms themselves are responsible for maintaining their own population levels. Volatile fatty acids (e.g., acetic, butyric and propionic acid) are produced by anaerobes as well as by some coliforms. These short-chain fatty acids reduce the intraluminal pH and suppress the growth of certain organisms, thereby serving to control proliferation. In addition, some organisms produce other substances that inhibit bacterial growth, called bacteriocins.

Thus far we have considered what the microorganisms are, where they are located, and how their numbers are controlled. We next examine the concept that the normal flora exert a profound influence on intraluminal constituents, including food, urea, bilirubin, bile salts, drugs and potential toxins. Bacteria ferment dietary carbohydrates, yielding short-chain fatty acids, hydrogen and carbon dioxide. Fatty acids from carbohydrates and those from fat in the diet are hydroxylated by the intestinal flora. The hydroxy fatty acids formed stimulate fluid secretion and are thus cathartics.

Similarly, bacteria alter protein and amino acids. Tryptophan is converted to indole compounds, glycine to ammonia, and methionine to hydrogen sulfide. Urea is converted to ammonia, a reaction that may contribute to hepatic encephalopathy. Bilirubin is metabolized to urobilinogen; bile salts may be deconjugated (removing glycine and taurine) and dehydroxylated (cholic acid becomes deoxycholic acid, and chenodeoxycholic acid becomes lithocholic acid). This deconjugation and dehydroxylation renders bile acids more insoluble and less capable of forming micelles. Bacteria also can affect vitamin synthesis and metabolism. Vitamin B_{12} may be bound, thereby becoming unavailable for absorption (hence the abnormal Schilling test in bacterial overgrowth) and vitamin K and folic acid produced.

The normal flora also affect drugs and other ingested materials. Sulfasalazine, a drug used in ulcerative colitis, is unabsorbed in its native form. Intestinal bacteria, however, convert the substance into two moieties, a therapeutically active aminosalicylic acid and an inactive sulfapyridine. The sulfa drug succinylsulfathiazole is itself inactive, but is converted by intestinal bacteria to sulfathiazole, which is an active antimicrobial agent. Another example is cyclamate, unabsorbed and inert in its native form. Intestinal bacteria produce cyclohexylamine, a potential carcinogenic agent. Thus, bacteria can activate pro-drugs and produce carcinogens.

TABLE 16.   Etiology of the bacterial overgrowth syndrome

Breakdown of normal defense mechanisms
Achlorhydria
Stasis: Anatomic (Crohn's disease, diverticula, lymphoma, strictures)
      Functional (scleroderma, diabetic autonomic neuropathy, pseudo-obstruction)
Loss of ileocecal valve

Contamination
Postinfection
Enteroenteric fistulas, gastrocolic fistulas

---

17. BACTERIAL OVERGROWTH SYNDROME

The bacterial overgrowth syndrome can result from any disease that interferes with the normal balance (ecosystem) of the small intestinal flora and brings about loss of gastric acidity; alteration in small bowel motility or lesions predisposing to luminal stasis; loss of the ileocecal valve; or overwhelming contamination of the intestinal lumen (Table 16).

The bacterial overgrowth syndrome gives rise to clinical abnormalities arising from the pathophysiological effects on the luminal contents and the mucosa. Bacteria can consume proteins and carbohydrates. In bacterial overgrowth there may be defective transport of sugars, possibly related to the toxic effect of deconjugated bile acids. Steatorrhea results from the deconjugation and dehydroxylation of bile acids; lithocholic acid is precipitated and free bile acids are reabsorbed passively, making them unavailable and incapable of performing micellar solubilization. Fats, cholesterol and fat-soluble vitamins are malabsorbed. Vitamin B_{12} is also malabsorbed as a result of the binding and incorporation of this vitamin into the bacteria. Folate deficiency, however, is not a common occurrence in bacterial overgrowth; unlike vitamin B_{12}, folate synthesized by microorganisms in the small bowel is available for host absorption. In patients with small bowel bacterial overgrowth, serum folate levels tend to be high rather than low. In addition to steatorrhea, patients with bacterial overgrowth frequently complain of watery diarrhea. Important mechanisms in producing this diarrhea include (1) disturbances of the intraluminal environment with deconjugated bile acids, and hydroxylated fatty and organic acids; and (2) direct changes in gut motility.

In some patients, symptoms of the primary disease predominate, and evidence of bacterial overgrowth may be found only on investigation. In others,

TABLE 17.   Diagnosis of the bacterial overgrowth syndrome

Jejunal culture

Tests of bile salt deconjugation
^{14}C-glycocholate breath tests
In vitro deconjugation assessment

Tests of malassimilation
Vitamin B_{12} (Schilling test)
D-xylose, glucose, lactulose

---

the primary condition is symptomless, and the patient presents with a typical malabsorption syndrome due to bacterial overgrowth (Table 17). Once diagnosis of bacterial overgrowth is suspected a careful history should be performed to identify possible causes. Physical examination may be normal or may demonstrate signs related to specific nutrient deficiencies.

A small bowel biopsy is of value in excluding primary mucosal disease as the cause of the malabsorption. Histologic abnormalities of the jejunal mucosa are usually not seen in patients with bacterial overgrowth. The sine qua non for the diagnosis of bacterial overgrowth is a properly collected and appropriately cultured aspirate of the proximal small intestine. Specimens should be obtained under anaerobic conditions and quantitative colony counts determined. Generally, bacteria concentrations of greater than 10^5 organisms per mL are highly suggestive of bacterial overgrowth. Alternatively, one can attempt to demonstrate a metabolic effect of the bacterial overgrowth, such as intraluminal bile acid deconjugation by the bile acid or ^{14}C-glycocholate breath test. Cholylglycine-^{14}C (glycine-conjugated cholic acid with the radiolabeled ^{14}C on the glycine moiety) when ingested circulates normally in the enterohepatic circulation without deconjugation. Bacterial overgrowth within the small intestine splits the ^{14}C-labeled glycine moiety and subsequently oxidizes it to ^{14}C-labeled CO_2, which is absorbed in the intestine and exhaled. Excess $^{14}CO_2$ appears in the breath. The bile acid breath test cannot differentiate bacterial overgrowth from ileal damage or resection where excessive breath $^{14}CO_2$ production is due to bacterial deconjugation within the colon of unabsorbed ^{14}C-labeled glycocholate. This creates clinical difficulties, since bacterial overgrowth may be superimposed on ileal damage in such conditions as Crohn's disease.

Another hallmark of bacterial overgrowth is steatorrhea, detected by the 72-hour fecal fat collection.

The Schilling test also is abnormal. ^{57}Co-B$_{12}$ is given with intrinsic factor following a flushing dose of nonradioactive B$_{12}$ given parenterally to prevent tissue storage of the labeled vitamin. In healthy subjects, ^{57}Co-B$_{12}$ combines with intrinsic factor and is absorbed and >8% excreted in the urine within 24 hours. In patients with bacterial overgrowth, the bacteria combine with or destroy intrinsic factor, the vitamin or both, causing decreased vitamin B$_{12}$ absorption. Following treatment with antibiotics the B$_{12}$ absorption returns to normal.

Breath hydrogen analysis allows a distinct separation of metabolic activity of intestinal flora of the host, since no hydrogen production is known to occur in mammalian tissue. Excessive and early breath hydrogen production has been noted in patients with bacterial overgrowth following the oral administration of either 50 g of glucose or 10 g of lactulose.

Treatment of bacterial overgrowth involves removing the cause, if possible. The addition of a broad-spectrum antibiotic (tetracycline 250 mg q.i.d., often accompanied by metronidazole 250 mg q.i.d., for 10 days) will often induce a remission for many months. If the cause cannot be eliminated and symptoms recur, good results can be achieved with intermittent antibiotics (e.g., one week out of every six).

18. PROTEIN-LOSING ENTEROPATHY

Protein-losing enteropathy describes a wide range of gastrointestinal disorders that are associated with an excessive loss of plasma protein into the gut lumen. Normal daily enteric loss of plasma protein corresponds to less than 1–2% of the plasma pool. The route of plasma protein loss across the normal mucosa is not well defined. It is likely that rapid shedding of epithelial cells from the mucosal surface is accompanied by loss of plasma proteins from the lamina propria at the site of cell extrusion.

In virtually any small intestinal disease, excessive transmural loss of plasma proteins may result from several mechanisms: in mucosal disease without ulceration but with increased permeability; in mucosal disease with erosion or ulceration (loss of inflammatory exudate that contains protein occurs); and in lymphatic obstruction with direct leakage of intestinal lymph from obstructed lacteals. Adaptive changes in endogenous synthesis of individual plasma proteins may compensate partially for excessive enteric loss.

Clinically, albumin loss may be manifested by dependent edema. A depression of the levels of thyroid and cortisol binding proteins will lower the total plasma level of these hormones, although normal levels of free hormone will maintain normal hormone function. Excessive enteric loss of plasma proteins other than albumin rarely leads to clinical problems; secondary hypogamma-globulinemia in these patients does not predispose them to infection, and the loss of blood clotting factors is rarely sufficient to impair hemostasis.

Patients with protein-losing enteropathy due to lymphatic obstruction, however, lose not only albumin and other plasma proteins but also intestinal lymph, with loss of long-chain triglycerides, fat-soluble vitamins and small lymphocytes.

Protein-losing enteropathy is considered in patients who exhibit hypoproteinemia and in whom other causes for hypoproteinemia (e.g., proteinuria, protein malnutrition and liver disease) are excluded. Fecal protein loss can then be quantitated using ^{51}Cr-labeled albumin or a_1-antitrypsin clearance into stool.

Management of protein-losing enteropathy involves the appropriate treatment of the disease(s) causing the protein loss. Enteral or parenteral feeding can be used to improve nutrition while the underlying disease is being treated. Enteric protein loss in patients with intestinal lymphangiectasia usually decreases with a low-fat diet. The normal absorption of long-chain triglycerides stimulates intestinal lymph flow; in their absence there is a decrease in the pressure within intestinal lymphatic vessels and hence a diminished loss of lymph into the lumen. Medium-chain triglycerides, which do not require intestinal lymphatic transport, can be substituted for the long-chain triglycerides and further decrease intestinal lymphatic pressure, with subsequent reduction in enteric lymph and protein loss.

19. MECKEL'S DIVERTICULUM

Meckel's diverticulum, an omphalomesenteric duct remnant, is a congenital outpouching usually located in the distal 100 cm of the ileum. Such diverticula are present in 1–3% of the general population. Of these, 30–40% are asymptomatic. Complications of Meckel's diverticulum include hemorrhage, intestinal obstruction, diverticulitis, umbilical discharge, perforation and peritonitis. Bleeding is the most common complication, resulting from ulceration of the ileal mucosa adjacent to atopic gastric mucosa located within the diverticulum. This is often painless and is usually encountered in children and young adults. Meckel's diverticulum accounts for nearly 50% of all lower gastrointestinal bleeding in children. Technetium-99m pertechnetate is normally taken by the ectopic gastric mucosa, providing the basis for the Meckel scan. Since only 60% of Meckel's diverticula contain ectopic gastric mucosa, false negative results occur.

20. CARCINOID SYNDROME

Over 90% of carcinoid tumors originate in the gastrointestinal tract. The most frequent sites are the appendix, terminal ileum and rectum. In general, non-metastasized carcinoid tumors are asymptomatic. The carcinoid syndrome is associated only with carcinoid tumors that have metastasized extensively to the liver or are extraintestinal (e.g., lung tumors). Metastasis is infrequent in carcinoids of the appendix, but is common in extra-appendiceal carcinoids.

Although carcinoid tumors differ in their ability to produce and store 5-hydroxytryptamine (5-HT), the excessive production of this substance and its metabolite 5-hydroxyindoleacetic acid (5-HIAA) remains their most characteristic chemical abnormality. Production of this hormone (as well as histamine, catecholamines, kinase and prostaglandins) causes the majority of symptoms. The symptom complex comprises diarrhea, flushing, wheezing, valvular heart disease (particularly pulmonary stenosis) and a pellagra-like skin rash. The carcinoid syndrome can be suspected clinically and confirmed biochemically by the demonstration of increased urinary 5-HIAA or platelet 5-HT.

Once the carcinoid syndrome is apparent, cure is usually impossible, since the tumor has metastasized by this time. Nevertheless, the intestinal origin of the tumor should be removed if it is causing obstruction. Serotonin antagonists (e.g., methysergide and cyproheptadine) can sometimes reduce symptoms. It is prudent to delay initiation of chemotherapy or radiation in the early metastatic stage of the disease, since the course is often indolent and patients survive many years with diffuse metastatic disease.

21. WHIPPLE'S DISEASE

Whipple's disease characteristically occurs in middle-aged men, who present with weight loss, fever, abdominal pain, arthralgias and intestinal symptoms of diarrhea and malabsorption. Small bowel biopsy characteristically demonstrates PAS-positive macrophages and bacilliform bodies plus an enteropathy with villous atrophy. Treatment with tetracycline improves the fever and joint symptoms within a few days; the diarrhea and malabsorption disappear within two to four weeks. Relapses may occur up to one or two years later and require repeat therapy.

22. IDIOPATHIC INTESTINAL PSEUDO-OBSTRUCTION

Idiopathic intestinal pseudo-obstruction is a disease of the muscular layer or of the enteric nervous system of the intestine. The myogenic form of idiopathic intestinal pseudo-obstruction is an autosomal dominant disease characterized by thinning of the intestinal musculature due to degeneration, fibrosis, malaligned smooth fibers and abnormal contractile filaments. All parts of the intestinal tract may be involved, but usually the small intestine, esophagus and colon are the most severely affected.

The neurogenic form of this disease is characterized by abnormal neuronal and glial cells. The damage may be in the spinal cord or in the splanchnic ganglia. When the splanchnic ganglia are involved, intranuclear inclusion bodies can be identified. The condition is characterized by abnormal systemic neural function, with an inappropriate blood pressure response to phenylephrine, Valsalva's maneuver, or achieving the upright posture. There is a lack of sweating on warming of the skin, pupillary denervation hypersensitivity, and lack of intestinal spike activity after small intestinal distention.

Treatment of both the myogenic and neurogenic forms of idiopathic intestinal pseudo-obstruction is generally unsuccessful. Anticholinergics and various promotility agents have been tried with only transient success. Associated bacterial overgrowth may worsen bloating and diarrhea, and should be treated with antibiotics. Surgery only aggravates the disorder and provides long intervals of severe ileus. Home parenteral nutrition may be the only alternative.

23. SMALL INTESTINAL VASCULAR DISORDERS

23.1 Acute Mesenteric Ischemia

The major causes of acute mesenteric ischemia are embolic obstruction thrombosis of the superior mesenteric artery (SMA), mesenteric venous thrombosis and nonocclusive ischemia. Embolic obstruction of the superior mesenteric artery is usually associated with cardiac arrhythmias, valvular disease, recent myocardial infarction or mycotic aneurysm. When an embolus lodges at the origin of the superior mesenteric artery, the entire small bowel and proximal colon are affected. Mesenteric venous thrombosis usually involves the superior mesenteric vein or its branches and the portal vein. It can be "primary" or "secondary" to a variety of hypercoagulable states (e.g., polycythemia rubra vera, carcinomatosis, oral contraception); to intra-abdominal sepsis (e.g., cholangitis, diverticular abscess); or to a condition in which blood flow is impaired (e.g., cardiogenic shock).

Nonocclusive bowel ischemia is the most common and lethal form of intestinal vascular insufficiency, accounting for at least 50% of all cases, with a mortality rate approaching 100%. It is commonly associated with reduced cardiac output, intra-abdominal sepsis and advanced malignant neoplasms. Digitalis constricts the splanchnic circulation and may aggravate or even precipitate mesenteric ischemia.

The typical patient is over 50 years of age, with arteriosclerotic or valvular heart disease, poorly controlled long-standing congestive heart failure, hypotension, recent myocardial infarction or cardiac arrhythmias. Abdominal pain is characteristically periumbilical and crampy. In the early stages, physical signs are often minimal. The abdomen is soft, sometimes slightly distended, with mild tenderness on palpation. Abdominal pain of any degree of severity associated with minimal abdominal findings and a high WBC (often over $20,000/mm^2$) is an important early clue to the correct diagnosis. Signs of advanced ischemia include nausea, vomiting, peritoneal irritation, leukocytosis and a progressive metabolic acidosis. In a minority, unexplained abdominal distention or gastrointestinal bleeding, or the rapid onset of confusion and acidosis in an elderly patient, may be the first manifestation of small bowel ischemia.

Initial resuscitation is directed at correcting the predisposing or precipitating cause(s). Restoration of cardiac output with IV fluid is paramount. Digitalis, diuretics and vasoconstrictors should be discontinued if possible. Plain radiographs, ultrasound or CT scans as appropriate should exclude other radiologically diagnosable causes of acute abdominal pain. After volume repletion, the key step in the management of acute mesenteric ischemia is abdominal angiography. Remember that angiography in a hypovolemic or hypotensive patient frequently shows mesenteric vasoconstriction; for such patients the technique loses its usefulness as a diagnostic tool. If the angiogram is normal, the patient should be carefully observed, and a diagnostic laparotomy performed only if peritoneal signs develop. If the angiogram shows a minor arterial occlusion and clinically there is no peritoneal irritation, papaverine can be infused into the superior mesenteric artery through the catheter used for angiography at a rate of 60 mg/hour. (The role of angioplasty or other angiographic techniques remains unproven.) If peritoneal signs occur at any time, a laparotomy with resection of the ischemic segment is indicated. If the angiogram shows a major obstruction at the origin of the superior mesenteric artery, laparotomy should be carried out immediately. An embolus can usually be easily removed, while thrombotic obstruction requires a bypass graft from the aorta to an area of the artery distal to the site of obstruction. After revascularization, any nonviable bowel should be resected. It is advisable to save all bowel that may be viable and to re-explore the patient 24 hours later. The decision to perform a "second look" operation is made at the initial laparotomy and should not be changed on the basis of a favorable postoperative course. Since acute occlusion of the superior mesenteric artery is associated with prolonged vasospasm, the artery should be perfused with papaverine for 24 hours postoperatively.

If nonocclusive splanchnic vasoconstriction is present, intra-arterial papaverine infusion should be started. If, in spite of the infusion, abdominal pain persists and signs of peritoneal irritation appear, a laparotomy must be performed without delay.

Venous thrombosis is characterized on the angiogram by a prolonged arterial phase and a lack of opacity in the venous system. If a firm diagnosis of venous thrombosis has been made, anticoagulants are appropriate. However, if the patient develops peritoneal signs, immediate laparotomy and resection are indicated.

This systemic approach to the management of ischemia originating in the superior mesenteric artery results in earlier diagnosis and avoidance of surgery. The overall mortality rate has been reduced to about 50%; 90% of the patients who have no peritoneal signs at the time of angiography survive.

23.2 Chronic Mesenteric Ischemia

This uncommon condition occurs in elderly patients with partial occlusion of at least two of the three principal mesenteric vessels. Epigastric or periumbilical abdominal pain beginning after a meal and lasting for one to three hours *("intestinal angina")* is the most characteristic clinical feature, although it is not often elicited. The pain may lead to a reduction in food intake (sitophobia) and secondarily a significant loss of weight. Bloating, flatulence and diarrhea are common, and steatorrhea is present in 50% of patients. The physical examination is usually not diagnostic. A systolic abdominal bruit is present in 50% of patients but is not pathognomonic. (Epigastric bruits are common.) Patients in whom the syndrome is suspected, and who have no other demonstrable abnormality to explain their symptoms, should have abdominal angiography. If angiography shows greater than 90% occlusion of at least two vessels, aorto-SMA graft is the procedure of choice. The mortality rate for this procedure is less than 10% and the majority of patients will be relieved of their postprandial intestinal angina.

24. SMALL BOWEL TUMORS

24.1 Benign Small Bowel Tumors

Adenomas, leiomyomas and lipomas are the three most frequently discovered primary tumors of the small intestine. Hamartomas, fibromas, angiomas and neurogenic tumors are much less common. As a general rule, benign tumors are least common in the duodenum and increase in frequency toward the ileum. Benign tumors often remain asymptomatic and are usually found incidentally.

Symptomatic benign tumors present primarily with obstructive features, giving rise to intermittent colicky abdominal pain or complete bowel obstruction. Bleeding may occur, particularly from leiomyomas that ulcerate centrally. Intussusception occurs with polypoid distal lesions.

24.2 Malignant Neoplasms of the Small Intestine

Adenocarcinomas, lymphomas, leiomyosarcomas and carcinoids are the most common primary small bowel malignant tumors. Metastatic cancer to the small intestine occurs rarely in patients with melanoma, breast cancer and lung cancer. Primary adenocarcinomas occur in the duodenal and proximal jejunum as annular lesions, narrowing the lumen and presenting with the signs and symptoms of obstruction. Leiomyosarcomas are evenly distributed along the small bowel. Symptoms are similar to those of adenocarcinoma – i.e., crampy abdominal pain and bleeding. Lymphoma of the small bowel must be carefully evaluated to determine whether the tumor has originated in the small intestine (primary lymphoma) or whether the small bowel is involved by a diffuse systemic lymphoma. Primary lymphoma of the small intestine is usually a histiocytic lymphoma. The lymphoma is most often proximal and presents with abdominal pain, weight loss, malabsorption, perforation and anemia. There is an increased incidence of primary lymphoma in patients with long-standing celiac disease or immunodeficiency states and in renal transplant patients receiving chronic immunosuppressive therapy.

A specific form of malignant lymphoma called immunoproliferative small intestinal disease occurs in people of Mediterranean descent. It is characterized by proliferation of mucosal B cells and has a high incidence of α-heavy chain paraproteinemia. It typically involves the duodenum and proximal jejunum, presenting with diarrhea and malabsorption.

OBJECTIVES

1. Discuss the intestinal fluid and electrolyte transport mechanisms.
2. Explain the normal digestion and absorption processes of fat, protein and glucose.
3. Describe the normal pathway of vitamin B_{12}, folate and iron absorption.
4. Locate the absorption sites of Fe, folate and B_{12}.
5. Utilize proper malabsorption screens in patients with chronic diarrhea.
6. Discuss normal enterohepatic circulation of bile acids.
7. Discuss normal assimilation of fat-soluble vitamins (A, D, E and K).

Diarrhea

1. Define diarrhea.
2. Classify the causes of diarrhea.
3. Discuss the pathogenic mechanisms of diarrhea.
4. Review diarrhea as altered fluid and electrolyte transport.
5. Differentiate between large and small bowel diarrhea.
6. Discuss diagnostic plans in patients with chronic diarrhea.
7. List conditions that are associated with typical small bowel lesions on biopsy.
8. List the complications of celiac disease.
9. List extraintestinal manifestations of celiac disease.
10. Outline the diagnosis and dietary management of celiac disease.
11. Give the differential diagnosis of "unresponsive" sprue.
12. Discuss the immunologic basis of celiac disease.
13. Recognize the principal manifestation of the carcinoid syndrome.
14. Discuss pharmacologic agents used in the carcinoid syndrome.
15. List biochemical tests used in diagnosing the carcinoid syndrome.
16. Discuss the management of traveler's diarrhea.
17. List the common causes of traveler's diarrhea.
18. Discuss the mechanisms of E. coli–induced diarrhea.
19. List the infectious causes of diarrhea and their management.
20. Discuss the use and mechanisms of antidiarrheal agents.
21. Give the differential diagnosis of abnormal terminal ileum.
22. Describe the radiographic features of small bowel obstruction.
23. Outline the etiology of vitamin B_{12} deficiency with the bacterial overgrowth syndrome.
24. List the underlying conditions associated with bacterial overgrowth.
25. Discuss the mechanisms of steatorrhea associated with the bacterial overgrowth syndrome.
26. Recognize the clinical presentations of the bacterial overgrowth syndrome.
27. Outline the management of the bacterial overgrowth syndrome.
28. Utilize appropriate diagnostic tests for the bacterial overgrowth syndrome.
29. Recognize complications of the short bowel syndrome and their mechanisms.
30. Discuss the adaptive mechanisms of the small bowel following resection.
31. Discuss the management of the short bowel syndrome.
32. Give the indications for the use of medium-chain triglycerides.
33. Outline the diagnosis and treatment of giardiasis.

34. Recognize the clinical presentations and treatment of amebiasis.
35. Describe typical features of Whipple's disease.
36. List the causes of protein-losing enteropathy.
37. List the possible mechanisms of diarrhea in patients with diabetes mellitus.
38. List the possible mechanisms of diarrhea in the Zollinger-Ellison syndrome.
39. List mechanisms of diarrhea following gastric surgery.
40. Discuss diagnostic tests for lactase deficiency/lactose intolerance.
41. List conditions associated with protein-losing enteropathy.
42. Recognize the features of intestinal lymphangiectasia and outline its treatment.

Skills
1. Give the indications for gastroscopy, small bowel biopsy, sigmoidoscopy and colonoscopy.
2. Arrange the proper sequences of GI diagnostic procedures, including radiographic examination (ultrasound, CT scan), and the appropriate order of investigational tests.
3. Utilize proper tests – including malabsorption screen, ^{14}C breath test, H_2 breath test, Schilling test, 72-hour stool collection, x-ray, small bowel biopsy and jejunal aspiration – in the investigation of chronic diarrhea.

Additional Objectives
1. Discuss different compositions of gastrointestinal gas.
2. Develop an awareness of types, availability, indications and complications of the following procedures:
   a. Upper endoscopy
   b. Sclerotherapy
   c. Small bowel biopsy
   d. Colonoscopy
   e. Polypectomy
   f. Sigmoidoscopy
   g. Papillotomy
   h. BICCP photocoagulation
   i. PEG
   j. ERCP
   k. Percutaneous transhepatic cholangiogram
   l. Liver biopsy

8
Gay Bowel Syndrome

R.N. Fedorak, P. Hallé and A.B.R. Thomson

1. INTRODUCTION

GAY BOWEL SYNDROME is the term recently developed to encompass the vast array of intestinal infections in homosexual men in addition to traumatic and other noninfectious problems. Homosexual men suffer the same health problems that afflict heterosexual men. However, they are also at risk for problems unique to their sexual orientation.

Noninfectious gastrointestinal health problems include those related to anorectal trauma and those gastrointestinal malignancies that have a higher incidence in the homosexual than in the heterosexual population (Table 1).

Infectious intestinal problems occur frequently and are often polymicrobial. In immunocompetent patients, they include enteric pathogens as well as the traditional venereal pathogens that also cause disease (Table 2A). In immunosuppressed patients with acquired immune deficiency syndrome (AIDS), additional opportunistic infections within the gastrointestinal tract often occur (Table 2B).

2. OBTAINING A MEDICAL AND SEXUAL HISTORY FROM THE HOMOSEXUAL MAN

2.1 Sexual Orientation
When seeing a patient with suspected gay bowel syndrome, a history of sexual activity and orientation is critical. Many physicians, however, have extreme difficulty in obtaining this part of the history.

It may be useful to preface the question with an explanation – e.g., "As you

TABLE 1. Noninfectious manifestations of the gay bowel syndrome

---

Anorectal trauma
Anal fissures and ulcers
Cryptitis and rectal abscess
Retained foreign bodies
Mucosal lacerations
Anal sphincter injury
Perforation of the rectosigmoid

Gastrointestinal malignancies
Carcinoma of the anal canal
Squamous cell carcinoma in situ
Lymphoma
Kaposi's sarcoma

---

are aware, many medical conditions and symptoms may be related to a person's sexual preference."

The physician may then proceed to ask whether the person is heterosexual, homosexual or bisexual. Since these formal phrases are avoided by much of the gay population, informal questioning as to whether the patient is gay, straight, bisexual or not sexually active might be preferred. Alternatively, one may ask whether the person prefers to have sex with men, women, both or neither.

If this direct questioning appears difficult, one can seek the answer indirectly when asking other questions about personal lifestyle. Questions relating to recent travel, sexual practices, diet or the use of drugs may be useful. Another indirect approach that is possible in the clinical context involves asking the patient whether it is possible that he could have gonorrhea of the anus or throat.

Both verbal and nonverbal communication can interfere with the patient–doctor relationship. A negatively phrased question conveys a judgmental attitude.

Sexual activity is also ascertained by asking about the number of male and female sexual partners over the previous 3–12 months and the number of regular and incidental sexual contacts during this period. Multiple sexual partners increase the risk of transmissible disease. Obtaining a history of sexual practices is as important as determining the risk factors for the presence of sexually transmitted disease and traumatic problems. A frank and open discussion of specific sexual practices is the only way to acquire this information.

The physician should also ask about the associated use of drugs and alcohol, and any past history of diseases associated with sexual intercourse.

TABLE 2. Infectious manifestations of the gay bowel syndrome

A. *Infections frequent in both immunocompetent and immunosuppressed hosts*
Shigella
Salmonella
Campylobacter
Giardia lamblia
Entamoeba histolytica
Neisseria gonorrhoeae
Chlamydia trachomatis
Treponema pallidum
Herpes simplex virus
Human papilloma virus

B. *Infections frequent only in immunosuppressed hosts*
Candida
Cryptosporidia
Isospora
Mycobacterium avium-intracellulare
Cytomegalovirus
Microsporidia

2.2 Diagnosis of AIDS in Homosexual Men

AIDS is the symptom complex that develops as a result of exposure to human immunodeficiency virus type 1 (HIV-1).

HIV-1 produces chronic, active, usually lifelong infection of CD4+ (helper) lymphocytes. After an incubation period of four to eight weeks, an acute mononucleosis-like syndrome may occur, with fever, malaise and lymphadenopathy. This syndrome resolves; however, the majority of HIV-positive individuals remain infected and are presumed to be persistently viremic and therefore potentially infectious to others. Between 70 and 90% of infected individuals develop late clinical features with the consequent syndromes. Nearly all (but not 100%) of HIV-infected people progress to AIDS, with the eventual development of opportunistic infections (e.g., Pneumocystis carinii pneumonia, Candida esophagitis) or tumors (e.g., Kaposi's sarcoma, lymphoma).

Voluntary HIV testing (with pre- and post-test counseling) of asymptomatic homosexual or bisexual males is recommended, since prophylactic therapy may prolong survival. Sexual contacts need to be made aware and "safe sex" practiced.

Should a physician ask a patient to sign a consent form before the test is ordered? This personal decision will depend upon the relationship established with each individual patient and should be made with a view to the social and/ or economic disadvantage or prejudice that may befall the patient as an indirect result of HIV antibody testing. Physicians should obtain the patient's informed consent before doing an HIV test. At all times, measures should be taken in the hospital and in the physician's office to ensure confidentiality.

3. TRAUMA AND NONINFECTIOUS PROBLEMS IN HOMOSEXUAL MEN

3.1 Anorectal Trauma
All men who present with anorectal trauma should be evaluated to determine the nature of the injury and evidence of perforation, peritonitis or bleeding. A frank history of sexual activities, drugs, past anorectal trauma and venereal disease should be sought.

3.1.1 *ANAL FISSURES AND ULCERS*
Lateral fissures, multiple fissures or associated proctitis point to a sexually related cause. Painful ulcers are commonly caused by herpes simplex virus or by trauma and less commonly caused by syphilis, lymphogranuloma venereum and amebiasis. Traumatic ulcers often relate to a specific event. Herpetic ulcers produce severe pain, paresthesias, inguinal lymphadenopathy and difficulty with urination. An infectious agent should always be sought. Serology, cultures for herpes simplex, and darkfield examination should be done. With associated proctitis, chlamydial culture and stool for culture, ova and parasites are required. Infections are treated with the appropriate antimicrobial agent. Fissures may respond to topical analgesics, sitz baths and bulk agents.

3.1.2 *CRYPTITIS AND RECTAL ABSCESSES*
The use of petroleum products (petrolatum jelly or mineral oil) during anal intercourse often causes cryptitis and mucosal granulomas. If these problems are left unattended, rectal abscesses may develop, presenting as firm, tender rectal or perirectal masses. Rectal abscesses in homosexual men respond to standard surgical drainage; however, special cultures should be obtained to rule out associated Neisseria gonorrhoeae, which requires specific antimicrobial therapy.

3.1.3 *RETAINED FOREIGN BODIES*
An array of objects (e.g., vegetables, fruit, bottles, billiard balls, light bulbs and vibrators) can become "lost in the colon" when they slip through the anal sphincter and advance into the upper rectum (or higher, if pushed).

Patients are usually embarrassed after having tried unsuccessfully to remove the foreign objects at home. Examination should exclude major complications of perforation, peritonitis or hemorrhage. The location and shape of the object is then determined by digital examination and/or x-ray (if radiopaque). Enemas and cathartics are avoided since they can push the object further into the colon or increase impaction and surrounding edema, respectively.

Visualization of the foreign body by anoscopy or sigmoidoscopy allows it to be grabbed directly with a uterine tenaculum and removed through the anoscope. If the foreign body cannot be removed without pain or trauma, the anal canal must be dilated under local or general anesthesia. Grasping blindly with an instrument can traumatize the bowel wall and lacerate it. Following removal of the foreign body it is mandatory to perform sigmoidoscopy and repeat the abdominal examination to exclude injury or peritonitis. Again, culture for Neisseria gonorrhoeae and syphilis serology are taken.

3.1.4 MUCOSAL LACERATIONS
Mucosal laceration typically presents with mild rectal bleeding and pain. Treatment is the same as for any other patient with rectal bleeding: signs of peritonitis are looked for and the patient is resuscitated with fluids as necessary. The site of bleeding is identified with sigmoidoscopy, colonoscopy or barium enema. The majority of lacerations stop bleeding spontaneously; endoscopic cautery or surgical repair rarely is required.

3.1.5 ANAL SPHINCTER INJURY
Permanent anal sphincter injury is uncommon. Primary surgical repair is the treatment of choice provided no secondary infection exists. When perirectal inflammation is present, a diverting colostomy with mucus fistula rests the area. The inflammation should respond to local therapy. A secondary surgical sphincter repair is then performed following resolution of the inflammation.

3.1.6 PERFORATION OF THE RECTOSIGMOID COLON
Transmural perforations of the rectosigmoid are infrequent. Free perforations above the peritoneal reflection present as sharp, severe abdominal pain and rectal bleeding. Most perforations of this type are in the anterior rectosigmoid wall just above the peritoneal reflection. The diagnosis is confirmed by demonstrating free interperitoneal air on x-ray. If the diagnosis is in doubt, a water-soluble enema can be performed. Free perforation is treated with laparotomy, repair or excision of the injured bowel, diverting colostomy and broad-spectrum antimicrobial agents.

Perforation below the peritoneal reflection results in severe pelvic cellulitis. The patient presents several days following injury with fever, rectal pain and discharge. Examination reveals perirectal induration and acute proctitis. Management of extraperitoneal perforation includes broad-spectrum antibiotics. Surgery is not usually required, except when a perirectal or supralevator abscess develops.

3.2 Gastrointestinal Malignancies

3.2.1 CARCINOMA OF THE ANAL CANAL

Homosexual men who practice anoreceptive intercourse may be at increased risk for developing squamous cell and transitional cell carcinoma of the anal canal. There is no alteration in the risk of adenocarcinoma of the rectum or colon, or in the risk of perianal squamous cell carcinoma. Carcinoma of the anal canal arises in transitional epithelium at the dentate line. Embryologically, this transitional epithelium has an origin similar to that found on the cervix. The association of carcinoma of the uterine cervix with sexual activity and with sexually transmitted herpes simplex 2 and condylomata acuminata has been documented. A similar association of anal canal carcinoma and anal sexual activity is thus likely.

Anal carcinoma, presenting as a mass with a fissure or fistula, causes anorectal pain and bleeding. The differential diagnosis includes benign, infectious etiology, such as syphilis, amebiasis, lymphogranuloma venereum and condylomata acuminata. The definitive diagnosis comes from biopsy of a highly suspicious lesion or one that fails to heal following successful treatment of a secondary infection. Radiation therapy combined with chemotherapy has effected cures while preserving anorectal function.

3.2.2 SQUAMOUS CELL CARCINOMA IN SITU

Squamous cell carcinoma in situ is often an incidental finding associated with condylomata acuminata and herpes simplex ulcers. Localized disease is treated with local incision. Multicentric disease requires topical 5-fluorouracil cream. The etiology of these lesions, although unknown, may relate to the human papilloma virus.

3.2.3 GASTROINTESTINAL LYMPHOMAS

B-cell lymphoma is the second most common neoplasm in AIDS. It is typically extranodal. The most common locations are the brain and the gastrointestinal tract. Most lymphomas are B-cell lymphomas; they include small- and large-cell types, with smaller subgroups of patients having Burkitt's lymphoma and Hodgkin's disease. These lymphomas develop secondarily to underlying immunosuppression from infection with the HIV-1 virus.

Most intestinal lymphomas in AIDS are aggressive, occurring in the mesentery with extension to the retroperitoneum and other viscera. The patients present with peripheral and abdominal lymphadenopathy and gastrointestinal symptoms, including diarrhea and abdominal pain. The diagnosis is usually made via ultrasound-guided biopsy or CT.

Lymphoma in AIDS is treated by combination chemotherapy.

3.2.4 KAPOSI'S SARCOMA

Kaposi's sarcoma is a multifocal neoplasm of the reticuloendothelial system. Since 1979, an aggressive form of Kaposi's sarcoma has been diagnosed with increasing frequency in patients with AIDS. These patients have a high incidence of gastrointestinal and visceral involvement.

Kaposi's sarcoma develops in one-third to one-half of AIDS patients. The GI tract is involved only when there is cutaneous and/or nodal involvement, and then only in about 40% of such patients. On endoscopy the lesion appears either macular (with intense submucosal hemorrhage) or nodular. Nodular lesions are violaceous, measuring 5–15 mm, and hemorrhage is less prominent. The majority of patients have no clinical symptoms related to gastrointestinal Kaposi's sarcoma. If symptoms do occur they are the cause of bulky lesions of the gingiva or palate that interfere with mastication, lesions of the hypopharynx that affect swallowing, lesions of the stomach or intestine that cause obstruction to luminal flow, lymphatic obstruction with diarrhea and GI bleeding from these relatively vascular tumors.

The tumor may be treated by local or systemic therapy. Local laser excision can be performed in the mouth, stomach and colon. The lesion is also responsive to radiation therapy and combination chemotherapy with doxorubicin hydrochloride, bleomycin and vincristine.

4. GASTROINTESTINAL INFECTIONS IN HOMOSEXUAL MEN

Infections in the homosexual population can be divided into those afflicting the immunocompetent population as well as the immunosuppressed population (particularly people with AIDS) (Table 2A) and those enteric infections almost exclusively specific to the AIDS group (Table 2B).

Since most of these infections have a predilection for specific segments of the gastrointestinal tract, symptomatic disease can conveniently be separated into distinct anatomic regions. These include the oropharynx and esophagus, the small intestine, the colon and the rectum and perianal region.

The spectrum of disease associated with each infection depends upon a variety of factors, including the individual's immunologic competence, the microorganism and the duration of the infection. Since intestinal infections in homosexual men are frequently polymicrobial, a careful selection of microbial and gastrointestinal studies needs to be conducted. The following discussion will review intestinal infections in homosexual men with and without AIDS. Treatment regimens for each infection are summarized in Table 3.

4.1 Oropharynx and Esophagus

4.1.1 *CANDIDA*

Oral candidiasis in homosexual men is a significant predictive factor for the later development of serious upper gastrointestinal infections. Esophageal candidiasis is one of the most frequent infections in AIDS patients. Predominant symptoms of invasive Candida esophagitis are dysphagia and/or odynophagia. Barium swallow can demonstrate findings ranging from a shaggy outline of the esophageal wall to ulceration, intramural filling defects and even segmental strictures. The lesions are most prominent in the distal third of the esophagus. On endoscopy, there are white, plaque-like pseudomembranes. The pseudomembranes are firmly adherent, so that any attempt to remove them with a brush for cytology or with biopsy forceps is accompanied by bleeding.

Although their endoscopic appearance may vary slightly, similar esophageal symptoms may be caused by herpes simplex virus or cytomegalovirus (CMV). Endoscopic biopsies or brushings may be required to distinguish among these various etiologies. If ulcerations are demonstrated at endoscopy, mycelia can be demonstrated growing within the epithelium on biopsies when stained with a silver methenamine stain. Routine cultures from the esophageal mucosa for Candida and serum agglutinin titers against Candida are of little value, as many normal individuals harbor these organisms within the gastrointestinal tract without tissue invasion.

In AIDS patients with oral candidiasis and accompanying dysphagia or odynophagia, it can be assumed that esophageal candidiasis exists and empirical treatment can be started. Endoscopy can then be performed at a convenient time to exclude herpetic or CMV infections. Treatment should be started with oral nystatin 500,000 units p.o. q4h × 7 days. Since its fungicidal action is a local effect requiring contact with nystatin, nystatin suppositories kept in the mouth until they dissolve are an alternative and probably better therapy. Ketoconazole 200 mg p.o. q.d. or low-dose intravenous amphotericin B can be used when nystatin fails. Odynophagia is treated with viscous Xylocaine® for symptomatic relief.

TABLE 3.   Treatment regimens for sexually transmitted diseases commonly seen in homosexual men

Infectious organism	Drug of first choice	Alternative treatments
Campylobacter	Erythromycin 500 mg po qid × 7 d	Tetracycline 500 mg po qid × 7 d
Candida albicans (oral)	Nystatin 500,000 U po q4h × 7 d	Ketoconazole 200 mg po qd × 7 d
(esophagitis)	Fluconazole 100–200 mg po qd × 14 d	
Chlamydia trachomatis Non-LGV	Tetracycline 500 mg po qid × 7 d	Erythromycin 500 mg po qid × 7 d
LGV	Tetracycline 500 mg po qid × 21 d	Erythromycin 500 mg po qid × 21 d
Condylomata acuminata	Podophyllum (25%) to lesion every other day × 7 d	Cryotherapy Surgery
Cryptosporidium	Supportive fluid therapy and octreotide 300–500 μg sq bid	Spiramycin 1 g po qid × 14 d
Cytomegalovirus	Ganciclovir 5 mg/kg IV q12h × 14–21 d	
Entamoeba histolytica	Metronidazole 750 mg po tid × 10 d plus iodoquinol 650 mg po tid × 20 d	
Giardia lamblia	Metronidazole 250 mg po tid × 5 d	Quinacrine hydrochloride 100 mg po tid × 5 d
Haemophilus ducreyi (chancroid)	Erythromycin 500 mg po qid × 14 d or ceftriaxone 250 mg IM once	Trimethoprim-sulfamethoxazole 160 mg/800 mg po bid × 14 d
Herpes simplex	Acyclovir 5 mg/kg IV/po q8h × 5 d Acyclovir ointment 5%, topical q4–6h × 5 d	Foscarnet 40 mg/kg IV q8h × 21 d
Isospora belli	Trimethoprim-sulfamethoxazole 160 mg/800 mg po qid × 10 d then bid × 21 d	Pyrimethamine 50–75 mg qd × 21 d

(cont'd)

TABLE 3.   Treatment regimens for sexually transmitted diseases commonly seen in
homosexual men (cont'd)

Infectious organism	Drug of first choice	Alternative treatments
Microsporidium	None	Octreotide (somatostatin analogue) (symptomatic relief of diarrhea)
Mycobacterium avium-intracellulare	Rifampin 600 mg po qd, plus ethambutol 15–25 mg/kg po qd, plus ciprofloxacin 750 mg po bid, plus clofazimine 100–200 mg po bid	
Neisseria gonorrhoeae		
Anal or urethral	Ceftriaxone (250 mg IM once)	Procaine penicillin G (PPG) 4.8 million U IM, plus probenecid (1 g po)
Pharyngeal	Ceftriaxone (250 mg IM once)	PPG 4.8 million U IM plus probenecid (1 g po)
Salmonella	Antibiotics not recommended except for severe or bacteremic cases	Chloramphenicol 500 mg IV q6h × 10 d Ampicillin 1 g IV q4h × 10 d Trimethoprim-sulfamethoxazole 160 mg/800 mg po bid × 10 d
Scabies, lice	1% permethrin shampoo 0.5% malathion	Piperonyl butoxide lotion Lindane lotion or shampoo
Shigella	Trimethoprim-sulfamethoxazole 160 mg/800 mg po bid × 7 d	Ampicillin 500 mg po qid × 7 d
Strongyloides stercoralis	Thiabendazole 50 mg/kg po bid × 2 d (disseminated disease × 5 d)	Ivermectin 200 µg/kg/d × 1–2 d Albendazole 400 mg qd × 3 d

4.1.2 HERPES SIMPLEX ESOPHAGITIS

Symptoms – dysphagia, severe odynophagia and occasionally hematemesis – are often identical to those of Candida esophagitis. In contrast to Candida, however, the whitish pseudomembranes seen at endoscopy tend to be smaller and more focal, with the central portions appearing denuded. Brushings and biopsies taken from the border of herpes simplex ulcers show multinucleated giant cells and epithelial inclusion bodies.

Oral or intravenous acyclovir therapy (5 mg/kg q8h) can effectively decrease shedding of the virus and heal virus-induced ulcerations. Because recurrent infection is common, chronic therapy becomes necessary in some patients. Odynophagia may respond symptomatically to viscous Xylocaine®.

4.1.3 CYTOMEGALOVIRUS (CMV)

More than 50% of Canadian adults and 90% of homosexual men have serological evidence of prior exposure to CMV. Organ involvement occurs almost exclusively in immunosuppressed persons with CMV infection, producing an acute or chronic inflammation all along the gastrointestinal tract. Autopsy studies of AIDS patients demonstrate classical CMV inclusion bodies in the gastrointestinal tract in 95% of cases.

CMV esophagitis ranges from asymptomatic disease to severe dysphagia and/or odynophagia. Endoscopically it appears as an extensive area of mucosal injury with inflammatory exudate and ulceration. The pathogenesis of CMV-associated ulceration is controversial: the virus may be a secondary invader colonizing previously damaged tissue, or the ulceration may be explained by a vasculitis precipitated by endothelial cell CMV infiltration. The diagnosis of localized disease is based upon the presence of intracellular inclusion bodies in a biopsy specimen. CMV cultured from the biopsy specimen further supports the diagnosis in the nonviremic patient. Systemic CMV infections are confirmed by viral cultures of white blood cell buffy coats, by a fourfold rise in antibody titer or by urine culture of excreted CMV.

Therapy with acyclovir, interferon or vidarabine has been ineffective against CMV. Recently, ganciclovir 5 mg/kg IV q12h × 14–21 days has induced clinical improvement and decreased the quantity of detectable virus in AIDS patients with CMV disease.

4.2 Small Intestine

4.2.1 GIARDIA LAMBLIA

In homosexual men, Giardia lamblia is the most frequent infectious agent involving the small bowel. It has a prevalence rate of 30% and is transferred through oral–anal contact.

Although it may be asymptomatic, Giardia lamblia is often accompanied by vague symptoms of abdominal cramps, bloating, nausea and diarrhea. Rarely, there is malabsorption and steatorrhea.

Diagnosis depends upon demonstrating Giardia in ova and parasite examinations of the stool, duodenal aspirate, duodenal biopsy or the string test (Enterotest®). Recently an enzyme-linked immunosorbent assay (ELISA) has been developed for the detection of Giardia antigen in stool specimens.

Treatment consists of metronidazole 250 mg p.o. t.i.d. × 5 days or, alternatively, quinacrine hydrochloride 100 mg p.o. t.i.d. × 5 days.

4.2.2 CRYPTOSPORIDIUM

Prior to the discovery of AIDS, Cryptosporidium, a protozoal parasite, was virtually unknown as a cause of gastrointestinal disease in humans. It is now well recognized as causing a short, self-limiting diarrheal episode in normal immunocompetent persons. In contrast, in immunosuppressed patients with AIDS, Cryptosporidia can cause a severe, debilitating, watery diarrhea with resultant dehydration and death.

Diagnosis of Cryptosporidium infection is based on detection in stool of Cryptosporidium oocysts. Additionally, the organism can be identified on the brush border of intestinal biopsies from the small intestine or colon. Since the infection may skip areas, and the organism may be located distally in the ileum and not proximally in the duodenum, multiple biopsies may be required.

Treatment is not generally required for the self-limiting disease in immunocompetent individuals. In AIDS patients with severe diarrhea, intravenous fluid administration may be required to prevent volume depletion. In a small study, spiramycin 1 g p.o. q.i.d. was found to be effective in several AIDS patients with Cryptosporidia-induced diarrhea; however, subsequent studies have not confirmed these findings. Continued experimental treatments with spiramycin, paromomycin and octreotide (the somatostatin analogue) are under investigation.

4.2.3 ISOSPORA BELLI

Isospora belli is another coccidium parasite that inhabits the small bowel of homosexual men. This normally rare intestinal protozoan has been identified in 15% of Haitian AIDS patients and less frequently in North American AIDS patients. The clinical features and diagnostic methods are identical to those for Cryptosporidium. Trimethoprim-sulfamethoxazole 160 mg tmp/800 mg smx p.o. q.i.d. × 10 days then b.i.d. × 21 days is usually effective therapy. The average recurrence rate of Isospora belli is high, 47%; in individual cases recurrence can depend upon the duration of therapy.

4.2.4 *MYCOBACTERIUM AVIUM-INTRACELLULARE*
Mycobacterium avium-intracellulare (MAI), an atypical microbacterium of environmental origin (probably ingested in contaminated water), occurs frequently in severely immunosuppressed patients with AIDS. It can infect and infiltrate the lining of the small and large intestine, producing a thickened mucosa with increased numbers of macrophages in the lamina propria. Additionally, it can involve intra-abdominal lymph nodes and the liver, spleen, blood and bone marrow.

Clinically, enteric involvement presents with diarrhea, malabsorption and progressive wasting, whereas systemic involvement presents with fever. The diagnosis depends upon culture of this atypical microbacterium from appropriate biopsy specimens. Unfortunately, therapy for this life-threatening infection has been unsuccessful, even with up to six antituberculous agents.

4.2.5 *MICROSPORIDIUM*
This intracellular protozoan, which measures 1–2 µg in size, has been identified by electron microscopy in AIDS patients with enteritis and diarrhea. The offending species in AIDS has been identified as Enterocytozoon bieneusi. Electron microscopy demonstrates that the organisms are localized to intestinal epithelial cells. Clinically, infection with Microsporidium resembles infection with Cryptosporidium. Endoscopically, the small intestinal mucosa ranges from normal to diffusely erythematous. Partial villous atrophy with malabsorption is usually seen. There is no known effective therapy for Microsporidium.

4.2.6 *STRONGYLOIDES STERCORALIS*
Strongyloides infects the host by penetrating the skin as filariform larvae. They travel through capillaries to enter the lungs. They are then coughed up, swallowed, and reach the small intestine, where they release eggs that develop into infective filariform larvae. During rectal intercourse, infective filariform larvae within the rectal lumen may penetrate the skin directly. Pruritus, papillary rashes and edema may occur at the site of skin entry. Involvement of the intestine results in fever, nausea, weight loss, vomiting, diarrhea and abdominal pain. Diagnosis is best made on an examination of duodenal secretions. One duodenal drainage is equal to 10 concentrated stool specimens as a means of diagnosing Strongyloides. Thiabendazole 50 mg/kg p.o. b.i.d. × 2 days is

the treatment of choice. In disseminated Strongyloides, thiabendazole should be continued for at least 5 days.

4.2.7. HUMAN IMMUNODEFICIENCY VIRUS
There are several reasons to suspect that HIV itself plays a role in intestinal disease. Unexplained gastrointestinal symptoms are prevalent in HIV-infected patients. HIV has been localized to the intestinal mucosa by a number of techniques, including molecular hybridization and immunohistologic techniques. HIV-induced intestinal injury may occur as a direct result of virus-induced cell injury, as an indirect effect of anti-HIV immunity, or as an innocent bystander in a systemic inflammatory response. Further studies will be required to define the exact role of the HIV virus on intestinal structure.

4.3 Colon
Infections with Campylobacter, Shigella, Salmonella, Entamoeba histolytica, Chlamydia trachomatis and CMV are frequently associated with colitis in the homosexual population. These organisms invade the colon, producing hemorrhagic ulcerations. Patients complain of low abdominal pain and bloody diarrhea. The diseases are usually limited to the colon (except in AIDS, when they often become systemic).

4.3.1 SHIGELLA
Shigella sonnei and Shigella flexneri account for most of the infections seen in homosexual men. They are characterized by an abrupt onset of bloody diarrhea, fever, nausea and lower abdominal cramps. An extensive list of extraintestinal complications may be associated with Shigella dysentery. Respiratory symptoms (e.g., cough and coryza), meningismus, hemolytic uremic syndrome, rash and arthritis can occur up to two or three weeks after onset of the intestinal infection. Diagnosis is made by culturing the organism from the stool.

Management of mild disease requires only supportive therapy. The treatment of choice for moderate or severe disease is trimethoprim-sulfamethoxazole 160 mg tmp/800 mg smx p.o. b.i.d. × 7 days, since ampicillin-resistant species are rapidly becoming prevalent. Curiously, amoxicillin, which is very well absorbed and achieves higher serum levels than ampicillin, is not effective therapy for shigellosis. Chronic carriers of Shigella are unusual; however, when one does present the individual is prone to intermittent attacks of the disease. This is in contrast to Salmonella carriers, who rarely become symptomatic from their own strain. Trimethoprim-sulfamethoxazole eradicates the carrier state in about 90% of patients.

4.3.2 SALMONELLA

Salmonella infections present as one of five clinical syndromes: gastro-enteritis, noted in 70% of Salmonella infections; bacteremia, with or without gastrointestinal involvement, in approximately 10% of cases; typhoid or "enteric fever," seen with all Salmonella typhi serotypes and in 8% of all other nontyphoidal Salmonella serotypes; localized infections (i.e., joints, bones and meninges) in 5% of cases; and a carrier state in asymptomatic individuals (the organism usually is harbored in the gallbladder).

Salmonella typhimurium (a specific serotype of the nontyphoidal Salmonella) is not a common enteric pathogen in homosexual men, but is at least 20-fold more prevalent in AIDS patients with diarrhea than in the general population. Diarrhea, weight loss, fever and bacteremia usually accompany this infection in patients with AIDS. Often both the gastroenteritis and bacteremia are recurrent and refractory to antibiotics to which the organism is sensitive in vitro. The diagnosis of nontyphoidal salmonellosis, including Salmonella typhimurium gastroenteritis, is made by culturing the organism from the stool. With nontyphoidal Salmonella, antibiotic therapy increases the incidence and duration of intestinal carriage of these organisms. Therefore, antibiotics should not be used unless there is evidence of systemic infection or immuno-suppression. In these cases, the drug of choice is ampicillin 1 g IV q4h × 10 days or trimethoprim-sulfamethoxazole (160 mg tmp/800 mg smx) p.o. b.i.d. × 10 days. If sensitivity testing reveals resistance to the above antibiotics (resistance to four or more drugs in 50% of isolates of S. typhimurium is common in the gay population) then chloramphenicol 500 mg IV q6h × 10 days should be used. With typhoidal Salmonella infections, chloramphenicol 500 mg IV q6h × 10 days remains the treatment of choice.

4.3.3 CAMPYLOBACTER

In addition to the typical Campylobacter organisms seen in the heterosexual population, recent studies have also identified an atypical form of Campylo-bacter, referred to as "Campylobacter-like organisms." They are frequently isolated from homosexual men with and without intestinal symptoms. These organisms resemble Campylobacter jejuni morphologically, but differ in sensitivity to cephalothin, growth temperature requirements and DNA homology.

Infection with Campylobacter organisms presents with fever, chills, myalgia, abdominal pain and diarrhea. The diarrhea is bloody in 50% of cases and often has a biphasic character, with initial diarrhea, slight improvement and then increasing severity. Diagnosis is confirmed by culturing the organism from stool. A selective isolation medium containing antibiotics must be used, and the plates grown at 40°C under conditions of reduced CO_2 and reduced O_2. The treatment of choice is erythromycin 500 mg p.o. q.i.d. × 7 days.

4.3.4 *ENTAMOEBA HISTOLYTICA*

In major urban centers, 40% of homosexual men are infected with Entamoeba histolytica. One-half of these individuals harbor an asymptomatic carrier state. In symptomatic patients, diarrhea, tenesmus, abdominal cramps and anorectal discharge are prominent. Sigmoidoscopy in this group may resemble inflammatory bowel disease. Extraintestinal symptomatology and disseminated disease can occur in the presence of AIDS.

Diagnosis is based upon demonstration of Entamoeba histolytica in the stool or in the biopsy of a rectal-mucosal lesion. Serology is useful only in cases of invasive amebiasis; it is not useful for the noninvasive forms commonly seen in homosexual men.

Asymptomatic carriers of Entamoeba histolytica are treated with iodoquinol 650 mg p.o. t.i.d. × 20 days. Effective treatment of mild to severe disease requires the combination of two drugs: metronidazole 750 mg p.o. t.i.d. × 10 days is effective only against intramural organisms but not against intraluminal organisms; therefore it must be combined with iodoquinol 650 mg p.o. t.i.d. × 20 days, to remove intraluminal organisms.

4.4 Anorectum

4.4.1 *NEISSERIA GONORRHOEAE*

Infection of the rectum with Neisseria gonorrhoeae may result in either symptomatic or asymptomatic disease. Asymptomatic infection of the rectum constitutes a major reservoir of gonococcal infection in homosexual men.

When present, symptoms are usually mild and consist of rectal discomfort, tenesmus and mucopurulent discharge. On sigmoidoscopy, the rectal mucosa may be normal or slightly erythematous. Diagnosis is made by Gram's stain and culture of materials swabbed from the rectal mucosa. The sensitivity of a Gram's stain of rectal exudate in anorectal gonorrhea is 80% when obtained through an anoscope, compared with 50% for swabs obtained without the aid of an anoscope. Since co-infection with other pathogens is frequent, stool culture and ova and parasites must be obtained.

The treatment of choice for homosexual men with anorectal gonorrhea is ceftriaxone 250 mg IM once. Pharyngeal gonorrhea is treated similarly.

4.4.2 *HERPES SIMPLEX VIRUS*

Anorectal herpes simplex virus infection is second only to gonorrhea in frequency in association with proctitis in homosexual men. Anorectal herpes is acquired by either anal intercourse or oral–anal contact with an individual who has oral herpes. Herpes infection may involve the perianal area, anal canal or rectum. The major clinical form of herpes simplex virus in AIDS is a chronic perineal ulcer that is painful, shallow and slow-spreading. If symptoms are prominent they will include localized pain, rectal paresthesias, constipation and rectal discharge. The initial anorectal herpes infection is usually self-limiting and resolves in two to three weeks. Recurrences are frequent but less symptomatic. In immunosuppressed AIDS patients, severe, progressive, destructive mucocutaneous herpes often develops. Diagnosis is based on the clinical appearance of the herpetic vesicles and on the recovery of herpes simplex virus on viral culture. Biopsy of rectal mucosa will demonstrate intranuclear inclusion bodies and a mononuclear cell infiltrate. A fourfold rise in antibody titer also confirms the diagnosis.

For non-AIDS patients, treatment includes analgesics, sitz baths and topical acyclovir to shorten the duration of symptoms and viral shedding. If herpes proctitis is present in addition to cutaneous lesions, then acyclovir 5 mg/kg IV or p.o. q8h × 5 days should be added. For AIDS patients, topical therapy is inadequate and intravenous acyclovir should be administered during the acute episode; the patient should then be placed on oral acyclovir q8h indefinitely to suppress recurrences.

4.4.3 CHLAMYDIA TRACHOMATIS
Chlamydia trachomatis infections occur with the lymphogranuloma venereum (LGV) serotypes and non-LGV serotypes.

Chlamydia proctitis with non-LGV serotypes is nearly identical to that described for Neisseria gonorrhoeae infection. The disease may be asymptomatic or mildly symptomatic, with anorectal discharge, tenesmus and perianal discomfort.

In contrast, Chlamydia proctitis with LGV serotypes is invasive and induces a severe proctocolitis. There is diffuse, severe anorectal pain, bloody discharge, tenesmus and diarrhea. Sigmoidoscopy demonstrates diffuse friability of the rectum and colon. Biopsies demonstrate granuloma formation. In chronic cases, strictures and fistulas develop in the anorectal region.

The diagnosis is based on isolating Chlamydia trachomatis from the rectum. Serology is useful only to diagnose the LGV serotypes.

Treatment consists of tetracycline 500 mg p.o. q.i.d. × 7 days for non-LGV serotypes and × 21 days for LGV infections.

4.4.4 CONDYLOMATA ACUMINATA
Condylomata acuminata (anal warts) are caused by human papilloma virus. They are easily transmitted during anal intercourse. Clinically they appear in clusters as raised pink to brown papules with warty surfaces in the perianal region. Perianal itching and discomfort are common symptoms.

Topical podophyllum (25%) applied with a cotton applicator to the lesion and left on for four to six hours before being washed off is usually effective therapy. Reapplication can be carried out at daily intervals if necessary. Cryotherapy, laser beam therapy and surgical excision are recommended for refractory cases.

4.4.5 SYPHILIS

Infection of the anorectal area by Treponema pallidum presents with a painless chancre approximately three weeks after exposure by rectal intercourse. Typically, anal chancres are undetected because of failure to examine the anal area, or misdiagnosed as traumatic lesions or anal herpes. If undiagnosed, these primary chancres disappear, and secondary syphilis becomes manifested in the form of condylomata acuminata or as discrete masses or mucosal ulcerations in the rectum.

Diagnosis of anorectal syphilis is based on serology. Darkfield examination is useful but not specific for rectal lesions since nonpathogenic treponemes may be present. Biopsies of the lesions should be processed for more specific silver staining or immunofluorescence.

Treatment of primary, secondary or latent syphilis is usually benzathine penicillin G, 2.4 million units IM once.

9
Inflammatory Bowel Disease

R.N. Fedorak and A.B.R. Thomson

1. CROHN'S DISEASE

CROHN'S DISEASE, or regional enteritis, is a chronic inflammatory disorder that can affect the small intestine and/or the large intestine. Inflammation, which may or may not be accompanied by noncaseating granulomas, extends through all layers of the gut wall to involve adjacent mesentery and lymph nodes. The inflammatory process is frequently discontinuous, with normal bowel separating portions of diseased bowel. This disease is characterized by an indolent variable course, by its diverse clinical manifestations, by its perianal and systemic complications, and by its tendency to recur after surgical resection.

1.1 Pathology

The key pathological feature of Crohn's disease is an inflammatory process that extends through all layers of the bowel wall. Microscopic examination reveals (1) hyperplasia of perilymphatic histiocytes, (2) diffuse granulomatous infiltration, (3) discrete noncaseating granulomas in the submucosa and lamina propria, (4) edema and lymphatic dilatation of all layers of the gut, and (5) monocytic infiltration within lymph nodules and Peyer's patches on the serosal surface of the bowel.

The mesentery in the vicinity of the diseased bowel is markedly thickened, fatty and edematous. Finger-like projections of thick mesentery characteristically extend over the serosal surface toward the antimesenteric border. The mucosal surface in the diseased segment has a characteristic "cobblestone"

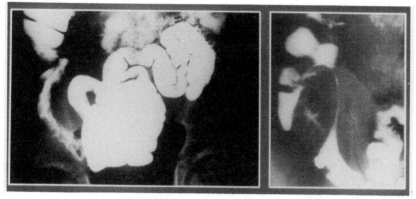

Ileitis   "String Sign"

FIGURE 1.   Crohn's disease. Barium contrast x-rays showing (a) ulcerations and narrowing characteristic of terminal ileal involvement and (b) the "string sign" as a consequence of stricturing following ulceration.

appearance, resulting from the combination of deep mucosal ulceration and nodular submucosal thickening. Ulcers are frequently elongated and tend to lie along the long axis of the bowel.

Since the serosa and mesentery are inflamed, a characteristic feature of Crohn's disease is the tendency for involved bowel loops to be firmly matted together by fibrotic bands. This adhesive process is often associated with the fistula formation characteristic of Crohn's disease. Fistulas begin as ulcerations and gradually burrow through the serosa into adjacent organs. Such fistulas communicate between the loops of small bowel themselves, as well as between loops of small bowel and colon, skin, perineum, bladder or vagina, or they may end blindly in indolent abscess cavities located within the peritoneal cavity, mesentery or retroperitoneal structures.

When the lesions of Crohn's disease are discontinuous, the intestine that lies adjacent to or between diseased segments (skip lesions) shows no gross or histological abnormalities.

1.2 Anatomic Distribution

Patients with Crohn's disease can be divided into those with small bowel disease alone (30%), those with both small and large bowel involvement (50%), and those with disease involving only the colon (20%) (Table 1). When Crohn's disease involves the small bowel, 80% of the time the terminal ileum is involved (Figure 1). In only 20% of cases are other areas of small bowel

TABLE 1. Anatomic distribution of Crohn's disease

Major site of involvement	Percentage
Small bowel only	30
Small bowel and colon	50
Colon only	20

also affected. When the colon is involved in Crohn's disease, all segments of the colon can be involved. Although absence of rectal disease is more characteristic of Crohn's disease than of ulcerative colitis, the rectum is involved in half those cases of Crohn's disease in which colonic disease exists.

1.3 Epidemiology
Crohn's disease occurs throughout the world, with a prevalence of 10 to 70 cases per 10^5 people. The disorder occurs most frequently among people of European origin, is 3 to 8 times more common among Jews than among non-Jews, and is more common among whites than nonwhites. Although the disorder can begin at any age, its onset most often occurs between 15 and 30 years of age. There appears to be a familial aggregation of patients with Crohn's disease such that 20–30% of patients with Crohn's disease have a family history of inflammatory bowel disease.

1.4 Etiology
The etiological agent responsible for inflammatory bowel disease has not yet been determined. The abnormalities of T cells and/or macrophages and their interaction still remains the most feasible hypothesis (1–4). In synthesizing existing literature, one could propose the following sequence of pathological events leading to the development of inflammatory bowel disease. The gastrointestinal immune system becomes exposed to a mucosal antigen, perhaps even an antigen normally present within the lumen – i.e., a bacterial constituent of normal flora. However, on this occasion the antigen does not evoke the typical antigen-specific suppressor T-cell activity, mucosal unresponsiveness. Rather, because of an antigen-specific immunoregulatory defect, it evokes helper T-cell activity and sets in play an ongoing immune response. This immune response as an epiphenomenon leads eventually to the development of self-antigens and appearance of autoantibodies. Subsequently, in an attempt to down-regulate the antigen-specific response, antigen-nonspecific suppressor T cells appear. Initially, these antigen-nonspecific suppressor T cells may prevent disease progression; however, they are gradually depleted, leaving the

unregulated antigen-specific helper T-cell activity to predominate. This unregulated antigen-specific immune response leads to the production of lymphokines, which stimulate migration of inflammatory and cytolytic cells to the region. Through this process the microscopic and gross morphological changes of inflammatory bowel disease are manifest.

The initiating antigen in the above process has yet to be identified. Mycobacteria have remained a contender as initiating antigen for a number of decades. However, recent studies have found no evidence for Crohn's disease–specific humoral or T-cell reactivity against a variety of mycobacterium species (5). Recent studies demonstrating an increase in intestinal permeability to polyethylene glycol (PEG-400) in healthy relatives of patients with Crohn's disease have proposed the hypothesis that Crohn's disease is caused by an epithelial permeability defect that allows exposure to an increased number of mucosal antigens (6). Whether the permeability abnormality is a genetic defect or of environmental origin remains to be determined. Furthermore, the pathways through which PEG-400 penetrates intestinal epithelium are poorly understood, require clarification, and may not truly reflect normal physiology.

1.5 Clinical Features

The typical patient with Crohn's disease is a young adult whose illness begins with right lower quadrant pain, diarrhea and a low-grade fever. Examination reveals tenderness, guarding and a palpable mass in the right lower quadrant. If the illness has come on acutely and diarrhea is not prominent, these findings, along with an elevated white blood cell count, often lead to a clinical diagnosis of appendicitis with consequent laparotomy and discovery of the Crohn's disease.

More often, however, the clinical picture is insidious. The patient has recurrent episodes of mild diarrhea, abdominal pain, and fever lasting from days to weeks, and then has a spontaneous improvement in symptoms. If disease is confined to a small segment of intestine, this can go on for many years before a correct diagnosis is made.

The abdominal pain of Crohn's disease is localized to the right lower quadrant. When the colon is involved, crampy pain may occur in one or both lower abdominal quadrants. Fever, in the absence of complications, rarely exceeds 38°C. Diarrhea tends to be moderate in severity, with five to six bowel movements per day when the disease is confined to the ileum. When the disease involves the colon, urgency, incontinence and rectal bleeding may also occur.

If the disease is not diagnosed, gradual deterioration will occur over a period of years; there will be shorter and shorter asymptomatic intervals,

TABLE 2.   Mechanisms responsible for malabsorption and malnutrition in Crohn's disease

---

Inadequate dietary intake (most important)
Anorexia
Specific dietary restrictions to avoid diarrhea/pain symptoms

Inflammatory involvement of small bowel
Decreased absorption of nutrients
Acquired disaccharidase deficiency
Protein-losing enteropathy
Iron deficiency due to chronic blood loss

Small bowel bacterial overgrowth due to strictures and fistulas
Malabsorption of cobalamin
Altered bile salt metabolism and fat malabsorption

Intestinal surgery
Loss of absorptive surface area due to resection
Ileal resection causing cobalamin malabsorption, bile salt deficiency, and steatorrhea

Diarrhea
Fluid and electrolyte losses

Combination of above factors

---

along with weight loss and increasing fatigue. A slow and persistent blood loss combined with poor food intake leads to anemia.

Malnutrition and malabsorption, with subsequent weight loss, are common at all stages of Crohn's disease. A variety of factors are responsible. Nevertheless, a voluntary decrease in food intake for fear of exacerbating abdominal symptoms is the primary cause of weight loss (Table 2).

Approximately 10–15% of individuals present without any of the above abdominal symptoms and are seen for the first time with perirectal disease, fever or one of the extraintestinal manifestations (Table 3).

Whatever the presenting clinical features, only 20% of patients will remain completely asymptomatic during the next 10 years. The remainder will have recurrent attacks of abdominal pain, diarrhea, and low-grade fever. If the disease progresses to the state where surgery is required, recurrence is common, particularly at the site of anastomosis. Seventy-five percent of patients operated on for small bowel Crohn's disease have recurrences within 5 years and require another operation within 15 years. Additionally, the interval between operations appears to be shorter after the second or third operation than after the initial resection.

TABLE 3. Extraintestinal manifestations of inflammatory bowel disease

	Crohn's disease	Ulcerative colitis
Local		
Perianal disease		
Anal fissures, rectovaginal fistulas, rectovesical fistulas	+++	+
Pararectal abscess	+++	+
Rectal prolapse	++	+
Hemorrhage		
Mild – may lead to anemia	+++	+
Massive – may be life-threatening	+	+++
Toxic megacolon	+	+++
Perforation		
Free, with or without toxic megacolon	+	+++
Walled-off	+++	–
Stricture		
Fibrous – permanent	+++	–
Muscularis mucosa hypertrophy – reversible	+	+++
Cancer	+	+++
Systemic		
Skin manifestations		
Erythema nodosum	+++	+
Aphthous ulcers of the mouth	+++	–
Pyoderma gangrenosum	+	+++
Eye lesions		
Conjunctivitis	+++	+
Iritis, uveitis, episcleritis	+++	+
Arthritis		
Peripheral joints – migratory, nondeforming, seronegative	+++	+
Ankylosing spondylitis, sacroiliitis	+	+++
Hepatic disease		
Biliary		
Pericholangitis	+	+
Primary sclerosing cholangitis	+	+++
Bile duct carcinoma	+	+
Gallstones	+++	–
Hepatocellular		
Chronic active hepatitis	+	+
Cirrhosis	–	+
Miscellaneous		
Fatty change (malnutrition)	+	+
Amyloidosis	+	–

(cont'd)

TABLE 3. Extraintestinal manifestations of inflammatory bowel disease (cont'd)

	Crohn's disease	Ulcerative colitis
Hematologic manifestations		
Megaloblastic anemia	+++	+
Iron deficiency anemia	+++	++
Autoimmune hemolytic anemia	++	+
Thrombocytosis	++	++
Clotting abnormalities (hypercoagulable state)	+	+++
Renal disease		
Nephrolithiasis	+++	–

1.6 Complications

1.6.1 *SMALL BOWEL OBSTRUCTION*
Small bowel obstruction is the most common reason for surgery when Crohn's disease involves the small intestine. The obstruction results from inflammation and edema in an already strictured segment of bowel. The obstruction is often partial and is transient once the edema and inflammation are treated and allowed to resolve. Progression to complete obstruction is often slow and results from fibrotic stricturing. Complete obstruction may, however, occur suddenly when the small bowel becomes kinked off as a result of an adhesive inflammatory process.

1.6.2 *FISTULAS AND FISSURES*
Perianal and perirectal fistulas and fissures are particularly common in Crohn's disease and may be so severe as to overshadow other intestinal manifestations. Enteroenteric fistulas can develop between loops of bowel and may contribute to nutritional problems if they cause ingested nutrients to bypass areas of small bowel absorptive surface. Additionally, the presence of enteroenteric fistulas may lead to recirculation of intestinal contents and stasis, thus causing bacterial overgrowth within the lumen. Fistulas between loops of bowel and the urinary bladder ultimately lead to chronic urinary tract infections. Fistulas can also occur between bowel and cutaneous surfaces, bowel and the vagina, or bowel and other internal organs.

1.6.3 *PERFORATION*
Free perforation is unusual in Crohn's disease. When free perforation does occur, it leads to frank peritonitis.

1.6.4 *GASTROINTESTINAL BLOOD LOSS*
Insidious blood loss occurs with small bowel disease and often leads to an iron deficiency anemia. Frank bleeding of bright red rectal blood occurs with colonic disease and with perianal fistulas.

1.6.5 *MALIGNANT NEOPLASMS*
Malignant neoplasms occur both in the involved bowel and in the noninvolved bowel of patients with Crohn's disease three times more frequently than in the general population. Nevertheless, the frequency of malignancy is much lower than that observed in patients with ulcerative colitis.

1.6.6 *EXTRAINTESTINAL MANIFESTATIONS*
Extraintestinal manifestations of Crohn's disease (Table 3) frequently develop alongside colonic involvement and perianal disease. Patients with one extraintestinal manifestation are at increased risk for developing a second.

Arthritis is the most common systemic manifestation and presents as migratory arthritis involving large joints, or as sacroiliitis or ankylosing spondylitis. Spondylitis or sacroiliitis may occur for many years prior to the manifestation of intestinal disease. There is no relationship between the course of spondylitis and sacroiliitis and the course of Crohn's disease. Migratory monoarthritis involves large joints and again runs a course independent of the intestinal disease.

Inflammation of the eye, skin and mucus membranes may also occur during the course of Crohn's disease. Iritis and episcleritis are frequent eye manifestations. Erythema nodosum and, less often, pyoderma gangrenosum are common skin conditions. Aphthous ulcerations of the buccal mucosa, tongue and lips are frequent, often refractory, problems.

Clinically important liver disease is not generally seen with Crohn's disease. Mild abnormalities in liver function studies may be observed in a few patients, and liver biopsy will often show a mild pericholangitis in these cases. Cholelithiasis occurs with a frequency of approximately 30% in patients with ileal disease and/or ileal resection. This high incidence is probably related to a bile salt deficiency that causes the production of a lithogenic bile conducive to cholesterol gallstone formation.

Nephrolithiasis occurs in 30% of patients with Crohn's disease. Oxalate stones and hyperoxaluria are common and are related to steatorrhea. Fat malabsorption increases the amount of dietary oxalate available for absorption in the colon.

1.7 **Diagnosis**
Diagnosis of Crohn's disease, as of ulcerative colitis, is made through the

TABLE 4. Differential diagnosis of Crohn's disease (includes
colonic and/or small bowel involvement)

Infectious
   Yersinia species
   Campylobacter species
   Salmonella species
   Amebiasis
   Tuberculosis
   Balantidium coli
   Cytomegalovirus
   Histoplasmosis
   Anisakiasis
Eosinophilic gastroenteritis
Vasculitis
Solitary rectal ulcer syndrome
Colonic cancer
Appendicitis
Appendiceal abscess
Appendiceal mucocele
Meckel's diverticulitis
Pelvic inflammatory disease
Ectopic pregnancy
Ovarian cysts or tumors
Cecal diverticulitis
Carcinoma of the cecum involving the ileum
Carcinoid tumor
Ileal plasmacytoma
Ischemic bowel disease
Intestinal lymphoma
Nongranulomatous ulcerative jejunoileitis
Pseudomembranous enterocolitis
Ulcerative colitis
Radiation enteritis
Small bowel tumors
Systemic vasculitis
Fabry's disease
Zollinger-Ellison syndrome
Benign lymphoid hyperplasia

---

accumulation of history and physical findings, as well as laboratory, radiologic, endoscopic and histologic findings.

Initially, other causes of bowel inflammation must be excluded (Table 4). In
the acute phase of Crohn's disease, viral gastroenteritis, appendicitis, Yersinia
enterocolitis and Salmonella gastroenteritis must be excluded. If the Crohn's

disease presents as a chronic recurrent illness, then culture of the stools and rectal mucosa for giardiasis, amebiasis, intestinal tuberculosis, nongranulomatous ulcerative jejunoileitis, fungal infections and pseudomembranous enterocolitis must be done. If the inflammatory state is limited to the colon or rectum, ulcerative colitis, ischemic colitis, diverticulitis, and occasionally cancer of the colon may simulate Crohn's disease.

1.7.1 *LABORATORY INVESTIGATIONS*

A complete blood count (CBC) will reveal leukocytosis, an elevated erythrocyte sedimentation rate and thrombocytosis, all of which suggest that an active inflammatory process is present. Indices may be microcytic hypochromic if an iron deficiency anemia exists, macrocytic megaloblastic if a vitamin B_{12} (absorbed in the terminal ileum) or folic acid deficiency exists. If both these states are present then the automated Coulter counter will present a normochromic, normocytic–type anemia that must then be investigated through peripheral smear and measurement of serum iron, total iron binding capacity (TIBC), ferritin, vitamin B_{12} and folic acid levels.

Urinalysis may demonstrate a urinary tract infection if a fistula is present and proteinuria if amyloidosis has developed. The serum albumin is a useful indication of the patient's overall condition. It is low in those patients not eating, those with extensive malabsorption, and those whose disease is causing significant enteric loss of proteins. Serum alkaline phosphatase activity is frequently elevated in patients with Crohn's disease who have no other indication of liver disease. Serum carotene, calcium, phosphorous, Schilling test and stool fat assessment are useful in determining whether or not frank malabsorption is present. Lactose hydrogen breath test and ^{14}C-labeled glycocholate breath test are useful in assessing the degree of lactose intolerance and bacterial overgrowth, respectively. Note that the ^{14}C-labeled glycocholate breath test will also be abnormal in the presence of ileal disease or ileal resection.

Endoscopy, flexible sigmoidoscopy, and/or colonoscopy are useful for identifying and performing biopsies on discrete mucosal ulcerations. These ulcers vary in size and may appear round and punched out, serpiginous or linear. Often islands of normal mucosa protrude into the colonic lumen as a result of submucosal inflammation and edema. When prominent islands of mucosa are separated by linear ulcerations, the intestine assumes a cobblestone appearance. This pattern is characteristically different from that seen in ulcerative colitis, where diffuse ulceration extends without patches of normal mucosa.

The decision to perform colonoscopy should take into account the specific

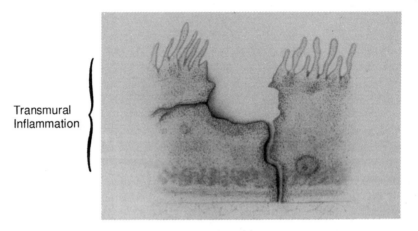

Transmural Inflammation

FIGURE 2. Crohn's disease. A transmural process.

diagnosis and/or therapeutic issues that the procedure may be asked to resolve. These include (1) establishing a diagnosis; (2) activity of disease; (3) extent of involvement; (4) type of disease; and (5) suspicion of cancer.

1.7.2 RADIOLOGIC FINDINGS

The plain x-ray of the abdomen will reveal dilatated bowel when a partial obstruction is present. Intra-abdominal masses resulting from matted inflamed loops of bowel or from abscesses can also be seen on the plain film.

An air contrast barium enema will demonstrate involvement of the colon and show narrowing, ulcerations, strictures or fistula formation. As with colonoscopy, a barium enema should be deferred in patients acutely ill with Crohn's colitis, since the examination is not critical for immediate management decisions and the risk of toxic megacolon and perforation is appreciable.

A barium enema may reveal disease of the terminal ileum as a result of reflux of barium past the ileocecal valve. However, determination of the extent of small bowel involvement requires administration of contrast medium orally or via enteroclysis. The small bowel abnormalities seen on x-ray are similar to those observed in the colon and include the characteristic cobblestone appearance, stenosis, and diseased segments separated by small bowel that appears normal (Figure 1).

It is important to note that changes in the appearance of both the large and small bowel on x-ray film correlate poorly with the course of the disease. There is thus no reason to take "routine" evaluative x-rays.

1.7.3 *HISTOLOGIC EXAMINATION*

Mucosal biopsies obtained from the rectum, colon, terminal ileum or duodenum at the time of colonoscopy or upper endoscopy provide histologic documentation. Granulomatous inflammation of bowel mucosa strongly supports a diagnosis of Crohn's disease (Figure 2).

1.8 Therapy

The management of Crohn's disease varies greatly depending upon the clinical status of the individual patient. No single therapeutic regime is considered routine for patients with Crohn's disease, and treatment must be individualized.

When the patient presents with acute Crohn's disease, the history and physical examination are critical in determining the severity of the disease, in addition to gathering evidence of intestinal obstruction, bowel perforation or abscess. The use of steroids or immunosuppressive agents in the presence of gross infection is disastrous. In mild cases, diarrhea and abdominal cramps can be treated effectively with codeine, diphenoxylate (Lomotil®) or loperamide (Imodium®). In moderate or severe cases, the patient should be admitted to hospital, remain n.p.o. and be maintained with intravenous fluids. When symptoms and findings suggest small bowel obstruction, nasogastric suction is usually required until edema and spasm of the bowel subside. If evidence of abscess formation, fever and leukocytosis suggests a systemic infection, broad-spectrum antibiotic coverage should be initiated after appropriate cultures of blood, urine, fistulas or other possible sources of infection have been collected.

1.8.1 *SUPPORTIVE THERAPY*

Symptomatic therapy may be necessary to control diarrhea in cases of chronic stable disease. As indicated above, diphenoxylate, loperamide and codeine are useful agents for controlling diarrhea, but they should be used carefully; they are potentially hazardous and should be promptly withdrawn if the patient's clinical status deteriorates.

Additionally, for patients with Crohn's disease, the diarrhea may be due to unabsorbed deconjugated bile acids that cause a cholerrheic diarrhea. Cholestyramine, an ion-exchange resin, effectively binds the unabsorbed bile salts and controls the diarrhea. Fat malabsorption may be treated with a low-fat diet supplemented with medium-chain triglycerides. Bacterial overgrowth proximal to areas of stenosis causes deconjugation of bile salts, again resulting in diarrhea; it responds well to courses of broad-spectrum antibiotics (e.g., tetracycline). Finally, lactase deficiency may occur secondary to the active inflammation and a trial of lactose-free diet is warranted.

The patient with Crohn's disease also requires continuous emotional support for this chronic, complicated illness; this support is necessary not only during acute attacks, but also during periods of remission. Although many consultants may be required to manage the varying aspects of complicated cases, one physician should be directly and continuously responsible for the overall care of the patient. Psychiatric consultation may occasionally be necessary for specific problems; however, successful management requires that continuous emotional support come from the physician who is directing the overall care of the patient.

1.8.2 NUTRITIONAL THERAPY

Nutritional deficiencies are frequent with Crohn's disease and often result from inadequate food intake by patients who have "learned" that ingestion of food aggravates diarrhea and abdominal pain. In addition, several pathophysiologic mechanisms contribute to nutritional problems in patients with Crohn's disease (Table 2). Nutritional problems may be further aggravated by surgical resection of diseased intestine, which decreases absorptive surface area; this decrease may be sufficient to interfere with an adequate absorption of multiple nutrients. Of particular importance, because of the distal small bowel involvement, is the malabsorption of bile salts and vitamin B_{12}, both of which have receptors located solely in the distal ileum.

Whatever the combination of mechanisms responsible for the impaired absorption and nutritional deficiencies in Crohn's disease, the physician must be attuned to assessing nutritional parameters, including ideal body weight, anthropometrics, serum proteins, and serum vitamin and mineral levels. The consequences of nutritional disturbances are particularly serious in children with Crohn's disease. Delayed growth and sexual maturation can and do occur, and if they are not corrected prior to closure of the epiphysis, permanent shortness of stature will result. Adjunctive nutritional therapy is, as well, required by patients who are malnourished at the time of their Crohn's exacerbation or who are unable to ingest adequate calories because of their disease.

Increasingly, patients with extensive and complicated Crohn's disease are being treated partially or completely with enteral or parenteral nutritional programs as a means of "resting" the gut, allowing fistulas to heal, inducing a positive nitrogen balance, and even causing weight gain. Short-term remission is often achieved through the use of "bowel rest"; however, relapse rates are high within a few months of discontinuing therapy. Recently, Greenberg et al. have demonstrated that disease remission could be induced provided the patient received an adequate number of calories. Furthermore, it did not mat-

TABLE 5.   Drug therapy in inflammatory bowel disease

Corticosteroids
Rectal
  Foam
  Suppositories
  Enemas
Oral

Sulfasalazine
Oral
Enemas

Mesalamine (5-ASA)
Oral
Rectal
Enemas
Suppositories

Metronidazole

Immunosuppressive agents
Azathioprine
6-mercaptopurine
Cyclosporine
Methotrexate

ter whether these calories were provided through oral intake, oral intake supplemented with enteral elemental feeding, or total parenteral nutrition (7).

1.8.3 DRUG THERAPY

Although a small percentage of patients with Crohn's disease enjoy prolonged symptom-free intervals when treatment is not required, the vast majority experience long periods of symptomatic active disease or frequent relapses that necessitate treatment of the disease with anti-inflammatory and immunosuppressive agents (Table 5). Evaluation of the efficacy of such agents is extremely difficult, given the fluctuating activity and unpredictable long-term course of Crohn's disease. Recently, randomized double-blind control studies have attempted to answer some of the questions relating to drug therapy.

1.8.3.1 *Corticosteroids*

1.8.3.1.1 *Rectal corticosteroid preparations*   Rectal instillation of steroid-containing preparations is useful when Crohn's disease involves the rectum and the sigmoid region. The topical application of steroids allows for rapid

TABLE 6.   Comparison of 5-ASA products and approximate monthly cost (May 1994)

5-ASA	Average dose per day	Approximate cost per month
Salazopyrin® (Azulfidine®)	4 g/d	$ 51.00
Asacol®	4 g/d	$121.00
Mesasal™	4 g/d	$142.00
Salofalk® (oral)	4 g/d	$130.00
Dipentum®	2 g/d	$124.00
Pentasa®	4 g/d	$151.00

healing of the area and restoration of the rectum and sigmoid to their stool reservoir capacity and, therefore, often leads to fewer episodes of diarrhea.

1.8.3.1.2 *Systemic corticosteroid preparations*   Corticosteroids are beneficial in the management of acute exacerbations of small and large intestinal Crohn's disease, in which they induce remission of symptoms and decrease disease activity indices. Although steroids continue to be used by many practitioners on a chronic basis in the management of Crohn's disease, there is little evidence to support administration to prevent disease relapse. Steroid therapy for acute disease is best begun at prednisone 40 mg/day (outpatient oral treatment in mild cases or inpatient intravenous therapy in severe cases). As improvement occurs, parenteral therapy may be replaced by oral administration of a dosage that is gradually reduced by 5 mg/week to the minimum level needed to suppress signs of the inflammatory process (20 mg) and then by 2.5 mg/week; the ultimate goal is to end steroid therapy. Unfortunately, this objective cannot always be achieved, and many patients become symptomatic when the dose of prednisone is reduced below 5–10 mg/day. This "steroid dependence" occurs frequently, and the amount necessary for maintenance varies from patient to patient. If possible, patients requiring long-term steroid therapy should be weaned onto an alternate-day regime; alternatively, the immunosuppressive therapy will allow steroid withdrawal or a lowering of the steroid dose.

1.8.3.2 *Mesalamine (5-aminosalicylic acid mesalazine [5-ASA])*
In Crohn's colitis, colon site–specific mesalamine (Table 6) is as effective as previously used sulfasalazine. Studies are continuing to determine whether mixed, slow-release and pH-dependent release mesalamine (Pentasa®) will be effective in small intestinal Crohn's disease or, indeed, will have a role in preventing disease relapse. Preliminary evidence would suggest that 5-ASA

delivered to the small bowel (Pentasa®, Mesasal™) may be effective in reducing small intestinal inflammation (8).

1.8.3.3 *Immunosuppressive agents*
Immunosuppressive agents are reserved for steroid-dependent or steroid-resistant patients. When combined with steroids, azathioprine (150 mg/day), its active metabolite, 6-mercaptopurine (1.5 mg/kg/day), cyclosporine (7.5–15 mg/kg/day), and methotrexate (15–25 mg/day) are useful in cases of both ileal and colonic Crohn's disease. A large number of case reports and open studies have found that immunosuppressive agents will induce remission in steroid-resistant or steroid-dependent patients in approximately 60–70% of cases; nevertheless, the relapse rate is high once the immunosuppressive agent is withdrawn (9–11). Methotrexate and cyclosporine appear to work more quickly than 6-mercaptopurine and azathioprine. Two ongoing multicenter Canadian studies are examining the effectiveness of cyclosporine and methotrexate in prevention of Crohn's disease relapse. The results of these studies will, it is hoped, be available within the next two to three years.

1.8.3.4 *Metronidazole*
Metronidazole (250 mg t.i.d.) is as effective as sulfasalazine in acute colonic disease if the patient has not received prior therapy, in patients whose disease does not respond to sulfasalazine, and in the treatment of perianal disease. Side effects include metallic taste, disulfiram-like effects with ingestion of alcohol, paresthesias and peripheral neuropathy. Most side effects are reversible upon withdrawal of the drugs; however, the peripheral neuropathy may persist.

1.8.4 *SURGICAL TREATMENT*
In view of the high rate of recurrence of Crohn's disease following resection of diseased bowel, operative therapy should be reserved for complications of the disease or for those cases where the disease unequivocally fails to respond to optimal medical management. Complications requiring surgery are (1) chronic obstruction; (2) symptomatic abscess or fistula formation; (3) enterovesical fistulas; (4) free perforation; and (5) retarded physical or sexual development in children with Crohn's disease. Removal of the diseased segment(s) in a young child will normally allow the child to grow and mature normally until the Crohn's disease recurs. Patients should be forewarned that surgery is not curative but is necessary for the treatment of complications. Patients should also be warned about the common recurrence of Crohn's disease after resection of the small bowel or after colonic disease. The recurrence rate is 40% within 5 years, 60% within 10 years and 85% within 15 years.

1.8.5 *TREATMENT FOR MAINTENANCE OR REMISSION OF INACTIVE CROHN'S DISEASE*

No therapeutic agents have been proven useful for maintaining a remission in Crohn's disease; therefore, once the active disease has been treated and controlled, there is no rationale for continuing medical therapy. Recently, preliminary evidence has become available to suggest that mesalamine (Pentasa®) may have some benefit in preventing Crohn's disease relapse. Ongoing multicenter placebo-controlled studies continue to examine the potential role for cyclosporine and Pentasa® in preventing Crohn's disease relapse.

1.8.6 *POSSIBLE NEW THERAPEUTIC APPROACHES*

In the past few years, a number of basic research studies have investigated the nature of the inflammatory process involved in inflammatory bowel disease. As a result, it is now known that several mediators, such as prostaglandins, leukotrienes, cytokines and platelet-activating factor, are involved in the inflammation. There is increasing evidence that 5-lipoxygenase products (leukotrienes) play a key role in causing and perpetuating mucosal inflammation, while cyclooxygenase products (prostaglandins) may provide a mucosal protective function (12,13). It has been recently shown that eicosapentaenoic acid, a fatty acid obtainable from marine fish, is metabolized by the lipoxygenase pathway to a less inflammatory leukotriene (LTB_5). Dietary supplementation with 3 g/day of eicosapentaenoic acid for 6 weeks reduced the capacity of neutrophils to produce LTB_4, and in a small open study, inflammatory bowel disease patients showed significant decrease in neutrophil inflammation and improvement in symptoms and histological appearance of rectal mucosa (14). Blocking the synthesis of leukotrienes with selective 5-lipoxygenase inhibitors in leukotriene B_4-receptor antagonists is another new approach to therapy. In a preliminary study the new specific 5-lipoxygenase inhibitor, A64077 (Zileuton®), has improved clinical, sigmoidoscopic and histological findings in 48 patients with colitis (15). Specific inhibitors of other cytokines have not yet reached the clinical stage.

2. ULCERATIVE COLITIS

Ulcerative colitis is an inflammatory disease of unknown etiology affecting the colonic mucosa from the rectum to the cecum. It is a chronic disease characterized by rectal bleeding and diarrhea, and given to remissions and exacerbations.

Ulcerative colitis is not a distinct entity, since most of the histological features of the disease may be seen in other inflammatory states of the colon,

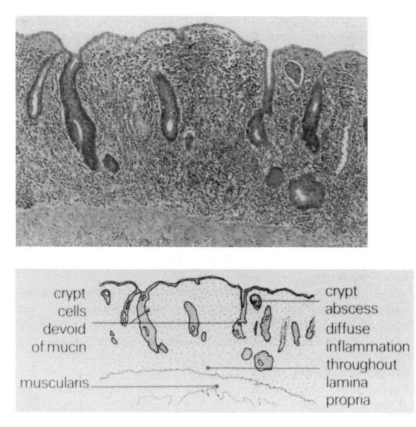

FIGURE 3. Cross-section of colonic mucosa showing typical crypt abscess seen in Crohn's disease.

such as those caused by bacteria or parasites. The diagnosis of ulcerative colitis, therefore, rests on discovery of a combination of clinical and pathological criteria, investigation of the extent and distribution of lesions, and exclusion of other forms of inflammatory colitis caused by infectious agents (Entamoeba histolytica, Clostridium difficile, Campylobacter, E. coli and Shigella).

2.1 Pathophysiology

Ulcerative colitis is an inflammatory state confined to the mucosa, unlike Crohn's disease, which extends into deeper muscle layers of the serosa. Since the inflammatory process involves only the mucosa, sharp localized abdominal pain, perforation and fistula formation are uncommon in ulcerative colitis;

this is in contrast to Crohn's disease, where they frequently appear. Under light microscopy, the colonic tissue displays small microabscesses, called crypt abscesses, which involve the crypts of Lieberkuhn. Polymorphonuclear cells accumulate in the crypt abscesses, and frank necrosis of the surrounding crypt epithelium occurs; thus the polymorphonuclear infiltrates extend into the colonic epithelium. These microabscesses in the crypts are not visible to the naked eye; however, several crypt abscesses may coalesce to produce a shallow ulceration visible on the mucosal surface (Figure 3). Occasionally, lateral extension of crypt abscesses may undermine the mucosa on three sides, and the resulting hanging fragment of mucosa will appear endoscopically and radiographically as a "pseudopolyp." Following this mucosal destruction, highly vascular granulation tissue develops in denuded areas, resulting in friability and bleeding. The two most prominent symptoms of ulcerative colitis – diarrhea and rectal bleeding – are related both to the extensive mucosal damage, which renders the colon less capable of absorbing electrolytes and water, and to the highly friable vascular granulation tissue, which bleeds readily.

Radiographically, evident foreshortening and narrowing of the colon, loss of haustral margins, and apparent stricture formation will often be seen. These findings, however, are often reversible, since they are due to hypertrophy and spasm of the muscularis mucosa and not to fibrosis.

2.2 Clinical Features

Ulcerative colitis typically occurs in patients between 20 and 50 years of age and may present as an early acute fulminating attack or may follow a rather indolent and often chronic course. Approximately 70% of patients will have complete symptomatic remissions between intermittent attacks. Ten percent of patients will have one initial attack and will experience no subsequent attacks, and 15–20% will be troubled by continuous symptoms that occur without remission.

The initial and most common symptom of ulcerative colitis is rectal bleeding. A blood stain on the toilet tissue or the appearance of bloody mucus on the surface of stools is usually the first symptom noticed. This initial bleeding is often mistaken for bleeding from hemorrhoids. Indeed, this first evidence of blood may follow a bout of constipation, which can sometimes be the presenting complaint. When constipation is the presenting complaint, the colitis is most often associated with disease limited to the rectum, where spasm prevents feces from entering the area involved. Hence, initial constipation or normal bowel habits may be the hallmark of ulcerative proctosigmoiditis.

Diarrhea occurs with more extensive colonic involvement, and blood is usually mixed with the feces. The principal mechanism responsible for diarrhea in ulcerative colitis is exudation with resultant secretion of interstitial fluids and loss of mucosal surface area for absorbing fluid and electrolytes and water. In addition, involvement of the rectum prevents this segment of the colon from acting as a reservoir for fecal contents prior to defecation. This rectal irritability causes frequent bowel evacuation of minute amounts of blood and mucus, an activity that can be termed "pseudodiarrhea."

Since the severity of the disease will affect the therapeutic approach and, indeed, the prognostic implications, it is important for the physician to assess the severity of the disease for every patient. The best indices of severity are clinical signs and symptoms. Large volumes of diarrhea indicate that the colonic mucosa has been involved to the extent that sodium and water absorption are significantly impaired. Frequency, however, is an unreliable indicator of severity because frequent bowel movements can indicate either large-volume diarrhea or rectal irritability. Large quantities of blood in the stools, a fallen hemoglobin concentration, and hypoalbuminemia as a consequence of loss of albumin into the stool are signs of widespread disease. Elevated erythrocyte sedimentation rate, fever, and abdominal pain and tenderness may point to transmural extension of the disease and the development of severe ulcerative colitis.

Ulcerative colitis can be classified according to the grade of clinical severity:

1. *Severe.* Diarrhea comprised of six or more movements per day, macroscopic blood in the stools, fever, tachycardia greater than 90/min, anemia and an elevated erythrocyte sedimentation rate.
2. *Moderate.* Diarrhea comprised of four or fewer movements per day, small amounts of macroscopic blood in stools, no fever, no tachycardia, mild anemia and a minimally elevated erythrocyte sedimentation rate.
3. *Mild.* Diarrhea comprised of fewer than four bowel movements per day without anemia, fever, tachycardia, weight loss or hypoalbuminemia.

2.2.1 SEVERE ULCERATIVE COLITIS

Severe ulcerative colitis, the least common form of the disease, occurs in 15% of all patients with ulcerative colitis. This form of the disease may be the initial presentation or may represent a progression from a less severe attack. Diarrhea is profuse and rectal bleeding is constant and severe. Fever is marked and sustained, and appetite and weight are both severely diminished. Abdominal cramps are severe and tenderness may be localized, indicating impending perforation. Leukocytes greater than 10,000, severe anemia, and hypoalbuminemia resulting from low protein intake (anorexia) and increased chronic loss of albumin are hallmarks of this form of the disease.

Medical therapy is often ineffective for this type of patient, and colectomy is often required.

2.2.2 MODERATE ULCERATIVE COLITIS

Moderate ulcerative colitis affects 25% of all patients with ulcerative colitis. Diarrhea is the major symptom, and it occurs three to four times per day. Invariably, the diarrhea contains macroscopic amounts of blood. Abdominal pain may occur and may awaken the patient at night; usually the cramps are relieved by defecation. Low-grade fever may exist, and the patient may complain of fatigue, anorexia and some mild weight loss.

Generally, moderate ulcerative colitis responds quickly to appropriate therapy. Immediate mortality in this group is low. However, the long-term prognosis is for repeated attacks of equal or greater severity, and the risk of ultimately developing cancer in the affected colon is appreciable. As well, at any time during the moderate attack of ulcerative colitis, the patient may become severely ill, developing a severe fulminant colitis characterized by high fever, profuse diarrhea, progressive dilatation of the colon (toxic megacolon) and rapid deterioration.

2.2.3 MILD ULCERATIVE COLITIS

Mild ulcerative colitis is the most common form of the disease, occurring in 60% of patients. In 80% of those affected with mild disease, the ulcerative colitis will be limited to the distal colon (sigmoid and rectum); in the other 20% the whole colon will be involved. The age, sex and familial incidence of ulcerative colitis are the same for mild disease as for severe disease. As well, the number of patients who have only one attack, intermittent attacks, or continuous disease is the same for both mild and severe ulcerative colitis.

In the case of mild disease limited to the rectal sigmoid, most often the disease will remain in this area; however, in 10% of these patients it will eventually involve the entire colon and bring about the simultaneous development of severe diarrhea and bleeding.

Neither colonic bleeding nor diarrhea is severe in mild ulcerative colitis, and the systemic complications of anorexia, weight loss and fatigue are not seen. Occasionally, the patient may suffer from a few days of crampy lower abdominal pain; however, hospitalization is usually not required and mild ulcerative colitis responds rapidly to therapy.

For patients who have mild ulcerative colitis, particularly proctosigmoiditis, the rate of colonic cancer is similar to that of control populations. Thus, colonic cancer occurs in mild cases of ulcerative colitis only one-fifth as often as in the more severe forms of the disease.

2.3 Diagnosis

The diagnosis of ulcerative colitis is made on the basis of the clinical symptoms listed above, on physical findings, and on the results of laboratory and endoscopic investigations.

2.3.1 *PHYSICAL EXAMINATION*

Physical examination during mild ulcerative colitis or between attacks may yield completely normal findings. In contrast to Crohn's disease, there are no palpable masses and no specific areas of tenderness, unless serosal involvement, peritoneal irritation or impending perforation (toxic megacolon) exists. Occasionally, the liver is palpable because of fatty infiltration or other hepatic abnormality. Auscultation of the abdomen may reveal increased bowel sounds and audible borborygmi. With toxic megacolon, bowel sounds are quiet or absent.

Rectal examination is usually painful and the anal sphincter is often spastic. The examiner may be able to detect gritty, coarse, granular changes in the rectal mucosa on digital palpation. Pseudopolyps may also be palpated, and a rectal stricture may be detected. In addition, it may be possible to feel a carcinoma. Rectal and perianal complications are far less frequent and destructive than they are in Crohn's disease and ordinarily consist only of minor fissures.

Examination of the skin and joints may confirm extracolonic complications (uveitis, stomatitis, pyoderma gangrenosum, erythema nodosum, large-joint arthritis, ankylosing spondylitis).

2.3.2 *LABORATORY INVESTIGATIONS*

There is no single laboratory test that will confirm ulcerative colitis. Anemia, leukocytosis and an elevated erythrocyte sedimentation rate often reflect the severity of the disease. Iron studies reflect iron deficiency anemia (low serum iron, high TIBC, low ferritin). Electrolyte abnormalities including hypokalemia, metabolic acidosis, hypocalcemia, hypomagnesemia and/or hypoalbuminemia may exist in patients with severe diarrhea. Liver function studies will demonstrate an elevated alkaline phosphatase as a manifestation of sclerosing cholangitis. Blood cultures may be positive in patients with toxic megacolon.

Examination of the stool will reveal abundant red and white blood cells. Stool cultures for Shigella, Campylobacter, Salmonella, Clostridium difficile (culture and toxin), E. coli 0157 and Entamoeba histolytica should be done in all cases to exclude the possibility of infectious colitis.

2.3.3 *ENDOSCOPIC FINDINGS*

The most useful method of establishing a diagnosis of ulcerative colitis is to assess the integrity of the mucosa directly. Since 97% of people with ulcer-

TABLE 7.   Endoscopic grading of activity in ulcerative colitis

Activity	Appearance
Quiescent	Distorted or absent mucosal vascular pattern Granularity
Mildly active	Continuous or focal erythema Friability (touch bleeding)
Moderately active	Mucopurulent exudate (mucopus) Single or multiple ulcers (<5 mm); fewer than 10 per 10 cm segment
Severe	Large ulcers (>5 mm); more than 10 per 10 cm segment Spontaneous bleeding

ative colitis have involvement of the rectum, simple sigmoidoscopy can be used to establish the diagnosis in the majority of cases.

The normal colonic mucosa is a smooth, glistening, pink surface. Seen underneath this smooth surface are the ramifying superficial submucosal blood vessels, which present a prominent vascular pattern. When brushed by a cotton swab, the normal colonic mucosa does not bleed because the mucosa is not friable.

Endoscopic examination of inactive or quiescent ulcerative colitis will show a distorted or absent mucosal vascular pattern with a mild granularity (Table 7). Mildly active disease will show continuous or focal erythema and friability. Moderately active disease will display mucopurulent exudate (mucopus) and ulcers less than 5 mm in diameter and fewer than 10 per 10 cm segment. Severe colitis will demonstrate ulcers larger than 5 mm and more than 10 per 10 cm segment; these ulcers are often accompanied by spontaneous bleeding.

Colonoscopy is rarely necessary in diagnosing a new case of ulcerative colitis. The rectal and distal sigmoid mucosa is almost always involved in cases of ulcerative colitis, and a carefully performed sigmoidoscopy with either a rigid or flexible instrument can usually lead to the correct diagnosis. Colonoscopy should never be performed in the case of acute, moderately severe or severe ulcerative colitis because of the risk of perforation during the procedure itself.

Colonoscopy for ulcerative colitis is, therefore, performed for specific indications only. These are (1) to determine the extent and/or activity of the disease in patients who are considered to be in poor symptomatic control; (2) to perform cancer surveillance or diagnosis; and (3) to determine the type of inflammatory disease, whether ulcerative colitis or Crohn's disease (Table 8).

TABLE 8. Inflammatory bowel disease: indications for colonoscopy

---

Differentiating IBD from other diseases and differentiating Crohn's from ulcerative colitis

Establishing the extent of the disease

Screening for malignancy and malignant precursors

Evaluation of abnormalities on radiographs
  Strictures
  Masses

Evaluation of patients not responsive to standard therapy or examination to explain recent flare; searching for complications

Examination prior to surgery
  Detection of intestinal involvement (active IBD) in fistulous disease
  Differentiation of ulcerative colitis from Crohn's colitis

2.3.4 RADIOLOGIC FINDINGS

A plain film of the abdomen should always be obtained, particularly with severe colitis, where the risk of toxic megacolon exists. The plain film may demonstrate foreshortening or loss of haustration; sufficient air in a segment of colon to silhouette the mucosa may reveal irregular mucosa, ulceration and mucosal tags. Patients with toxic megacolon will have mid-transverse colon dilatation to a diameter of 6 cm or more.

An air contrast barium enema examination can be used for the same indications as for colonoscopy: to determine disease extent and/or activity, examine for cancer, or differentiate from Crohn's disease. Barium enema examination should thus be performed on all patients with ulcerative colitis, but only at an appropriate time. During the active disease phase, the colonic preparation, and even the barium enema itself, may precipitate a toxic megacolon. It is therefore prudent to delay the barium enema examination until the disease has been brought under medical control.

Radiologic features vary according to the location and state of the disease. There may be a loss of haustration on the left side of the colon (this can be the normal appearance of the colon in elderly patients) (Figure 4). Additionally, the radiolucent filling defects of pseudopolyps may be seen scattered throughout the colon.

Despite significant advances in radiography, comparisons of results from colonoscopy and double contrast barium enema suggest that the extent of the disease is often considerably underestimated with the barium enema. Nevertheless, colonoscopy is best reserved for investigating the disease of patients who have considerable symptoms of colitis yet have minimal changes on

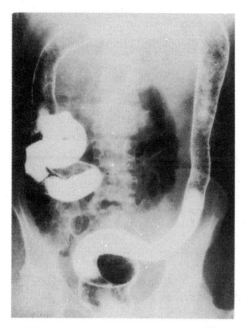

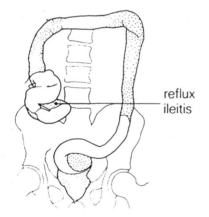

reflux
ileitis

FIGURE 4. "Instant" double-contrast barium enema in total ulcerative colitis. The distal ileum is dilatated with a granular surface indicating reflux or "backwash" ileitis.

TABLE 9.   Differential diagnosis of ulcerative colitis

Infectious
  Viral
    Cytomegalovirus
    Herpes

  Bacterial
    Salmonella species
    Shigella species
    Yersinia enterocolitica
    Vibrio parahaemolyticus
    Aeromonas hydrophila
    Neisseria gonorrhoeae
    Chlamydia trachomatis
    Syphilis
    Staphylococcus aureus
    Escherichia coli

  Protozoan
    Amebiasis
    Balantidiasis
    Schistosomiasis

  Fungal
    Histoplasmosis
    Candidiasis

  Other
    Clostridium difficile

Radiation colitis

Crohn's colitis

Medication/drugs
  Enemas
  Laxatives
  Local nonsteroidal anti-inflammatory drugs
  Sulfasalazine
  Penicillamine
  Gold
  Methyldopa

Eosinophilic gastroenteritis

Behçet's syndrome

Colitis in graft-versus-host disease

TABLE 10.   Clinical differentiation of ulcerative colitis from Crohn's colitis

Feature	Ulcerative colitis	Crohn's colitis
Clinical features		
Rectal bleeding	Very common – 90%	Uncommon: may be occult
Diarrhea	Early, frequent, small stools	Less prevalent or absent
Abdominal pain	Predefecatory, urgency	Colicky, postprandial
Fever	Uncommon if uncomplicated	Frequent
Palpable mass	Rare	Frequent, right lower quadrant
Recurrence after resection	Rare	Frequent
Clinical course	Relapses/remissions 65%	Usually slowly progressive;
	Chronic/continuous 20–30%	fulminant
	Acute/fulminating 5–8%	
Endoscopic features		
Proctosigmoidoscopy	Diffuse pinpoint ulcerations, continuous lesions	Discrete aphthoid ulcerations, patchy lesions
Radiologic features		
Rectal involvement	Invariable	Infrequent
Distribution	Continuous	Segmental, discontinuous
Mucosa	Fine ulcerations	"Cobblestones"
Strictures	Rare	Frequent
Fistulas	Rare	Frequent
Histologic features		
Distribution	Mucosal	Transmural
Cellular infiltrate	Polymorphs	Lymphocytes
Glands	Mucin depletion	Gland preservation
	Gland destruction	
	Crypt abscesses	
Special features	None	Granulomas, aphthoid ulcers, histiocyte-lined fissures

sigmoidoscopy and in barium enema results, and for obtaining biopsies of suspicious areas.

2.4 Differential Diagnosis

The disorder from which ulcerative colitis needs to be distinguished is Crohn's disease of the colon. In addition, a host of other diseases may resemble ulcerative colitis. The possibility of these diseases must also be excluded (Table 9).

Methods of distinguishing between ulcerative colitis and Crohn's colitis are illustrated in Table 10. It is important to note that, because of the anatomic distribution of ulcerative colitis, proctosigmoidoscopic examination is abnormal in virtually all cases. By contrast, even when Crohn's disease affects the colon, it often does not involve the rectum. In addition, perianal disease is much more characteristic of Crohn's disease. Although diarrhea and weight loss occur with approximately equal frequency in both diseases, abdominal pain is more evident with Crohn's disease. Extraintestinal manifestations occur in about the same proportion with both diseases.

2.5 Therapy

2.5.1 HOSPITALIZATION
Hospitalization is indicated for the following reasons:

1. Failure of mild disease to improve significantly within four weeks of the start of outpatient treatment. Hospitalization removes the patient from an aggravating environment and provides the physician with the opportunity to initiate more effective and intensive therapeutic measures.
2. Severe illness with anorexia, nausea, vomiting, fever and uncontrollable bloody diarrhea (severe ulcerative colitis). Early hospitalization is critical for such patients so that they may be provided with therapy to control the disease and prevent complications, especially toxic megacolon.
3. Development of local or systemic complications including massive hemorrhage, persistent anemia, severe hypoalbuminemia, and/or cancer. Hospitalization at this time provides for assessment of the need for surgical therapy.

2.5.2 SUPPORTIVE THERAPY
Supportive therapy consists of medications that improve the patient's general state of health or alleviate symptoms. Chronic losses of potassium, sodium and water must be replaced with oral and/or intravenous fluids, since uncorrected fluid and electrolyte deficits have been implicated in the development of toxic megacolon and renal calculi. Blood loss due to severe disease should be replaced with transfusions. With mild disease, oral iron replacement is indicated. The use of antidiarrheal agents – e.g., diphenoxylate (Lomotil®) or loperamide (Imodium®) – for patients with ulcerative colitis is generally contraindicated. In severe disease where the colonic mucosa is severely damaged, antidiarrheal agents are generally ineffective, since there is a loss of absorbing capacity. Furthermore, they may contribute to the development of toxic megacolon. Similarly, anticholinergics can also precipitate toxic megacolon and thus should not be prescribed for patients with ulcerative colitis.

2.5.3 NUTRITIONAL THERAPY

Neither total parenteral nutrition nor enteral nutrition has yet been shown to have any beneficial effect in inducing remission of ulcerative colitis.

2.5.4 DRUG THERAPY

2.5.4.1 Corticosteroids

Corticosteroids should be used to treat active ulcerative colitis. They have no role in maintenance treatment to prevent relapse. The dosage and routes of administration vary with the severity and location of ulcerative colitis.

2.5.4.1.1 *Rectal corticosteroid preparations* These are available as hydrocortisone 100 mg in a 60 mL aqueous suspension (Cortenema®), as hydrocortisone acetate 80 mg in a propylene glycol gel (Cortifoam®), and as hydrocortisone acetate 10 mg or 40 mg in an ointment base (Cortiment®). Budesonide enemas (Entocort® 0.02 mg/mL) have now been released for use in Canada. They are effective, the cost is competitive, and the adverse-effect profile is favorable. In general, enema preparations will cover a larger surface area of the colon, while the effect of foam and ointment preparations is generally limited to the rectum. With mild disease, especially that of the distal colon, rectal instillation of steroids will induce or maintain remission for a high percentage of patients. With mild to moderately severe ulcerative proctitis, twice-daily rectal steroids combined with systemic therapy will promote remission and more quickly return the rectum to its normal functional reservoir capacity. Patients should instill the solution while in the left lateral decubitus position and then change their position to right decubitus followed by prone for at least 20 minutes after each position, to allow for maximal topical coverage. Studies indicate that up to one-half of rectally administered steroids is absorbed. Even though systemic absorption does occur, adrenal cortical responsiveness is not adversely affected.

2.5.4.1.2 *Systemic corticosteroid preparations* In active pancolonic disease of mild to moderate severity, prednisone should be started in a dose of 40 mg/day. A single daily dose of prednisone is most convenient; however, such a dose does produce adrenal suppression. No significant difference in healing between groups given single daily doses or divided daily doses of oral steroids has been detected. For patients whose disease responds promptly to oral steroids, withdrawal should be undertaken at 5 mg/week until a dose of 20 mg/day is reached; then the drug should be tapered by 2.5 mg/week to off. In the case of severe ulcerative colitis, the patient requires hospitalization, and intravenous steroids (prednisone 40 mg equivalent/day) should be started. The tapering off protocol is as outlined above.

Once the disease is in remission, further steroid treatment should be avoided until a subsequent exacerbation occurs. Treatment is then reinstituted at a level appropriate to the severity of exacerbation (steroid enemas for mild to moderate exacerbations of proctosigmoiditis, oral or intravenous steroids for moderate to severe pancolonic relapses). If, however, symptoms recur with the attempted withdrawal of steroids, then long-term steroid therapy may be necessary until the patient experiences remission. The use of high doses of steroids to maintain the patient relatively symptom-free is not recommended, however, in view of the potential side effects of steroid therapy. If a patient requires more than 15 mg of oral prednisone daily for many months in order to keep the colitis in control, elective colectomy should be considered as an alternative means of treatment.

Steroids, particularly steroids in the high doses necessary for severe cases, may "mask" a perforation of the colon and lead to peritoneal soiling and death; therefore, careful monitoring of the patient on such high doses is vitally important.

2.5.4.2 Mesalamine derivatives

Mesalamine (5-aminosalicylic acid mesalazine, or 5-ASA) has been shown to be the active part of sulfasalazine and is effective in the treatment of active disease and in maintenance therapy to prevent relapse.

2.5.4.2.1 Mesalamine (5-ASA) rectal preparations

During the past decade mesalamine has been developed in the form of rectal enemas and suppositories. Mesalamine enemas have an overall efficacy of about 80% in patients with active left-sided colitis. Side effects occur in less than 2% of ulcerative colitis patients, many of whom would have had previous allergic reactions to sulfasalazine. In comparison studies, mesalamine enemas are as effective as corticosteroid enemas in the treatment of proctitis and proctosigmoiditis (16). In patients with distal proctitis, mesalamine suppositories (500 mg b.i.d.) are rapidly effective without side effects (17).

2.5.4.2.2 Mesalamine (5-ASA) oral preparations

5-ASA is available as sulfasalazine (Salazopyrin®) or as second-generation 5-ASA products that deliver the active ingredient (5-ASA) to the colon without the toxic sulfapyridine moiety (Asacol®, Dipentum®, Mesasal™, Pentasa®, Salofalk®).

Sulfasalazine is metabolized by colonic flora, thus releasing sulfapyridine, an absorbable antibiotic, and 5-aminosalicylic acid (5-ASA), the active ingredient. The sulfapyridine acts only to carry the 5-ASA to the colon and, when released by bacterial metabolism, it is absorbed and is responsible for the dose-related side effects of sulfasalazine. The acetylation rate of sulfapyridine is genetically determined; slow acetylators develop side effects at lower dose levels of sulfasalazine than fast acetylators. The most common dose-related symptoms are anorexia, nausea, dyspepsia and diarrhea. Common hematological complications include impairment of folate absorption (thus supplemental folate therapy is a requirement for all patients on sulfasalazine) and Heinz-body hemolytic anemia. Hypospermia may occur and is reversible through withdrawal of the drug. Hypersensitivity reactions are rare; symptoms include fever, rash, bone marrow suppression, infiltrative lung disease, a lupus-like syndrome, pancreatitis and hepatic toxicity. Sulfasalazine is inferior to corticosteroids in the treatment of acute, moderately severe colitis. For this reason, sulfasalazine is used as an adjunctive to steroid therapy and not as the first line of therapy for acute attacks of ulcerative colitis. Therefore, once steroids have been started and the patient is tolerating oral fluids well, sulfasalazine can be started at a dose of 1 g/day and gradually increased to 4–6 g/day within 7 days. The second-generation site-specific compounds capable of delivering mesalamine to the colon appear to have less systemic toxicity than sulfasalazine. Patients doing well on sulfasalazine are usually not changed to mesalamine product. Nevertheless, new patients presenting with ulcerative colitis are often started on second-generation mesalamine product rather than sulfasalazine.

The two main pharmacological approaches of the second-generation mesalamine compounds adopted are (1) the creation of azo-derivative compounds similar to sulfasalazine but linked with mesalamine through a diazo-bond with another mesalamine molecule (olsalazine, as in Dipentum®); and (2) the incorporation of mesalamine either into pH-dependent delivery capsules such as Asacol® (pH 7.0) or Mesasal™ and Salofalk® (pH 6.0), or into a mixed slow-release pH-dependent polymer (Pentasa®). These second-generation compounds have shown comparable efficacy to sulfasalazine, with generally fewer side effects (18). Comparative studies assessing which compound might favor a higher mesalamine release into the colon and thus would be more suitable for patients with colonic inflammation are yet to be finalized. Comparison of mesalamine product dose and cost is presented in Table 6.

Once remission has been induced by either corticosteroid or mesalamine therapy, the risk of ulcerative colitis relapse can be reduced from 60% to approximately 20% with maintenance mesalamine therapy in approximately one-half the active treatment dose.

2.5.4.3 *Immunosuppressive agents*
In general, the use of immunosuppressive agents (azathioprine, 6-mercaptopurine and cyclosporine) have been disappointing in ulcerative colitis. Encouraging preliminary results with methotrexate in severe ulcerative colitis have been published (19).

2.5.4.4 *Metronidazole*
Unlike Crohn's disease, ulcerative colitis does not respond to metronidazole.

2.6 Complications
Ulcerative colitis may be complicated by a variety of associated conditions. These are (1) local complications arising in and around the colon, and (2) systemic complications arising at sites distant from the colon (Table 11).

2.6.1 *MINOR LOCAL COMPLICATIONS*
Minor local complications in ulcerative colitis, unlike those in Crohn's colitis, are infrequent and generally heal with conservative management. Enteroenteric perianal fistulas develop in a very small number of patients with ulcerative colitis. In these instances the physician must be certain that he or she is not dealing with Crohn's colitis, in which enteroenteric fistulas are common.

2.6.2 *MAJOR LOCAL COMPLICATIONS*

2.6.2.1 *Toxic megacolon*
Toxic megacolon is characterized by an acute dilatation of all or part of the colon to a diameter greater than 6 cm (measured in the mid-transverse colon) and is associated with severe systemic toxicity. Toxic megacolon occurs in 1–2% of patients with ulcerative colitis. Histological examination reveals extensive deep ulcerations and acute inflammation that involves all muscle layers of the colon and often extends to the serosa. This widespread inflammation accounts for toxic megacolon's systemic toxicity (fever, tachycardia, localized abdominal pain and leukocytosis). The loss of colonic muscular tone results in the dilatation of the colon.

Though the association between a barium enema and toxic megacolon has not been experimentally proven, there are many reports of toxic megacolon developing after the patient has undergone a barium enema. Thus, a barium enema should not be performed on patients who are acutely ill with ulcerative colitis.

Clinically, the patient with toxic megacolon presents as severely ill with a

TABLE 11.   Complications of ulcerative colitis

Local complications	Frequency (%)
Minor	
Hemorrhoids	20
Pseudopolyps	15
Anal fissures	12
Anal fistulas	5
Perianal abscess	5
Rectal prolapse	2
Rectovaginal fistulas	2
Major	
Toxic megacolon	2
Colonic perforation	3
Massive colonic hemorrhage	4
Colonic carcinoma	–
Colonic stricture	5

Systemic complications	Frequency (%)
Hepatic	
Biliary	
Pericholangitis	30
Sclerosing cholangitis	1
Bile duct carcinoma	0.5
Hepatocellular	
Fatty infiltration	30
Chronic active hepatitis	5
Cirrhosis	3
Amyloidosis	1
Hematologic	
Anemia	
Iron deficiency	
Autoimmune hemolytic anemia	
Microangiopathic hemolytic anemia	
Heinz-body hemolytic anemia	
(with sulfasalazine therapy)	
Thrombocytosis	
Thromboembolic disease	
Joint	
Peripheral arthritis, migratory, nondeforming, large-joint,	
seronegative	20
Ankylosing spondylitis, sacroiliitis	20

(cont'd)

TABLE 11.   Complications of ulcerative colitis (cont'd)

Systemic complications	Frequency (%)
Skin	
Erythema nodosum	3
Pyoderma gangrenosum	4
Ocular	
Episcleritis, uveitis	5
Iritis	5

TABLE 12.   Diagnosis of toxic megacolon

Signs of toxicity (three of the following criteria are required)
Fever >38.6°C
Tachycardia >120 beats per minute
Leukocytosis >10,000/mm^3
Anemia <60% of normal
Hypoalbuminemia <3 g/dL

Associated signs (one of the following criteria is required)
Dehydration
Mental confusion
Hypotension
Electrolyte disturbance

Signs of dilatation
Colonic diameter >6 cm or progressive distention with abnormal haustral pattern

fever, tachycardia, dehydration, abdominal pain and distention (Table 12). Examination reveals absent bowel sounds, tympany and rebound tenderness. Leukocytosis (greater than 10,000), anemia and hypoalbuminemia are often present. A plain x-ray of the abdomen will reveal dilatation of a colonic segment or of the entire colon. On plain supine x-ray, dilatation of the transverse colon is most often seen. This distention of the transverse colon does not indicate severity of disease in this segment of the colon; rather, the distention is determined by the anterior position of the transverse colon. Repositioning the patient to a prone position will redistribute the gas to the more posterior descending colon and will dramatically decrease gaseous tension in the transverse colon.

If toxic megacolon is the presenting symptom of ulcerative colitis, diagnosis may be difficult, since a history of rectal bleeding and diarrhea is sometimes obscured by toxic megacolon. Most often, toxic megacolon complicates chronic intermittent ulcerative colitis and the diagnosis is not difficult. Occasionally, however, a patient seriously ill with ulcerative colitis and the resultant profuse bloody diarrhea will experience a sudden decrease in the frequency of bowel motions upon development of toxic megacolon. This decrease in stool frequency represents diminished colonic evacuation rather than improvement in the patient's status. In this instance, a delay in diagnosis could result in perforation and death.

Treatment of toxic megacolon consists of general supportive measures, including replacement of fluid and electrolyte deficits, correction of hypokalemia, transfusions and nasogastric suction. Intravenous steroids (prednisone equivalent 60–80 mg/day) should be utilized for 48 to 72 hours. If there is insufficient response, surgery should be seriously considered. If the systemic symptoms subside and the abdominal signs improve, high-dose steroids should be continued for 10 to 14 days, after which the dose should be gradually tapered off.

Patients whose disease does not respond to appropriate intensive medical therapy within three days have a risk of colonic perforation of 50%. Mortality in the face of recognized or unrecognized perforation is approximately 85%; thus, surgery should be considered at an early stage rather than at a later.

2.6.2.2 Cancer of the colon

Carcinoma of the colon afflicts patients with ulcerative colitis 7 to 30 times more frequently than it does the general population. The risk of colon cancer in ulcerative colitis is related to two factors: (1) duration of the colitis, and (2) extent of colonic involvement. The risk of colon cancer for patients who have had the disease less than 10 years is low, but this risk steadily increases. The cancer risk for patients who have had disease activity for 10 to 20 years is 23 times that of the general population, while a disease duration of more than 20 years is associated with a cancer risk 32 times greater than that of the general population. The extent of colonic involvement in colitis also influences the risk of cancer. The incidence of cancer when ulcerative colitis is limited to the rectum or to the left side of the colon is much lower than when ulcerative colitis involves the entire colon.

The colonic malignancy associated with ulcerative colitis is generally an adenocarcinoma evenly scattered throughout the colon. The adenocarcinoma is often flatter than cancers in the general population and has fewer overhanging margins. It is generally considered extremely aggressive.

Because of this high cumulative risk of cancer, prophylactic diagnostic procedures have been employed in an attempt to detect early malignant changes in the colon of patients with ulcerative colitis. Colonoscopy and biopsy have revealed that colorectal dysplasia is associated with colonic malignancy. However, areas of dysplasia can be missed at the time of biopsy, and the interpretation of dysplasia in the presence of active inflammatory disease is difficult, since regenerative epithelium may exhibit many of the features of dysplasia.

In summary, no test or group of diagnostic tests (not even frequent colonoscopies and biopsies) can absolutely guarantee that the patient with long-term ulcerative colitis is free of focal malignancy.

Patients with ulcerative colitis should have a colonoscopy and multiple biopsies performed after 5 years of disease. If no dysplasia is revealed by multiple colonic biopsies, repeat colonoscopy can be performed every 2 years thereafter. For patients with moderate or severe dysplasia on colonoscopic biopsies, repeat colonoscopy every 6 months to 1 year is recommended. Until more diagnostic tools are available to identify those patients at risk for cancer, colectomy at 10 years to cure the ulcerative colitis and prevent colonic cancer is highly recommended.

2.6.2.3 *Colonic stricture*
Colonic stricture occurs infrequently but may mimic colonic adenocarcinoma clinically and radiologically. If there is any question regarding the diagnosis, surgical removal is advocated.

2.6.2.4 *Massive colonic hemorrhage*
Although rectal bleeding is universal in cases of ulcerative colitis, massive, life-threatening colonic hemorrhage is rare. For most patients, massive colonic hemorrhage can be medically managed with blood transfusions, steroids and 5-ASA products. Hemorrhage usually resolves spontaneously.

2.6.3 *SYSTEMIC COMPLICATIONS*

2.6.3.1 *Hepatocellular disease*
Pericholangitis is seen in 30% of patients with ulcerative colitis. It tends to occur more often in patients with pancolitis than in those with ulcerative colitis limited to the distal colon. This liver lesion is characterized by periportal inflammatory infiltrates, degenerative changes in bile ductules, and varying degrees of periportal edema and fibrosis. The lesion of pericholangitis is patchy; therefore, sampling error on needle biopsy of the liver often occurs. Clinical manifestations of pericholangitis or its progression to cirrhosis are exceedingly rare, and many patients have only minor abnormalities in serum alkaline phosphatase.

Sclerosing cholangitis develops in less than 1% of patients with ulcerative colitis. In this disorder, the bile duct becomes severely narrowed and resultant recurrent attacks of jaundice, right upper quadrant pain, fever and leukocytosis occur. This lesion must be distinguished from other causes of obstruction of the common bile duct. Sclerosing cholangitis does not respond to any therapy.

Fatty infiltration of the liver is seen in 30% of patients with ulcerative colitis. The etiology of the fat deposition is unknown, but it may be due to malnutrition and protein depletion resulting from diarrhea and protein-losing enteropathy. Liver function studies are normal or only mildly abnormal in patients with fatty infiltration.

2.6.3.2 Hematologic abnormalities

The most common hematologic abnormality in ulcerative colitis is iron deficiency anemia secondary to gastrointestinal blood loss. Most often this can be treated with oral ferrous sulfate (325 mg t.i.d.). However, for some patients, gastrointestinal intolerance of ferrous sulfate will necessitate parenteral iron injections (Imferon®).

Heinz-body hemolytic anemia can be seen in patients receiving sulfasalazine. This type of hemolytic anemia is directly related to the sulfasalazine and resolves when the offending agent is withdrawn. Additionally, autoimmune hemolytic anemia and microangiopathic hemolytic anemia, with or without disseminated intravascular coagulation, can occur.

Secondary thrombocytosis may appear. It is not associated with coagulation defects. However, in addition to thrombocytosis, increased levels of factor V and fibrinogen can be seen, together with reductions in levels of antithrombin III. In rare instances, pulmonary embolism and thrombosis of mesenteric or cranial vessels due to thromboembolic disease can occur. Repeated pulmonary embolisms in spite of adequate anticoagulation therapy or massive colonic hemorrhage during anticoagulation therapy will necessitate a vena cava ligation with colectomy.

2.6.3.3 Joint manifestations

The arthritis of ulcerative colitis may antedate the colonic symptoms. It tends to be migratory and affect the larger joints, is associated with a synovitis and swollen painful joints, and is nondeforming with no involvement of adjacent cartilage or bone. Rheumatoid factors are negative in these patients. Arthritis usually subsides with control of the colitis.

There is a high incidence of ankylosing spondylitis and sacroiliitis in patients with ulcerative colitis. Unlike peripheral arthritis, the ankylosing spondylitis in ulcerative colitis is chronic, progressive, deforming and generalized. It does not respond to corticosteroids and will progress in the face of quiescent colitis. The incidence of sacroiliitis is higher than that of ankylosing spondylitis in patients with ulcerative colitis. However, the sacroiliitis is often asymptomatic and can be identified only through appropriate x-rays of the pelvis.

2.6.3.4 *Skin manifestations*
Erythema nodosum with raised tender erythematous swellings on the extensor surfaces of the legs and arms is less frequent with ulcerative colitis than with Crohn's disease.

Pyoderma gangrenosum complicates severe ulcerative colitis but is rarely seen with mild disease. This skin lesion begins as a small, elevated nodule, which gradually becomes gangrenous, thus resulting in progressive necrosis of the surrounding skin. It tends to ulcerate deeply, involving underlying soft tissue and sometimes bone.

Usually both erythema nodosum and pyoderma gangrenosum will respond to control of the colitis. Occasionally, despite control of the colonic disease, the pyoderma gangrenosum will progress. Persistent severe pyoderma gangrenosum is thus an indication for colectomy.

2.6.3.5 *Ocular manifestations*
Iritis occurs in 5% of patients with ulcerative colitis and presents as blurred vision, eye pain and photophobia. The attack may be followed by atrophy of the iris, anterior and posterior synechiae, and pigment deposits on the lens. Episcleritis and other ocular lesions are only rarely seen with ulcerative colitis.

REFERENCES

1. Mayer L, Eisenhardt D. Lack of induction of suppressor T-cells by intestinal epithelial cells from patients with inflammatory bowel disease. J Clin Invest 1990; 86:1255–1260.
2. Saxon A, Shanahan F, Landers C, Ganz T, Targan S. A distinct subset of antineutrophil cytoplasmic antibodies is associated with inflammatory bowel disease. J Allergy Clin Immunol 1990; 86:202–210.
3. Gitnick G. Etiology of inflammatory bowel disease: Where have we been? Where are we going? Scand J Gastroenterol 1990; 25(Suppl 175):93–96.
4. Das KM, Vecchi M, Sakamaki S. A shared and unique epitope(s) on human colon, skin, and biliary epithelium detected by a monoclonal antibody. Gastroenterology 1990; 98:464–469.
5. Seldenrijk CA, Drexhage HA, Meuwissen SG, Meijer CJ. T-cellular immune

reactions (in macrophage inhibition factor assay) against Mycobacterium para-tuberculosis, Mycobacterium kansasii, Mycobacterium tuberculosis, Mycobacterium avium in patients with chronic inflammatory bowel disease. Gut 1990; 31:529–535.

6. Katz KD, Hollander D, Vadheim CM, et al. Intestinal permeability in patients with Crohn's disease and their healthy relatives. Gastroenterology 1989; 97:927–931.

7. Modigliani R, Mary YJ, Simon JF, et al. Clinical, biological, and endoscopic picture of attacks of Crohn's disease: evolution on prednisolone. Gastroenterology 1990; 98:811–818.

8. International Mesalazine Study Group. Coated oral 5-aminosalicylic acid versus placebo in maintaining remission of inactive Crohn's disease. Aliment Pharmacol Ther 1990; 4:55–64.

9. Present DH. 6-Mercaptopurine and other immunosuppressive agents in the treatment of Crohn's disease and ulcerative colitis. Gastroenterol Clin North Am 1989; 18:57–71.

10. Present DH, Meltzer SJ, Krumholz MP, Wolke A, Korelitz BI. 6-Mercaptopurine in the management of inflammatory bowel disease: short- and long-term toxicity. Ann Intern Med 1989; 111:641–649.

11. Brynskov J, Freund L, Rasmussen SN, et al. A placebo-controlled, double-blind, randomized trial of cyclosporine therapy in active chronic Crohn's disease. N Engl J Med 1989; 321:845–850.

12. Fedorak RN, Empey LR, MacArthur C, Jewell LD. Misoprostol provides a colonic mucosal protective effect during acetic acid–induced colitis in rats. Gastroenterology 1990; 98:615–625.

13. Wallace JL, Keenan CM. An orally active inhibitor of leukotriene synthesis accelerates healing in a rat model of colitis. Am J Physiol 1990; 258:G527–534.

14. Salomon P, Kornbluth AA, Janowitz HD. Treatment of ulcerative colitis with fish oil n-3-omega-fatty acid: an open trial. J Clin Gastroenterol 1990; 12:157–161.

15. Laursen LS, Naesdal J, Bukhave K, Lauritsen K, Rask-Madsen J. Selective 5-lipoxygenase inhibition in ulcerative colitis. Lancet 1990; 335:683–685.

16. Campieri M, De Franchis R, Bianchi Porro G, Ranzi T, Brunetti G, Barbara L. Mesalazine (5-aminosalicylic acid) suppositories in the treatment of ulcerative proctitis or distal proctosigmoiditis: a randomized controlled trial. Scand J Gastroenterol 1990; 25:663–668.

17. Campieri M, Gionchetti P, Belluzzi A, et al. Topical treatment with 5-aminosalicylic in distal ulcerative colitis by using a new suppository preparation: a double-blind placebo controlled trial. Int J Colorectal Dis 1990; 5:79–81.

18. Riley SA, Turnberg LA. Sulphasalazine and the aminosalicylates in the treatment of inflammatory bowel disease. Q J Med 1990; 75:551–562.

19. Kozarek RA, Patterson DJ, Gelfand MD, Botoman VA, Ball TJ, Wilske KR. Methotrexate induces clinical and histologic remission in patients with refractory inflammatory bowel disease. Ann Intern Med 1989; 110:353–356.

SUGGESTED READING LIST

Calkins BM. A meta-analysis of the role of smoking in inflammatory bowel disease. Dig Dis Sci 1989; 34:1841–1854.

Delpre G, Avidor I, Steinherz R, Kadish U, Ben-Bassat M. Ultrastructural abnormalities in endoscopically and histologically normal and involved colon in ulcerative colitis. Am J Gastroenterol 1989; 84:1038–1046.

Ekbom A, Helmick C, Zack M, Adami HO. Ulcerative colitis and colorectal cancer: a population-based study. N Engl J Med 1990; 323:1228–1233.

Gyde S. Screening for colorectal cancer in ulcerative colitis: dubious benefits and high cost [Editorial]. Gut 1990; 31:1089–1092.

Hamilton PW, Allen DC, Watt PCH. A combination of cytological and architectural morphometry in assessing regenerative hyperplasia and dysplasia in ulcerative colitis. Histopathology 1990; 16:59–68.

Lashner BA, Kane SV, Hanauer SB. Colon cancer surveillance in chronic ulcerative colitis: historical cohort study. Am J Gastroenterol 1990: 85:1083–1087.

Lennard-Jones JE, Melville DM, Morson BC, Ritchie JK, Williams CB. Precancer and cancer in extensive ulcerative colitis: findings among 401 patients over 22 years. Gut 1990; 31:800–806.

10
The Colon

G.K. Turnbull, M. Burnstein and B. Vair

THIS CHAPTER OUTLINES specific diseases that primarily involve the colon. The student is referred to the recommended textbooks and the Suggested Reading List for more detailed information on each of these conditions. In addition, an overview of lower gastrointestinal tract bleeding and diseases specifically involving the anal canal is given in this chapter.

1. SPECIFIC COLONIC DISEASES

1.1 Colon Polyps and Cancer

Colon cancer is the second most common cancer (after lung cancer) in men and women combined in Canada. Unlike lung cancer, it has a high survival rate in patients diagnosed before it has spread beyond the confines of the bowel wall. Since it is a very common cancer, has a high survival rate with early curative surgery and is poorly responsive to other forms of cancer therapy, a high index of suspicion must be maintained in approaching patients with symptoms of colonic dysfunction (Table 1), especially if they are over the age of 40, when the incidence of colon cancer begins to rise. Increased colon cancer risk is also seen in patients with ulcerative colitis, a history of female genital or breast cancer, or a family history of colon cancer or adenoma (including familial polyposis syndromes).

The Dukes' classification is used to stage colon cancer after surgical resection. It is based on the pathological extent and invasion of the primary colonic tumor (adenocarcinoma) at the time of resection (Table 2). Dukes' A stage is adenocarcinoma confined to the mucosa and submucosa; the cure rate for this stage of adenocarcinoma with surgery is about 90%. Dukes' B stage has two

TABLE 1.   Presenting features of colon cancer

Abdominal pain, including symptoms of bowel obstruction
Change in bowel habit
Abdominal mass
Vague abdominal complaints of recent onset
Hypokalemia
Iron deficiency anemia

subdivisions: B1 for adenocarcinomas that have invaded the muscularis pro-pria, and B2 for tumors that have invaded through to the circular longitudinal muscle although regional lymph nodes are free of cancer. Dukes' C stage is adenocarcinoma that has spread to regional lymph nodes, and Dukes' D stage is adenocarcinoma that is metastatic to distant sites, usually the liver and beyond. Cure rates with stage C and D adenocarcinoma of the colon are very low with surgery; as well, both chemotherapy and radiotherapy have limited success, reinforcing the need to make an early diagnosis. Table 2 also describes the newer TNM colorectal adenocarcinoma staging system, which is similar to the Dukes' A–D staging system. The TNM staging system includes stage 0 when the carcinoma is limited to the mucosa and is called "in situ."

Early recognition is of the utmost importance to try to identify early cancer at a curative stage. Therefore, patients with intermittent symptoms are as important to investigate as patients with persistent symptoms, and the story of occasional blood in the stool in a patient over 40 years of age should not be attributed to local anorectal disease without excluding a more proximal lesion. Many patients may present with no gastrointestinal symptoms, but rather an iron deficiency anemia due to chronic bleeding from the tumor. Patients may not see blood in the stool or note a melena stool, particularly when there is a right-sided colonic lesion. A change in bowel habit, often with constipation alternating with diarrhea, may be the first sign of obstructive symptoms from a colon cancer, and should never be ignored in a patient over 40 years of age with a recent onset of these symptoms. Some patients may present with prima-rily diarrhea if they have a high output of mucus and fluid from the tumor; in this instance the tumor may be a villous adenoma, and some patients may have hypokalemia due to large amounts of potassium lost with the mucus secretion from the tumor.

1.1.1 POLYP–CARCINOMA SEQUENCE
It is now agreed that the majority of colon cancer patients have a colonic adenocarcinoma arising from an adenomatous polyp. Polyps of 2 cm or

TABLE 2. Colorectal adenocarcinoma staging

Dukes' stage	TNM stage	Tumor invasion	5-year survival
	0	Mucosa	
A	I	Submucosa No lymph node or distant metastases	90%
B	II	B1: Circular muscle B2: Longitudinal muscle No lymph node or distant metastases	70–75%
C	III	C1: 1–4 lymph nodes positive C2: > 4 lymph nodes positive	45%
D	IV	Distant metastases (e.g., liver)	20% or less

greater have about 50% incidence of cancer, compared to 1% in adenomas of 1 cm or less. Therefore, adenomatous polyps are a premalignant condition, and their identification and removal before becoming malignant prevents the development of colon cancer. These polyps can arise anywhere in the colon, but (as is the case for colon cancer) they are more frequently seen in the left colon. The majority of polyps are completely asymptomatic, but the occurrence of occult bleeding does increase in frequency as they grow. Unfortunately, however, polyps can still be missed, even with occult blood testing of the stool, since the blood loss may be intermittent.

Three histologic types of adenomatous polyps occur: tubular, tubulovillous and villous. The malignant potential is greatest in villous polyps (40%) and lowest in tubular polyps (5%), with an intermediate risk in tubulovillous polyps (22%). The malignant potential may also be described pathologically as the degree of "dysplasia": the more severe the dysplasia, the greater the rate of malignancy. These tubular, tubulovillous and villous polyps can often be completely removed by snare polypectomy at colonoscopy if they are pedunculated on a stalk, but sessile polyps that carpet a wide area of colonic mucosa (often villous polyps) can usually be completely removed only by resection surgery. Since polyps precede cancer and removal of polyps "cures" the cancer, it has been hoped that screening colonoscopy may help reduce the incidence of cancer. Other polyps as well may be present at the initial or index colonoscopy, and polyps and cancer tend to recur. This sets the stage for the rationale for performing follow-up surveillance colonoscopies (colon cancer surveillance program). The best time interval for this surveillance is probably every three years; longer intervals between surveillance colonoscopies may be safe but have yet to be tested. The cost-effectiveness of screening all patients over the age of 40 has not been proven, and until particular subgroups of patients likely to have polyps are identifiable, routine colonoscopy screening is not indicated.

Particular conditions have been associated with an increased risk of colon cancer. The polyposis syndromes of familial polyposis and Gardner's syndrome are manifested by early onset (usually before age 30) of innumerable colonic adenomatous polyps that eventually and invariably lead to colon cancer (usually before age 40). Since the colon has too many polyps to remove by endoscopy-guided polypectomy these patients are referred at an early age for total colectomy to remove the risk of colon cancer. There are other families (site-specific colorectal cancer, family cancer syndrome) that have a high risk of colon cancer (autosomal dominant inheritance), with more than two first-degree relatives having had colon cancer. It would be prudent to enter such patients into a colon cancer surveillance program of colonoscopy and/or air contrast barium enema if they have colonic polyps when screened at age 40. Other groups of patients with other malignancies such as breast cancer and ovarian cancer appear to be at increased risk of colon cancer, but there are currently no recommendations for these patients to be screened regularly for colonic polyps.

Also at a high risk for colon cancer are patients with total colon involvement with chronic ulcerative colitis for more than 10 years; this risk also appears to be present, but to a lesser extent, in patients with Crohn's pancolitis. The patients at highest risk are those who have had total colon involvement and those with left-sided disease, up to and including the hepatic flexure; patients with proctosigmoiditis are at least risk – probably not greater than the general population. Curiously, the risk of cancer does not correlate with the degree of disease activity. Therefore, patients with just one bout of proven subtotal ulcerative colitis would have an increased risk of cancer after 10 years of disease, and the younger the patient at the time of onset of his or her disease, the greater the cumulative risk of cancer will be for that patient. Unlike those who experience the "polyp–carcinoma sequence," patients with colitis do not develop adenomatous polyps before they develop cancer; therefore they require colonoscopy about once every one to two years, with endoscopic biopsies of the colon performed to identify dysplasia of the mucosa. Particular attention should be paid to "elevated" or "flat" lesions seen at colonoscopy where the incidence of early colon cancer is high. If there is high-grade dysplasia, colectomy should be recommended to the patient.

1.2 Diverticulosis

In Western societies diverticulosis occurs in at least one person in two above the age of 50 years. The frequency increases with age. Diverticulosis or diverticular disease of the colon is due to pseudodiverticula in that the wall of the diverticulum is not full-thickness colonic wall, but rather outpouchings of colonic mucosa through points of weakness in the colonic wall where the blood vessels penetrate the muscularis propria. These diverticula are prone to infection or "diverticulitis" presumably because they trap feces with bacteria. If the infection spreads beyond the confines of the diverticula in the colonic wall, an abscess is formed. Patients present with increasing left lower quadrant pain and fever, often with constipation and lower abdominal obstructive symptoms such as bloating and distention. Some patients with severe obstructive symptoms may actually describe nausea or vomiting.

With diverticulitis, both with and without abscess formation, the above symptoms can develop. On physical examination the patient often has localized tenderness in the left lower quadrant, and with severe infection and an abscess may have rebound tenderness in the left lower quadrant. A palpable mass is often identifiable where the sigmoid colon (the most common site of diverticulitis) is infected. Treatment consists of intravenous fluids and bowel rest by placing the patient on no oral intake or just a clear liquid diet; intravenous antibiotics are administered. Generally broad-spectrum antibiotics are used to cover gram-negative enteric bacteria and anaerobic bacteria that are normally found in the colon.

Many complications can occur in diverticulitis. These are listed in Table 3. Colonic stricture after resolution of diverticulitis is described further in Section 1.6.

Bleeding occurs in less than 5% of diverticulosis patients; is abrupt in onset, painless, and often massive; and often occurs from the right colon. It is rare for patients with diverticulosis to have significant bleeding. Over 80% of diverticulosis patients will stop bleeding, but the rest will continue and require investigation and treatment (see Section 3). Segmental colonic resection is reserved for that small group of patients who continue bleeding or have recurrent bleeding.

1.3 Irritable Bowel Syndrome

Most commonly, patients exhibiting symptoms from the GI tract are suffering

TABLE 3. Complications of diverticulitis

Abdominal abscess/Liver abscess
Colonic obstruction
Fistulas
    Colovesical
    Colovaginal
    Colocutaneous

---

from the irritable bowel syndrome. This is a condition that may be a variant of normal function. Causes of irritable bowel are still being evaluated. It appears that patients have no organic disease of the gastrointestinal tract, yet they experience frequent symptoms from the bowel. Large epidemiologic studies would suggest that the condition occurs in at least 15% of the population.

The commonest symptom that brings a patient to a doctor is abdominal pain. Criteria have been developed to identify with more certainty those patients who have the irritable bowel syndrome. A more positive diagnosis can be made, particularly in women, if the abdominal pain is not localized and tends to have been present for at least three months. The pain is associated with bowel movements and relieved after defecation. Abdominal pain is also associated with increased looseness of stool as well as increased frequency. For a "strict" diagnosis of the irritable bowel syndrome, along with the above criteria it is felt that three of the following symptoms should also be present: (1) patients have difficult defecation; (2) patients complain of abdominal bloating or distention; (3) mucus is present in the stool; (4) there is increased stool frequency; (5) there is increased looseness of the stool at the onset of the abdominal pain.

Patients who have difficulty with defecation can have the following complaints. There can be "urgency," with the sudden urge to pass stool and a fear of incontinence if defecation is not performed immediately. Many patients with this symptom will relate that they always identify where the toilet is when they are away from home. The fear of incontinence can often greatly limit a patient's ability to function normally in society. Other patients with difficult defecation may have to strain – defined as having to hold their breath and push when attempting defecation. Straining is defined as "constipation" when a patient must strain 25% or more of the time when trying to defecate. Finally, some patients describe a feeling of incomplete emptying after passing stool. This symptom has to be asked for specifically, as most patients will not spontaneously report it. Nevertheless, the symptom is commonly reported by patients with an irritable bowel.

The presence of mucus in the stool can be alarming to some patients, since they may interpret this to mean they have "colitis." In the past, some doctors used to refer to irritable bowel as "mucus colitis," which is a misnomer since there is no "colitis" or inflammation of the colon in irritable bowel. Mucus is a normal product of the colon, and only if mucus and blood are seen together should other diagnoses such as "colitis" be considered.

The typical stool pattern described by patients with an irritable bowel is the change in stool character and frequency with the onset of abdominal pain. Typically, patients will pass a normally formed stool (sometimes even a constipated stool) first thing in the morning. Then with the attacks of abdominal pain the stools become more frequent and looser, sometimes becoming just liquid diarrheal stools. Once bowel movements cease the pain is relieved, but it can recur again later in the day, often precipitated by eating high-fat foods or other gut stimulants (e.g., coffee).

There have been reports that in men the above criteria (called the Manning Criteria) may not be as helpful as they are in women. It is also important to note that the vast majority of people with an irritable bowel have their symptoms begin in young adult life. One should consider other colonic diseases in patients over the age of 40 who develop these symptoms for the first time without previous episodes suggesting irritable bowel. Sometimes later in life patients can develop irritable bowel after severe infectious diarrhea, but in this population as well, further investigations are warranted to ensure no other cause for the change in bowel function.

The irritable bowel syndrome is a disorder affecting the entire gut, and although many of the symptoms appear to arise from the colon, these patients frequently have symptoms from other parts of the GI tract as well as from other organs. Upper GI symptoms are very common in irritable bowel; these consist of increased frequency of esophageal reflux. As well, nonulcer dyspepsia is associated with irritable bowel. Dyspepsia symptoms in general occur more commonly than lower bowel symptoms, but are obviously due to many other causes, including reflux esophagitis, gastritis, peptic ulcer disease and, less commonly, biliary tract and pancreatic disease. When upper GI symptoms are associated with irritable bowel, other underlying diseases must be considered. Other associated symptoms include frequent headaches and urinary symptoms that are similar to bowel symptoms, in that patients can have urgency and frequency of urination. These symptoms are often worse at times when the bowel symptoms are troublesome. In women, irritable bowel symptoms can often be exacerbated or worsened around the time of menstruation. Studies suggest that bowel symptoms associated with menstruation occur in at least 50% of the normal female population.

When assessing a patient complaining of irritable bowel symptoms, remember that only a small proportion of patients with an irritable bowel present to doctors with these symptoms. Recent studies would suggest that patients who see doctors about their symptoms often have psychological problems, with increased levels of distress and depression as common findings. It is important to inquire about these problems, as successful treatment often consists of dealing with the distress and/or depression that accompanies the irritable bowel symptoms. They may often be the reason that the patient has sought medical attention in the first place.

1.3.1 DIFFERENTIAL DIAGNOSIS

The Manning Criteria provide a more positive diagnosis of irritable bowel: abdominal pain with the association of increased frequency and increased looseness of stool, relief of abdominal pain with defecation, abdominal bloating, mucus in the stool and defecation difficulties such as a sensation of incomplete rectal emptying after defecation. However, lactose intolerance is a common cause of change in bowel habit in young adults, particularly if their racial background is not northern European. Therefore, investigating for lactose intolerance in patients who present with increased frequency and looseness of stool is worthwhile, since the ingestion of lactose-containing foods may be the reason for their symptoms. All patients should have a thorough physical examination, in particular for evidence of disease in other organ systems such as the thyroid, which can present with a change in bowel habit. Patients with an irritable bowel will often have pain over the colon, particularly the sigmoid colon, on palpation. The identification of an enlarged liver or spleen or other abdominal masses necessitates further investigations. A barium enema is rarely required in a young healthy adult with new onset of irritable bowel symptoms. However, a patient over the age of 40 presenting with symptoms that may be irritable bowel yet of new onset and without previous complaints would warrant at least a barium enema and a sigmoidoscopic examination. The barium enema should also evaluate the terminal ileum if there is pain on palpation in the right lower quadrant. A complete blood count with platelet count should be done, as an elevated platelet count is often a sensitive finding for underlying inflammation and in the presence of bowel symptoms could mean the presence of early inflammatory bowel disease. Crohn's disease is more likely to present this way than irritable bowel. The persistence of the abdominal pain, even though lessened after bowel movements, would suggest possible underlying inflammation of the gut rather than an irritable bowel. Ulcerative colitis usually presents with rectal bleeding. Rectal bleeding is not a symptom of irritable bowel and its cause must always be investigated.

The presence of nocturnal symptoms, particularly with diarrhea waking the patient at night, is almost never due to an irritable bowel. Occasionally patients with depression who have early morning waking report this symptom, but in general further investigations are indicated.

1.3.2 THERAPY

The therapeutic approach in irritable bowel is as much reassurance as any specific therapies, as most patients do not have any "disease." It is most important to do a thorough history and physical examination to ensure that the complaints are not due to any underlying disease. Once this has been confirmed, explain to the patient how the bowel can produce these symptoms and that there is no cause for concern. Since patients presenting with irritable bowel symptoms frequently have more distress and tend to be more prone to seek medical attention for other minor medical conditions than other patients (so-called illness behavior), these patients may require considerable reassurance to convince them that they do not have serious disease. Part of this reassurance will be provided by screening blood tests such as a complete blood count with platelet count. Sigmoidoscopic examination will rule out most underlying early inflammatory bowel disease and any rectal pathology, particularly in patients complaining of defecation difficulties or a sensation of being unable to empty the rectum adequately. The stool should be analyzed for pathogens if diarrhea is present. Following these initial screening tests emphasis should be placed on the stresses present in the patient's life. Evaluating the level of stress and taking steps to correct it will often be helpful. Many patients, particularly those who have symptoms of constipation, may be helped with a high-fiber diet.

Drug treatment for irritable bowel is generally discouraged. There is no single drug that treats all the varied symptoms in irritable bowel, but occasional patients will continue to have intractable symptomatology. In this situation selected medications for specific symptoms may be helpful. Table 4 outlines some drugs that may be useful for specific symptoms. Drug therapy for irritable bowel should always by restricted to short periods during exacerbation of symptoms, and patients should be taken off medications when well. As irritable bowel is a chronic condition and is probably "normal" for these patients, the chronic use of medications often reinforces the notion that they have a "disease." Reassuring the patient that there is no association between irritable bowel symptoms and the development of more serious bowel disease such as colon cancer or inflammatory bowel disease can often alleviate some of the unreasonable yet very real concerns of many patients who present to doctors with these symptoms.

TABLE 4. Drug therapy in irritable bowel syndrome

Symptom	Drug	Dosage
Abdominal pain	Anticholinergics	
	Hyoscyamine	0.125 mg q4h prn
	Dicyclomine	10–20 mg po tid–qid before meals
	Antidepressants	
	Amitriptyline	10–25 mg hs (increase by 10–25 mg increments weekly)
	Enteric opioids	
	Trimebutine	100–200 mg po tid
Constipation	High-fiber diet	> 30 mg qd, plus 2 L liquid qd
	Osmotic laxatives	
	Milk of magnesia	15–30 mL po bid–tid prn
	Prokinetic agent	
	Cisapride	20 mg po bid
Diarrhea	Binding agent (resin)	
	Cholestyramine	4 g po qd–qid
	Antimotility agent	
	Loperamide	2–4 mg po qid prn
Abdominal bloating, "gas"	Simethicone	≤ qid prn
	Peppermint oil, enteric coated	1 cap po qid prn
	? motility agent	
	Cisapride	10–20 mg po bid–qid
	Domperidone	10 mg po qid

1.4 Fecal Incontinence

Understanding fecal incontinence requires knowledge of the normal function of the anorectum. Anatomically, it consists of the internal anal sphincter surrounded by the external anal sphincter and puborectalis muscles. The internal anal sphincter consists of smooth muscle and is a continuation of the circular smooth muscle of the rectum. The external anal sphincter is made up of skeletal muscle and surrounds the internal anal sphincter, whereas the puborectalis (also consisting of skeletal muscle) is a large U-shaped muscle that wraps around the upper anal canal at the anorectal junction above the external anal sphincter and loops anteriorly to attach to the pubic bone. This creates an anatomical sling of muscle that pulls the anorectal junction forward when it tight-

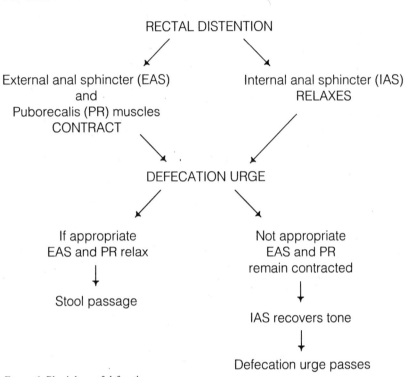

RECTAL DISTENTION

External anal sphincter (EAS)
and
Puborecalis (PR) muscles
CONTRACT

Internal anal sphincter (IAS)
RELAXES

DEFECATION URGE

If appropriate
EAS and PR relax

Stool passage

Not appropriate
EAS and PR
remain contracted

IAS recovers tone

Defecation urge passes

FIGURE 1. Physiology of defecation.

ens, thus closing the upper anal canal and creating the anorectal angle that is vital to the maintenance of fecal continence.

When stool (or gas or liquid) enters the rectum or sigmoid colon, a normal rectoanal inhibitory reflex (RAIR) or rectosphincteric reflex is initiated – that is, the internal anal sphincter relaxes and, if voluntary muscle action occurs, the rectum empties through the anal canal (Figure 1). Fecal continence is maintained by contraction under voluntary control of the striated-muscle sphincters – i.e., the external anal sphincter (EAS) and puborectalis (PR) – until the rectal pressure rise decreases and the resting tone of the internal anal sphincter is restored. Thus, the "voluntary" sphincters (i.e., the EAS and PR) have the ability to be maximally contracted for approximately one minute, beyond which fecal continence is lost as a result of fatigue in the muscle if the tone of the internal anal sphincter has not recovered.

The patient with fecal incontinence will often describe the problem as "diarrhea" rather than loss of control of bowel function. All patients with a complaint of diarrhea should be asked if they have lost control of stool, as this may indicate where the problem actually lies. Once fecal incontinence has been noted, it is then necessary to identify the frequency of the incontinence, whether both liquid and solid stool have been leaked and whether the individual has an urge to defecate before the leakage occurs. A history of previous anorectal trauma (surgical or otherwise) is important to note, as is the strength of voluntary anal canal tone on digital rectal exam.

Most patients presenting with fecal incontinence have "idiopathic" fecal incontinence, but recent investigations in females with this complaint indicate they have suffered damage to the pudendal nerves during childbirth and, with time, this has led to gradual striated-muscle anal sphincter weakness. Surgical trauma is the next most common cause of fecal incontinence; it should be remembered that surgery (e.g., a vaginal hysterectomy) can put excess stretch on the pelvic floor nerves and muscles, causing injury that may lead to weakness of the anal sphincters. Another common source of fecal incontinence is disruption of the internal anal sphincter, either during a lateral internal sphincterotomy to treat an anal fissure or, more commonly, with the older "Lord's" procedure of forceful three- or four-finger dilation of the anal sphincter under anesthetic, where the extent of damage to the sphincters is not predictable. The finding of perineal descent can be noted on examination of the perineum when the patient is asked to strain and appears to be associated with weakness of the pelvic floor muscles as well as loss of the normal anatomy. This gives rise to a mechanical disadvantage affecting the sphincter mechanism. Perineal descent may be associated with a rectocele or, in female patients, with a uterine prolapse. Rectal prolapse can also accompany weakness of the pelvic floor muscles and give rise to fecal incontinence.

Therapy of fecal incontinence has improved over the past decade, primarily because of the introduction of biofeedback training. This technique allows the patient to practice tightening of the striated-muscle portion of the anal sphincter, usually with a surface electromyography (EMG) plug electrode held in the anal canal with audio and visual feedback that the patient can see and hear to encourage maximal contraction of these muscles. Attention should also be given to improving dietary fiber to help reduce the amount of liquid stool. Other drug therapy is limited, but loperamide has been shown to increase the resting tone of the anal sphincters and is a useful adjunct, especially if the stool frequency is increased (loperamide reduces this contributing factor). Cholestyramine may be useful when the patient has diarrhea or loose stool(s) since cholestyramine can make stool more solid (constipating effect). Surgery is sometimes required and is of greatest benefit in those patients who appear to have a mechanical problem such as rectal prolapse or disruption of the sphincter. Surgery to correct perineal descent is often less helpful, since the problem of muscle weakness that gives rise to the descent is not satisfactorily reversed by any of the surgical procedures currently used, and attempts to "suspend" the pelvic floor muscles cannot strengthen these muscles. Patients should refrain from excess straining if they have significant perineal descent, since this will serve only to worsen the pelvic floor muscle weakness.

1.5 Constipation

In the approach to a patient with constipation, it is first necessary to define what the patient means by the term. Many definitions exist, but the best clinical definition is that over 95% of the North American population has a stool frequency from three times a day to three times a week: therefore, patients who have a bowel frequency less than three times a week would be defined as being constipated. Many patients will describe their stool as "constipated," usually meaning that the stool is hard or in pellets (scybalous), while other patients may have a stool frequency that falls within the "normal" range yet feel that their bowels have not completely emptied. This latter symptom is a frequent complaint of the irritable bowel syndrome, and many patients with this disorder will describe a constipated bowel habit. Those constipated patients who have infrequent stool alternating with occasional diarrheal stool have the most common presentation of irritable bowel syndrome. Yet there are a great many patients, almost all female, who have infrequent stool passage, and this group must be considered as separate from the usual irritable bowel syndrome patient for they may be among those rare patients with a secondary cause of constipation.

In Western culture the most frequent cause of constipation is a lack of dietary fiber. The concept of "fiber" has become quite confusing to many patients with the increased emphasis on "oat fiber" for elevated cholesterol treatment. Many foods that patients consider to be high in fiber (e.g., salads, lettuce, tomatoes and celery) are in fact mainly water, and some vegetables may aggravate their symptoms. Fiber is complex carbohydrates that are incompletely digested by the small bowel and are then "digested" by colonic bacteria, liberating fermentation gases and short-chain fatty acids that may provoke and aggravate many of the associated abdominal symptoms (e.g., abdominal pain, "gas" and bloating). It should be emphasized that cereal grain fibers that have more insoluble fiber (as opposed to soluble oat bran fiber) are best to increase stool frequency, but should be added gradually over 8 to 12 weeks to a daily dose of about 30 g. Other fibers in the form of "bulk laxative" preparations containing psyllium, methylcellulose Sterculia or isphagula may be added to wheat bran fiber to accomplish this level of fiber without completely altering a patient's diet. Many patients who are constipated continue to pass dry, hard stool despite an increase in dietary fiber because they do not increase the water content of their diet. Fiber works in the gut by holding onto water and keeping the stool soft; to achieve this effect, the intake of liquids must be increased. For a 30 g/day fiber diet, it is recommended that patients drink eight 8 oz. glasses (i.e., 2 L) of non–caffeine-containing beverages per day.

Secondary causes of constipation must be excluded. The patient with bowel obstruction can present with constipation, and this possibility should always be considered in a patient with the onset of constipation after the age of 40 years (when the incidence of colon cancer rises). A rarer cause of constipation is hypothyroidism; not infrequently, patients with an underactive thyroid will present with a primary symptom of constipation. Hypercalcemia rarely reaches levels that produce constipation but should always be considered, since it can be a life-threatening disorder; constipation in this setting is always resistant to therapy until the hypercalcemia is treated. Proctitis can present with a complaint of infrequent stool passage due to the functional obstruction caused by the inflammation of the rectum; the colon more proximally continues to produce formed stool, which cannot pass easily through the inflamed rectum. Proctitis will usually be associated with excess mucus production, with or without blood in the stool, and proctosigmoidoscopy will always diagnose this entity.

Another cause of constipation is diabetes mellitus, often as a result of impaired motility; dietary factors may also play a role, along with autonomic neuropathy of the enteric nervous system. A small proportion of these diabetic patients with constipation can go on to develop diarrhea, which again has been linked to the autonomic neuropathy seen with long-standing diabetes mellitus.

Inactivity from whatever cause seems to increase the likelihood of a patient's complaining of a constipated bowel habit. This is presumed to be secondary to reduced colonic activity but could be aggravated by a low fiber intake in many of these patients. Severe cardiopulmonary diseases of whatever cause that limit activity can result in constipation. Neurologic disorders that cause the patient to have a reduced ability to ambulate can have constipation as a feature. Some patients with diseases of the nervous system may have impaired awareness of rectal distention to signal a need to defecate, and nerve dysfunction (both peripheral and central) may impair normal colonic propulsion. Finally, the elderly may develop problems with defecation, and although constipation with fecal impaction occurs they may complain of "diarrhea" or "soiling" due to overflow incontinence of stool from the fecal impaction of the rectum inhibiting the normal resting tone of the anal sphincter. Not surprisingly, many of these patients may respond to laxative therapy after the fecal impaction is removed, since this prevents the recurrence of the fecal impaction with overflow incontinence. Some patients can aggravate long-standing constipation with regular laxative abuse, and some theoretical concerns remain that this practice may indeed damage the normal innervation of the colon, rendering it atonic and nonfunctional.

The physical findings are often minimal in the majority of patients with constipation, but specific secondary causes must be looked for. Signs of hypothyroidism may be present; signs of dehydration should be sought, as this may be an early indicator of hypercalcemia. Thorough cardiopulmonary and neurologic examinations are necessary to pick out associated diseases that may be treated, thereby improving the patient's overall health and thus improving bowel function. On abdominal examination, inspection for evidence of distention or hyperperistalsis or masses may point out the source of the impaired stool passage. Localized tenderness of the abdomen must be noted, along with any evidence of liver, spleen or renal enlargement. A complete rectal examination and proctosigmoidoscopy is required in any patient with constipation so that the presence or absence of a fecal impaction, dilatation or enlargement of the rectum or the presence of proctitis can be determined.

1.5.1 MEGARECTUM
When the rectum is enlarged, further investigations are required to exclude other causes, particularly Hirschsprung's disease (Section 1.5.2). The majority of patients with constipation and a dilatated rectum and/or colon at proctosigmoidoscopy or barium enema have idiopathic or acquired megarectum. A useful guideline for the diagnosis of a "megarectum" is a rectal diameter of greater than 6 cm on a lateral film at the level of the S2 vertebral body. These patients can often present in childhood (many of them presenting with encopresis) and in the elderly with a fecal impaction. The cause of the megarectum is unknown, but if the onset is in childhood it may be the result of chronic stool holding by the child, leading to progressive distention of the rectum and eventual loss of awareness of rectal distention. Once this has occurred the patient can no longer recognize when stool is present in the rectum; the distention of the rectum causes chronic inhibition of the resting tone of the internal anal sphincter. This leads to the loss of control of liquid or semisolid stool that passes by the fecal impaction without the patient being aware of it.

1.5.2 HIRSCHSPRUNG'S DISEASE
The majority of patients with this disorder present soon after birth or in early childhood. This is a lesion, present at birth, where variable lengths of distal

colon have no myenteric plexus. The distal colon remains contracted and the normal proximal colon dilatates as it fills with stool. Most of these patients present early in life with obstipation and colonic obstruction, and require surgery. However, a few patients have a very short segment of denervated distal colon, so that they can overcome the obstruction and force stool out of the rectum. They usually have lifelong constipation; the normal rectum proximal to the denervated segment dilatates over time so that the patient presents with constipation and a "megarectum." These patients rarely have fecal incontinence or fecal "soiling" as seen with idiopathic megarectum, since the internal anal sphincter and denervated distal rectum maintain a high resting tone. This condition can be diagnosed by anorectal manometry in that a normal rectoanal inhibitory reflex cannot be identified (Figure 1). However, a definite diagnosis requires deep rectal biopsy from the denervated segment, which will show absence of the myenteric plexus ganglion cells and hypertrophy of nerve fiber bundles. It should be added that an identical condition can be acquired with Chagas' disease from South America, which attacks the myenteric plexus and other autonomic ganglion cells; patients with this condition can also present with achalasia or intestinal pseudo-obstruction as well as cardiac arrhythmias.

1.5.3 PELVIC FLOOR DYSSYNERGIA

The majority of patients with constipation have a form of irritable bowel syndrome, but there is a small subgroup of patients who may have a specific disorder in colonic and/or anorectal function that produces constipation. These patients are almost all female, may have delayed colonic transit or present with anorectal dysfunction with impaired awareness to rectal distention (without a megarectum), or may demonstrate a phenomenon of rectal outlet obstruction due to inappropriate contraction of the voluntary anal sphincters during defecation. This has been termed pelvic floor dyssynergia or anismus. These patients can present major therapeutic dilemmas and warrant further investigation in specialized coloproctology units involved in the care of such patients.

1.6 Colonic Obstruction

Acute colonic obstruction is a surgical emergency that must be recognized early and dealt with expeditiously in order to avoid the high fatality rate due to colonic perforation. The highest risk patients for colonic perforation are those with an intact ileocecal valve that does not allow air to reflux back into the small bowel from the obstructed colon. The cecum is the most frequent site of perforation, because wall tension is highest in the bowel with the largest diameter (Laplace's law).

Patients with colonic obstruction usually have pain as a prominent symptom, with constipation often preceding the complete obstruction. Patients may initially present with diarrhea as the bowel distal to the obstruction empties, but diarrhea may be persistent, especially with a partial obstruction, because of the increased intestinal secretion proximal to the obstruction. The small intestine is the most common site of intestinal obstruction because of the narrower caliber of the bowel, and therefore the left colon is the most common site for colonic obstruction, especially since stool is often more formed in the left colon and less able to pass through a narrowed lumen.

On physical examination the general state of the patient depends upon the duration of the obstruction. With a recent sudden obstruction the patient will be in extreme pain, will often have distention of the abdomen if the ileocecal valve is intact and may describe initially diarrheal stool as the bowel distal to the obstruction is emptied. Abdominal palpation can often discern a mass lesion at the site of the obstruction. Prompt identification of the site of obstruction is mandatory, with the use of supine and erect abdominal x-rays. An urgent surgical consultation is required if the rectum is empty of air with dilatation of more proximal colon, indicating a complete colonic obstruction.

Many patients may present with a more gradual history. If they have had protracted diarrhea up to the point of obstruction, the amount of abdominal pain may be less; they may have abdominal distention, but be less tender on abdominal exam; and they will often show signs of dehydration. Fever and an abdominal mass is particularly common in patients with diverticulitis and a resulting colonic obstruction. A third type of colonic obstruction can be seen that is actually a form of ileus limited to the colon and is sometimes referred to as Ogilvie's syndrome. These patients are most often seen in intensive care units, but the condition can also occur postoperatively (even when no bowel surgery has been performed). As with a "mechanical" bowel obstruction described above, patients with Ogilvie's syndrome may have marked abdominal distention, but frequently they have little abdominal pain and the abdominal x-rays show a picture of dilatated colon with impaired movement of air into the distal colon.

Once a diagnosis of colonic obstruction has been made, the site of obstruction should be determined by plain abdominal x-rays and/or with a water-soluble contrast enema (such as iothalamate meglumine) to identify whether urgent surgery is indicated. Urgent colonoscopy is being done increasingly in this setting, especially if a colonic ileus or Ogilvie's syndrome is suggested, since the excess colonic air can be aspirated via the colonoscope and colonic decompression tubes can be placed in the colon to prevent dangerous reaccumulation of air until the ileus resolves.

TABLE 5. Causes of colonic obstruction

Common
Left-sided cancer
Diverticulitis
Ogilvie's syndrome

Others
Hernia
Strictures
    Crohn's
    Postischemic
    Postsurgical
Intussusception
Volvulus
Adhesions

There are many causes of colonic obstruction (Table 5). Colon cancer and diverticulitis are the most common causes. Most colon cancers that obstruct are in the left colon. They cause circumferential disease or "apple-core" lesions (so called because of the irregular mucosal appearance with luminal narrowing seen at x-ray). Diverticulitis commonly occurs in the sigmoid colon, where diverticular disease is most common; the acute abscess formation with swelling of the inflamed diverticulum compresses and obstructs the affected sigmoid colon. Ogilvie's syndrome may initially have been considered to be due to a cancer or diverticulitis, but contrast x-ray or colonoscopy demonstrates a patent lumen and the diagnosis appears to be clear.

Less common causes of colonic obstruction are hernias, in which a loop of colon (usually sigmoid) becomes strangulated and the bowel is acutely obstructed. This is a much more common cause of small bowel obstruction. Strictures in the colon can also be associated with obstruction, especially when they occur in the left colon. These can occur with Crohn's colitis, after a bout of ischemic colitis or at the site of anastomosis following colonic surgery. This latter cause of obstruction should always be visualized endoscopically if possible, since most colonic resections are for cancer and the possibility of a local cancer recurrence can complicate a postsurgical stricture.

Intussusception can occur in the colon, and in adults it almost always occurs at the site of a polyp, which "leads" the intussusception. Typically, this will cause intermittent acute bowel obstruction associated with severe pain and often rectal bleeding from the vascular compromise produced in the intussuscepting bowel. Because of the intermittent nature of the obstruction, a diagnosis may not made be until after repeated attacks. A barium enema should always be considered in this setting, as it identifies the mucosal lesion "leading" the intussusception and can occasionally be used to reduce the intussusception without the need for urgent surgery.

Volvulus of the colon tends to happen in the cecum and/or the sigmoid colon, because the mesentery can be long and redundant in these areas and cause the bowel to rotate upon itself. This can be a surgical emergency, since the affected bowel will strangulate if the volvulus is not relieved quickly. Again, an urgent barium enema may be able to reduce the volvulus, thus allowing a more elective surgical procedure to correct the problem. A sigmoid volvulus will usually be reduced by this approach, and success with colonoscopic decompression of a sigmoid volvulus has been reported. A cecal volvulus may not be easily treatable with either a barium enema or colonoscopic therapy; thus, surgical advice should be sought urgently if the cecal volvulus will not reduce after these attempts.

Adhesions are often described as a common cause of bowel obstruction, but this is probably true only for small bowel obstruction. Since much of the colon is retroperitoneal or on a limited mesentery, adhesive disease with obstruction of the colon is rare. However, it can occur, particularly in the sigmoid colon if the mesentery is quite long, and particularly after pelvic operations.

1.7 **Diarrhea**
Intestinal fluid and electrolyte absorption has been described and the clinical problem of diarrhea has been considered earlier in Chapter 7, "The Small Intestine." A brief overview of how the colon functions and an approach to diarrhea will be presented here.

1.7.1 *PHYSIOLOGY OF COLONIC FUNCTION*
The colon works to reabsorb the liquid from the ileal effluent presented to it and to form solid feces to expel at the anus. This function is important for normal fluid balance, yet it is possible to live without a colon, as evidenced by the many people with an ileostomy following a colectomy.

The colon reabsorbs 90% of the 1–1.5 L of fluid presented to it daily, and can increase this amount fourfold if required. The colon cannot concentrate stool, but is very efficient at reabsorbing electrolytes and other additions, particularly sodium, along with the short-chain fatty acids that arise from carbohydrate digestion by colonic bacteria. It is also very efficient at reabsorbing water passively. The pathways for electrolyte reabsorption include an Na^+/K^+ exchange with preferential reabsorption of Na^+. A specific Na^+ pump with Cl^-

following passively is also present. These mechanisms of electrolyte reabsorption explain why patients with diarrhea may have hypokalemia (due to preferential Na^+ absorption with K^+ loss) and a nonanion gap acidosis (due to excess bicarbonate loss). Normal colonic reabsorption requires normal calcium and magnesium levels, so hypocalcemia or hypomagnesemia may result in or contribute to a diarrheal state.

The colon has an important function in salvaging carbohydrates and incompletely digested fats that escape normal small intestinal absorption. When malabsorption occurs in the small intestine, the colon can increase the salvage of these foods presented to it.

From a "motility" viewpoint, the colon is actually two organs. The right colon and proximal transverse colon appear to function as a "brake" to the propulsion of stool. Here it is common to see wave-form patterns moving the fecal stream toward the ileocecal valve. This movement facilitates fluid and electrolyte absorption in the right colon by delaying the passage of stool through the colon to increase contact time. In the left colon, the smooth muscle responds differently, with more caudad peristaltic waves that appear to facilitate the movement of stool along the left colon and into the sigmoid colon. The sigmoid colon also functions as a brake to the movement of feces, with increased contraction in the sigmoid colon being paradoxically associated with constipation, while decreased contraction is associated with diarrhea. Very little fluid or electrolyte reabsorption occurs in the rectum, which appears to serve primarily a reservoir function. Our present understanding of colonic motility is limited. Since the luminal contents vary from liquid in the right colon to solid in the left colon, methods of studying whole gut function have been limited.

1.8 Ulcerative Colitis

Ulcerative colitis is an idiopathic inflammatory bowel disease that is limited to involvement of the colon. The other common idiopathic inflammatory bowel disease is Crohn's disease, which is described in Chapter 9, "Inflammatory Bowel Disease."

The cause of ulcerative colitis is unknown, and treatment at this time is directed toward symptom improvement and reduction of the inflammatory response in the colon. Patients present with rectal bleeding, usually with mucus or slime in the stool. With increasing involvement of the colon, diarrhea becomes a prominent symptom and patients frequently also have to get up at night to pass stool. Abdominal pain is often minimal, but if the patient has a desire to pass stool, cramping can be quite prominent if the individual is not close to a toilet. This is also termed "urgency." Abdominal cramping and urgency are usually followed by relief of the cramps once the bowel movement has been passed.

On physical examination patients with milder attacks of colitis are often outwardly not in marked distress. However, 20% of patients can present with acute attacks of colitis along with dehydration due to the diarrhea. Patients with acute pain can be quite ill and have profound blood loss from rectal bleeding. Abdominal pain is often not a prominent feature of this disease; localized areas of significant tenderness should alert the examiner to possible impending colonic perforation due to severe toxic exacerbation of ulcerative colitis. Microscopic examination of the stool identifies large numbers of leukocytes and neutrophils present. On digital exam the examining finger is often coated with blood from the inflamed rectum. Masses should not be palpable on rectal examination.

In a patient with chronic recurrent attacks, a diagnosis of ulcerative colitis is made by a biopsy that shows the characteristic pathological changes under the microscope. However, these pathological findings are very similar to the changes that occur with acute exacerbations of colitis due to bacterial infection. Bacterial causes of diarrhea must be excluded before a diagnosis of ulcerative colitis is made; the causes of bacterial infections with dysentery are discussed in Chapter 7, "The Small Intestine." Amebiasis is a rare cause in North America of bloody diarrhea, but is encountered more frequently in individuals who have traveled to tropical or subtropical areas where the E. histolytica parasite is endemic. As well, outbreaks of amebiasis have been described in male homosexual patients. All patients with ulcerative colitis, even if a diagnosis has been confirmed, should have stool analysis for C. difficile and cytotoxicity during an exacerbation. Exacerbations of ulcerative colitis have been described in patients who have not taken antibiotics and will respond to the usual treatment given for pseudomembranous colitis. Because of the pre-existing colitis, one cannot rely on the characteristic endoscopic appearance of pseudomembranous colitis to rule out this diagnosis, and cultures should be done in any exacerbation.

Treatment should always be directed toward controlling symptoms. It is accepted that all patients with ulcerative colitis should be on a "remittive" agent that has 5-aminosalicylic acid in it. Only patients allergic to this drug should be taken off it, since all ulcerative colitis patients will be expected to have more frequent exacerbations of their colitis off the 5-aminosalicylic acid. The drugs available in Canada that are approved for use in colitis with release primarily of 5-aminosalicylic acid in the colon are sulfasalazine (Salazopyrin®), mesalamine (Asacol®) and olsalazine (Dipentum®). Other mesalamine compounds that dissolve at pH 6 (Salofalk®, Mesasal™) as opposed to pH 7 do release medication into the colon, but are also commonly used for Crohn's disease because of release of the medication in the small intestine.

Corticosteroids (prednisone) are often used for exacerbations of the disease. Patients should be tapered off prednisone once the exacerbation is brought under control and the 5-aminosalicylic acid restarted if it has been discontinued during the exacerbation. Corticosteroids are very effective for controlling flare-ups of the disease, but have no role in preventing relapses. More recently, the use of immunosuppressant drugs has been considered in ulcerative colitis. Because surgery is curative for the disease, these agents are often used only in patients who refuse surgery or because of other medical conditions are a poor risk for surgery. One of the newer immunosuppressants that has been reported to have significant beneficial effects in colitis is cyclosporine. This drug, in early studies, has shown dramatic resolution of acute colitis exacerbations unresponsive to intravenous glucocorticoids in patients who are being considered for surgery. Long-term benefits and complications of this drug are still not clear, but cyclosporine may be used in some patients where surgery is deemed to be inappropriate or in a patient not responding to glucocorticoids.

Complications from ulcerative colitis include perforation of the colon in acute exacerbation and flare-up of the disease. Generally, most attacks of acute colitis if treated promptly with glucocorticoids will settle within five days. A patient who is not responding to high-dose intravenous steroids and in whom investigations for infectious causes of colitis have been negative should be considered for surgical therapy, as the mortality rate rises very rapidly if a patient is not treated surgically before colon perforation. This necessitates that all patients with acute flare-ups of ulcerative colitis who are not improving after 48 hours on high-dose intravenous steroids be transferred to a center where colectomy can be performed safely.

Longer term complications generally relate to some of the drugs' side effects. Because glucocorticoids have significant side effects with long-term therapy it is to be emphasized that all patients with colitis should be tapered off prednisone if their disease is under control and kept in remission with 5-aminosalicylic acid preparations. Patients whose disease does not remain under control should be considered for surgery, as the side effects of glucocorticoids will often lead to more disabling problems for the patients than the disease itself. Other longer term risks include an increased risk of colon cancer. To attempt to reduce the risk of colon cancer developing in ulcerative colitis patients, yearly or biannual colonoscopy is generally recommended with biopsies to evaluate the presence of dysplasia in the colon. Ulcerative colitis patients do not have the typical polyp–carcinoma sequence seen in other forms of colonic adenocarcinoma. Rarer complications include complications in the liver, where sclerosing cholangitis and pericholangitis develop. These complications can precede the development of ulcerative colitis or appear years later. It would appear that the liver complications are not prevented by colectomy, although all the other complications related to colitis are "cured" by colectomy. Some patients with ulcerative colitis will develop cholangiocarcinoma, a tumor that is often unresponsive to all forms of chemotherapy. At present there are no specific recommendations for surveillance for this cancer, as it occurs very infrequently, even in ulcerative colitis patients, but one should be alert to any new symptoms suggesting liver involvement and investigate early.

2. THE ANAL CANAL / M. Burnstein

2.1 Functional Anatomy of the Anal Canal and Anorectal Spaces

2.1.1 *THE ANAL CANAL*
The anal canal begins where the terminal portion of the large bowel passes through the pelvic floor muscles, and it ends at the anal verge. It measures roughly 4 cm in length. The wall of the anal canal is formed by a continuation of the circular muscle of the rectal wall; the smooth muscle is thickened in this area to form the internal anal sphincter. This smooth-muscle sphincter is wrapped by skeletal muscle, the external anal sphincter. The top of the external anal sphincter is formed by the U-shaped puborectalis muscle, which loops around the anus, arising and inserting on the pubis. This is felt posteriorly and laterally as the anorectal ring on digital examination. The longitudinal muscle coat of the rectum descends in the plane between the sphincters as the conjoined longitudinal muscle, and it sends fibers across the lower part of the external anal sphincter to insert on the skin (corrugator cutis ani, responsible for the anocutaneous reflex or "anal wink"). These fibers also traverse the internal anal sphincter to insert on the submucosa ("mucosal suspensory ligament").

In approximately the mid-anus there is a rolling line of demarcation called the dentate line. Above the line is columnar epithelium; below it is squamous epithelium without appendages (the anoderm). The demarcation does not really occur at a line, but at a transitional zone of 0.5–1 cm in length.

As the rectum narrows into the anal canal, the mucosa develops 6 to 14 longitudinal folds, Morgagni's columns. Between the distal ends of the columns are small crypts. Anal glands open into the crypts. There are 4 to 10 glands, and they are lined by stratified columnar epithelium. About half of these tubular glands end in the intersphincteric plane.

Blood is supplied to the anus via the inferior rectal artery, a branch of the internal pudendal artery. The inferior rectal artery crosses the ischiorectal fossa. The superior rectal vein drains the upper part of the anal canal via the inferior mesenteric vein to the portal vein. The middle and inferior rectal veins drain the upper and lower anal canal into the systemic circulation via the internal iliac and internal pudendal veins, respectively.

Lymphatic drainage above the dentate line is via the superior rectal lymphatics (accompanying the superior rectal vessels) to the inferior mesenteric nodes, and laterally along the middle and inferior rectal vessels to the internal iliac nodes. Lymphatic drainage from the anal canal below the dentate line may be in a cephalad or lateral direction, but is primarily to the inguinal nodes.

Motor innervation of the external anal sphincter is via the inferior rectal branch of the internal pudendal nerve and the perineal branch of the fourth sacral nerve. The internal anal sphincter has sympathetic (motor) and parasympathetic (inhibitory) innervation. Parasympathetic supply is from the nervi erigentes (S2, S3, S4). Sympathetic innervation is from the first three lumbar segments via the preaortic plexus. Fibers from the preaortic plexus ultimately join the nervi erigentes to form the pelvic plexuses. Sensation below the dentate line (and for up to 1.5 cm above the dentate line) is carried by the inferior rectal nerve. Above the level of the inferior rectal nerve sensory distribution, there are only dull perceptions, mediated by parasympathetic fibers.

2.1.2 ANORECTAL SPACES

Around the anorectum are a number of potential spaces filled with fat or connective tissue. These may become the sites of abscess formation. The perianal space is at the anal verge, and is continuous with the intersphincteric space. The pyramid-shaped ischiorectal fossa is medially bounded by the external anal sphincter and the levator ani muscles. The lateral wall is the obturator internus muscle and fascia. The inferior boundary is the skin of the perineum, and the apex is the origin of the levator ani from the obturator fascia. Posteriorly is the gluteus maximus muscle, and anteriorly the transverse perinei muscles. On the obturator fascia is Alcock's canal, containing the internal pudendal vessels and pudendal nerve. The fossa is filled with fat and also contains the inferior rectal nerve and vessels, and the fourth sacral nerve. The two ischiorectal spaces communicate with one another behind the anal canal.

2.2 Evaluation of Anorectal Complaints

This section will review the symptoms associated with anorectal pathology and the techniques of anorectal examination.

2.2.1 HISTORY

As in most of medicine, taking a careful history is the most productive step in leading to a diagnosis. In the evaluation of the patient with anorectal complaints, there is a limited number of questions to be asked:

2.2.1.1 Pain

There are three common lesions that cause anorectal pain: fissure in ano, anal abscess and perianal hematoma (also called "thrombosed external hemorrhoid"). If the pain is sharp and occurs during, and for a short time following, bowel movements, a fissure is likely. Continuous pain associated with a perianal swelling probably stems from a perianal hematoma, especially when there is an antecedent history of straining, either at stool or with physical exertion. An anal abscess will also produce a continuous, often throbbing pain, which may be aggravated by the patient's coughing or sneezing. Anorectal abscesses are generally associated with local signs of inflammation. The absence of an inflammatory mass in the setting of severe local pain and tenderness is typical of an intersphincteric abscess; the degree of tenderness usually prevents adequate examination, and evaluation under anesthesia is necessary to confirm the diagnosis and to drain the pus.

Anal pain of any etiology may be aggravated by bowel movements. Tenesmus, an uncomfortable desire to defecate, is frequently associated with inflammatory conditions of the anorectum. Although anal neoplasms rarely produce pain, invasion of the sphincter mechanism may also result in tenesmus. Tenesmus with urgency of evacuation suggests proctitis.

Transient, deep-seated pain that is unrelated to defecation may be due to levator spasm ("proctalgia fugax").

Anorectal pain is so frequently, and erroneously, attributed to hemorrhoids, that this point bears special mention: pain is *not* a symptom of uncomplicated hemorrhoids. If a perianal vein of the inferior rectal plexus undergoes thrombosis, or ruptures, an acutely painful and tender subcutaneous lump will appear. This is the "thrombosed external hemorrhoid." Internal hemorrhoids may prolapse and become strangulated to produce an acute problem of anorectal pain, tenderness, and mucous, bloody discharge. Gangrene and secondary infection may ensue.

2.2.1.2 Bleeding

The nature of the rectal bleeding will help determine the underlying cause. However, the historical features of the bleeding cannot be relied upon to define the problem with certainty. Bright red blood on the toilet paper or on the outside of the stool, or dripping into the bowl, suggests a local anal source, such as a fissure or internal hemorrhoids. Blood that is mixed in with the stool, or that is dark and clotted, suggests sources proximal to the anus. Melena is always due to more proximal pathology. The associated symptoms are very helpful. A history of local anal bleeding, as described above, associated with painful defecation, suggests a fissure. The same bleeding pattern without pain indicates internal hemorrhoids; this may be associated with some degree of hemorrhoidal prolapse. Bleeding and diarrhea may occur with inflammatory bowel disease. When bleeding is associated with a painful lump and is not exclusively related to defecation, a perianal hematoma is likely. Bleeding associated with a mucopurulent discharge and tenesmus may be seen with proctitis, or possibly with a rectal neoplasm.

Bleeding per rectum is an important symptom of colorectal cancer, and although this is not the most common cause of hematochezia, it is the most serious and must always be considered. This does not mean that every patient who passes blood must have contrast radiography of the colon or total colonoscopy. If the bleeding has an obvious anal source, it may be prudent not to proceed with a total colon examination, especially in a patient at low risk for colorectal neoplasms (i.e., age under 50 years; no history of Crohn's or ulcerative colitis; no family history of colon cancer; and no personal history of colorectal neoplasms, or breast or gynecologic malignancies). However, if bleeding persists after treatment of the anal pathology, more ominous lesions have to be excluded.

2.2.1.3 Prolapse

In evaluating protrusion from the anal opening, there are several relevant questions: Is the prolapse spontaneous or exclusively with defecation? Spontaneous prolapse is less characteristic of internal hemorrhoids than of hypertrophied anal papillae or complete rectal prolapse. Does the prolapsing tissue reduce spontaneously (as may be the case with second-degree internal hemorrhoids) or does it require manual reduction (as with third-degree internal hemorrhoids or complete rectal prolapse)? The patient may be able to describe the size of the prolapsing tissue, and this may suggest the diagnosis.

Complete rectal prolapse (procidentia) must be distinguished from mucosal prolapse or prolapsing internal hemorrhoids. Procidentia occurs mainly in women (female:male = 6:1), with a peak incidence in the seventh decade. Procidentia is often associated with fecal incontinence. In later stages, protrusion occurs even with slight exertion such as coughing or sneezing. The extruded rectum becomes excoriated, leading to tenesmus, mucus discharge and bleeding. (Examination of the patient with procidentia usually reveals poor anal tone, and with the tissue in a prolapsed state, the mucosal folds are seen to be concentric, whereas with prolapsed hemorrhoids there are radial folds.) Rarely, a large polypoid tumor of the rectum may prolapse through the anal canal.

2.2.1.4 Perianal mass

A painful perianal lump may be an abscess or a thrombosed external hemorrhoid. Knowing whether there has been a discharge of blood or pus may be helpful. An intermittent mass suggests a prolapsing lesion.

External or "skin" tags are very common deformities of the anal margin. They may be the result of previous or active fissure disease, or the sequelae of a perianal hematoma. Condylomata acuminata – or venereal warts – are caused by a sexually transmitted virus. The perianal skin is frequently affected, and the condition occurs with greatest frequency in gay men.

The differential diagnosis also includes benign and malignant neoplasms.

2.2.1.5 Pruritus

Itching is a common associated feature of many anorectal conditions, especially during the healing phase or if there is a discharge. But pruritus ani may also be an isolated symptom or the patient's primary complaint. As a chief complaint, pruritus may be caused by infections (e.g., pinworms, condylomata, Candida) or skin conditions (e.g., contact dermatitis, psoriasis). More commonly, no specific underlying pathology is identified, and the problem is idiopathic.

Idiopathic pruritus ani is more common in men, and is typically worse at night. When chronic, the characteristic changes of hypertrophy and lichenification, nodularity, scarring and fissuring of the skin become apparent.

2.2.1.6 Discharge

Although mucus is a normal product of the colorectal mucosa, it is not normally seen in the stool. Increased mucus may be the result of proctocolitis or a colorectal neoplasm, especially a villous adenoma of the rectum. Both inflammatory and neoplastic conditions may present with mucus and blood. Phosphate enemas are irritating and often elicit copious mucus production.

Mucus staining of the underclothes may be associated with prolapsing tissue. When the staining has a fecal component, or when there is associated inability to control gas or to discriminate gas from solids within the rectum, a disturbance of the continence mechanism exists. A history of "accidents," or the need to wear pads during the day or night, will help indicate the magnitude of the problem. The discharge may arise from an obvious external lesion – e.g., blood from a perianal hematoma, or pus from an abscess, from the external opening of a fistula, from a pilonidal process or from perianal hidradenitis suppurativa.

Other issues that will prove helpful in coming to a diagnosis of anorectal pathology include bowel habits, associated medical conditions and medications, sexual practices, travel history and family history.

2.2.2 EXAMINATION

The patient about to undergo examination of the anorectum may be embarrassed, and afraid of impending pain and discomfort. Explanation of the examinations to be performed, and reassurance, will lessen the patient's anxiety and contribute greatly to patient cooperation.

The four steps in anorectal evaluation are inspection, palpation, anoscopy and proctosigmoidoscopy.

2.2.2.1 Positioning

The patient is placed either in the left lateral position or (preferably) in the prone-jackknife position. The prone-jackknife position requires a special table that tilts the head down and raises the anorectal region, with the buttocks tending to fall apart. This provides the best and easiest access for the examiner, although patient comfort may be slightly less.

The left lateral (Sims') position has the advantages of patient comfort and of being suitable for any examining table, bed or stretcher. The patient's buttocks are allowed to protrude over the edge of the table, with hips flexed and knees slightly extended. The examiner may sit or stand.

The patient is unable to see "what's going on back there," and it is important to continually explain what you are doing and what can be expected.

2.2.2.2 Inspection

Looking at the anal area may reveal obvious external pathology. The resting anal aperture should be observed: a patulous opening may be seen with procidentia, sphincter injury or neurologic abnormality.

Gentle spreading of the buttocks may elicit pain in a patient who has an anal fissure. Asking the patient to strain down may provide information: internal hemorrhoids may protrude or procidentia may be seen. However, if procidentia is suspected, it should be sought with the patient squatting or sitting at the toilet.

2.2.2.3 Palpation

A disposable plastic glove and water-soluble lubricant are required. The patient is told that a finger will be gently placed into the rectum. While one hand separates the buttocks, the index finger is placed on the anal verge, and with the patient bearing down, thereby relaxing the anus, the digit is advanced into the anal canal.

A methodical approach is best. Palpation anteriorly checks the prostate in males, and the cervix in females. The finger then sweeps backward and forward to palpate the rest of the circumference of the anorectum. This may be the only part of the examination that identifies submucosal lesions, which may easily go undetected by endoscopy. Resting tone and ability to squeeze should also be assessed.

2.2.2.4 Anoscopy

The anoscope is the optimal instrument for examining lesions of the anal canal. It is not a substitute for proctosigmoidoscopy, and the proctosigmoidoscope does not provide as satisfactory a view of the canal as does the anoscope. Many anoscopes are available; the best instrument is end-viewing, with an attached fiberoptic light source.

2.2.2.5 Proctosigmoidoscopy

The rigid 25 cm sigmoidoscope (or proctoscope) is the best instrument for examining the rectum. Barium enemas, and even flexible endoscopes, are not as efficient at evaluating the rectal ampulla.

A variety of rigid sigmoidoscopes are available: disposable or reusable, in a range of diameters (1.1 cm, 1.9 cm, 2.7 cm) and with proximal or distal lighting. The 1.9 cm instrument provides good visibility with minimal patient discomfort. The instrument includes a 25 cm tube, a magnifying lens, a light source, and a bulb attachment for air insufflation. Long swabs may be helpful in maintaining visibility, but suction is best.

A single Fleet® enema provides excellent preparation of the distal bowel and should be used just before the examination. The Fleet® enema may produce transient mucosal changes, and if inflammatory bowel disease is suspected, it should be avoided.

The digital examination has set the stage for instrumentation by permitting the sphincter to relax. With the tip well lubricated, the sigmoidoscope is inserted and passed quickly up the rectum. As always, the patient is informed of what is being done, and is reassured that the sensation of impending evacuation is caused by the instrument, and that the bowels are not about to move.

Air insufflation should be kept to a minimum, as it may cause discomfort, but it is of value both on entry and on withdrawal in demonstrating the mucosa and lumen. Advancement should occur only with the lumen clearly in sight. When the lumen is "lost," withdraw and redirect to regain it.

As the rectosigmoid is reached (approximately 15 cm along), the patient should be warned of possible cramping discomfort that will disappear as the scope is removed. Frequently, even with experience, the rectosigmoid angle cannot be negotiated, and the examination should be terminated. Most importantly, the patient should not be hurt or caused significant discomfort. The scope should be withdrawn making large circular motions, carefully inspecting the circumference of the bowel wall, flattening the mucosal folds and valves of Houston. The posterior rectal wall in the sacral hollow must be specifically sought out, or it will be missed.

In most large studies, the average depth of insertion is 18–20 cm; the full length of the instrument is inserted in less than half the patients.

Perforation of the normal rectum by the sigmoidoscope is extremely rare (1 in 50,000 or less). However, advancing the instrument or insufflating air may be hazardous in settings such as inflammatory bowel disease, radiation proctitis, diverticulitis and cancer. Of course, biopsy and electrocoagulation have to be performed with care and with knowledge of the technique and equipment.

The incidence and significance of bacteremia following anorectal manipulations is controversial, and has been reported in 0–25% of proctoscopies. Prophylactic antibiotics should be considered in patients with prosthetic heart valves.

2.3 Specific Anorectal Problems
This section will briefly review some of the more common anorectal problems.

2.3.1 HEMORRHOIDS

2.3.1.1 Background
The upper anal canal has three sites of thickened submucosa containing arterioles, venules and arteriovenous communications. These three vascular "cushions" are in the left lateral, right anterior and right posterior positions. Minor cushions may lie between the three main ones. The cushions are held in the upper anal canal by muscular fibers from the conjoined longitudinal muscle of the intersphincteric plane.

Hemorrhoids exist when the anal cushions prolapse after disruption of their suspensory mechanism, or there is dilatation of the veins and arteriovenous anastomoses within the cushions. Various theories can be put forward: raised intra-abdominal pressure, pressure on the hemorrhoidal veins by an enlarging uterus, poor venous drainage secondary to an overactive internal anal sphincter, straining at stool with a resultant downward displacement of the cushions, etc.

Skin tags are projections of skin at the anal verge. They may be the result of previous thrombosed external hemorrhoids, fissure in ano, or inflammatory bowel disease.

External hemorrhoids are dilatated veins of the inferior hemorrhoidal (rectal) plexus. This plexus lies just below the dentate line and is covered by squamous epithelium.

Internal hemorrhoids are the symptomatic, enlarged submucosal vascular cushions of the anal canal. The cushions are located above the dentate line and are covered by columnar and transitional epithelium. The patient's history allows internal hemorrhoids to be subdivided. First-degree hemorrhoids produce painless bleeding but do not protrude from the anal canal; at anoscopy, they are seen to bulge into the lumen. Second-degree hemorrhoids protrude with bowel movements, but reduce themselves spontaneously. Third-degree hemorrhoids prolapse outside the anal canal, either spontaneously or with bowel movements, but require digital reduction. Fourth-degree hemorrhoids are always prolapsed, and cannot be reduced.

2.3.1.2 Diagnosis and treatment

2.3.1.2.1 Thrombosed external hemorrhoids As a rule, external hemorrhoids are asymptomatic until the complication of thrombosis (intravascular clot) or rupture (perianal hematoma) supervenes. In either case, the presentation is severe pain with a perianal lump, often after straining. The natural history is one of continued pain for 4 to 5 days, then slow resolution over 10 to 14 days. The treatment depends on the severity of the pain and the timing of presentation. A patient who presents within 24 to 48 hours and with severe pain is best dealt with operatively. Under local anesthesia, the involved vein and clot are excised. The wound may be left open or may be closed. Simple evacuation of the thrombus is less effective. A patient presenting later, after 3 to 4 days, is advised to take frequent warm baths, a bulk laxative, a surface-active wetting agent, and oral analgesics. This regimen is also prescribed post-excision.

2.3.1.2.2 Internal hemorrhoids Painless, bright red rectal bleeding (usually with or following bowel movements) is the most common symptom of this condition. Blood appears on the toilet paper or on the outside of the stool, or drips into the bowl. Although the volume of blood loss may occasionally be sufficient to explain iron deficiency anemia, further workup is indicated.

Prolapse with defecation or other straining activities is also common. Chronic prolapse is associated with mucus discharge, fecal staining of the underclothes and pruritus.

Anal sphincter spasm may result in thrombosis and strangulation of pro-lapsed hemorrhoids. This presents as an acute problem of a painful, discharg-ing, edematous mass of hemorrhoids.

Inspection will identify the later stages of the disease, especially when the patient is asked to bear down. Digital examination can rule out other pathol-ogy, as well as assess the sphincters. A palpable abnormality suggests some other process. Anoscopy provides a diagnosis in first- and second-degree dis-ease. With the anoscope in place, the patient is once again asked to strain, and the degree of prolapse observed. Proctosigmoidoscopy should always be per-formed to exclude other diseases, particularly rectal neoplasms and inflamma-tory bowel disease.

If the symptoms are at all atypical, or the physical findings leave any doubt about the source of blood, a colon-clearing examination (either colonoscopy or barium enema) should be performed.

In patients over the age of 50, it is reasonable to take the opportunity to screen (or to practice "case-finding") for colorectal cancer by performing sigmoidos-copy with the 60 cm flexible instrument. If risk factors for colorectal neoplasia are present, then colonoscopy or barium enema should certainly be performed.

Occasional bleeding, especially if it is related to hard stools or straining, should be managed by improving bowel habits using high-fiber diet and bulk agents (e.g., psyllium). If bleeding persists or is frequent, intervention is indi-cated, and in most cases should take the form of rubber-band ligation. Prolaps-ing hemorrhoids that reduce spontaneously, or can be easily reduced, are also nicely treated by rubber-band ligation. If prolapsing tissue is not easily reduced, or if there is a significant external component, surgical hemorrhoid-ectomy offers the best cure. Similarly, prolapsed, thrombosed internal hemor-rhoids should be surgically excised.

2.3.1.2.3 *Rubber-band ligation*   In this technique, rubber rings are placed on the insensitive mucosa above the dentate line. This repositions the vascular cushions in the upper anal canal and decreases their size by causing scarring. It is a simple office procedure, requiring an anoscope and ligator. In general, only one or two areas are banded at a time, so that several treatments are usu-ally undertaken.

2.3.1.2.4 *Hemorrhoidectomy*   Since the popularization of rubber-band liga-tion, excisional hemorrhoidectomy has been much less frequently performed. The important principles of all excisional procedures are removal of all exter-nal and internal hemorrhoids, protection of the internal anal sphincter from injury, and maintenance of the anoderm, so as to avoid anal stenosis.

2.3.2 *FISSURE IN ANO*

This is a linear crack in the lining of the anal canal, extending from the dentate line to the anal verge. It is seen equally in men and women, and at all ages, but is a common entity in young adults. It is encountered mainly in the posterior midline, but also occasionally in the anterior midline. If a fissure persists, secondary changes occur. These include the "sentinel pile" at the distal end of the fissure and the "hypertrophied anal papilla" at the proximal end. They are due to edema and low-grade infection.

2.3.2.1 *Pathogenesis*

Fissure in ano is probably the result of trauma during the passage of hard stool, but not all patients with fissure in ano give a history of "constipation." While most fissures will readily heal with an appropriate change in bowel habits, some will persist. This may be due to continued trauma or to spasm of the internal anal sphincter.

There is an association between fissures and inflammatory bowel disease, particularly Crohn's disease, and this should be kept in mind.

2.3.2.2 *Diagnosis*

Pain with defecation is the chief complaint. The pain may persist for minutes to hours. Bright red blood is often seen on the toilet paper and on the stool. The patient with an edematous, tender skin tag (sentinel pile) may complain of a painful hemorrhoid. The patient may be constipated in response to painful defecation.

With gentle separation of the buttocks, most fissures will be visible. The sentinel pile of a chronic fissure may be the initial finding. With acute fissures, digital and anoscopic examination are usually not possible because of local tenderness. However, these examinations should be performed later to rule out other pathology. With chronic fissures, anoscopy reveals the defect in the anoderm, with exposed muscle fibers of the internal anal sphincter at the fissure base. The hypertrophied anal papilla may be seen.

Fissures off the midline should raise the possibility of other diseases. Ulcerative colitis, and especially Crohn's disease, may be associated with atypical-looking fissures that are off the midline and have atypical symptoms. Anal and rectal carcinoma should be palpably different from fissures, but if any doubt exists, a biopsy should be done. A syphilitic chancre may occasionally look like an idiopathic fissure.

2.3.2.3 *Treatment*

The mainstay of therapy for acute fissures is to achieve daily soft bowel movements. This will prevent further tearing and relieve the anal spasm, allowing most acute fissures to heal within one to two weeks. Warm tub baths are soothing and cleansing, and may also reduce spasm. A high-fiber diet supplemented with bulk agents and surface-active wetting agents will accomplish the desired effect.

If the history is longer than a few weeks and the physical findings suggest chronicity (i.e., exposed sphincter fibers, hypertrophied papilla, sentinel pile and palpable induration), this conservative therapy may not help. If symptoms warrant, such a fissure should be treated operatively, generally by lateral internal sphincterotomy. This relieves the internal anal sphincter spasm and allows the fissure to heal.

2.3.3 FISTULA-ABSCESS DISEASE

Anorectal abscess and fistula are the acute and chronic phases, respectively, of the same disease. The disease begins as an infection in the anal glands and initially presents as an abscess. When the abscess is surgically drained, or drains spontaneously, a communication (i.e., a fistula) exists between the gland of origin and the perianal skin.

The infection begins in the intersphincteric plane, where many of the anal glands terminate. The infectious process may remain in this plane as an intersphincteric abscess, or, more commonly, it may track downward in the intersphincteric plane to present as a perianal abscess. Similarly, infection may penetrate the external sphincter to enter the ischiorectal fossa. Many complex variations are seen, determined by the direction of spread and sometimes by inappropriate intervention. The infection may track circumferentially from one side of the anal canal to the other to cause a "horseshoe" abscess. Perianal and ischiorectal abscesses account for at least three-quarters of anorectal abscesses.

The classical signs of inflammation are generally present, although with an intersphincteric abscess there may be nothing to see. In the case of intersphincteric abscess, the patient will be too tender for adequate examination, and examination under anesthesia will be necessary.

Management of the abscess consists of incision and drainage, and this can usually be accomplished under local anesthesia. To ensure adequate drainage, a cruciate or elliptical incision is made. For the one-half to two-thirds of patients who go on to develop a fistula in ano, a fistulotomy, or laying-open, with curettage of the track is required. The wound heals secondarily. Nonhealing or recurrence of the fistula usually indicates a failure to destroy the gland of origin. In performing fistulotomy, the utmost attention must be paid to the anatomic relationship between the fistula track and the sphincter mechanism. Excessive division of muscle contained within the fistula can lead to partial or complete fecal incontinence.

2.3.4 PILONIDAL DISEASE

This is an acquired condition in which body hair is drilled into the skin of the natal cleft by the back-and-forth motion of the buttocks. This produces a primary midline opening or track, from which abscesses and secondary tracks and openings may form.

The disease is mainly seen in young, hirsute males. It commonly presents as an acute abscess, but may also present as a chronic "sinus," usually with multiple openings.

The abscess stage is treated by incision and drainage, usually under local anesthesia. After the abscess has healed, some of these patients will require definitive surgery to deal with the primary and secondary tracks. The preferred treatment consists of opening the anterior wall of the tracks and suturing the edge of the track to the skin edge. This technique is called "marsupialization."

2.4 Sexually Transmitted Diseases of the Anorectum

There is an increasing incidence of venereal infections of the anorectal region, mainly accounted for by sexual practices among gay men. Many of these diseases may mimic nonvenereal conditions of the anorectum, and multiple venereal infections may coexist.

While immunocompetent gay men are subject to infection with the usual venereal pathogens, AIDS patients may additionally suffer from opportunistic infections of the gut.

The common anorectal venereal infections seen in North America are discussed here.

Condylomata acuminata, or venereal warts, are seen in the perianal region and anal canal, as well as the vulva, vagina and penis. They are most often seen in male homosexuals. The causative agent is believed to be a papilloma virus with an incubation period of one to six months. Symptoms are generally minor – itching, and occasionally bleeding. Perianal warts are frequently accompanied by warts within the anal canal, and these must be looked for at anoscopy.

Many treatments exist. None has a better than 70% chance of eradicating the disease by a single application. For perianal and anal canal warts, electrocoagulation or laser destruction is preferred. For extensive persistent disease, immunotherapy with an autologous vaccine has been very successful.

Squamous cancer has been seen to arise in condylomata acuminata.

Neisseria gonorrhoeae may produce proctitis. The incubation period of *gonococcal proctitis* is five to seven days. Gonococcal proctitis is most often asymptomatic; symptoms may include mucopurulent discharge and tenesmus. Proctoscopy reveals a thick, purulent discharge on a background of mild, non-ulcerative inflammation of the distal rectum. Gram's stain is unreliable, but culture of the pus confirms the diagnosis. Serologic testing for syphilis should be carried out. Treatment for homosexual men is ceftriaxone, 250 mg IM once.

Syphilis can affect the anal region. The incubation period ranges from 9 to 90 days. The primary lesion is a chancre, and because it is painful, it may be mistaken for a fissure. However, chancres are off the midline, are often multiple, and have an atypical appearance. Bilateral inguinal lymphadenopathy may be present. The chancre regresses over 6 weeks. Treponema pallidum is demonstrated from the primary lesion by darkfield microscopy. Serologic testing will be positive within a few weeks of the appearance of the chancre. If untreated, the secondary stage of syphilis may involve the anal area 6 to 8 weeks after healing of the chancre. This takes the form of a rash or of condylomata lata – flat, wart-like lesions teeming with Treponema pallidum. Treatment of primary and secondary syphilis is with benzathine penicillin G, 2.4 million units IM once. Sexual contacts should be treated prophylactically.

Herpes simplex 2 may infect the anorectum. The incubation period is 4 to 21 days. Constitutional symptoms are followed by severe anorectal pain. Small vesicles and aphthous ulcers are seen perianally and in the anal canal and lower rectum. Examination may reveal tender inguinal lymphadenopathy. Viral cultures of the vesicular fluid will be positive and rectal biopsy has a characteristic appearance. Spontaneous resolution occurs over several weeks. Recurrences are frequent but less severe. Immunosuppressed patients may develop a severe, destructive process. Treatment is with tub baths and analgesics. Topical acyclovir q8h × 5 days shortens the symptomatic period and the duration of viral shedding. Intravenous acyclovir is used when there is proctitis in addition to anal and perianal disease. In the AIDS patient, acyclovir is used intravenously in the acute phase, followed by oral acyclovir for 6 months.

Chlamydia proctitis with non-LGV (lymphogranuloma venereum) serotypes is almost identical to gonococcal proctitis. However, the LGV serotypes are invasive and produce a severe proctocolitis with pain, tenesmus, discharge and diarrhea. Chlamydia is isolated from the rectum. Treatment is with tetracycline.

3. LOWER GASTROINTESTINAL BLEEDING / B. Vair

Abrupt passage of frank blood or melena from the lower gastrointestinal tract is an alarming symptom with a wide spectrum of etiology and clinical significance. The causes of intestinal bleeding vary with the age of the patient. Congenital lesions and inflammatory conditions make up the majority of cases in the pediatric population. In the adult, acquired conditions become more prominent. Gastrointestinal bleeding may be considered as either occult (presenting as iron deficiency anemia and guaiac-positive stools) or overt (with fresh or altered blood passed from the lower tract in noticeable quantities). Most occult bleeding is a result of benign or malignant neoplasia, inflammatory disease in the proximal gastrointestinal tract and ulcerogenic medications. Diagnosis and treatment of these etiologies is usually elective and straightforward. The management of overt bleeding is often more urgent and warrants specific consideration.

In all cases of bleeding from the lower gastrointestinal tract, an origin from more proximal sources in the stomach and duodenum as well as the biliary tract should be considered. Peptic ulceration is the most common cause of melena and if associated with active bleeding can present as fresh blood passed per rectum. Most of these lesions are readily visible with upper gastrointestinal endoscopy. Hemobilia, although rare, should always be considered, especially with a previous history of trauma or surgery and a triad of upper abdominal pain, jaundice and melena. Arteriography is often required to define the origin of bleeding from the liver and biliary tract.

The vast majority of rectal bleeding is a result of benign perianal disease. Minor ulcerated or thrombosed hemorrhoids and anal fissure are the most common of these and are readily evident on rectal and proctoscopic examination. A bloody discharge may be a result of a fistula in ano or an ulcerated perianal neoplasm. These conditions are easily recognized and the associated bleeding responds readily to appropriate treatment.

Vascular ectasias are now believed to be the most common cause of lower gastrointestinal bleeding in older patients. These benign arteriovenous malformations are acquired degenerative lesions of aging and are most commonly found in the right colon as a result of increased intraluminal pressure and intramural venous obstruction. They usually present as copious dark bleeding in elderly patients; the bleeding is usually self-limited and rarely results in hemorrhagic shock. Bleeding, however, recurs in most individuals and requires prompt diagnosis and appropriate treatment. These lesions are usually readily identifiable on mesenteric angiography and can also be visualized endoscopically. Although most common in the right colon as a result of the pressure effects dictated by Laplace's law, these lesions can also be found throughout the gastrointestinal tract. They are distinct from the congenital lesions of Osler-Weber-Rendu disease, which are associated with cutaneous telangiectasias and bleeding most prominently from the upper intestinal tract. Diverticular disease of the intestines is now recognized as the second most prominent cause of lower intestinal bleeding. Meckel's diverticulum, which is a true diverticulum on the antimesenteric border of the distal ileum, may be associated with bleeding if acid-secreting gastric epithelium is present within the pouch. Bleeding occurs subsequent to adjacent mucosal ulceration and presents as dark bleeding from the lower tract, usually in small intermittent quantities. Most Meckel's diverticula are not visible on contrast radiography but can be detected using scanning with technetium, which binds to parietal cells.

Acquired diverticula of the pulsion type occur throughout the entire sigmoid. The outpouchings of the intestinal wall arise from areas of weakness between the mesenteric teniae, where penetrating blood vessels produce an area of weakness and allow for mucosal and submucosal herniation. Stretching of the vasa recta over the diverticulum predisposes to hemorrhage into the intestinal lumen. Although more numerous in the left colon, those diverticula that bleed most commonly arise on the right side of the bowel. Diverticular bleeding is usually copious and bright red and may proceed to hemorrhagic shock. It is unusual for occult bleeding to be a result of diverticular disease, and diverticulitis is rarely associated with gross bleeding. Most bleeding of diverticular origin is self-limited, and rebleeding occurs in approximately 25% of patients.

Inflammatory bowel disease, especially ulcerative colitis and proctitis but also Crohn's disease involving the colon, commonly presents as rectal bleeding. While not as commonly associated with bleeding as ulcerative colitis, Crohn's disease can result in more profuse hemorrhage as the transmural inflammation erodes the larger muscular arteries. The complication of toxic megacolon can also result in profuse bleeding as a result of the transmural nature of the inflammation. These conditions are usually readily evident on proctosigmoidoscopic examination. Infectious colitis (most notably those types involving Shigella, Campylobacter and Yersinia) is frequently associated with rectal bleeding. Although uncommon in Canada, amebic colitis should also be considered in any patient with a history of foreign travel. These causes usually become evident after appropriate stool culture and testing for ova and parasites.

Vascular causes for gastrointestinal bleeding distinct from arteriovenous malformations include ischemic colitis and radiation proctitis. Ischemic colitis is usually seen in older individuals with a compromised splanchnic circulation or in those taking medications with vasoconstrictor effects. The most common area of the bowel to be involved is the splenic flexure region, where the anastomosis between the middle colic and left colic arteries through the marginal artery of Drummond is prone to compromise. Most cases of ischemic colitis resolve spontaneously; however, a number of patients progress to free perforation and peritonitis. Thumb-printing on plain abdominal x-rays as a result of submucosal edema and hemorrhage is a pathognomonic diagnostic finding. Radiation proctitis usually follows external irradiation for pelvic malignancies. Ischemic mucosal changes result from endarteritis obliterans and usually lead to diarrhea in association with frank rectal bleeding.

Neoplastic lesions of the intestine very rarely result in severe hemorrhage and usually present as occult bleeding. Lesions in the distal colon, however, may present with recognizable bleeding, usually as bright red blood rather than melena. Neoplastic polyps and carcinomas associated with bleeding are usually readily identified by endoscopic means and contrast studies. Rare causes of lower intestinal bleeding include foreign-body–related trauma and postoperative anastomotic hemorrhage.

The severity of hemorrhage and the presence of associated hemodynamic instability dictate whether resuscitative measures or diagnostic measures take priority in management. Once the circulation has been stabilized with appropriate crystalloid and red cell transfusions, a systematic approach to diagnosis is indicated. Essential features to be obtained in the history include a history of previous bleeding episodes, a change in bowel pattern and other abnormalities in gastrointestinal function. Any history of previous surgery, radiation and medication use should be carefully sought. A careful physical examination with attention to the presence of abdominal tenderness, postural hypotension, tachycardia, palpable masses and organomegaly, as well as digital rectal examination, is important. Baseline laboratory studies should include CBC, coagulation parameters and platelet count, and measures of renal and hepatic function. Electrolyte loss in association with diarrhea may be significant and should be promptly corrected. The presence of hypotension should suggest a loss of intravascular volume approximating 4 units, and appropriate crossmatch should be obtained. Associated cardiorespiratory disease should be ruled out with a chest x-ray and electrocardiogram.

As many patients with rectal bleeding have underlying causes in the upper gastrointestinal tract, an initial diagnostic measure should be the passage of a nasogastric tube into the stomach. The presence of clear fluid including bile in the nasogastric aspirate excludes a bleeding source proximal to Treitz's ligament. A clear gastric aspirate not containing bile does not reliably rule out a source of bleeding within the duodenum. In addition to a diagnostic function, nasogastric intubation prevents gastric dilatation and pulmonary aspiration.

Once resuscitation has begun and the patient has been stabilized, endoscopic visualization of the distal gastrointestinal tract should be attempted. The presence of melena would suggest a more proximal source within the intestinal tract not potentially visualized by rigid sigmoidoscopy. Sigmoidoscopic examination should be carried out in any patient with frank rectal bleeding to rule out inflammatory proctitis and bleeding neoplasms. As well, lesions within the anal canal can occasionally present with profuse hemorrhage. Rectal varices in patients with portal hypertension are a rare but important cause of profuse bright red rectal bleeding. If sigmoidoscopic examination suggests a bleeding source more proximally in the intestinal tract, colonoscopy should be attempted. This may on occasion be futile in the face of profuse bleeding; however, the cathartic effect of blood may effectively prepare the large bowel for visualization by the experienced examiner. Colonoscopy offers the additional advantage of therapeutic options, including electrocoagulation and snare cauterization of polyps.

If colonoscopy is not feasible or is unsuccessful and if bleeding continues to be active, the next diagnostic step is nuclear scanning. Either technetium sulfur colloid or technetium-labeled red blood cells are available for a relatively noninvasive attempt to visualize the bleeding source. In contrast to angiography, which requires a rate of bleeding of 0.5–1 cc per minute, nuclear studies can detect active bleeding with as little as 0.1 cc per minute. Technetium sulfur colloid studies have the disadvantage of background uptake in liver and spleen; technetium-labeled red blood cells (which have a longer half-life) may permit visualization of intermittent bleeding sources as extravasated contrast accumulates in the intestinal tract on delayed scanning.

If either endoscopic measures or nuclear scanning locates the source of bleeding, the need for surgery is dictated by the ability to control the bleeding source endoscopically and by the stability of the patient. In the presence of profuse hemorrhage and a hemodynamically unstable patient, the best choice is to proceed with surgery once the bleeding source has been localized. A stable or high-risk patient or a patient in whom the bleeding source has not been identified should be considered for mesenteric angiography. Selective catheterization of the mesenteric vessels not only confirms the source of bleeding as suggested by nuclear scan, but may be more anatomically precise and offers the therapeutic option of vasopressin infusion with or without absorbable gelatin sponge occlusion. Vasopressin acts as a local vasoconstrictor and effectively controls intestinal hemorrhage in up to 90% of patients when infused into the bleeding site via the catheter. The potential of vasopressin to induce coronary and splanchnic vasoconstriction with resulting myocardial and intestinal ischemia should be considered. As well, bleeding commonly recurs once the vasopressin infusion has been discontinued. Vasopressin may, however, allow for stabilization of the patient while associated medical illnesses are brought under control and the large bowel is prepared for less urgent surgery.

Failure to visualize the source of bleeding or failure of vasopressin infusion in the presence of continued hemorrhage dictates an urgent surgical approach. Fortunately, most cases of lower gastrointestinal bleeding resolve spontaneously, allowing for an elective diagnostic workup and elective therapy. In patients over the age of 60 in whom an upper gastrointestinal source has been excluded, the procedure of choice is a blind subtotal colectomy – which, although associated with high morbidity and mortality, carries a risk of rebleeding of less than 10%. Ideally, preoperative diagnostic measures will allow accurate localization of the bleeding source and direct a limited resection of the offending area of intestine.

The prognosis of patients presenting with a frank gastrointestinal hemorrhage originating in the lower tract remains poor as a result of the often prolonged period prior to diagnosis and appropriate treatment. An understanding of the possible etiologies and a systematic approach to diagnosis and therapy will, it is hoped, improve this picture in the future.

SUGGESTED READING LIST

Sleisenger MH, Fordtran JS (eds.). Gastrointestinal disease: pathophysiology, diagnosis, management. 5th ed. Philadelphia: WB Saunders, 1993.

Phillips SF, Pemberton JH, Shorter RG (eds.). The large intestine: physiology, pathophysiology and disease. New York: Raven Press, 1991.

OBJECTIVES

1. Discuss the normal intestinal microflora.
2. Discuss the role of the colon in the intestinal transport of fluid and electrolytes.
3. Discuss the mechanism of defecation.
4. Give a definition of acute and chronic diarrhea.
5. Classify the causes of diarrhea.
6. Differentiate between large and small bowel diarrhea, and between organic and functional diarrhea.
7. Outline the investigations of a patient with chronic diarrhea.

8. Discuss the value of 72-hour stool collection, ^{14}C breath test, H_2 breath test, Schilling test, D-xylose test, jejunal aspiration and small bowel biopsy in patients with chronic diarrhea.
9. Discuss the value of quantitative and qualitative stool fat determinations.
10. Discuss the pathophysiology of diarrhea.

Rectal Bleeding
1. Give the differential diagnosis of rectal bleeding in a 10-/30-/70-year-old person.
2. Outline a plan of management of rectal bleeding.

Carcinoma of the Colon
1. List the predisposing causes for colonic carcinoma. Discuss the epidemiology of colonic carcinoma.
2. Discuss the role of CEA in the diagnosis and follow-up of patients with carcinoma of the colon.
3. Discuss the Dukes' classification of carcinoma of the colon and then give average survival rate (in years) for each classification.
4. Discuss the role of diet in the etiology of colon cancer.
5. Discuss the role of chemotherapy and radiation in colon cancer.
6. Discuss the use of stool occult blood testing in the early detection of cancer.
7. Determine the malignant potential of colonic polyps.
8. Classify colonic polyps.
9. Recognize the polyposis syndrome.
10. Discuss the roles of various diagnostic tests used in patients with rectal bleeding.
11. Discuss the value of rectal biopsy in patients with bloody diarrhea.
12. List the etiological causes of colitis.

Inflammatory Bowel Disease
1. Differentiate between Crohn's disease (CD) and chronic ulcerative colitis (CUC).
2. Recognize the reasons for making the distinction between CD and CUC.
3. List the possible mechanisms of diarrhea in patients with Crohn's disease.
4. Discuss the significance of dysplasia in ulcerative colitis and outline the management of such patients.
5. List the determining factors of colonic carcinoma in patients with ulcerative colitis.
6. List the extraintestinal manifestations of inflammatory bowel disease (CD or CUC).

7. Discuss the pathophysiologic mechanisms of gallstone and kidney stone formation in patients with Crohn's disease.
8. List the side effects of corticosteroids, azathioprine, metronidazole, sulfasalazine and 5-ASA.
9. Discuss the mechanisms of action of corticosteroids, azathioprine, metronidazole, sulfasalazine and 5-ASA in the treatment of Crohn's disease and ulcerative colitis.
10. Recognize the activity of Crohn's disease using the Crohn's Disease Activity Index (CDAI).
11. Perform a nutritional assessment in patients with Crohn's disease.
12. Discuss the role of nutritional support in patients with inflammatory bowel disease (IBD).
13. List the gastrointestinal complications of IBD.
14. Describe the fluid and electrolyte contents of ileostomy output.
15. List the complications of ileostomy.
16. Recognize the complications of total parenteral nutrition.
17. Discuss the management of IBD in pregnancy and in childhood.
18. Outline the mechanisms responsible for malabsorption and malnutrition in Crohn's disease.
19. List the causes of anemia in Crohn's disease and ulcerative colitis.
20. Discuss the medical management of Crohn's disease and ulcerative colitis.
21. Discuss the indications for surgery in Crohn's disease and ulcerative colitis.
22. Recognize the clinical presentation and laboratory findings of toxic megacolon.
23. Discuss the management of toxic megacolon.
24. Discuss the investigation of patients with suspected antibiotic-associated colitis.
25. Outline the management of patients with pseudomembranous colitis.
26. Recognize the symptoms of radiation-induced enteropathy.

Perianal Disease
1. Discuss the principles of management of patients with symptomatic hemorrhoids.
2. Recognize the symptoms of hemorrhoids.
3. Describe the physical examination of a patient with internal hemorrhoids.
4. Define fissure in ano.
5. Describe the symptoms of patients with fissure in ano.
6. Outline the principles of management of patients with fissure in ano.

Obstruction

1. List the signs and symptoms of large bowel obstruction.
2. List four causes of large bowel obstruction in adult patients.
3. Outline the diagnostic approach to patients with large bowel obstruction.
4. Describe the radiographic findings in patients with partial bowel obstruction.

Constipation

1. Discuss the etiological classification of constipation.
2. Outline the management of constipation.
3. Recognize the clinical entity "laxative abuse."
4. List four causes of solitary rectal ulceration.
5. Recognize the features of irritable bowel disorders.
6. Discuss the investigation and management of patients with functional bowel disorders.
7. Discuss the pathophysiology of diverticular disease.
8. Discuss the management of complications of diverticular disease.
9. Define gastrocolic reflex and ileal break.
10. List the differential diagnosis of the irritable bowel syndrome.

Ischemia

1. Describe the colonic blood supply.
2. Describe the clinical presentations of intestinal ischemia.
3. Outline the diagnostic approach to management of a patient with ischemic bowel disease.
4. Discuss the indications for surgery in ischemic bowel disease.
5. Recognize GI conditions occurring in association with homosexuality and/or the gay bowel syndrome.

Skills

1. Elicit all the symptoms associated with colonic disease.
2. Demonstrate the ability to do proper rectal examination for occult blood testing.

11
The Pancreas
F. Habal

1. ANATOMY AND PHYSIOLOGY

THE PANCREAS IS an endocrine and exocrine organ located retroperitoneally in the upper abdomen overlying the spine. The head and uncinate process lie within the curve of the duodenum, while the body and tail extend to the gastric border of the spleen. The pancreas is supplied by the gastroduodenal arteries and by branches of the splenic artery. The splenic vein and artery run superiorly and posteriorly; the mesenteric vein lies in the angle between the head and body of the gland. At this point the superior mesenteric vein and splenic vein join to form the portal vein (Figure 1).

The islets of Langerhans, clumps of cells scattered throughout the gland, produce the *endocrine* secretion of the pancreas. Their hormones, secreted directly into capillaries, include insulin, which is produced by the beta cells, and glucagon, pancreatic peptide, somatostatin and other hormones secreted by nonbeta cells.

The *exocrine* portion of the pancreas accounts for about 80% of the total glandular volume. It consists of at least two functional units: *acinar cells*, which secrete primarily digestive enzymes; and *centroacinar* or *ductal cells*, which secrete fluids and electrolytes (Figure 2). Pancreatic secretion is regulated by several peptides that are released from the gastrointestinal tract. Some of these peptides, such as secretin and cholecystokinin (CCK), stimulate pancreatic secretion, whereas somatostatin and pancreatic polypeptide inhibit their release. The pancreas secretes about 20 digestive enzymes and cofactors. Some enzymes are activated in the duodenum by enterokinases and calcium (Figure 3). These enzymes account for most of the intraluminal digestion of

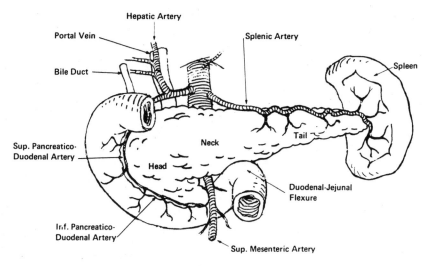

FIGURE 1. Relationships and blood supply of pancreas.

dietary proteins, triglycerides and carbohydrates. They are also important in the cleavage of certain vitamins (such as A and B_{12}) from carrier molecules, thereby allowing them to be absorbed efficiently. Because pancreatic enzymes are secreted in great excess, maldigestion and serious nutritional deficiencies occur only when over 90% of the gland has been destroyed.

2. PANCREATIC SECRETION

2.1 Bicarbonate Secretion
The pancreas secretes an isosmotic juice at a daily rate of 1,500–3,000 mL. It has a pH of 8.3 and contains enzymes, water and electrolytes. The principal anions are Cl^- and HCO_3^-, whereas Na^+ and K^+ are the major cations. Chloride is secreted by the acinar cells and bicarbonate is actively secreted by the ductal cells. The total concentration of both anions approaches 150 mEq/L (Figure 4). At maximum output, as would be observed following a meal, HCO_3^- concentration reaches 150 mEq/L, whereas Cl^- concentration is less than 50 mEq/L. This ratio is reversed at low flow rates. The high pH of the postprandial juice neutralizes acidic gastric chyme and raises duodenal contents to an optimal pH for enzymatic digestion. Pancreatic juice also contains Ca^{++} and traces of Mg^{++}, $HPO_4^=$ and $SO_4^=$, although the role of these electrolytes is not known.

Pancreatic Lobule

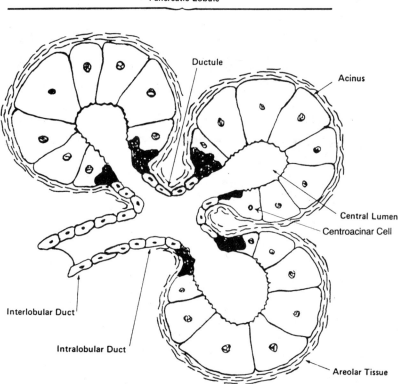

FIGURE 2.   Schematic representation of acinar structure of exocrine pancreas.

2.2 Enzyme Secretion

Four classes of enzymes are secreted by the pancreas. Proteolytic enzymes in the form of proenzymes are activated by enterokinases that are secreted by the mucosa of the proximal intestine. Trypsin and chymotrypsin constitute the largest component and act by cleaving the peptide bonds of dietary protein, producing oligopeptides and amino acids. Other enzymes include carboxy-peptidases A and B, and elastase.

Lipolytic enzymes are secreted in active form. Lipase is the major compo-nent. This enzyme hydrolyzes triglycerides to diglycerides, monoglycerides and fatty acids. Lipase acts as the oil–water interface of fat droplets. Its action is thus facilitated when the fat droplets are emulsified by bile salts and fatty acids. Bile salts also form molecular aggregates, micelles, to solubilize the products of lipolysis in the aqueous duodenal juice, removing them from the

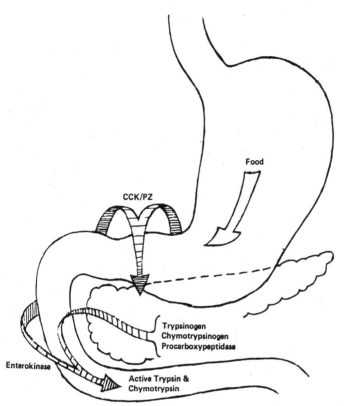

FIGURE 3. Role of cholecystokinin/pancreozymin and of enterokinase activation in pancreatic secretion.

oil–water interface and so enhancing lipase activity. Colipase, a small-molecular-weight cofactor, is secreted by the pancreas. It combines with lipase to prevent the latter from being inhibited and removed from the oil–water interface by bile salts. Colipase also lowers the pH optimum of lipase from 8.5 to 6.5, which is the normal pH in the proximal intestine.

Amylase hydrolyzes starch to form maltose, maltotrioses and dextrins. The fourth class of enzymes comprises nucleolytic enzymes, which hydrolyze the phosphodiester bonds that unite nucleotides in nucleic acid.

2.3 Regulation of Pancreatic Secretion

There are two patterns of pancreatic secretion. The first pattern is *basal secretion*, which is punctuated every 1 to 2 hours by bursts of increased bicarbonate

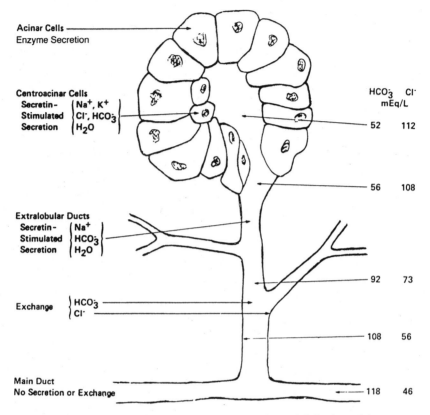

FIGURE 4.   Secretion by centroacinar cells and by cells of the extralobular ducts of the pancreas. Chloride concentrations (right) were determined on fluid collected by micropuncture, and bicarbonate concentrations were inferred from the fact that the fluid is isotonic. These data are for the cat pancreas, but other species seem to be similar.

SOURCE: Adapted from Lightwood R, Reber HA. Micropuncture study of pancreatic secretion in the cat. Gastroenterology 1977; 72:61.

and enzyme secretion that last 10 to 15 minutes. The second pattern is the *postprandial stage*, which results from a complex interaction of neural and hormonal mechanisms. It is divided into three phases. The cephalic phase occurs in response to the sight or taste of food and is probably mediated by the vagus nerve. The stimulation of cholinergic nerve fibers results in the production of enzymes and bicarbonate. The gastric phase occurs partially in response to distention of the stomach, which may stimulate gastrin release, probably by vagal reflexes. The released gastrin and neural reflexes stimulate acid secretion by the gastric parietal cells and pancreatic enzyme secretion.

The intestinal phase, which is the most important, is initiated in response to acid entering the duodenum. When the pH of duodenal contents falls to 4.5 or below, secretin is released from the intestine; secretin in turn stimulates the pancreatic ducts to secrete bicarbonate. The presence of fatty acids, oligopeptides and amino acids results in the release of cholecystokinin (CCK), which stimulates the secretion of pancreatic enzymes. It appears that CCK and secretin each augments the action of the other on the secretion of both bicarbonate and enzyme.

The ultimate result of these interactions is food digestion and then absorption. Although secretin and cholecystokinin induce pancreatic secretion, other hormones – such as pancreatic polypeptide (PP) and peptide YY – inhibit basal and stimulated pancreatic secretion. Produced by the intestinal mucosa, they appear to act as a feedback mechanism to inhibit pancreatic production of further enzymes and electrolytes.

Stimulation of the vagus nerve induces bicarbonate secretion by the pancreas. This activity is thought to be in part mediated by vasoactive intestinal peptide (VIP). VIP hormone is present in vagal nerve endings and throughout the entire gastrointestinal tract. Its physiological role has not been established.

3. PANCREATIC FUNCTIONS

3.1 Secretory Studies

It is easy to diagnose pancreatic insufficiency in the presence of the clinical triad of pancreatic calcification, diabetes and steatorrhea. Most pancreatic diseases, however, remain clinically silent until approximately 90% of the gland is destroyed. Lipase secretion appears to decrease earlier than trypsin secretion; hence, steatorrhea appears earlier than azotorrhea in patients suffering from pancreatic disease. Earlier recognition of pancreatic dysfunction may improve the management of the patient's disease and his or her quality of life.

Pancreatic function tests may be divided into two main groups: direct (duodenal intubation) and indirect (Table 1).

3.2 Direct Tube Tests

The direct tube tests involve intubating the duodenum and collecting pancreatic juices. The pancreas can be stimulated directly by hormones (e.g., secretin test) or indirectly by a meal (e.g., Lundh test meal). A double-lumen tube is commonly used to aspirate juices from the stomach, thus preventing contamination of the duodenum with acidic gastric contents, as well as aspirating from the duodenum. The collection period varies from 45 to 120 minutes.

TABLE 1.   Exocrine pancreatic function

Direct invasive intubation tests
CCK/secretin stimulation
Lundh meal
ERCP and pancreatic aspiration

Indirect noninvasive tests
Stool fats and nitrogen
Stool trypsin and chymotrypsin
Breath tests
Oral function tests (bentiromide test and pancreolauryl test)

Blood determination
Trypsinogen
Lipase
Pancreatic amylase

The stimulation of the pancreas can be accomplished directly by infusing secretin alone or in combination with cholecystokinin. The combination allows the assessment not only of bicarbonate secretion (with secretin) but also of enzyme secretion, mainly trypsin.

A more physiological stimulation test of the pancreas by a meal is called the Lundh test. It assesses the response of the pancreas to endogenous secretin and pancreozymin (or CCK) released in response to a test meal of protein, fat and carbohydrates. The concentration of trypsin and the volume of secretion are measured in samples obtained in the duodenal aspirate. The Lundh meal is virtually always abnormal in pancreatic insufficiency. Unfortunately there is a borderline zone of abnormal values that are uninterpretable. In addition, many other factors influence the results of a Lundh meal, including small bowel mucosal disease, rate of gastric emptying, and surgical interruption of gastroduodenal anatomy. Although this is a more physiological test, its sensitivity and specificity are lower (70–80%) than the direct hormonal stimulation.

Cannulation of the pancreatic duct during endoscopic retrograde cholangiopancreatography (ERCP) has been combined with direct stimulation of the pancreas. This technique allows the measurement of pure pancreatic juice uncontaminated by biliary or intestinal secretions, but this method is possibly no more sensitive than other tests in the diagnosis of pancreatic disease.

3.3 Indirect Pancreatic Function (Tubeless) Tests
The intubation tests tend to be unpleasant for the patients; they are also time-consuming and expensive and are performed mostly in specialized centers.

Indirect tests of pancreatic function detect the result of pancreatic disease. The standard indirect test is the 72-hour fecal fat determination. The patient is placed on a 100 g/day fat diet and the stool is collected daily for three days. Individuals with normal pancreatic functions excrete less than 7% of the total amount of fat ingested, whereas those with pancreatic insufficiency excrete greater than 20%. Although steatorrhea occurs in mucosal malabsorption, it is not as great as that encountered with pancreatic insufficiency. Measurements of stool nitrogen and stool chymotrypsin have not proved superior to fecal fat determinations. The major drawbacks to stool fat estimations are the lack of specificity and the inconvenience of collecting and analyzing the specimens. Attempts to screen for steatorrhea with less offensive tests (such as urine oxalate levels, ^{14}C-triolein/^{3}H-oleic acid assimilation test tripalmitate or palmitic acid breath tests) are promising but not generally accepted. After a rice-flour challenge, breath hydrogen is negligible in normal individual subjects but is dramatically increased in those with pancreatic insufficiency, in whom it is in turn reduced when the challenge rice flour is given with pancreatic enzymes.

There are two oral function tests available for assessing pancreatic functions: the bentiromide test and the pancreolauryl test.

The bentiromide test is useful in discriminating patients with pancreatic steatorrhea from those with normal fat absorption. Bentiromide, a synthetic compound attached to para-aminobenzoic acid (PABA), is hydrolyzed by pancreatic chymotrypsin in the duodenum. This yields a low-molecular-weight substance, para-aminobenzoic acid, which is absorbed in the proximal small bowel and is partially conjugated in the liver. Metabolic byproducts of PABA are excreted in the urine. The excretion of less than 50% of the ingested dose in six hours indicates pancreatic exocrine insufficiency. Thus, the urine output of PABA should reflect duodenal chymotrypsin activity. Low output is an indirect assessment of normal infants, presumably due to immaturity of the exocrine pancreas. Falsely abnormal results also occur in patients with intestinal mucosal, liver or renal disease as a result of abnormalities of absorption, conjugation or excretion of PABA. A two-stage test has therefore been proposed in which PABA excretion following bentiromide is compared with the urine recovery of an equivalent dose of free PABA given on a subsequent occasion. PABA may also be measured in plasma instead of urine, and the plasma test may be more reliable in identifying patients with pancreatic insufficiency. The greatest use of this test may be in excluding pancreatic disease as a cause of diarrhea, steatorrhea, or weight loss.

The pancreolauryl test, using fluorescein dilaurate, has been extensively evaluated in Europe. It can detect only severe pancreatic insufficiency. This test is rarely used.

Chronic pancreatitis may give rise to an abnormal Schilling test, but rarely causes B_{12} deficiency. Vitamin B_{12} is released from food by gastric hydrochloric acid. This B_{12} is bound to an R factor that is present in the saliva and the gastric juices. In the upper intestine, pancreatic enzymes release the R factor from B_{12}, which is then bound to intrinsic factor; the complex is subsequently absorbed in the terminal ileum. The Schilling test is relatively simple, but unfortunately it is not predictably abnormal except in instances of obvious pancreatic insufficiency.

3.4 Miscellaneous Tests

Differentiating pancreatic carcinoma from chronic pancreatitis can at times be difficult; many tests have been described to aid diagnosis, but none are of proven value. Assay of carcinoembryonic antigen (CEA) in serum or from pure pancreatic juice obtained during ERCP has not proved to be a useful discriminator. The pancreatic oncofetal antigen has proved to be of uncertain significance. Serum galactosyl II transferase activity has recently been shown to be a reasonably specific indicator of pancreatic carcinoma in some patients. A sophisticated assay, it is unlikely to be suited to widespread use.

Trypsinogen, a proteolytic proenzyme, is exclusively produced in the pancreas. This enzyme can be detected by radioimmunoassay. It is elevated during an attack of pancreatitis and in renal failure, and is decreased in severe pancreatic insufficiency, cystic fibrosis and insulin-dependent diabetes without exocrine insufficiency. The levels of trypsinogen in cystic fibrosis decrease with age if the pancreas is involved. Low levels are found in about 60% of patients with pancreatic insufficiency. Patients with pancreatic insufficiency who have ongoing inflammation may have normal or raised levels. This fact, in addition to low levels in non–insulin-dependent diabetes, casts some doubt on the usefulness of this test in diagnosing pancreatic insufficiency. It may be useful in patients with steatorrhea that is due to nonpancreatic causes.

3.5 Tests Suggestive of Active Disease

When faced with a patient with hyperamylasemia, it is necessary to exclude disease involving many organs other than just the pancreas (Table 2).

Amylase is produced and released from a variety of tissues, including the salivary glands, intestine and genitourinary tract. Normal serum contains three types of isoamylases as identified by isoelectric focusing. The pancreatic gland secretes one amylase at an isoelectric point of 7.0 that constitutes 33% of the total serum amylase. The parotid secretes several isoamylases with isoelectric points of about 6.4 and 6.0. Electrophoresis on polyacrylamide gel can

TABLE 2. Conditions associated with hyperamylasemia

Pancreatic amylase
(Pancreatic pancreatitis/carcinoma/trauma, including surgical
  and post-ERCP complications of pancreatitis)
Intra-abdominal
Drugs
Diabetic ketoacidosis

Salivary amylase
Malignant neoplasms
Pulmonary diseases/pneumonia/tuberculosis/carcinoma
Diabetic ketoacidosis/ruptured ectopic pregnancy/ovarian cyst

Mixed or unknown
Renal insufficiency
Thermal burns
Macroamylasemia

---

separate five isoamylases on the basis of electrode mobility. Amylases originating in the fallopian tubes, tears, mucus and sweat have the same mobility as salivary amylase. All amylases have similar molecular weight and amino acid composition, but vary in terms of their glycosylation or deamination.

Amylase is filtered through the glomerular membrane and is reabsorbed in the proximal tubule. In healthy individuals, the amylase clearance parallels creatinine clearance. During acute pancreatitis, there is an increase in amylase clearance as opposed to creatinine clearance. Although this ratio was once thought to be specific to acute pancreatitis, other conditions that produce hyperamylasemia (such as diabetic ketoacidosis, burns, renal failure and perforated duodenal ulcer) may demonstrate a similar elevation. Occasionally, the serum amylase may be markedly increased in the absence of pancreatic or salivary diseases, whereas the urinary amylase is normal. In this instance, one must suspect either renal disease or macroamylasemia.

Frequently physicians are faced with a patient who has no overt salivary gland disease but has hyperamylasemia and no specific abdominal findings. As a rule, the level of amylase in pancreatitis usually is elevated to greater than 3 times the upper limit of normal and returns to normal within 2 to 10 days. If the amylase continues to be elevated in the absence of pancreatic complications, other causes (such as malignancy and macroamylasemia) should be investigated.

A rapid rise and fall in serum amylase in a patient with abdominal pain suggests the passage of a stone through the ampulla of Vater. When the serum amylase remains elevated for several days, the gallstone disease is usually complicated by pancreatitis.

Marked hyperamylasemia has been observed in patients with metastatic disease with ovarian cysts and tumors, and ruptured ectopic pregnancy. Isoamylase analysis reveals that the amylase has the same electrophoretic mobility as salivary-type isoenzyme. Macroamylase consists mostly of salivary amylase complexed with globulins, being therefore too large to be filtered at the glomerulus. Therefore these individuals have elevated serum amylase and low urinary amylase, with a low amylase-to-creatinine clearance ratio.

While the amylase levels in serum and urine are usually used as a measure of acute pancreatitis, measurements of lipase may be more specific and sensitive than total serum amylase. The assay of lipase is as accurate as the pancreatic isoamylase assay, and is likely to replace the amylase assay. Measuring both offers no advantage. Amylase and lipase measurements are readily available clinically, whereas radioimmunoassays are still being developed for other pancreatic enzymes (such as trypsin, chymotrypsin and elastase). Their role in the diagnosis of pancreatic disease needs to be established.

4. PANCREATITIS

4.1 Etiology and Pathogenesis
Inflammatory disease of the pancreas is a common problem in North America, with gallstones and alcohol being the major causes (Table 3). Pancreatitis tends to present with abdominal pain, which may improve with no sequelae or may run a more severe course that can lead to death. When the pancreas is continuously injured, such as with alcohol, a chronic condition results in obstruction and fibrosis of the gland, which leads to pancreatic insufficiency and chronic pain. Even one attack of pancreatitis from alcohol use can lead to some residual pancreatic damage.

Pancreatitis results from an autodigestive process. The release of pancreatic digestive enzymes results in problems that range from simple edema to severe hemorrhage and necrosis. Trypsin and chymotrypsin are the initiating enzymes; their release can in turn result in the release and activation of other proenzymes (including proelastase, procollagenase and phospholipases). Trypsin damages endothelial cells and mast cells, resulting in the release of histamine. This major inflammatory mediator enhances vascular permeability, leading to edema, hemorrhage and the activation of the kallikrein system, which in turn results in the production of vasoactive peptides or kinins. The latter are thought to cause pain and further aggravate the inflammatory

TABLE 3.   Causes of acute pancreatitis

Alcoholism

Gallstones

Postoperative

Traumatic

Penetrating duodenal ulcer

Metabolic
   Hyperlipoproteinemia, especially types I, IV and V
   Hypercalcemia
   Renal failure
   Acute fatty liver of pregnancy

Infections
   Mumps
   Viral hepatitis
   Other viral infections (e.g., Coxsackie)
   Ascariasis

Drug-associated
   Diuretics (e.g., thiazides, furosemide)
   Tetracycline
   Sulfonamides
   Estrogens
   Azathioprine

Miscellaneous
   Hereditary
   Regional enteritis
   Connective tissue disorders with vasculitis
   Systemic lupus erythematosus
   Polyarteritis
   Thrombotic thrombocytopenic purpura
   Duodenal diverticulum

Undetermined

response. The other released enzymes destroy the supporting matrix of the gland and the plasma membrane of the acinar cell, precipitating further release of digestive enzymes, which in turn leads to further damage. Lysolecithin, which is released by the action of phospholipase on lecithin (a phospholipid found in bile), has also been implicated in the pancreatic damage, because of its cytotoxic and hemolytic properties. Although these enzymes result in pancreatic damage, the triggering mechanism is not well known. In the case of gallstones, the major theories include (1) reflux of bile into the pancreatic duct; (2) reflux of duodenal content into the pancreatic duct; and (3) distal obstruction of the pancreatic duct, with continued pancreatic secretion leading to increased ductal pressure and resulting in pancreatitis.

Although alcohol has been implicated as a major cause of acute pancreatitis, there is no evidence that an occasional bout of excessive alcohol intake can lead to an acute attack. It is suggested that chronic ingestion may lead to chronic damage and sensitization, which may lead to acute pain even with small amounts of alcohol. Alcohol can cause direct damage to acinar cells in a manner similar to that in which it damages liver cells.

Hyperlipoproteinemia types I, IV and V are associated with the majority of lipid-associated cases of pancreatitis. The incidence of pancreatitis varies from 15–40% of patients. Hypercalcemia and hyperparathyroidism may also induce pancreatitis. Although the incidence of pancreatitis in patients with hyperparathyroidism was at one time shown to vary from 7–19%, recent findings suggest this variation to be closer to 1.5%. This discrepancy can be accounted for by the difference in the degree or duration of the hyperparathyroidism and by the earlier treatment of hypercalcemia. Other causes of pancreatitis are shown in Table 3.

4.2 Acute Pancreatitis

4.2.1 CLINICAL MANIFESTATIONS
The clinical spectrum of acute pancreatitis ranges from mild, self-limiting disease to fulminant lethal disease. Up to 80% of patients will have an uneventful recovery; the remainder will have serious complications with a high mortality rate. Objective measurements such as Ranson's criteria (Table 4) show a good correlation with the risk of major complications and death. The overall mortality rate of acute pancreatitis ranges from 7–20%. The mortality rate correlates well with complications such as shock and hemorrhage.

4.2.2 SYMPTOMS
Pain from acute pancreatitis is a knife-like, steady, sharp pain that starts suddenly and reaches its zenith rapidly. It is commonly localized to the epigastric area and may radiate directly to the back. It improves on leaning forward and is frequently associated with nausea or vomiting. Depending on the location of the inflammation, the pain may be referred to either the left upper quadrant or the right upper quadrant. When the pancreatitis is severe, it may result in shock and lead to death. Frequently the pain is dyspeptic in quality and aggravated by food. This is due partially to the fact that eating stimulates secretion.

TABLE 4. Poor prognostic signs in acute
pancreatitis

Age over 55
Shock, fever, hypotension, tachycardia
Hypoxemia, respiratory failure
Hemoconcentration
Elevated serum creatinine, AST, LDH
Amylase >1,000
Hyperglycemia
Hypocalcemia

Classically the pain lasts between three and four days. When the pancreatitis is severe, it may result in peripheral circulatory failure; under these conditions, the mortality rate approaches 60%.

Recurrent nausea and vomiting may be due to a reflex mechanism secondary to pain and occurs in over 90% of the cases. Other causes include pseudo-obstruction secondary to ileus and distention or obstruction secondary to a pancreatic mass or pseudocyst. Since the common bile duct traverses the pancreatic head before entering the duodenum, jaundice may occur, often transiently.

4.2.3 SIGNS
Depending on the severity of pancreatitis, the patient may appear in distress or be in shock. Jaundice may be caused by edema of the head of the pancreas or by an obstructing stone. Tachycardia could be secondary to pain, volume depletion or the inflammatory process. Low-grade fever could be secondary to the inflammation in the pancreas or from such complications as abscess formation.

Abdominal examination may reveal epigastric and abdominal tenderness with guarding or rigidity. Bluish discoloration of the flanks (Grey Turner's sign) or of the periumbilical area (Cullen's sign) indicates that blood from hemorrhagic pancreatitis has entered the fascial planes. The signs are not specific and may occur in any condition that causes retroperitoneal hemorrhage. Tender red and painful nodules that mimic erythema nodosum may appear over the extremities. These are due to circulating lipases.

4.2.4 COMPLICATIONS
Since the signs and symptoms of acute pancreatitis mimic those of surgically correctable intra-abdominal disorders, the diagnosis of acute pancreatitis is

often one of exclusion. Other diseases to be considered are a perforated peptic ulcer, mesenteric thrombosis, intestinal obstruction, dissecting aneurysm, peritonitis, acute cholecystitis and appendicitis. The diagnostic process is complicated by the fact that hyperamylasemia can occur in disorders other than pancreatic inflammation (such as ectopic pregnancy, parotiditis, carcinoma of the lung, posterior penetrating ulcer, ruptured aortic aneurysm and opiate administration). Although amylase values greater than 1,000 units have been said to occur principally in conditions requiring surgery (e.g., biliary tract disease), this distinction is not absolute.

Complications are divided into local and systemic. Local involvement includes phlegmon (18%), pancreatic abscess (3%), pancreatic pseudocyst (10%) and thrombosis of the central portal system. Phlegmon is an area of edema, inflammation and necrosis without a definite structure (unlike an abscess). This results from the ischemic insult caused by decreased tissue perfusion and release of the digestive enzymes. When this damage is not cleared, further inflammation ensues, declaring itself by increased pain, fever and tenderness. A pseudocyst develops as a result of pancreatic necrosis and the escape of activated pancreatic secretions through pancreatic ducts. It contains blood and debris. This fluid coalesces and becomes encapsulated by an inflammatory reaction and fibrosis. These patients usually have pain and hyperamylasemia, but may be asymptomatic. They may present with an abdominal mass, which can cause compressive symptoms. If a superimposed infection occurs with acute pancreatitis, a pancreatic abscess develops. This complication occurs in about 3% of acute pancreatitis cases and has a high mortality rate.

Systemic complications of acute pancreatitis are numerous (Table 5) and correlate well with the severity of the inflammatory process. They may be manifested by circulatory collapse, respiratory and renal failure and profound metabolic disturbances.

4.2.5 DIAGNOSTIC EVALUATION
The diagnosis of acute pancreatitis is based on a combination of clinical findings and elevated serum amylase and serum lipase. Elevation of serum amylase in acute pancreatitis is short-lived. Amylase is rapidly cleared by the renal tubules and may return to normal within 24 hours from the time of onset. Although amylase-to-creatinine clearance was used in the past to diagnose pancreatitis, it is now rarely used.

Recently radioimmunoassays for pancreatic lipase have become available, whereas the trypsinogen assay remains experimental. These assays may add to the accuracy of the diagnosis of pancreatitis.

TABLE 5.   Systemic complications of pancreatitis

Metabolic
   Hypocalcemia, hyperglycemia,
      hypertriglyceridemia, acidosis

Respiratory
   Atelectasis, effusion, pneumonitis
   Acute respiratory diseases (ARDS)

Renal
   Renal artery or vein thrombosis
   Renal failure

Circulatory
   Arrhythmias
   Hypovolemia and shock; myocardial infarct
   Pericardial effusion, vascular thrombosis

Gastrointestinal
   Ileus
   GI bleed
   GI obstruction

Hepatobiliary
   Jaundice
   Portal vein thrombosis

Neurologic
   Psychosis or encephalopathy
   Cerebral emboli
   Blindness, retinal artery thrombosis

Hematologic
   Anemia
   DIC (disseminated intravascular coagulopathy)
   Leukocytosis

Dermatologic
   Painful subcutaneous fat necrosis

4.2.6 RADIOLOGIC EVALUATION

A plain film of the abdomen is very helpful. It may reveal calcification of the pancreas (indicative of a chronic process) or it may reveal gallstones (if calcified). The presence of free air suggests perforation, whereas the presence of thumb-printing in the intestinal wall may indicate a mesenteric ischemic process. A localizing ileus of the stomach, duodenum or proximal jejunum (all of which are adjacent to the pancreas) suggests pancreatic inflammation. When the transverse colon is also involved, air fills the transverse colon but not the descending colon (colon "cut-off" sign) and a diagnosis of acute pancreatitis can be confidently made. The chest x-ray can show atelectasis or an effusion, more often involving the left lower lobe.

Although clinical, biochemical and simple radiographic evaluation suffice for the diagnosis of pancreatitis, ultrasonographic and computed tomography (CT) imaging are essential. These confirm the diagnosis, provide an early assessment regarding the course of the disease and detect complications such as phlegmon, pseudocyst and abscess formation. A cyst or an abscess may also be drained percutaneously under CT or ultrasound guidance.

The most common ultrasonographic and CT finding in patients with acute pancreatitis is diffuse glandular enlargement. Ultrasonographically there is a decrease in echogenicity of the organ; on CT scan there is decreased attenuation from edema of the tissues. Frequently intravenous contrast is given, and this may demonstrate a uniform enhancement in the pancreatic parenchyma. A normal examination does not rule out the presence of acute disease. In up to 30% of the uncomplicated cases of acute pancreatitis CT scan may be normal; these patients usually have a mild form of pancreatitis. When a stone or an obstruction of the distal common bile duct is present, the common bile duct and the intrahepatic biliary tree may be dilatated.

Endoscopic retrograde cholangiopancreatography (ERCP) involves visualizing, cannulating the ampulla of Vater and then injecting contrast material. This procedure is usually contraindicated during the acute phase, except when the pancreatitis is caused by an impacted common bile duct stone. Under those conditions a sphincterotomy and stone removal may be performed. If performed as early as 24 hours following admission, this procedure may result in significant improvement in morbidity and mortality.

4.2.7 TREATMENT

The aims of therapy of acute pancreatitis are (1) hemodynamic stabilization, (2) alleviation of pain, (3) stopping the progression of the damage, and (4) treatment of local and systemic complications. As yet there are no specific medical therapies capable of reducing or reversing the pancreatic inflammation. Hence therapeutic interventions are aimed at the complications of the disease.

Once the diagnosis is established with certainty, the patient's intravascular volume is replenished, and electrolytes, calcium, magnesium and blood sugar are closely monitored. Depending on the severity of the attack, an indwelling urinary catheter and close monitoring of urinary output may be necessary. Analgesics such as meperidine should be administered regularly during the first several days of the attack. This may alleviate the pain, decrease the patient's apprehension and improve respiration, thus preventing pulmonary complications such as atelectasis. The risk of narcotic addiction is minimal during the first days; most patients settle within 72 hours. The patient is kept off oral feeding; nasogastric suctioning is maintained if the disease is severe and complicated by ileus. Mild cases with minimal symptoms may be managed without suctioning. The rationale behind nasogastric suctioning is to place the pancreas at rest by removing the acidic gastric juices. This suppresses secretin release and decreases pancreatic stimulation. The validity of this postulate has not been substantiated. Similarly, the use of acid-suppressive medications such as cimetidine has failed to show benefit in the treatment of acute pancreatitis. The use of enzyme inhibitors such as soybean trypsin inhibitor to prevent further damage is controversial, as is the use of prostaglandins and corticosteroids.

The routine administration of antibiotics does not improve the course of mild to moderate disease. However, when the development of pancreatic abscess is suspected from an increase in fever and abdominal pain, antibiotic therapy should be instituted using an aminoglycocide and cephalosporin.

Respiratory insufficiency may occur in up to 40% of the cases, usually in patients with severe or recurrent pancreatitis. In such patients, arterial oxygen saturation should be monitored and corrected. Fluid overload should be avoided. Intubation and ventilation may be required.

Peritoneal lavage has been advocated in patients with severe disease, such as those with marked hypovolemia or hypotension or those who continue to deteriorate despite appropriate medical therapy. Although this technique reduces the circulatory and renal complications, it does not seem to alter the local complications.

Intravenous hyperalimentation has been advocated in patients who continue to have pain and whose symptoms are aggravated postprandially. If during a trial of six weeks or longer complications develop (such as an abscess or an enlargement of phlegmon), a surgical debridement may be warranted, albeit as a last resort.

4.3 Chronic Pancreatitis

Chronic pancreatitis is defined as a continued inflammation characterized by irreversible morphologic changes. These changes include fibrosis, ductal abnormality, calcification and cellular atrophy. Alcohol is the major etiologic factor, accounting for about 75% of the cases. Repeated attacks of gallstone-related pancreatitis rarely if ever result in chronic pancreatitis. Other causes include diabetes, protein-calorie malnutrition, hereditary pancreatitis, cystic fibrosis and idiopathic causes.

Alcohol presumably causes pancreatic injury by the intraductal formation of protein plugs secondary to increased protein concentration and precipitation, with or without calcification. These plugs lead to obstruction and secondary pancreatic damage caused by autodigestion. The length of time between alcohol ingestion and the development of clinical manifestations is 10 to 12 years for females and 17 to 18 years for males. Men predominate over women, with a median age of onset ranging from 38 to 49 years.

4.3.1 CLINICAL MANIFESTATIONS

Recurrent or persisting pain is one of the commonest manifestations of chronic pancreatitis. The pain is localized to the upper abdomen, with radiation to subcostal regions and to the back. The pain is aggravated by meals and improves with fasting.

Malnutrition and weight loss are common. The reason for the weight loss is secondary to postprandial pain and hence decreased food ingestion (sitophobia). Steatorrhea and azotorrhea from exocrine insufficiency result in maldigestion and diarrhea in addition to diabetes mellitus. These patients frequently present with loss of adipose tissues – judged by hanging skin folds, and more objectively by demonstrating that the skin fold at the mid-triceps is less than 8 mm in males and less than 12 mm in females. In addition, they manifest muscle wasting and edema, indicating protein deficiency.

4.3.2 COMPLICATIONS

4.3.2.1 Pancreatic pseudocyst

Pancreatic pseudocyst is an encapsulated collection of necrotic debris, blood and pancreatic secretions surrounded by a non-epithelial wall. Its frequency varies from 10–50% of patients experiencing severe pancreatitis. When a pseudocyst is present for less than six weeks, it is considered acute; after that it becomes chronic. The pseudocyst may be asymptomatic or may present as an acute exacerbation of pancreatitis, with abdominal pain, nausea, vomiting and weight loss. These pseudocysts may obstruct intra-abdominal viscera, cause pancreatic ascites, rupture into viscera or the abdominal cavity, hemorrhage or become infected. Spontaneous resolution occurs in 20% of the cases within the first six weeks of the pseudocyst's development. Chronic pseudocysts or pseudocysts greater than 5 cm rarely improve. Successful drainage may be accomplished by CT- or ultrasound-guided drainage techniques. Surgical drainage is sometimes necessary. If the pseudocyst is in the head of the pancreas, drainage can be done via ERCP.

4.3.2.2 *Pancreatic ascites*

Pancreatic ascites results from the leakage of pancreatic juices into the peritoneal cavity through a fistula or ruptured pseudocyst. It presents with gradually increasing massive ascites, high levels of amylase, abdominal pain and weight loss. Subcutaneous fat necrosis with painful lesion results from the high levels of circulating pancreatic lipase.

4.3.2.3 *Common bile duct obstruction*

Common bile duct compression is another manifestation of chronic pancreatitis, but it rarely results in significant obstruction. As the distal common bile duct traverses the head of the pancreas, it may be narrowed secondary to inflammation, with edema or fibrosis of the gland.

Although pancreatic carcinoma was formerly thought to be more common in chronic pancreatitis, the incidence is now believed to be the same as in the general population. Pancreatic carcinoma may present as pancreatitis.

4.3.3 DIAGNOSTIC EVALUATION

The diagnosis of chronic pancreatitis is often one of exclusion. When 90% of the pancreas is damaged and pancreatic insufficiency results, the diagnosis is not difficult to make, especially when a plain film of the abdomen reveals pancreatic calcification. These patients usually present with abdominal pain, weight loss and steatorrhea.

Diagnostic evaluation includes a direct tube test that measures the bicarbonate concentration and volume of pancreatic juice in response to secretin stimulation. The commonest manifestation is a decreased bicarbonate concentration (< 50 mEq/L) and decreased volume of secretion. The indirect tube method uses the Lundh meal, which is infused into the duodenum, following which the levels of trypsin and lipase are measured in the aspirate. The bentiromide test also can be positive.

4.3.4 RADIOGRAPHIC EVALUATION

A plain film of the abdomen may reveal calcification, which is demonstrable when at least 80% of the exocrine pancreas is damaged; such calcification is frequently associated with alcoholic pancreatitis. Calcification may also be detected by CT scans or by ultrasonography. The latter may show enlargement of the gland, dilatation of the ducts and, at times, large concretions and calcification.

Cannulation of the pancreatic duct and injection of contrast dye at ERCP may reveal narrowing and dilatation of the duct, stenosis and filling of side ductules. It also may reveal obstruction of the common bile duct. This test is not as accurate as pancreatic function studies for diagnosing chronic pancreatitis. Its use is warranted prior to pancreatic surgery in order to delineate the ductal anatomy and the site of stenosis or obstruction. It may also demonstrate the presence of a pseudocyst.

4.3.5 TREATMENT

The treatment of chronic pancreatitis is directed toward pain relief and correction of diarrhea, steatorrhea, azotorrhea and weight loss.

The mechanism of pain in chronic pancreatitis is not known. Abstinence from alcohol may decrease the frequency and severity of painful attacks in patients with alcoholic pancreatitis. Large meals with foods rich in fat should be avoided. Analgesics should be given prior to meals, since the pain is maximal postprandially. The continuous use of narcotics often leads to addiction to the drug(s), which makes the management of pain more difficult. Large doses of pancreatic extracts may reduce the frequency and severity of the pain in patients with no demonstrable duct obstruction. These enzymes appear to suppress pancreatic exocrine output, thus putting the pancreas at rest and resulting in pain relief. Pancreatic replacement is given with meals and at bedtime. Patients who respond to this therapeutic regimen tend to be middle-aged women with idiopathic pancreatitis who suffer from mild or moderate disease. These patients tend to have a bicarbonate output greater than 55 mEq/L and normal fat absorption. Patients with more severe disease, whose peak bicarbonate output is less than 50 mEq/L, tend not to respond to this regimen.

Patients who continue to be symptomatic and are found to have an obstruction of the duct with proximal dilatation frequently benefit from a longitudinal pancreatojejunostomy. Similarly, pain that is caused by a pseudocyst often responds to either percutaneous or surgical drainage. When there is no ductal obstruction and the disease is subtotal, pancreatectomy may be beneficial. Despite surgical intervention, pain may recur within five years of the operation, especially in patients who continue to ingest alcohol and/or narcotics. Frequently the improvement in pain correlates with the progression of pancreatic dysfunction.

Octreotide, a long-acting somatostatin analogue, appears to decrease the pain of chronic pancreatitis. Its action is mediated by suppressing pancreatic secretion, hence resting the pancreas. The role of octreotide has not been fully proven.

Steatorrhea and azotorrhea result when pancreatic enzyme output is

TABLE 6.   Causes of failure of pancreatic replacement

Incorrect diagnosis (nonpancreatic causes of steatorrhea, such as sprue, bacterial overgrowth)

Poor compliance

Incorrect timing of the medications (should be given with meals)

Variability in the enzyme content of the pancreatic replacement or loss of potency of the enzyme (inadequate amount of enzymes)

Inactivation of the enzymes by gastric juices or by sunlight

reduced to less than 10% of normal. Pancreatic extract therapy may alleviate the pancreatic maldigestion and its sequelae. Azotorrhea is more easily reversed than steatorrhea, since trypsin is more resistant to acid inactivation than lipases. It seems that the most important barrier preventing correction of steatorrhea is the destruction of enzymes in the stomach, which prevents the delivery of enough active enzyme to the duodenum.

Replacement pancreatic enzymes are made from hog pancreas and contain a mixture of proteases, lipase and amylase, along with a variety of enzymes normally present in pancreatic secretions. Different preparations vary in the amount of lipase activity and the method of enzyme delivery (e.g., tablets, capsules or enteric-coated microspheres). Treatment with these enzymes is lifelong. Pancreatic enzymes are inactivated by pH 4 or below; hence, enteric-coated preparations such as Pancrease™ or Cotazym® may be appropriate. In patients who do not respond well, the use of histamine H_2-receptor antagonists (cimetidine, ranitidine or famotidine) or antacids with meals may overcome the detrimental effect of acid on the enzymes. The causes of failure to respond to pancreatic enzyme supplementation are shown in Table 6.

Hypersensitivity to pancreatic enzymes has been reported in patients who have hypersensitivity to pork proteins. Hyperuricosuria may occur in patients receiving high doses of pancreatic extracts, although recent reports have questioned this relationship. There appears to be a relationship between urinary urate concentration and the severity of pancreatitis. It appears that oral pancreatic enzymes may bind to folic acid, thereby impairing its absorption, but the clinical significance of this is not clear. Fat-soluble vitamins (e.g., vitamins A and E) are poorly absorbed when steatorrhea exceeds 20 g of fat loss per day. Vitamin D and calcium malabsorption leads to osteopenia with tetany. Vitamin K is also malabsorbed, but bleeding is rare. Malabsorption of vitamin B_{12} occurs in up to 40% of patients with chronic pancreatitis, although vitamin

TABLE 7.   Commonest sites of metastases from pancreatic carcinoma

Local nodes
Liver
Peritoneum
Adrenal glands
Lung
Kidneys
Spleen
Bone

B_{12} deficiency is rare. This malabsorption is thought to be due to the failure of R factor to cleave from the vitamin B_{12}–intrinsic factor complex, resulting in nonabsorbable vitamin B_{12}.

5. CARCINOMA OF THE PANCREAS

The incidence of cancer of the pancreas has increased steadily over the past 25 years. In males it is the fourth commonest cancer causing death, exceeded only by cancers of the lung, colon and rectum, and prostate. In females it is the fifth commonest cause of death, with only cancers of the breast, colorectum, lung and ovary/uterus being more frequent. The incidence is higher in males, with a sex ratio of two males to each female; peak incidence occurs in the fifth through seventh decade.

The overall five-year survival rate is less than 1%, and most patients who develop carcinoma of the pancreas die within six months of diagnosis. The poor prognosis in this condition is secondary to the inability to diagnose the carcinoma at an early stage. When symptoms present, the tumor is far advanced and often has metastasized to regional lymph nodes and to adjacent and distant organs, as shown in Table 7.

Ductal cell adenocarcinoma accounts for 90% of pancreatic tumors. Approximately 5% of adenocarcinomas of the pancreas are of islet cell origin; the rest consist of cystadenocarcinoma, giant cell carcinoma and epidermoid carcinoma. The head of the pancreas is the commonest site of involvement, accounting for 70% of the cases, whereas the body and tail account for 20% and 10% of the cases, respectively.

Several etiological agents have been invoked in the pathogenesis of pancreatic carcinoma. The incidence in smokers appears to be twice that of nonsmokers. The mechanism causing carcinoma is not proven and has been explained on the basis of the presence of a carcinogen in tobacco smoke. High-fat or high-protein diets tend to stimulate CCK release from the duodenum, which in turn can cause pancreatic hypertrophy and may predispose to carcinoma, although the evidence is not convincing. Diabetics are at twice the risk of developing carcinoma of pancreas as the general population. The mechanism of this is not known. There is no evidence to suggest that alcoholic chronic pancreatitis predisposes to carcinoma.

Some epidemiological studies have suggested an increased rate of pancreatic carcinoma in patients who drank chlorinated water; this remains to be proven. Genetic defects have also been invoked, such as oncogenes and 53 p tumor suppressor mutation, in addition to some evidence suggesting an increase in epidermal growth factor receptor activity.

5.1 Clinical Manifestations

The major symptoms of pancreatic carcinoma include pain, jaundice and weight loss.

Rapid and progressive weight loss is probably the commonest symptom of carcinoma of the pancreas, and is not related to the location or to the extent of the tumor.

Most (up to 90%) of the patients suffer from pain during the course of the disease. The pain frequently is a dull aching or boring. Located in the epigastrium, it radiates to the back and increases in severity at night. Depending on the site of the tumor, the pain may radiate to the right or left upper quadrant. Unrelenting pain results from retroperitoneal extension, with invasion of the neural plexuses around the celiac axis.

Jaundice may be the presenting symptom in up to 30% of the patients, and the incidence increases as the disease progresses. It may be associated with pain and pruritus. Jaundice is more common when the head of the pancreas is involved, but obstruction or jaundice can occur secondary to spread to the liver or to lymph nodes around the bile duct. Other nonspecific symptoms include bloating, nausea and vomiting, weakness and fatigue, and diarrhea.

5.2 Signs

The commonest finding in carcinoma of the head of the pancreas is jaundice, with abdominal tenderness and an enlarged liver. Less common signs include a palpable gallbladder, an abdominal mass and edema. Thrombophlebitis occurs in less than 10% of the patients.

The development of diabetes in a middle-aged man or elderly patient with no family history of diabetes should suggest pancreatic carcinoma, especially when this is associated with abdominal pain or weight loss.

5.3 Diagnostic Evaluation

Laboratory tests are often normal or nonspecific. Serum alkaline phosphatase and bilirubin are elevated when the bile duct is obstructed or there are hepatic metastases. Serum amylase may be moderately elevated but also may be normal. Pancreatic secretory studies are not often helpful, since findings overlap with chronic pancreatitis.

Several tumor markers have been detected in the sera of patients with pancreatic carcinoma. These include pancreatic oncofetal antigen, α-fetoprotein (AFP), carcinoembryonic antigen (CEA) and pancreatic cancer associated antigen. Certain serum tumor markers such as CA 19-9 and CA 242 have been useful in following the progression of pancreatic cancer but not in its diagnosis. These tests are nonspecific and not sensitive enough for screening purposes. Cytologic specimens can be obtained by percutaneous needle aspiration under ultrasound or CT guidance and by aspiration of duodenal or pancreatic juices at ERCP. Positive cytology may guide further management; on the other hand, negative cytology does not rule out the disease.

Ultrasonography is the procedure of choice for detecting pancreatic cancer. Its usefulness is dependent on the examiner's expertise. Examination may be less than optimal in the presence of increased bowel gas. The sensitivity of this test in pancreatic cancer is reported to be 76–94%, with a specificity of 96%. Once a lesion is detected, a guided biopsy may be helpful in establishing the diagnosis. When obstructive jaundice is present, ultrasound may reveal the presence of hepatic lesions or obstruction of the biliary tree. This procedure is simple and involves no radiation exposure.

Computerized tomography (CT) is more accurate and gives more information than ultrasonography. However, it is also more expensive and involves low radiation exposure; also, small centers may not have the equipment. With this technique, bowel gas does not interfere with the visualization of the pancreas. There is better identification of any retroperitoneal invasion. A guided biopsy of the lesion is also possible. However, small early lesions (especially in the head of the pancreas) may be missed on CT scan; hence, its usefulness in early diagnosis is not clear.

When there is a clinical suspicion of a pancreatic lesion and the ultrasound or CT scan is normal, an ERCP is helpful. It has the advantage of combining gastroduodenoscopy, cholangiography and pancreatography. The papilla may also be examined and cytologic sampling may be obtained. When obstruction is present, therapeutic drainage via stents may be attempted. Nuclear magnetic resonance is a novel technique, but its role in pancreatic diseases is limited. Angiography is no longer used for diagnosing pancreatic carcinoma, but is still useful to evaluate patients who have known carcinoma for resectability, by outlining vascular anatomy. Newer diagnostic tools such as endoscopic ultrasound may further improve selection of patients who might benefit from curative surgery.

5.4 Treatment

At the time of presentation, 75–80% of patients have unresectable tumor. Pancreatectomy or pancreatoduodenal resection for localized disease is the only treatment that carries a potential for cure. Despite this intervention, the disease carries a poor long-term prognosis, with a survival rate of 4% at five years. Complications can occur in up to 20% of patients following pancreatico-duodenectomy. This includes delayed gastric emptying, pancreaticojejunal leak, intra-abdominal sepsis, biliary anastomotic leak, gastrointestinal bleeding and other intra-abdominal hemorrhage. Factors favoring longer survival include jaundice at presentation, a small tumor mass, early tumor stage and a well-differentiated tumor. Palliative operations for unresectable tumor offer some relief, such as alleviating biliary or duodenal obstruction. Operative intervention is frequently associated with high morbidity and mortality; hence, nonsurgical intervention may be preferable. Biliary obstruction can be relieved by percutaneous drainage or by endoscopic stenting of the bile duct. Unfortunately these stents tend to occlude and may require frequent changes.

6. PANCREATIC ISLET CELL TUMORS

Several pancreatic islet cell tumors have been identified. These tumors tend to elaborate a variety of biologically active peptides, resulting in a variety of clinical presentations. These peptides include glucagon, gastrin, vasoactive intestinal peptide (VIP), somatostatin and pancreatic polypeptide (PP).

Glucagon-secreting tumors *(glucagonomas)* arise from the alpha cells of the pancreas. Patients commonly present with mild diabetes, delayed gastric emptying, ileus and constipation. A migratory necrotizing erythematous eruption may develop, commonly over the lower extremities. The diagnosis is established by the demonstration of elevated plasma glucagon levels that increase, paradoxically, with challenge by intravenous tolbutamide.

Gastrin-secreting tumors *(gastrinomas*; Zollinger-Ellison syndrome) arise from nonbeta islet cells. They are frequently malignant and tend to be multiple. They commonly present with recurrent severe peptic ulceration with marked gastric acid hypersecretion and occasionally diarrhea. The diagnosis is established by the demonstration of marked fasting hypergastrinemia and marked gastric acid hypersecretion. In patients who have borderline increases in gastrin, provocative testing with secretin is indicated. Following secretin stimulation, gastrin levels increase in patients with gastrinoma, whereas in patients with common duodenal ulcer, gastrin levels may show a minimal increase, a decrease or no change. High levels of gastrin may be present in a condition known as G-cell hyperplasia. This can be distinguished from gastrinoma by the sharp rise of gastrin level (>200%) in response to meals. Patients with gastrinoma show minimal or no rise in gastrin levels.

Vasoactive intestinal peptide–secreting tumors (*VIPoma*; Werner-Morrison syndrome) produce the pancreatic cholera syndrome, which is characterized by severe diarrhea, hypokalemia and hypochlorhydria or achlorhydria. Fluid secretion may exceed 3–5 L, with a loss of 200–300 mEq of potassium daily. Although the diagnosis is established by the demonstration of high levels of VIP, other substances, such as prostaglandins and secretin-like substances, may contribute to this syndrome.

Somatostatin-producing tumors *(somatostatinomas)* tend to be malignant and have usually metastasized by the time of diagnosis. They commonly present with mild diabetes mellitus, gallstones and a dilatated gallbladder, anemia, hypochlorhydria and malabsorption. The diagnosis is established by the demonstration of high levels of serum somatostatin.

Pancreatic polypeptide–producing tumors have not been shown to produce any clinically defined syndrome.

6.1 Treatment
Pancreatic endocrine tumors are ideally treated by resection. Unfortunately, despite all our available techniques up to 40% of these tumors tend to escape localization. These tumors tend to be single or multiple and may be located in any portion of the pancreas or ectopically in the duodenum or any other part of the gastrointestinal tract. It appears that endoscopic ultrasonography may play an important role in tumor localization, but this technique is operator dependent and is not widely used.

7. PANCREAS DIVISUM

Pancreas divisum is the most common variant of human pancreas, occurring in nearly 10% of the population. This anomaly results from the failure of fusion of the dorsal and ventral pancreatic ducts, which usually occurs in the second month of fetal life. This results in the drainage of the main pancreatic duct (including the superior-anterior aspect of the head, the body and the tail) into the dorsal duct via the accessory papilla. The ventral duct, which drains the posterior-inferior aspect, joins the common bile duct and empties into the

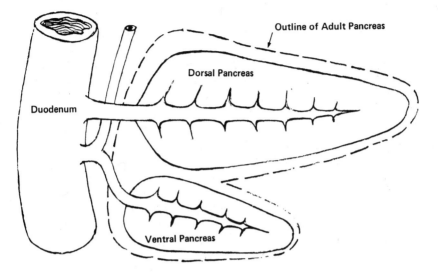

FIGURE 5. Pancreas at approximately 7 weeks fetal life.

major papilla (Figure 5). The diagnosis of this condition is made by ERCP.

Most patients having this anomaly are symptom-free, although some reports have suggested a high incidence of abdominal pain and pancreatitis. It has been suggested that the relative stenosis of the accessory papillary orifice, the major outflow tract for pancreatic secretions, is the cause of problems.

Endoscopic sphincterotomy or transduodenal sphincteroplasty has been advocated as the operation of choice in these individuals. The results obtained with this intervention have been controversial. Some studies have reported a success rate of 90% in patients with pancreas divisum pancreatitis after two years, whereas other reports did not support such findings. From the available literature, surgical intervention in pancreas divisum is as controversial as its causative relationship in abdominal pain and pancreatitis.

8. CYSTIC FIBROSIS IN THE ADULT

Cystic fibrosis (CF) is no longer solely a pediatric disease. CF is the most common potentially lethal genetic disease affecting Caucasians. Its incidence shows regional variations, but overall incidence in Caucasians is approximately 1 per 2,500 live births; it is inherited as an autosomal recessive trait. CF is also the most common cause of chronic lung disease and pancreatic insufficiency in patients under the age of 20.

Over the past decade the fundamental biochemical defect in CF has been identified. The gene has been cloned and up to 300 alleles have been discovered. The gene product is the cystic fibrosis transmembrane conductance regulator. This regulator, the main chloride transport system, is defective in individuals with CF. The regulator is localized on the apical membrane of the epithelial duct cells of the proximal pancreatic duct. In addition to cystic fibrosis transmembrane conductance regulator, these cells contain "Cl^-/ HCO_3^- exchangers," which are responsible for bicarbonate secretion and are dependent on luminal chloride, which is supplied by the cAMP-activated Cl^- channel. Thus, in CF, altered chloride secretion results in decreased bicarbonate production and ultimately failure to adequately hydrate and alkalinize the concentrated protein secretions of the acinar cells. This proteinaceous material becomes inspissated, resulting in ductal obstruction and ultimately acinar cell destruction, fibrosis and malabsorption. The decrease in bicarbonate secretion also results in failure to neutralize duodenal acid, thus leading to further malabsorption by decreasing lipase activity and altering the bioavailability of enteric-coated enzyme supplement.

The "classic" picture of a chronically malnourished child with a progressive lung disease and pancreatic dysfunction culminating in early death is an oversimplification. CF should now be regarded as a syndrome with a heterogeneous assortment of presentations involving variable degrees of organ dysfunction and damage. Pulmonary disease and its complications still dominate the clinical picture in most patients, and are the primary determinants of overall morbidity and mortality. However, as many as 20% of CF patients are not diagnosed until after the age of 15 because they have atypical presentations (e.g., recurrent sinusitis, nasal polyps, chronic bronchitis, recurrent abdominal pain, loose, foul-smelling stools, cirrhosis and infertility).

The advent of vigorous physiotherapy, more effective antibiotics, improved pancreatic extracts and continuing care in specialized CF clinics has resulted in a median survival of at least 18 years. Indeed, in many CF centers, half the patients survive 26 years, and up to 90% of patients may live more than 18 years after the diagnosis has been made. With such increased survival, gastrointestinal complications are becoming increasingly common.

Abnormalities have been identified in glycoproteins, mucus secretions, circulating proteases and cell transport mechanisms. Biliary dyskinesia may also be a factor. Abnormal electrolyte concentrations (due to impaired reabsorption of sodium chloride in secretions) lead to heat prostration, cardiovascular collapse and death. The abnormally thick mucus produced obstructs ductules and tubules, and results in distal organ damage, which leads to chronic obstructive lung disease, pancreatic insufficiency, hepatic fibrosis and intestinal obstruc-

TABLE 8. Nonpulmonary complications in adult CF patients

Steatorrhea, diarrhea
Impaired nutritional status
Meconium ileus equivalent, intussusception
Gallbladder disease
Cirrhosis
Glucose intolerance, diabetes mellitus
Pancreatic exocrine dysfunction
Psychological problems

tion. The mucosal and submucosal glands of the small intestine are dilatated, with acidophilic concretions. Steatorrhea results from exocrine pancreatic failure and perhaps also impaired absorption of fatty acids. Carbohydrate malabsorption relates to disaccharidase deficiency and impaired absorption due to retarded diffusion across the intestinal unstirred water layer.

Abdominal pain is common in CF patients. It may be related to steatorrhea, constipation, meconium ileus equivalent, intussusception, cholelithiasis, duodenal ulcer or pancreatitis. In contrast to infants and children, adults are less affected by malabsorption, although close questioning may reveal that they experience cramps, flatulence and frequent, greasy, foul-smelling, bulky stools.

8.1 Complications
There are a number of nonpulmonary complications of CF in adults (Table 8). Most CF patients have height and weight levels that are less than the mean for their age and sex. Although during adulthood nutritional status declines progressively with advancing age, not all patients are malnourished at the time of diagnosis or in early adulthood. In early adulthood, some 10% of patients are above the 90th percentile, while others are even overweight.

There is no correlation between the patient's nutritional status and the severity of the steatorrhea or gastrointestinal symptoms, or age at diagnosis. The height and weight attained seem to correlate only with the severity of the pulmonary disease; those individuals with the least pancreatic insufficiency tend to have better preservation of pulmonary function.

Pancreatic insufficiency markedly overshadows the other complications of CF. In spite of the clinical impression of a voracious appetite, overall energy intake in the CF patient is usually inadequate. Maldigestion and malabsorption, along with the increased energy requirements associated with pulmonary disease, further compound the energy problem.

CF patients also show biochemical evidence of essential fatty acid deficiency. Improvement may be achieved with oral linoleic acid monoglyceride or with total parenteral nutrition. Essential fatty acid deficiency is associated with impaired intracellular oxygenation, decreased membrane fluidity and impaired transport mechanisms. It has not yet been established, however, what benefit will be derived by treating and preventing essential fatty acid deficiency.

In addition to the problems of essential fatty acid and energy deficiency, there is a third major problem in the nutrition of the CF patient: deficiency of fat-soluble vitamins. Even with a standard supplementation of vitamin A 4,000 IU/day, vitamin A levels, retinol binding protein levels and serum carotene may remain low. Approximately 25% of patients have evidence of vitamin D deficiency.

The management of pancreatic insufficiency in adults with cystic fibrosis is similar to the management of pancreatic insufficiency due to other conditions. About half of the adults with CF show some degree of glucose intolerance. Diabetes mellitus is easy to control with insulin; because glucagon levels are decreased, ketoacidosis is extremely uncommon. The presumed pathogenesis of the pancreatic islet cell dysfunction is fibrosis-induced islet cell disarray and strangulation.

Meconium ileus is seen in approximately 10% of neonates with CF and is primarily related to the secretion of abnormal mucinous (glycoprotein) material by the intestinal glands. Children, adolescents and adults have a counterpart, termed *meconium ileus equivalent,* that is characterized by recurrent episodes of intestinal obstruction. Typically, there is colicky abdominal pain, a palpable, indentable right lower quadrant mass and evidence of mechanical obstruction. Constipation is considered a milder form of this disorder, and must be differentiated from intussusception, which occurs in a small number of CF patients. There is usually a history of precipitating cause, such as immobilization, use of antidiarrheal agents, dietary indiscretions, or reduction or abrupt discontinuation of oral enzyme therapy.

The diagnosis of meconium ileus equivalent is suggested by the presentation. Plain abdominal radiographs may show an empty colon with bubbly granular material proximally, and ileal distention with air fluid levels. It is necessary to confirm the diagnosis by early Gastrografin® enema studies because of the high mortality of this condition and the need to rule out intussusception. Nasogastric suction and correction of electrolyte imbalance result in resolution of the obstruction in 80% of cases. Decompressive surgery may be necessary if medical management fails.

Pancreatitis is relatively uncommon in CF patients, but tends to occur in those patients (some 15%) whose pancreatic function is initially normal. The pathophysiology of the pancreatitis is presumably related to precipitation of abnormal secretions in the tubules, with subsequent damage. Biliary tract disease and alcohol are other possible causes of pancreatitis in these patients.

An increase in the incidence of duodenal ulcer might be expected in CF patients because of the loss of pancreatic bicarbonate buffer, but in fact duodenal ulcer is uncommon.

Patients with untreated pancreatic insufficiency commonly have profound malabsorption of bile acids in the terminal ileum and fecal losses of bile acids. This interrupts the normal enterohepatic circulation of bile acids. The etiology of bile acid wastage is unknown, but it probably relates to the presence of steatorrhea, with bile acid binding to undigested fat, fiber and other intraluminal contents. As a result of the excessive fecal bile acid loss, there is a decrease in the total bile acid pool; the bile becomes saturated with cholesterol. Up to 60% of adolescents and adults with CF have gallbladder abnormalities (e.g., cholelithiasis, nonvisualization, microgallbladder, and marginal filling defects or septations). There is a high incidence of both gallbladder abnormalities and abdominal pain in these patients, but there is not necessarily a cause–effect relationship between the cholelithiasis or gallbladder abnormalities and the clinical symptoms. The hazards of surgery must be weighed against the hazards of nonoperative intervention. The structure and function of the gallbladder may be evaluated by ultrasonography and oral cholecystography.

Treatment of pancreatic insufficiency with oral enzymes will decrease bile acid loss, thus correcting the lithogenic nature of the bile. However, the abnormal glycine:taurine ratio and the preponderance of cholic and chenodeoxycholic acid persist despite enzyme replacement. Ursodeoxycholic acid therapy remains experimental.

With increased age and survival, liver disease is becoming increasingly prevalent in CF patients. The most common hepatic lesion in CF is steatosis, secondary to decreased circulating lipoprotein levels and decreased hepatic triglyceride clearance. Other hepatic lesions include nonspecific portal changes, excessive biliary ductal mucus, mild ductal proliferation and focal biliary cirrhosis. A small number of these patients will develop multilobular biliary cirrhosis, the progression remaining clinically silent until portal hypertension supervenes with classical presentation of ascites, hypersplenism or variceal bleeding. Hepatic decompensation and portal-systemic encephalopathy are extremely uncommon because of the relative hepatic parenchymal integrity and the overall focal nature of the pathology. The only clinical clue is the development of a hard, knobby liver, while liver biochemical tests remain relatively normal. The results of therapeutic portacaval anastomoses are encouraging, with no development of portal-systemic encephalopathy.

8.2 Diagnosis

Classical CF in infants and children is easy to diagnose. However, diagnosis of CF is more difficult in adults and in mild or atypical cases. The cornerstone of diagnosis is the quantitative pilocarpine iontophoresis sweat chloride test. This should be performed on two separate occasions, using a sample of 100 mg of sweat or more. Chloride levels that are continually above 60 mEq/L are virtually diagnostic. Such levels are not found with other chronic pulmonary or gastrointestinal tract diseases. Sweat chlorides may, however, occasionally reach 60 mEq/L or more in a variety of other disorders, including untreated adrenal insufficiency, hereditary nephrogenic diabetes insipidus, hypothyroidism and a variety of genetic mucopolysaccharide disorders.

Sweat chloride testing should be performed in infants and children with chronic pulmonary disease, meconium ileus, steatorrhea, rectal prolapse, failure to thrive, heat prostration or pansinusitis, and in siblings of affected individuals. In addition, children, adolescents and young adults should be screened if they have any type of chronic liver disease, long-standing gastrointestinal complaints, childhood or cryptogenic cirrhosis, aspermia or malabsorption.

8.3 Treatment

Pancreatic enzyme replacement is the mainstay of treatment in patients with CF who suffer from pancreatic insufficiency. Enteric-coated enzymes ideally should be used, since they are not inactivated by gastric acids. Ultimately these enzymes could be used in combination with an H_2 blocker. At least 30,000 USP units of lipase should be administered and taken together with food.

Hyperuricosuria may occur in these patients secondary to the large purine content in the enzyme preparation. This complication can be controlled by decreasing the dose of the enzymes.

OBJECTIVES

Pancreatitis

1. Classify pancreatitis on the basis of the severity of injury to the organ.
2. List four etiologies of pancreatitis.
3. Discuss at least five potential early complications of acute pancreatitis.
4. Discuss four potential adverse outcomes of chronic pancreatitis.
5. Describe the clinical presentation of a patient with acute pancreatitis.

6. Outline the appropriate diagnostic approach for a patient with acute pancreatitis, emphasizing the timing, interpretation and reliability of various studies.
7. Discuss the management of acute pancreatitis, including the specific medical management of the initial phase and indications for surgical intervention.
8. Discuss the criteria used to predict the prognosis for acute pancreatitis.

Pancreatic Pseudocysts
1. Discuss the mechanism of pseudocyst formation with respect to the role of the pancreatic duct.
2. List and discuss five symptoms and physical signs of pseudocysts.
3. Given a patient with a pancreatic mass suspected to be a pseudocyst, discuss the indications for and sequence of diagnostic methods, including laboratory, radiological and invasive studies.
4. Discuss the natural history of an untreated pancreatic pseudocyst.
5. Describe the medical and surgical treatment of a pancreatic pseudocyst.

Carcinoma of the Pancreas
1. List four pancreatic neoplasms; describe the pathology of each with reference to cell type and function.
2. Describe the symptoms and physical signs of pancreatic cancer on the basis of the location of the tumor in the pancreas.
3. Outline the diagnostic approach for pancreatic masses, including laboratory, radiological and invasive methods.
4. List the laboratory tests that would be expected to be abnormal in a patient with a large cancer of the head of the pancreas.
5. Describe the surgical treatment for pancreatic neoplasms.
6. On the basis of pathology and cell type, discuss the long-term prognosis for pancreatic cancers.

Skills
1. Demonstrate the ability to perform a complete abdominal examination of a patient with an upper abdominal mass.
2. Given a patient with suspected pancreatitis, interpret a plain abdominal x-ray and identify pertinent positive and negative findings.
3. Given a patient with obstructive jaundice and a mass in the head of the pancreas, accurately interpret the transhepatic cholangiogram.

12
The Biliary System
E.A. Shaffer

1. GALLSTONE DISEASE

GALLSTONES (CHOLELITHIASIS) are the most common cause of biliary tract disease in adults, afflicting 20–30 million persons in North America. Between one-fifth of men and one-third of women will eventually develop cholelithiasis. In Canada, calculous disease of the biliary tract is also a major health hazard, accounting for about 130,000 admissions to hospital and 80,000 cholecystectomies annually. Cholecystectomy is the second most common operation in Canada and the United States, where it is performed six to seven times as often as in the United Kingdom or France. Although the frequency of gallstone disease does vary between countries and regions, it is high in both Western Europe and North America (Table 1). Such variance suggests overuse of our health-care system, particularly as few (20%) ever become symptomatic.

1.1 Classification of Gallbladder and Bile Duct Stones
Two major types of gallstones exist (Table 2).

1. *Cholesterol stones* are hard, crystalline stones that contain more than 50% cholesterol plus varying amounts of protein and calcium salts. They predominate (>85%) in the Western world.
2. *Pigment stones* consist of several insoluble calcium salts that are not normal constituents of bile.

Pigment stones can be further divided into (a) black pigment stones, which consist of a linear polymer of bilirubin, large amounts of calcium salts such as

TABLE 1. Frequency of gallstone disease in different countries

Very common (30–70%)	Common (10–30%)	Intermediate (<10%)	Rare (≈0%)
American Indians	United States (whites)	United States (blacks)	East Africa
Sweden	Canada (whites)	Japan	Canada (Inuit)
Chile	Russia	Southeast Asia	Indonesia
Czechoslovakia	United Kingdom	Northern India	West Africa
	Australia	Greece	Southern India
	Italy	Portugal	

phosphates and carbonates (making 50% of these radiopaque) and only trace amounts of cholesterol; and (b) brown pigment stones, which are predominantly calcium bilirubinate (an amorphous polymer) and calcium salts of fatty acids – hence their earthy friability.

1.2 Basis for Gallstone Formation

1.2.1 CHOLESTEROL STONES
Cholesterol gallstones form in three stages.

1.2.1.1 Chemical stage
Bile secreted by the liver becomes supersaturated with cholesterol. Such abnormal bile contains an excess of cholesterol relative to the solubilizing agents, bile salts and the phospholipid, lecithin. This stage may develop as early as puberty and is often associated with obesity. The liver produces supersaturated bile by a decreased secretion of bile salts, an increased secretion of cholesterol, or both. Obesity is associated with excess cholesterol production. With ileal disease or loss, bile salt malabsorption breaks the enterohepatic circulation, decreasing its hepatic return and thus decreasing secretion. Reduced bile flux through the liver produces lithogenic bile with excess cholesterol.

1.2.1.2 Physical stage
The excess cholesterol precipitates out of solution as solid microcrystals. A nucleating factor secreted in bile hastens this relatively rapid precipitation. Conversely, there may be a deficiency of antinucleating factors.

1.2.1.3 Gallstone growth
The cholesterol microcrystals precipitate from bile, are retained, aggregate and grow into macroscopic stones. Retention occurs in the gallbladder

TABLE 2. Classification of gallstones

		Pigment	
	Cholesterol	Black	Brown
Composition	Cholesterol	Pigment polymer Calcium salts (phosphates, carbonates)	Calcium bilirubinate Calcium soaps (palmitate, stearate)
Consistency	Crystalline	Hard	Soft, greasy
Location	Gallbladder +/– common duct	Gallbladder Bile ducts	Common duct
Radiodensity	Lucent (85%)	Opaque (50%)	Lucent (100%)
Clinical associations	Metabolic	Hemolysis Cirrhosis	Infection Inflammation Infestation

because its epithelium secretes excess mucus (consisting of mucin, a glyco-protein). This mucus gel forms a colloidal shell that entraps cholesterol microcrystals, preventing it from being ejected from the gallbladder. Mucin also creates a scaffold for the addition of more crystals. A defect in the contractile function of the gallbladder smooth muscle fails to properly evacuate the solid material.

"Biliary sludge" consists of calcium bilirubinate, cholesterol microcrystals and mucin. On ultrasound, biliary sludge is echogenic material that layers but does not cast an acoustic shadow (unlike gallstones). Sludge develops in association with conditions causing gallbladder stasis, such as pregnancy or total parental nutrition. Though frequently asymptomatic and prone to disappear, sludge in the gallbladder can produce biliary-type pain and progress to overt gallstones.

1.2.2 PIGMENT STONES
In North America, black pigment stones constitute about 15% of gallstones found at surgery (cholecystectomy). They are frequently associated with hemolysis or alcoholic cirrhosis (Table 3). The basis for their formation is excessive bilirubin excretion in bile. Brown pigment stones are associated with stagnation and infection (often from a stricture) or infestation (e.g., liver flukes) of the biliary tract. Such conditions predispose to chronic cholangitis and eventually cholangiocarcinoma. Infection and inflammation increase β-

TABLE 3. Risk factors for gallstone formation

Factor	Pigment stone	Cholesterol stone
Demography		
Race	Asian	American Indian
Female sex	?	++
Age	+	++
Familial	Hemoglobinopathies	++
Diet	+	Obesity (high calorie)
		Weight reduction
		High animal fats
		Low fiber
Gallbladder stasis	+	++
	Total parenteral nutrition	Reduced meal frequency
		Vagotomy
		Pregnancy
Female sex hormones		
Parity/fertility	—	Early menarche
Oral contraceptives	—	+
Estrogens	—	+
Associated disease	Cirrhosis	Cystic fibrosis
	Hemolytic anemia	Ileal disease or loss
	Biliary infections	Diabetes mellitus
Drugs	Clofibrate	

++ = definite; + = probable; ? = questionable; — = unknown

glucuronidase, an enzyme that deconjugates bilirubin; the resultant free bilirubin then polymerizes and complexes with calcium, forming calcium bilirubinate in the bile duct system.

1.3 Natural History of Gallstone Disease

Gallstones grow at about 1–2 mm per year over a 5- to 20-year period before symptoms develop. They frequently are clinically "silent," being incidentally detected on routine ultrasound performed for another purpose. Most patients (80%) with gallstones never develop symptoms. Problems, if they do occur, usually arise in the form of biliary pain during the first 5 to 10 years. Complications are from stones obstructing

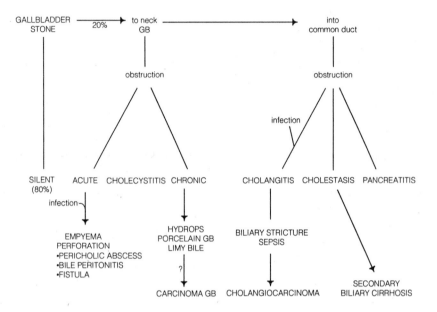

FIGURE 1.   Potential complications of cholelithiasis. Migration of the stone in the gallbladder to impact in the neck of the gallbladder or the bile duct can cause obstruction and result in complications. Cystic duct obstruction results in cholecystitis. Chronic calculous cholecystitis may be associated with carcinoma of the gallbladder, but causality is unproven. Common duct obstruction leads to cholangitis, cholestatic jaundice and/or pancreatitis. Chronic cholestasis not only results in malabsorption but also predisposes to secondary biliary cirrhosis. Chronic duct obstruction and injury may lead to cholangiocarcinoma.

1. the cystic duct, leading to cholecystitis: this begins as a chemical inflammation and later may become complicated by bacterial invasion; or
2. the common duct, causing biliary obstruction (cholestasis), sometimes accompanied by bacterial infection in the ductal system (cholangitis) (Figure 1).

1.4 Clinical Features
Biliary colic pain ensues when an obstructing stone causes sudden distention of the gallbladder and/or the biliary tract. "Colic" is a poor term, as biliary pain typically does not increase and decrease spasmodically. Rather, abdominal pain onsets suddenly, quickly becomes severe, remains steady for 1 to 3 hours and then gradually disappears over 30 to 90 minutes, leaving a vague ache. Its duration may be less than an hour, but is not as brief as 30 minutes.

TABLE 4. Comparison of biliary colic to acute cholecystitis

	Biliary colic	Acute cholecystitis
Pain	Constant	Constant
Duration	Hours	Hours to days
Vomiting	Yes	Yes
Onset	Rapid	Variable
Jaundice	No	Later (20%)
Tenderness	RUQ	RUQ
Fever	No	Yes
Leukocytosis	Minimal	Marked
Resolution	Spontaneous	Spontaneous (≈66%)

Although biliary pain can follow a fatty or spicy meal, such "fatty food intolerance" is not specific for biliary tract disease. Its location usually is the epigastrium or right upper quadrant. Mediated by splanchnic nerves, biliary pain may radiate like angina to the back, right scapula or shoulder tip, down the arm or into the neck. The pain may also be confined to the back. Analgesics are usually required for relief. Episodes of pain occur irregularly, being separated by pain-free periods lasting from days to years. Severity of pain also varies. Being a visceral pain, biliary colic is not aggravated by movement but is deep-seated. The patient is usually restless and may exhibit vasomotor features such as sweating and pallor. Nausea and vomiting often accompany a severe attack. Fever and rigors are absent unless infection supervenes.

Findings consist of right upper quadrant or epigastric tenderness, perhaps with some guarding. During an attack or often soon after one, the pain disappears. There are no peritoneal signs. Often the examination is completely normal.

Laboratory tests are usually normal. In 10–20% of cases, there may be a slight elevation of serum bilirubin, alkaline phosphatase, aminotransferases (AST and ALT) or γ-glutamyl transpeptidase (GGT).

Between attacks the patient feels well. Liver biochemistry is normal. Over long periods the activity of the disease remains fairly constant. If having frequent episodes of biliary pain, the patient will probably continue to experience this pattern.

Pain lasting more than 6 to 12 hours, especially if accompanied by persistent vomiting or fever, suggests another process such as cholecystitis or pancreatitis (Table 4). Conversely, abdominal pain and bloating relieved by defecation suggests the irritable bowel syndrome.

1.5 Diagnosis

Diagnosis of the gallstones (but not symptomatic disease) is radiological. Plain abdominal x-ray will identify the 10–15% with a high calcium content as radiopaque densities in the right upper quadrant. Ultrasonography is the most sensitive and specific method for detecting gallstones (appearing as echogenic objects that cast an acoustic shadow) or a thickened gallbladder wall (indicating inflammation). If the gallbladder is not identified (perhaps being obscured by bowel gas or scarred and contracted by cholecystitis), then an oral cholecystogram should be performed in suspected cases. This technique also determines gallbladder function (the ability to fill and concentrate the radiographic agent). Persistent failure to opacify after two days of oral contrast agent is 95% diagnostic for gallbladder disease.

1.6 Management

1.6.1 MEDICAL THERAPY

1.6.1.1 Expectant

Management should be expectant in asymptomatic adults with gallstones, as most will never develop problems. In minimally symptomatic patients without major complications or those unfit for or unwilling to undergo surgery, medical therapy has offered a wide array of new techniques for dissolving, fragmenting or extracting stones.

1.6.1.2 Dissolution

1.6.1.2.1 *Bile acids* Administered orally, bile acids can dissolve cholesterol gallstones. Two bile acids, chenodeoxycholic acid and ursodeoxycholic acid, work to reduce cholesterol saturation of bile. The stones must be radiolucent and hence presumably composed of cholesterol, and the gallbladder must function for the unsaturated bile to bathe the stones. The reported success rate varies from 13–80% over one to two years. Gallstone size largely determines the success rate. Stones must be less than 1.5 cm in diameter. Small stones with a relatively great surface area have the best result. Ideal cases have tiny (<0.5 cm) gallstones that float on oral cholecystography (floating indicates a low calcium content); here, dissolution has a success rate greater than 80%. Large stones in obese individuals have less favorable results. Chenodeoxycholic acid (15 mg/kg/day), though cheaper, has significant side effects in terms of dose-related diarrhea and liver damage. Ursodeoxycholic acid (8–10 mg/kg/day) is therefore the drug of choice. Combination therapy with both agents at lower doses appears to be equally effective and safe. About 15–20% of patients are candidates for ursodeoxycholic acid therapy. Even after successful dissolution, 50% will experience gallstone recurrence, although most are asymptomatic. Prevention of gallstone formation is possible in those at high risk, such as obese people after gastric bypass surgery or while on a very restrictive caloric diet.

1.6.1.2.2 *Direct-contact dissolution*   This form of dissolution is feasible in those who are quite symptomatic but poor candidates for surgery. Under ultrasound guidance, a catheter is placed through the skin and liver into the gallbladder. A potent solvent, methyl tert-butyl ether, is cyclically instilled and withdrawn using an automated pump. In experienced hands, the success rate has been good for the several hundred patients treated to date, but the technique remains experimental and is done in only a few centers.

1.6.1.2.3 *Shock-wave lithotripsy*   The surface area of gallstones is so critical to successful dissolution that stone fragmentation has been undertaken with shock-wave lithotripsy that is then followed by bile acid therapy to dissolve the residual fragments. Ultrasonic fragmentation has a low complication rate: 1% develop pancreatitis, 40% develop biliary pain. The cystic duct must be patent. This is determined either by a radiologically functioning gallbladder filling with contrast agent or by ultrasonography showing a decrease in gallbladder volume in response to a fatty meal. Within a year, 60–80% will go on to successful clearance of debris from the gallbladder using oral bile acids to dissolve the remnants. Best results (up to 95% success) occur with a single gallstone 2 cm in diameter. Again, only about 20% of patients overall are eligible. Gallstones can recur, although the rate is low at 15%.

1.6.2 CHOLECYSTECTOMY

1.6.2.1 *Open cholecystectomy*
The term "open" connotes the need for an incision to open the abdominal cavity for direct visualization and operation. In contrast, the laparoscopic technique uses endoscopy and tiny incisions. Cholecystectomy is the "gold standard" for treating gallstone disease. The operation is relatively safe, with mortality less than 0.5% when electively performed for biliary colic. Mortality reaches 3% for emergency surgery in acute cholecystitis or for common duct procedures, and is higher in the elderly.

1.6.2.2 *Laparoscopic cholecystectomy*

This technique views the abdominal contents through a laparoscope (with the peritoneal cavity insufflated with gas) and uses instruments inserted through three trocars in the abdominal wall to perform surgical manipulation. In 5% of cases the procedure must be converted to an open cholecystectomy because of technical problems. There is overwhelming enthusiasm for this procedure because it is as safe as the open technique, it leaves the patient with less postoperative pain and tiny scars, and it allows for an early discharge from hospital (about two days) and return to work. It has a higher complication rate, particularly from common duct injury and retained common duct stones. Laparoscopic cholecystectomy is now the standard for elective surgery and for some cases of acute cholecystitis.

Surgery is indicated in those with significant symptoms (e.g., repeated visits to the emergency room for narcotic relief) or with complications. Prophylactic cholecystectomy is not warranted except for rare cases suspected of developing/harboring carcinoma of the gallbladder (e.g., very large stones >3 cm or a calcified gallbladder wall). It generally should not be done on asymptomatic people with gallstones.

2. CHOLECYSTITIS

2.1 Chronic Calculous Cholecystitis

Chronic inflammation of the gallbladder is the most common pathologic process in this organ. Some degree of chronic inflammation inevitably accompanies gallstones, but stones develop first. Even transient obstruction of the cystic duct will produce biliary colic. Yet there is little correlation between the severity and frequency of such biliary episodes and the pathology found in the gallbladder. There may be only modest round cell infiltration with marked symptoms. Conversely, symptoms may be minimal while gallbladder scarring is marked. Prolonged obstruction can lead to acute cholecystitis (Figure 1). Chronic inflammation may follow acute cholecystitis or evolve insidiously. The inflammatory process is chemical in origin.

2.1.1 *CLINICAL FEATURES*

The clinical features are those of either biliary colic or a previous episode of acute cholecystitis that has resolved, leaving the gallbladder chronically inflamed. The pain characteristically is a constant dull ache in the right hypochondrium and epigastrium, and sometimes also in the right shoulder or back. Nausea is frequent. There may be local tenderness in the right upper quadrant of the abdomen. Flatulence, fatty food intolerance and dyspepsia occur, but are equally frequent in patients without gallstone disease. Fever or leukocytosis suggests acute cholecystitis or another entity.

2.1.2 DIAGNOSIS

Diagnosis largely depends upon detecting gallstones by plain film of the abdomen (10–15% are calcified), ultrasound or oral cholecystogram. The latter two are more than 95% accurate. If the gallbladder is fibrotic and shrunken, visualization may be difficult. This is considered a positive finding, given the accuracy of these tests. Merely identifying calculi in the gallbladder confirms biliary tract disease but *does not* necessarily mean that gallstones were responsible for the symptoms. Nuclear medicine scanning helps. Cholescintigraphy normally demonstrates filling of a healthy gallbladder. Nonvisualization in suspected cases of acute cholecystitis is diagnostic. The test is much less sensitive for chronic cholecystitis, in which the gallbladder commonly fills. If no filling occurs, then biliary tract disease is likely.

2.1.3 MANAGEMENT

Once symptoms begin, they are likely to recur. Medical management depends upon gallstone size, gallbladder function and any co-morbid conditions (e.g., age, obesity, diabetes). Cholecystectomy provides definitive treatment, removing the stones and the gallbladder.

2.2 Acute Cholecystitis

Here the gallbladder becomes acutely inflamed. In most, a stone obstructs the cystic duct, resulting in a vicious cycle of increased secretion of fluid, causing distention, mucosal damage and the release of chemical mediators of the inflammatory process. Inflammatory damage results from agents such as lysolecithin, derived from the hydrolysis of lecithin by phospholipase, and prostaglandins whose synthesis increases. Any role that bile salts and regurgitated pancreatic enzymes may have is unclear. Bacterial infection is a late complication.

Obstruction of the cystic duct results in the gallbladder becoming distended with bile, an inflammatory exudate or even pus. The gallbladder wall can go on to necrosis and perforation. If resolution occurs, the mucosal surface heals and the wall becomes scarred, but the gallbladder may not function (i.e., fill with contrast agent) on oral cholecystography. If the inflammation subsides but the cystic duct remains obstructed, the lumen becomes distended with a clear mucoid fluid (hydrops of the gallbladder). The hydropic gallbladder is evident as a right upper quadrant mass that is not tender. Cholecystectomy is indicated.

2.2.1 CLINICAL FEATURES

Acute cholecystitis onsets like biliary colic (Table 4). The abdominal pain rises to a plateau and remains constant. Its location is usually the right upper quadrant or epigastrium, sometimes radiating to the back or the right shoulder. There may be a previous history of biliary pain. Pain in acute cholecystitis, unlike biliary colic, persists for more than 6 to 12 hours. As the gallbladder becomes inflamed, the visceral pain is replaced by parietal pain that is aggravated by movement. Anorexia and vomiting are common. Fever is usually low-grade. If rigors occur, suspect bacterial invasion.

Abdominal examination characteristically shows tenderness in the right upper quadrant. During palpation of the right upper quadrant, a deep breath during the inspiratory effort worsens the pain, which suddenly ceases (Murphy's sign). Severe cases exhibit peritoneal signs: guarding and local rebound tenderness. A reflex paralytic ileus may be present. Patients appear unwell and are reluctant to move with such parietal pain. An enlarged gallbladder is palpable in one-third of cases, particularly with the first attack.

2.2.2 DIAGNOSIS

Jaundice with mild hyperbilirubinemia and elevated liver enzymes (including aminotransferase) occurs in about 20% of cases, even in the absence of common duct stones. The higher the bilirubin level, the more likely is a common duct stone. Transaminases also may be elevated in acute cholecystitis. Serum amylase can be mildly raised (up to 10-fold) without pancreatitis. If higher, suspect a common duct stone. Leukocytosis is common. If the patient is febrile, blood cultures may be positive. Cholangitis suggests a common duct stone.

Diagnosis is best confirmed by ultrasound, which detects the stone(s) and a thickened gallbladder wall. In doing the procedure, the physician can elicit tenderness ultrasonographically when pressing over the gallbladder (the ultrasonographic Murphy's sign). A plain film may reveal calcification of the stone(s). Cholescintigraphy typically fails to visualize the gallbladder at one hour, a feature highly accurate for acute cholecystitis. Conversely, a normal scan filling the gallbladder virtually eliminates acute cholecystitis, but cannot detect gallstones. Late visualization (after one hour) sometimes occurs in chronic cholecystitis.

2.2.3 MANAGEMENT

Treatment is surgical and is performed in hospital. General measures include rehydration, observation, analgesia and antibiotics. In mild or resolving acute cholecystitis, cholecystectomy can be delayed for two to three months after remission, but increasingly surgery is performed early, once the patient has been stabilized during the current admission.

2.2.4 COMPLICATIONS

Acute cholecystitis normally resolves spontaneously, usually within three days. Inflammation may progress to necrosis, empyema or perforation in about one-third of cases. These complications will be heralded by (1) a continuation of the pain, along with tachycardia, fever, peritoneal signs and leukocytosis; (2) features of a secondary infection, such as empyema or cholangitis; or (3) a suspected perforation. Then, urgent surgery becomes mandatory.

Empyema is suppurative cholecystitis with an intraluminal abscess (i.e., an inflamed gallbladder containing pus). It develops from continued obstruction of the cystic duct leading to secondary infection. The abdominal findings of acute cholecystitis are accompanied by systemic features of bacteremia, with a hectic fever and rigors. Treatment consists of antibiotics and surgery.

Perforation of the gallbladder occurs when unresolved inflammation leads to necrosis, often in the fundus, which is relatively avascular. Gallstones also may erode through a gangrenous wall. If localized, the perforation spawns an abscess, clinically evident as a palpable, tender mass in the right upper quadrant. Free perforation with bile peritonitis is uncommon, fortunately, as the mortality reaches 30%. With perforation the gallbladder, if enlarged, suddenly disappears. The pain and temperature may also transiently resolve, only to be replaced by acute peritonitis. Both localized and free perforations demand surgical drainage of the abscess. Rupture into adjacent viscera (e.g., the small intestine) creates an internal biliary fistula. Large stones can produce a mechanical small intestine obstruction *(gallstone ileus)*. Obstruction usually occurs at the terminal ileum, rarely at the duodenal bulb or the duodenojejunal junction. This is a rather common cause of distal small bowel obstruction in the elderly. Radiologic diagnosis comes from finding air in the biliary system, a small bowel obstruction and perhaps a calcified gallstone ectopically located. Urgent surgery with appropriate antibiotic coverage is imperative.

Limy bile occurs when prolonged gallbladder obstruction causes loss of the pigment material from bile and the residual calcium salts precipitate. The hydropic, obstructed gallbladder secretes calcium into the lumen. Calcium can also accumulate in the wall of the gallbladder, producing a *porcelain gallbladder.* The mural calcifications are easily identified on plain films of the abdomen. Although presumably there has been at least one episode of acute cholecystitis in the past, most patients with a porcelain gallbladder are asymptomatic. Half will develop carcinoma of the gallbladder, making prophylactic cholecystectomy necessary.

2.3 Choledocholithiasis (Common Duct Stones)

Stones in the common duct are classified according to their site of origin: *primary stones* are formed in the bile ducts; *secondary stones* originate in the gallbladder and then migrate into the common duct. In North America, virtually all cholesterol stones and most pigment stones are considered secondary when the gallbladder is intact. Thus, more than 85% of patients with common duct stones also have stones in the gallbladder. Conversely, about 10% of patients undergoing cholecystectomy for chronic cholecystitis also have common duct stones. *Residual stones* are those missed at the time of cholecystectomy; *recurrent stones* develop in the ductal system more than three years after surgery. The composition of stones also varies with their site of origin. Stones are predominantly (approximately 80%) cholesterol when situated in the gallbladder and in the common duct. After cholecystectomy, the proportion of ductal stones that are pigment rises with time: most recurrent ones (more than three years after surgery) are pigment stones. These brown stones result from stasis (e.g., a postoperative stricture) and infection. Bacteria and inflamed tissues release ß-glucuronidase, an enzyme that deconjugates bilirubin. The result is calcium bilirubinate, which polymerizes and precipitates along with calcium soaps. Biofilm, a glycoprotein produced by bacteria as its glycocalyx, then agglomerates this pigment material, leading to brown stones.

2.3.1 CLINICAL FEATURES

Common duct stones may be asymptomatic, but usually cause biliary colic, obstructive jaundice, cholangitis or pancreatitis (Figure 1). Biliary colic results from sudden obstruction of the common duct, which increases biliary pressure. The abdominal pain is steady, located in the right upper quadrant or epigastrium, and often bores through to the back. Cholangitis results when duct obstruction leads to infection. Obstruction and ductal damage permit bacteria to regurgitate across the ductal epithelium into the hepatic venous blood, causing a bacteremia with chills and a spiking fever. The raised intrabiliary pressure also initiates abdominal pain. The third component of "Charcot's triad," jaundice, results from the mechanical obstruction of the ducts plus a component of intrahepatic cholestasis due to sepsis (endotoxin, for example, impairs hepatic bile formation). Pain and fever are common, though jaundice is often less apparent on presentation. Most patients are toxic. There is abdominal tenderness and a large, tender liver. Hypotension, confusion and a septic picture predominate in critical cases.

2.3.2 DIAGNOSIS

Leukocytosis and abnormal liver biochemistry are common. Urine may be positive for bilirubin. Blood cultures reveal the causal microorganisms, which are usually enteric (e.g., E. coli or Klebsiella) in origin. Ultrasound will show dilatated ducts and, in advanced cases, liver abscesses. Cholangiography (by endoscopy from below or via percutaneous transhepatic catheterization from above) is necessary to locate the site and cause of obstruction.

2.3.3 MANAGEMENT

The presence of cholangitis necessitates urgent decompression of the biliary system. In the past, laparotomy was the only recourse. Now, endoscopic surgery (using the ERCP procedure – endoscopic retrograde cholangiopancreatography) is routinely performed under antibiotic coverage (usually requiring coverage for enteric gram-negative organisms, enterococci and anaerobes). ERCP also allows sphincterotomy followed by extraction of the stone and, if needed, placement of a stent through a stricture. Large common duct stones may need fragmentation, either by mechanical means using a basket for crushing, or by energy delivered as shock or laser waves. This allows cholecystectomy to be done electively. Another option is open cholecystectomy with common duct exploration, removing the gallbladder and all stones.

Pancreatitis can result from gallstones impacting at the ampulla of Vater. Acute biliary pancreatitis does not differ clinically from other forms of acute pancreatitis. Biliary pancreatitis tends to be more commonly associated with jaundice and higher serum levels of bilirubin, alkaline phosphatase and transaminase than alcohol-induced pancreatitis, but there is significant overlap. Ultrasound should detect any gallstones and the inflamed pancreas. In patients unfit for surgery, early ERCP with papillotomy may be done, but its role as the definitive procedure is unproven. Most will come to elective cholecystectomy to prevent recurrent pancreatitis. Unlike alcoholic pancreatitis, gallstone-related disease does not progress to chronic pancreatitis.

3. NONCALCULOUS GALLBLADDER DISEASE

3.1 Congenital Anomalies

Congenital abnormalities of the gallbladder and biliary system result from embryonic maldevelopment and are most interesting for the surgeon attempting to identify biliary anatomy at cholecystectomy. Agenesis of the gallbladder is rare. Curiously, it is associated with common duct stones.

3.2 Acalculous Cholecystitis

3.2.1 ACUTE ACALCULOUS CHOLECYSTITIS

Inflammation of the gallbladder can occur in the absence of gallstones. Though uncommon in adults, acute acalculous cholecystitis may appear associated with AIDS, pregnancy, trauma, burns, sepsis or following major surgery. In young children, acute cholecystitis frequently occurs without gallstones and follows a febrile illness, although no definite infectious agent is identified. Biliary stagnation sometimes accompanied by sludge appears to be a factor. Impaired blood flow to the gallbladder, coagulation factors and prostaglandin may also have roles. Cytomegalovirus or Cryptosporidia can cause gangrenous cholecystitis in AIDS.

Clinical presentation is identical to that of acute cholecystitis, with pain, fever and abdominal tenderness in the right upper quadrant. These features are often obscured by the patient's underlying critical condition. Diagnosis is then revealed at laparotomy, but sometimes can be determined preoperatively by nonvisualization of the gallbladder on cholescintigraphy (although nonvisualization is less sensitive here because of the prolonged fast many are on) or by ultrasonographic evidence of a thickened gallbladder wall. Perforation, gangrene and empyema are all too frequent complications. The best treatment is prompt cholecystectomy.

3.2.2 CHRONIC ACALCULOUS CHOLECYSTITIS
Recurrent biliary colic in the absence of gallstones has been associated with rather modest inflammation. The basis is presumed to be a motility disorder, impaired gallbladder evacuation; hence the alternative term "biliary dyskinesia." Relief can follow cholecystectomy. Difficulties arise in attempting to make this diagnosis: the symptoms are often not clear-cut (sometimes having features of irritable bowel syndrome or nonulcer dyspepsia), and there are no gallstones to detect. Abnormal gallbladder evacuation in response to CCK (cholecystokinin) may be evident on cholecystography or cholescintigraphy. Sensitivity and specificity of these tests remain unclear. CCK infusion alone can reproduce the biliary pain, but the value of this provocative test is unclear. The entity remains poorly defined.

3.3 Cholecystoses
Cholesterolosis consists of deposits of cholesterol esters and triglycerides within the gallbladder wall. These submucosal deposits produce a fine yellow reticular pattern on a red background of mildly inflamed mucosa, providing an appearance like a strawberry: hence the term "strawberry gallbladder." Some of the cholesterol deposits protrude like polyps; these can be detected on ultrasound. There is no well-defined symptom complex linked to this entity: although frequently an incidental finding at post mortem, it is sometimes associated with vague dyspeptic complaints, the irritable bowel syndrome or recurrent right upper quadrant abdominal pain. The importance of cholecysto-

kinin (CCK) provocative tests to reproduce the pain or demonstrate reduced gallbladder emptying on cholescintigraphy in response to CCK is unclear.

Adenomyosis is characterized by hyperplasia of the gallbladder mucosa and by deep clefts. The meaning of any biliary-type symptoms is moot.

3.4 Postcholecystectomy Syndrome

Cholecystectomy relieves the symptoms of most, but definitely not all, patients with biliary calculi. The occasional patient will experience diarrhea following cholecystectomy, perhaps the result of unmasking a malabsorption of bile acids, which leads to a cholerrheic (bile acid–induced) diarrhea. Symptoms persist or recur in 5–50%, depending upon selection bias. Most often the original complaint was not true biliary pain, but rather reflux esophagitis, peptic ulcer disease or the irritable bowel syndrome. There may be recurrent biliary tract problems such as biliary stricture, a retained common duct stone or even pancreatic disease. In suspected cases, ERCP is indicated. Occasionally, narrowing (papillary stenosis) or altered motility (sphincter of Oddi dysfunction) will produce recurrent biliary-type pain, often with abnormal liver biochemistry tests or increased serum amylase. Nuclear medicine scanning (cholescintigraphy) and sphincter of Oddi pressure measurements (manometry) provide diagnostic clues. Endoscopic sphincterotomy relieves pain in selected patients.

3.5 Neoplasms of the Gallbladder

Carcinoma of the gallbladder is fortunately uncommon, as its prognosis is extremely poor. Adenocarcinoma is generally cured only when incidentally discovered after cholecystectomy for cholelithiasis. Gallstones are present in most (75%) cases, probably as innocent bystanders rather than as causal agents (Figure 1). Any risk is too low to advocate prophylactic cholecystectomy in the many people with asymptomatic gallstones. Porcelain gallbladder with calcifications in the wall predisposes to adenocarcinoma and calls for cholecystectomy. Large gallstones (>3 cm) are also a risk factor for carcinoma.

The clinical features of gallbladder carcinoma consist of pain, a hard mass in the right epigastrium, jaundice, pruritus and weight loss. Ultrasound and CT scan help define the mass and metastases. Prognosis is grim, as it is common for the cancer to spread. The five-year survival is less than 5%. Therapy is palliative; most are not resectable unless removed incidentally at the time of cholecystectomy.

Benign tumors of the gallbladder are uncommon. Adenomas are asymptomatic, being detected on ultrasound or found incidentally at surgery. Small masses in the wall of the gallbladder, however, are relatively common findings on ultrasound; most particularly when multiple they represent cholesterol polyps or adherent gallstones. Polypoidal masses warrant a repeat ultrasound in six months. If these are larger than 1 cm, surgery is necessary to exclude a carcinoma.

4. DISEASES OF THE BILE DUCTS

4.1 Congenital

Caroli's disease (congenital intrahepatic biliary dilatation) is a rare condition in which saccular, dilatated segments of the intrahepatic bile ducts lead to stone formation, recurrent cholangitis and hepatic abscesses with sepsis. Episodes of abdominal pain, fever and jaundice may onset at any age, most commonly in childhood or young adult life.

Cholangiography reveals the irregularly dilatated segments of the intrahepatic bile ducts that connect with the main ducts. The common duct is normal. Endoscopy (or surgery) can remove some stones but does little for the process that affects small bile ducts in the liver. If involvement is unilateral, partial hepatectomy can be curative. Otherwise, management is conservative, using antibiotics for infectious complications of the duct system, or cholangitis. The recurrent episodes of cholangitis sometimes progress to secondary biliary cirrhosis, portal hypertension and eventually cholangiocarcinoma.

Congenital hepatic fibrosis frequently accompanies Caroli's disease (perhaps reflecting a developmental defect of the small interlobular ducts). It clinically presents as portal hypertension with esophageal varices in children. Liver biopsy is diagnostic, revealing broad bands of fibrous tissue entrapping bile ducts but no cirrhosis.

Choledochal cyst is a congenital dilatation of a portion of the common bile duct, which may form a diverticulum in the intraduodenal segment. This congenital cystic anomaly can be associated with Caroli's disease: both represent a spectrum of defective budding and cannulation from the primitive foregut. Presentation may be as cholestasis in infants, or intermittent jaundice, pain and fever (cholangitis) later in young adults. Complications include chronic obstruction leading to biliary cirrhosis and the development of ductal carcinoma. Diagnosis is provided by ultrasound or CT scan and verified by endoscopic cholangiography. Surgery involves excising the cyst and re-establishing biliary drainage with a biliary-enteric anastomosis.

Biliary atresia is a common cause of neonatal cholestatic jaundice. Although congenital (appearing at birth), it is not inherited. Complete absence of bile ducts reflects either an arrest in remodeling of the ductal plate in utero or, more probably, inflammatory destruction of the formed bile ducts during the postpartum period. The latter process is evident by an inflammatory infiltrate in the portal tracts and, in some, features of neonatal hepatitis. Large duct obstruction then leads to small duct injury within the liver and hence biliary cirrhosis. Severe cholestasis develops in the neonatal period. The stools are pale and the urine is dark and devoid of urobilinogen. Cholestatic features predominate, with the development of steatorrhea, skin xanthoma, bone disease and failure to thrive. Surgery is usually necessary to confirm the diagnosis and attempt some form of biliary drainage. In some, existence of a patent hepatic duct or dilatated hilar ducts potentially allows correction of the obstruction by anastomosis to the small intestine (e.g., a Roux-en-Y choledochojejunostomy). Much more common is an absence of patent ducts; dense fibrous tissue encases the perihilar area and precludes conventional surgery. Such obliteration of the proximal extrahepatic biliary system requires the Kasai procedure. A conduit for biliary drainage is fashioned by resecting the fibrous remnant of the biliary tree and anastomosing the porta hepatis to a Roux-en-Y loop of jejunum. With either surgery, most children eventually develop chronic cholangitis, hepatic fibrosis/cirrhosis and portal hypertension. When the child is larger, hepatic transplantation dramatically improves the prognosis.

4.2 Inflammatory

4.2.1 *CHOLANGITIS*
Cholangitis is any inflammatory process involving the bile ducts, but common usage implies a bacterial infection, usually above an obstructive site. The presence of bacteria in the biliary tree plus increased pressure within the system results in severe clinical features of cholangitis *(suppurative cholangitis).* Any condition producing bile duct obstruction is liable to cause bacterial infection of bile. Most commonly, this takes the form of a common duct stone (Section 2.3), a benign biliary stricture (trauma from biliary surgery, ischemia following liver transplantation or sclerosing cholangitis), stasis in a congenital biliary cyst (Section 4.1), a parasite residing in the ducts, an occluded biliary stent or extrinsic compression from a diseased papilla or pancreas. A less likely cause of infection is neoplastic obstruction. The difference relates to the high-grade, fixed obstruction of neoplasms versus the intermittent blockage with a stone or an inflammatory stricture. Such intermittent blockage allows retrograde ascent of bacteria; the stone may act as a nidus for infection. The bacteria are commonly thought to ascend the biliary tree (hence the term "ascending cholangitis"), but may enter from above via the portal vein or from periductular lymphatics.

In acute bacterial cholangitis, particularly if severe, the classical Charcot's triad of intermittent fever and chills, jaundice and abdominal pain may be followed by septic shock. Most cases are less severe and life-threatening; jaundice may be absent. Mild cases may respond to antibiotics and conservative measures. Investigation and decompression of the biliary system are mandatory in all patients, whether by ERCP, percutaneous transhepatic cholangiography or surgery.

4.2.2 SCLEROSING CHOLANGITIS

Primary sclerosing cholangitis is a chronic cholestatic syndrome of unknown etiology characterized by progressive inflammation of the intra- and extrahepatic bile ducts. The entity may appear either alone or in association with inflammatory bowel disease, particularly ulcerative colitis. Primary sclerosing cholangitis may precede inflammatory bowel disease and it runs a separate course, not being cured by colectomy. The patchy scarring (sclerosis) leads to fibrotic narrowing and eventually obliteration of the bile ducts. Like other organs, the biliary tract exhibits a limited number of responses to injury: here it responds with diffuse strictures and segmental dilatations. Periductal inflammation and fibrosis in the portal areas, termed "pericholangitis," probably represents the intrahepatic extension of this process. The basis may be an infectious agent, an enterohepatic toxin or an immunological attack on the biliary epithelium.

Diffuse stricturing also occurs in *secondary sclerosing cholangitis*, which may complicate a biliary obstruction from a common duct stone, biliary stricture or cholangiocarcinoma, or some AIDS-related infections.

The presentation in primary sclerosing cholangitis is insidious in most cases, with fatigue, pruritus or just an elevated alkaline phosphatase level. In others, acute cholangitis develops with obstructive jaundice, pruritus, abdominal pain and fever. Biliary stagnation leads to pigment stones. Eventually, secondary biliary cirrhosis supervenes with portal hypertension, pronounced cholestasis and progressive liver failure. Antimitochondrial antibody is negative. ERCP provides the diagnosis, showing thickened bile ducts with narrowed, beaded lumens.

Therapeutic trials of corticosteroids and immunosuppressive agents (for the presumed immunologically mediated inflammatory process), penicillamine (to mobilize copper, because this toxic material accumulates in cholestasis) and proctocolectomy in patients with inflammatory bowel disease have all failed. As some patients may be asymptomatic for a decade, only careful observation is warranted early on. Recurrent bacterial cholangitis requires antibiotics. Predominantly large-duct strictures respond to endoscopic or transhepatic dilation and stent placement. Evaluation of ursodeoxycholic acid (which helps the pruritus but may not change the disease process), cyclosporine, methotrexate and colchicine awaits good clinical trials. Some 10–15% of patients develop cholangiocarcinoma, creating a diagnostic challenge. Primary sclerosing cholangitis is a frequent indication for liver transplantation with a good outcome.

4.3 Neoplasia (Including Cholangiocarcinoma)

Benign tumors (adenomas, papillomas, cystadenomas) are rare causes of mechanical biliary obstruction.

Adenocarcinoma, the most common malignancy, is uncommon in the Western world. Predisposing factors are chronic parasitic infestations of the biliary tract (e.g., a liver fluke, such as Clonorchis sinensis or Opisthorchis viverrini), congenital ectatic lesions (Caroli's disease, choledochal cyst) and primary sclerosing cholangitis.

Jaundice and pruritus are common, but the presentation is varied. Cholestasis and weight loss eventually develop. There may be a deep-seated, vague pain localized in the right upper quadrant of the abdomen, in contrast to the severe pain of biliary colic and the septic picture of cholangitis. Indeed, cholangitis is not a feature if no biliary manipulations have been performed, such as an ERCP-placed stent. Hepatomegaly is frequent. A distended, nontender gallbladder may occasionally be palpated, feeling like a small rubber ball, if the common duct is obstructed below the entry of the cystic duct ("Courvoisier's sign"). Obstruction produces dilatation of the biliary tree that can be readily detected on ultrasound or CT scan. Cholangiography, usually by ERCP, should reveal the diagnosis. This slow-growing tumor presents late. The terminal event is usually hepatocellular failure. Palliation using biliary stents placed across strictures sometimes helps. Occasionally, a distal common duct lesion is amenable to curative surgery. Transplantation does not provide a good outcome.

OBJECTIVES

1. Describe the physicochemical characteristics of normal bile, its production and the physiologic mechanism of bile salt reabsorption.
2. Discuss the mechanisms for the stimulation of bile secretion and the hormonal mediators of this response.
3. Recognize the normal anatomy of the biliary tree.

Acute and Chronic Gallbladder Disease, Carcinomas of the Biliary Tract
  1. Identify the common types of gallstones and describe the pathophysiology involved in their formation.
  2. List several diseases known to predispose to gallstones.
  3. List the tests commonly used in the diagnosis of calculous biliary tract disease. Describe the indications for, limitations of and potential complications of each.
  4. Describe the probable natural history of a young patient with asymptomatic gallstones.
  5. List the complications that can occur from biliary calculi and describe the history, physical examination and laboratory findings for each.
  6. Outline the management of a patient with acute cholecystitis.
  7. Describe the symptoms and signs of choledocholithiasis; describe the management of this problem.
  8. Outline a diagnostic and management plan for a patient with acute right upper quadrant pain.
  9. Describe the diagnostic evaluation and management of a patient with fever, chills and jaundice.
 10. Describe the following:
     a. Murphy's sign
     b. Courvoisier's sign
     c. Gallstone ileus
 11. Contrast carcinomas of the gallbladder, bile duct and ampulla of Vater with regard to presenting features and survival.

Diagnostic Studies in Biliary Tract Disease
  1. Contrast the liver enzyme abnormalities in cholestasis and viral hepatitis.
  2. Identify the most common bacteria found in cholecystitis and cholangitis.
  3. Describe the indications for and risks of oral cholecystogram, transhepatic cholangiogram and ERCP.
  4. Accurately interpret an abnormal oral cholecystogram, transhepatic cholangiogram and ERCP.

Skills
  1. Given a patient with acute cholecystitis, demonstrate the right upper quadrant physical findings that indicate this diagnosis.

13
The Liver

L.J. Worobetz, R.J. Hilsden, E.A. Shaffer, J. Simon, P. Paré,
L.J. Scully, G. Minuk, F. Wong, L. Blendis, P. Adams,
J. Heathcote, S.S. Lee, I. Altraif and G.A. Levy

1. LIVER STRUCTURE AND FUNCTION / R.J. Hilsden and E.A. Shaffer

1.1 Liver Morphology

THE LIVER IS the largest and most metabolically complex organ in humans. Anatomically, it consists of two main lobes, right and left, separated by the round and falciform ligaments, plus two smaller lobes, the caudate lobe located on the posterior surface and the quadrate lobe on the inferior surface. The liver is functionally divided into eight segments based on the distribution of the portal and hepatic veins. Each segment receives a pedicle of the portal vein and is an independent functional unit. The caudate lobe (segment 1) differs from other segments in that it receives blood from both the right and left branches of the portal vein and drains directly into the inferior vena cava.

At a microscopic level, the liver consists of myriads of individual functional units, traditionally called lobules. Each lobule is bounded by four to five portal triads (supplied from the portal vein and hepatic artery) and has a central terminal hepatic venule (central vein). A more physiologically sound concept is the unit termed the acinus. At the center is the portal triad, while the terminal hepatic venules are at the periphery. The acinus is divided into three zones based upon the distance from the feeding vessels (Figure 1).

The liver receives a dual blood supply. The portal vein drains the splanchnic circulation and provides 75% of the total blood flow (1,500 mL/min). The hepatic artery provides the remaining 25%. Small branches of each blood vessel (the terminal portal venule and the terminal hepatic arteriole) enter the acinus at the portal triad (zone 1). Blood then flows through sinusoids between plates of hepatocytes toward the terminal hepatic venule (zone 3), where

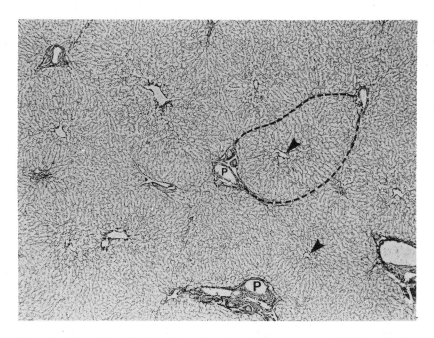

FIGURE 1. Normal liver. This liver biopsy shows the orderly arrangement of the liver cell plates, central veins (arrowheads) and portal tracts (P). A hepatic lobule is outlined. (Retic. stain, original magnification × 370)

blood from several adjacent acini merges. The sinusoidal lining is fenestrated; this porosity allows nutrients to gain access to the intervening Disse's space and from it to the hepatocyte. The terminal hepatic venules coalesce to form the hepatic vein, which carries all efferent blood to the inferior vena cava. A rich supply of lymphatic vessels also drains the liver.

Hepatocytes make up the bulk of the organ. They are arranged in plates that radiate out from each portal triad toward adjacent central veins. Those hepatocytes surrounding the portal tract form an interface between the connective tissues of the portal tract and the hepatic parenchyma, termed the limiting plate.

The bile canaliculus is formed by grooves on the contact surface of adjacent liver cells. Bile forms in these canaliculi and progressively flows into ductules, interlobular bile ducts and then larger hepatic ducts. Outside the porta hepatis, the hepatic duct joins the cystic duct from the gallbladder to form the common bile duct, which drains into the duodenum.

Sinusoidal lining cells comprise at least four distinct populations: endothelial cells, Kupffer's cells, perisinusoidal fat-storing cells and pit cells. Endothelial cells differ from the vascular endothelium elsewhere in the body in that they lack a basement membrane and contain numerous fenestrae that permit hepatocytes ready access to nutrients and macromolecules in plasma. Endothelial cells are also responsible for endocytosis of molecules and particles, and play a role in lipoprotein metabolism.

Spindle-shaped Kupffer's cells are tissue macrophages. They form an important part of the body's reticuloendothelial system. Their major functions include phagocytosis of foreign particles, removal of endotoxins and other noxious substances, and modulation of the immune response through the release of mediators and cytotoxic agents.

Perisinusoidal fat-storing cells (Ito cells) store vitamin A and transform into fibroblasts in response to hepatic injury. They may contribute significantly to hepatic fibrosis.

Pit cells, the least common sinusoidal lining cells, are large, granular lymphocytes, which function as natural killer cells.

The extracellular matrix of the liver includes its reticulin framework and several molecular forms of collagen, laminin, fibronectin and other extracellular glycoproteins.

1.2 Hepatobiliary Function

1.2.1 METABOLISM
The liver plays a central role in carbohydrate, protein and fat metabolism. It maintains a stable blood glucose level by taking up and storing glucose as glycogen (glycogenesis), breaking this down to glucose (glycogenolysis) when needed, and forming glucose from noncarbohydrate sources such as amino acids (gluconeogenesis). Hypoglycemia occurs only late in the course of severe liver disease because the liver has a large functional reserve; glucose homeostasis can be maintained with only 20% of the liver functioning. The liver synthesizes the majority of proteins that circulate in the plasma, including albumin and most of the globulins other than gamma globulins. Albumin provides most of the oncotic pressure of plasma and is a carrier for drugs and endogenous hydrophobic compounds such as unconjugated bilirubin. Globulins include the coagulation factors: fibrinogen, prothrombin, and factors V, VII, IX and X. Factors II, VII, IX and X are vitamin K–dependent. Availability of vitamin K, a fat-soluble vitamin, requires adequate bile salts for the vitamin's absorption. These factors decrease with fat malabsorption (as with prolonged cholestasis) and with the reduced synthetic function of hepatocellular disease. (In hepatocellular diseases, deficiency of these coagulation factors

is not corrected by vitamin K administration.) The liver is also the site of most amino acid interconversions and catabolism. Amino acids are catabolized to urea. During this process ammonia, a product of nitrogen metabolism and a possible neurotoxin, is utilized and therefore detoxified. Fatty acids are taken up by the liver and esterified to triglycerides. The liver packages triglycerides with cholesterol, phospholipids and an apoprotein into a lipoprotein. The lipoprotein enters blood for utilization or storage in adipocytes. Most cholesterol synthesis takes place in the liver.

1.2.2 DRUG DISPOSITION
The liver's rich enzyme system allows the metabolism of many drugs, including alcohol. The liver detoxifies noxious substances arriving from the splanchnic circulation, preventing them from entering the systemic circulation. It converts some lipophilic compounds into more water-soluble agents, which are then easily excreted in the urine or bile. Others are metabolized to less active agents.

1.2.3 BILE FORMATION
Bile provides the main excretory pathway for toxic metabolites, cholesterol and lipid waste products. Bile is also necessary for the efficient digestion and absorption of dietary fats. Bile salts are synthesized exclusively in the liver from cholesterol and are the driving force behind bile formation. After excretion by the liver, bile is stored in the gallbladder during periods of fasting.

Cholecystokinin (CCK), released from the small intestine during digestion by fatty acids and amino acids, stimulates gallbladder evacuation. When the bile reaches the duodenum it aids in fat absorption by acting as a biologic detergent. Bile salts are reabsorbed predominantly in the ileum and return to the liver via the portal vein to be taken up and secreted once again. This is the enterohepatic circulation (intestine-to-liver).

2. APPROACH TO THE PATIENT WITH LIVER DISEASE / J. Simon

Because of the liver's complexity, liver disease is often reflected by abnormalities of different hepatic "systems" – i.e., hepatocytes (hepatocellular dysfunction), the biliary excretory apparatus (cholestasis) and the vascular system (portal hypertension). In addition, the liver often is involved in systemic disease by virtue of its rich metabolic and reticuloendothelial activity and its large blood supply.

Patterns of disproportionate involvement often provide an important clue to

TABLE 1. Major clinical manifestations of liver disease (asterisk implies chronicity)

Systemic
    Anorexia, malaise, fatigue
    Fever
    *General deterioration, weight loss, "cirrhotic habitus"
    Cholestasis: pruritus, *xanthelasma/xanthomas, *malabsorption problems

Jaundice

Hepatomegaly ± pain

Portal hypertension

Fluid derangements
    *Ascites ± edema
    Electrolyte disturbances
    Functional renal failure ("hepatorenal syndrome")

Hepatic encephalopathy (portal-systemic encephalopathy)

*Cutaneous and endocrine changes
    Spider nevi, palmar erythema, Dupuytren's contractures
    Gynecomastia, testicular atrophy, impotence
    Amenorrhea
    Parotid enlargement

Coagulopathy
    Hypoprothrombinemia
    Thrombocytopenia
    Dysfibrinogenemia

Circulatory changes
    Hyperdynamic circulation
    *Arterial desaturation, clubbing

the underlying disorder. For example, viral hepatitis characteristically produces predominant hepatocellular dysfunction; primary biliary cirrhosis, predominant cholestasis; cryptogenic cirrhosis, predominant portal hypertension; and alcoholic liver disease, variably predominant dysfunction of any of these three systems. The clinician can usually take advantage of these general patterns to help establish a diagnosis, though overlap and exceptions are frequent.

2.1 Clinical Features of Liver Disease

Table 1 lists the most important clinical manifestations of liver disease. Most can be seen in both acute and chronic hepatic disorders; features marked by an asterisk usually denote chronicity. This distinction can be of diagnostic value at the bedside. For example, a clinical diagnosis of acute hepatitis should be reconsidered if physical examination reveals spider nevi and palmar erythema.

2.1.1 *SYSTEMIC FEATURES*

Nondescript anorexia, malaise and fatigue are common manifestations of both acute and chronic liver disease. An abrupt onset often reflects acute viral or drug-induced hepatitis, whereas insidious development typifies alcoholic liver disease, chronic active hepatitis and other chronic disorders.

Fever is another nonspecific feature of some liver conditions, especially the prodromal phase of acute viral hepatitis, severe alcoholic hepatitis and (sometimes) malignancy. However, frank rigors and chills are rare in these conditions, and instead strongly suggest acute cholangitis, usually secondary to common duct stone.

Patients with advanced chronic liver disease, especially alcoholic cirrhosis, often develop deterioration of general health, weight loss and a characteristic "cirrhotic habitus" in which wasted extremities and shoulder girdle contrast with a bloated belly from ascites.

Generalized pruritus is a hallmark of cholestatic disorders, especially if chronic. When cholestasis is prolonged – for example, in primary biliary cirrhosis – this may be accompanied by cutaneous lipid deposits (xanthelasma, xanthomas) and by features of malabsorption.

2.1.2 *JAUNDICE*

This cardinal feature of liver disease indicates hyperbilirubinemia. Bilirubin arises primarily from the physiologic breakdown of senescent red blood cells, with a minor contribution from other heme sources. It is not water-soluble and is therefore transported in plasma loosely attached to albumin. This form of the pigment is called *unconjugated* or *indirect-reacting bilirubin*. The molecule is then taken up by hepatocytes and conjugated in microsomes with glucuronic acid to form bilirubin diglucuronide; the reaction is catalyzed by the enzyme glucuronyl transferase. Other minor conjugates are also formed; their clinical significance is unknown.

Transformed bilirubin is then secreted into the bile canaliculus along with the other constituents of bile. A small amount normally enters the blood as *conjugated* or *direct-reacting bilirubin*. In contrast to unconjugated bilirubin, this form of the pigment is water-soluble and is therefore excreted into urine, though a portion becomes tightly bound to circulating albumin (the so-called albumin-bound fraction of conjugated bilirubin).

After reaching the gut through the biliary tree, bilirubin is transformed by intestinal bacteria into pigmented breakdown products collectively called urobilinogen; these impart the normal brown color to stool. With impairment of biliary secretion (cholestasis) the stools are therefore often pale, but this is a relatively crude and unreliable diagnostic feature. Some urobilinogen is absorbed from the intestine and recycled through the liver (the enterohepatic circulation), with a portion escaping into the urine.

Various derangements in the above metabolic steps can result in jaundice. An increased bilirubin load from hemolysis may overwhelm the liver's conjugating capacity, resulting in unconjugated hyperbilirubinemia. This is invariably mild, however, unless there is also concomitant hepatic dysfunction. Isolated unconjugated hyperbilirubinemia also occurs in some specific defects of bilirubin metabolism, though these are rare except for Gilbert's syndrome (see Section 3 below).

In the vast majority of cases, jaundice is due to either hepatocellular disease or biliary obstruction. Both produce multiple defects in the pathway of bilirubin metabolism, including impaired hepatocellular uptake and transport, defective conjugation, decreased canalicular secretion, and "leakage" of conjugated bilirubin into the circulation. The resultant hyperbilirubinemia is a mixture of unconjugated and conjugated pigment; usually the latter predominates, but the exact proportion varies widely and has no specific diagnostic value.

Clinically, mild jaundice can usually be detected when serum bilirubin is about twice the upper limit of normal, and is best diagnosed by inspecting the patient's sclerae in natural daylight. More advanced cases are often apparent at a glance. Patients with severe long-standing jaundice sometimes have a generalized muddy-yellow appearance.

2.1.3 HEPATOMEGALY WITH OR WITHOUT PAIN

A readily palpable liver is not necessarily enlarged, for it may merely be low-lying – as, for example, in emphysema. Thus the upper border should be percussed when the edge is palpable.

The "quality" or feel of the liver is at least as important diagnostically as its size. For example, the liver usually retains its rubbery, relatively sharp edge when enlargement is due to fatty infiltration, acute hepatitis and passive congestion, whereas chronic fibrosis typically produces a blunt, indurated edge. Individual cirrhotic nodules are rarely detectable clinically. Palpable lumpiness instead favors malignant infiltration. It is important to remember that major liver disease – including a high proportion of cirrhosis – may not be associated with hepatomegaly.

Abdominal pain is common in biliary or pancreatic disease that might secondarily affect the liver – for example, common duct stone or pancreatic carcinoma – but pain is relatively uncommon in primary hepatic disorders. True hepatic pain is usually due to distention of the liver capsule, typically felt as a deep-seated right upper quadrant ache. This is often accompanied by hepatic tenderness on physical examination, best elicited by compression of the rib cage or fist percussion over the liver. The commonest causes are acute hepatitis, passive congestion from cardiac failure, and malignancy. Pain from malignancy is sometimes pleuritic in character and may be accompanied by a hepatic friction rub or bruit on auscultation. The liver edge when palpable can produce discomfort; this has no special significance and should not be interpreted as hepatic tenderness.

2.1.4 CUTANEOUS AND ENDOCRINE CHANGES
These findings as listed in Table 1 are important clues to chronic liver disease. Their pathogenesis is still poorly understood, but altered metabolism of sex hormones by the diseased liver appears important. The abnormalities may be seen in any chronic hepatic disorder, but are especially prevalent in alcoholic liver disease; this probably relates in part to a direct toxic effect of ethanol on gonadal function.

2.1.5 COAGULATION DISTURBANCES
The liver synthesizes most clotting factors, including vitamin K–dependent factors II, VII and IX. Severe hepatocellular dysfunction is therefore often accompanied by an enhanced bruising and bleeding tendency and by abnormal coagulation studies, particularly a prolonged prothrombin time. Malabsorption of the fat-soluble vitamin K in prolonged cholestasis can also produce an abnormal prothrombin time.

Thrombocytopenia is common in patients with cirrhosis, primarily as a result of portal hypertension with hypersplenism, but usually the platelet counts are not low enough to induce clinical bleeding. In patients with alcoholic liver disease, thrombocytopenia may also be due to direct marrow suppression by alcohol and/or nutritional folate deficiency.

Dysfibrinogenemia also sometimes contributes to coagulopathy in cases of severe hepatic dysfunction.

2.1.6 CIRCULATORY CHANGES
A hyperdynamic circulation and relatively low blood pressure are sometimes seen in patients with severe liver disease, especially fulminant hepatitis and advanced cirrhosis. The mechanism may relate to the accumulation of vasoactive agents normally cleared by the liver, which reduce tone. Occasional patients with cirrhosis develop intrapulmonary A–V shunting, with resultant arterial desaturation and (rarely) clubbing.

A number of topics will be discussed in later sections, including portal hypertension (Section 11), fluid derangements (Sections 12 and 14) and hepatic encephalopathy (Section 13).

2.2 Laboratory, Radiologic and Histologic Evaluations

No single test can assess overall hepatic function, as the liver is a complex organ with interdependent metabolic, excretory and defense functions. Thus a number of laboratory tests are usually combined to detect hepatobiliary abnormalities and to assess their severity, follow the course of the disease, and help establish an etiology. Diagnosis is often based on patterns of abnormality that help distinguish hepatocellular dysfunction from excretory impairment (cholestasis), though overlap is great. In only a minority of cases does a specific laboratory test establish the diagnosis.

Radiologic imaging techniques and liver biopsy often provide essential diagnostic information, but their use should be tailored to the specific clinical circumstances.

2.2.1 SERUM BIOCHEMICAL TESTS

2.2.1.1 Bilirubin

This is a relatively insensitive indicator of liver disease, but it provides a clue to the overall assessment of hepatic function. The degree of bilirubin elevation often correlates poorly with clinical severity, but serial values are useful for following the course of the illness. Direct/indirect (conjugated/unconjugated) fractionation is *not* of diagnostic value in most cases of jaundice, and cannot distinguish hepatocellular disease from biliary obstruction. Measuring the presence of unconjugated hyperbilirubinemia is useful only in cases of mild, isolated bilirubin elevation to corroborate hemolysis or Gilbert's syndrome.

Urine bilirubin has little diagnostic value except in early hepatitis, when bilirubinuria precedes clinical jaundice, and in isolated unconjugated hyperbilirubinemia, when bilirubinuria is absent despite jaundice. (Unconjugated bilirubin is not cleared into urine.) Otherwise bilirubin is commonly present in urine with hepatobiliary jaundice of any cause.

2.2.1.2 Aminotransferases (transaminases)

These liver enzymes include alanine aminotransferase (ALT), found primarily in liver cytosol, and aspartate aminotransferase (AST), also found in several other tissues, most notably skeletal and cardiac muscle. Both are exquisitely sensitive indicators of hepatocellular injury and provide the best guide to hepatocellular necrosis/inflammation.

The magnitude of elevation covers a very wide range. Levels <100 IU are common and nonspecific, and often have no clinical significance; levels of 100–300 IU are seen in numerous mild/moderate inflammatory processes. In acute viral or drug hepatitis transaminase levels are typically in the 500–1,500 IU range, but in alcoholic hepatitis they are usually <300 IU, even if severe. Values >3,000 IU usually are seen only in acute toxic necrosis or severe hypoxia ("shock liver," "ischemic hepatitis"); in both disorders levels typically plummet within two to three days, whereas values fall more slowly in viral hepatitis. Transaminase levels are variable in biliary obstruction but usually remain <200 IU, except with acute passage of common duct stone, characterized by a sudden rise to hepatitic levels and a rapid fall over the next one to two days.

The AST to ALT ratio is usually <1 in most circumstances, but typically >1.5 in alcoholic liver disease; though not absolute, this is diagnostically helpful for alcoholic injury. Alcohol consumption lessens the ALT rise.

2.2.1.3 Alkaline phosphatase (ALP)

A bile canalicular enzyme disproportionately increased in impaired bile excretion, this is a hallmark of cholestasis. Elevations in its level are due to enhanced synthesis rather than hepatocytic leakage; thus, levels usually rise slowly over days or weeks rather than abruptly. Levels are also disproportionately elevated in infiltrative disorders, especially malignancy.

ALP isoenzymes also are present in bone and placenta. If the source of an isolated increase in ALP is not clinically clear, the concomitant elevation of γ-glutamyl transpeptidase (GGT) indicates a hepatobiliary origin. A form of ALP specific to the liver is 5′-nucleotidase (5′NT).

2.2.1.4 Gamma-glutamyl transpeptidase (GGT)

Levels of GGT usually parallel ALP, but an elevated level is easily inducible – for example, by ethanol and numerous drugs. Thus, GGT is often disproportionately elevated in alcoholic liver disease, although this rise is too nonspecific for diagnostic reliability.

2.2.1.5 Proteins

2.2.1.5.1 *Albumin*   Synthesized by the liver, albumin is the major contributor to oncotic pressure in the serum. Decreased levels usually develop only in severe hepatic dysfunction, and most often in advanced cirrhosis, and therefore imply a relatively poor prognosis. Albumin usually remains normal in acute hepatitis; falling values in this setting imply an unusually severe course.

2.2.1.5.2 *Globulins*   Nonspecific diffuse elevation is common in chronic liver disease, and of no consequence. Sometimes there is disproportionate elevation of IgG in chronic active hepatitis, especially of the autoimmune type. IgM rises in primary biliary cirrhosis; IgA can be quite high in alcoholic liver disease.

2.2.1.6 *Prothrombin time*
The prothrombin time is a valuable index of the liver's ability to synthesize vitamin K–dependent clotting factors – a time "function" test. Prolongation implies relatively severe dysfunction, analogous to low serum albumin. Prolongation in acute hepatitis is especially worrisome. An abnormal value may be found in chronic cholestasis due to vitamin K malabsorption rather than impaired hepatic synthesis of clotting factors. Improvement after parenteral administration of vitamin K therefore favors a diagnosis of cholestasis over hepatocellular failure, but there are too many exceptions for diagnostic reliability.

2.2.1.7 *Lipids*
Complex lipoprotein derangements are common in liver disease, though usually not routinely studied. Cholesterol is often low in acute or chronic liver failure, whereas hypercholesterolemia is associated with prolonged cholestasis. Striking triglyceride elevations occasionally occur in alcoholic liver disease ("alcoholic lipemia").

2.2.2 SERUM IMMUNOLOGIC TESTS

2.2.2.1 *Hepatitis serology*
Serology is crucial for the specific diagnosis of hepatitis A, B, C and D. See Section 4 for details.

2.2.2.2 *Antimitochondrial antibody*
This is actually a complex series of antibodies directed against mitochondrial membranes of various tissues. Nevertheless, it serves as a valuable marker for primary biliary cirrhosis, as it is present in >90% of cases. The antimitochondrial antibody is uncommon in other disorders, though there is some overlap with autoimmune chronic active hepatitis.

2.2.2.3 *Antinuclear factor and antismooth muscle antibody*
Such nonspecific immune markers are seen relatively commonly in autoimmune chronic active hepatitis; they are infrequent in other hepatic diseases.

2.2.2.4 *Alpha-fetoprotein*
This normal hepatic fetal protein disappears soon after birth. Detection

reflects hepatic dedifferentiation. Levels >250 ng/mL serve as a relatively specific marker for hepatocellular carcinoma, though they are also seen occasionally in other tumors. Values <100 ng/mL are nonspecifically seen in hepatic regeneration – e.g., recovering from hepatitis.

2.2.3 IMAGING PROCEDURES

In general, radiologic imaging is essential for the accurate diagnosis of biliary disease, important for focal liver disease (e.g., tumor), but overused and of relatively little value for diffuse hepatocellular disease (e.g., hepatitis, cirrhosis).

2.2.3.1 Ultrasonography (US)

Ultrasound is now the most widely used imaging procedure. Highly reliable for diagnosis of gallstones (>95% sensitivity), it has replaced oral cholecystography. US is less accurate in detecting common bile duct stones (<40% sensitivity), but reliably establishes the presence of a dilatated biliary tree, which implies mechanical obstruction. It is therefore the primary initial tool to distinguish intrahepatic from extrahepatic cholestasis. It also detects focal hepatic lesions (e.g., tumor, cysts), sometimes with characteristic diagnostic features. It is less useful in detecting diffuse hepatocellular disease, as features are usually nonspecific.

Ultrasonography can also provide important ancillary information relevant to hepatobiliary disease – e.g., splenomegaly and pancreatic mass. Doppler US is valuable in establishing the patency of hepatic vessels, especially the portal vein; it has largely replaced splenoportography.

2.2.3.2 Computerized tomography (CT)

An expensive alternative to US, CT sometimes provides additional hepatic information. Generally less valuable than US for biliary disease, CT has proven more valuable for assessing the pancreas.

2.2.3.3 Direct biliary visualization

2.2.3.3.1 Endoscopic retrograde cholangiopancreatography (ERCP) Upper endoscopy allows direct cannulation of the common bile duct and/or pancreatic duct; the injection of contrast agent yields excellent definition of ductal anatomy. ERCP permits definitive visualization of the biliary tree for common duct stone, sclerosing cholangitis and other conditions. It also allows therapeutic intervention – e.g., removal of common duct stones via endoscopic papillotomy or stenting a stricture.

2.2.3.3.2 Percutaneous transhepatic cholangiography (PTC) In PTC, direct contrast visualization of the biliary tree is obtained via percutaneous needle puncture of liver. This is done less often than ERCP, but is especially useful if there is high biliary obstruction – e.g., a tumor at the bifurcation of the hepatic ducts. It also permits therapeutic intervention such as stent insertion to bypass a ductal malignancy.

ERCP and PTC require considerable technical expertise and have significant risks. They should not be undertaken lightly, but are highly valuable in selected cholestatic situations and may obviate laparotomy.

2.2.3.4 Radionuclide scanning

The liver–spleen scan using 99mTc-sulfur colloid can reveal space-occupying lesions and diffuse parenchymal disease, but such scans are much less sensitive than US or CT; therefore, their use is rapidly waning. The 99mTc-labeled RBC scan can clarify suspected vascular lesions, especially hemangiomas. Cholescintigraphy using 99mTc-iminodiacetic acid derivatives (termed HIDA scan) can reveal cystic duct obstruction, especially in acute cholecystitis. The HIDA scan also assesses biliary excretion/patency and anatomy, but results often are less than ideal or misleading. Occasionally 67Ga-citrate scans are used to help detect liver abscess or tumor.

2.2.3.5 Nuclear magnetic resonance imaging (NMR)

NMR is an expensive new imaging technique, not yet widely available. It can detect some lesions poorly seen by US or CT; it will probably become an increasingly important tool.

2.2.4 LIVER BIOPSY

Percutaneous liver biopsy provides important diagnostic information at relatively low risk, but is needed in only a minority of cases with hepatic dysfunction. A small core of liver tissue is obtained at the bedside by needle aspiration under local anesthesia. This usually provides a surprisingly reliable reflection of the underlying disorder, though sampling error occurs in focal disease and some cases of cirrhosis.

The major indications are shown in Table 2. Transient right upper quadrant pain is not uncommon after biopsy, but significant hemorrhage, bile peritonitis or other major complications are rare if cases are properly selected.

Relative contraindications include a clinical bleeding tendency or prothrombin time more than three seconds greater than control, severe thrombocytopenia, marked ascites, and high-grade biliary tract obstruction. A

TABLE 2. Indications for liver biopsy

Unexplained liver function abnormalities
Hepatosplenomegaly of unknown cause
Diagnosis and staging of alcoholic liver disease
Cirrhosis – diagnosis and etiology
Chronic hepatitis
Unexplained cholestasis
Acute necrosis, if cause unclear
Suspected infiltrative disorder, especially malignancy
Unexplained systemic illness – fever of unknown origin, suspected granulomatous disease, etc.

transjugular approach can be used with relative safety in cases of coagulopathy or severe ascites.

Fine-needle aspiration of specific hepatic lesions can be obtained under US or CT guidance. This provides a cytologic sample, but is usually inadequate for full histologic assessment.

2.3 Clinical Approach

When faced with a patient with known or suspected liver disease, the physician should attempt to answer several central questions: (1) Is the disorder acute or chronic? (2) Is it primarily a hepatocellular problem (e.g., hepatitis), a disorder of hepatobiliary secretion (cholestasis) or a vascular problem (e.g., portal hypertension)? (3) If hepatocellular, is alcohol, a virus or a drug responsible? If cholestatic, is it an intrahepatic problem, or is it due to mechanical biliary obstruction? If vascular, is it due to cirrhosis or to a less common cause? (4) Is this actually a systemic disorder involving the liver rather than a primary hepatic problem? (5) Are there complications that require specific treatment? These and other pertinent questions are approached by bedside clinical judgment coupled with ancillary tests.

Broadly speaking, the most important diagnostic tool is a complete history and physical examination. Laboratory tests, imaging techniques and liver biopsy are valuable and sometimes essential for diagnosis, but in most cases clinical acumen provides the most important diagnostic information. Moreover, clinical judgment determines what additional studies should be undertaken and how to interpret the results. *Diagnostic errors most often arise from an inadequate history and physical examination with undue reliance on ancillary tests.*

The clinical assessment should emphasize aspects discussed above in Section 2.1. Inquire about ethanol, drugs (prescribed, over-the-counter and illicit) and epidemiologic factors relevant to viral hepatitis, especially in cases of suspected hepatocellular injury. In addition, pursuit of systemic illness is often necessary. A family history of liver disease is occasionally important – e.g., in hemochromatosis.

The extent and nature of laboratory investigations are guided by the initial clinical evaluation. Broadly speaking, a minimal initial study will include CBC plus bilirubin, AST and/or ALT, and ALP. These few simple tests usually clarify whether the problem is primarily a hepatocellular injury (disproportionate aminotransferase elevations) or an excretory problem (predominant ALP elevation). If the former is clinically apparent but the etiology is not, viral hepatitis markers may help, especially if the disorder is acute. If a cholestatic problem seems most likely, early US (or CT) should help distinguish intrahepatic from extrahepatic causation. If US indicates extrahepatic obstruction, direct biliary visualization by ERCP (or PTC) should be considered, whereas liver biopsy may be warranted if the process appears intrahepatic.

As yet there is no reliable biochemical marker of liver fibrosis. Thus laboratory indicators of hepatic dysfunction are often normal or only mildly deranged in cases of inactive cirrhosis; this is a common circumstance. It is well to remember that alcoholic liver disease is the commonest cause of chronic hepatocellular injury, even in patients who initially deny heavy ingestion.

With appropriate evaluation, a diagnosis can readily be established in the large majority of patients with hepatobiliary dysfunction. In many circumstances, however, especially if the hepatic abnormalities are minor, the wisest approach is simply to follow the patient's progress with periodic clinical and laboratory assessments.

3. CONGENITAL HYPERBILIRUBINEMIA / P. Paré

The importance of recognizing congenital hyperbilirubinemia lies mainly in distinguishing it from other, more serious hepatobiliary disease: congenital conjugated hyperbilirubinemia or hepatobiliary diseases. Except for Crigler-Najjar syndrome, congenital hyperbilirubinemia does not impair either the quality of life or the life expectancy of affected subjects. By definition, patients with familial hyperbilirubinemia have normal standard liver tests, and the liver histology is also normal (except for the pigment accumulation in Dubin-Johnson syndrome). With the exception of Gilbert's syndrome, these syndromes are uncommon and are divided into two groups on the basis of the type of the serum hyperbilirubinemia.

3.1 Unconjugated Hyperbilirubinemia

3.1.1 GILBERT'S SYNDROME
Gilbert's syndrome is the most common congenital hyperbilirubinemia syndrome, occurring in about 5% of Caucasians. It is probably transmitted through an autosomal dominant mode. Its pathogenesis is related to a partial deficiency in hepatic UDPglucuronyl transferase, the enzyme responsible for the glucuronidation of bilirubin. In addition, some patients have reduced bilirubin uptake by the hepatocytes, as observed with diagnostic substances (BSP, indocyanine green) and drugs (tolbutamide). The syndrome is usually detected in adolescents and young adults. Complaints leading to the diagnosis are various (fatigue, nausea, vague abdominal discomfort) and unrelated to the condition. Scleral icterus may be present and fluctuating, but the physical examination is otherwise normal. Liver tests and hemogram (to exclude hemolysis) are normal except for unconjugated serum bilirubin, which is elevated between 20 and 100 $\mu M/L$ and conjugated bilirubin, which is often unrecordably low. Diagnostic tests are available but usually not necessary: fasting for two days or intravenous administration of nicotinic acid significantly increases serum unconjugated bilirubin, while phenobarbital significantly decreases it. No treatment is warranted and prognosis is excellent.

3.1.2 CRIGLER-NAJJAR SYNDROME
This syndrome may present in two types. Type I is a very rare and serious disease characterized by unconjugated hyperbilirubinemia often greater than 400–500 $\mu M/L$. It is due to an absolute deficiency of UDPglucuronyl transferase. Jaundice occurs almost immediately after birth and may lead to kernicterus with consequent neurologic damage and mental retardation. The syndrome is inherited in an autosomal recessive fashion, often with a family history of consanguinity. Phenobarbital treatment is ineffective in inducing UDPglucuronyl transferase activity; an early death occurs. The treatment of choice appears to be hepatic transplantation.

Crigler-Najjar syndrome type II is a much more benign condition in which the unconjugated hyperbilirubinemia usually does not exceed 400 $\mu M/L$. Kernicterus rarely develops in these patients (except with prolonged fasting, in which bilirubin can rise). Hepatic UDPglucuronyl transferase activity is very low or undetectable, but phenobarbital therapy lowers serum bilirubin levels. (Phenobarbital presumably induces even the low levels of this enzyme.) Prognosis is very good despite a lifelong persistent unconjugated hyperbilirubinemia.

3.2 Conjugated Hyperbilirubinemia

Two conditions characterized by congenital conjugated hyperbilirubinemia without cholestasis have been described. Both syndromes are inherited as autosomal recessive traits. Both are uncommon disorders believed to result from specific defects in the hepatobiliary excretion of bilirubin. These conditions are benign, and their accurate diagnosis provides reassurance to the patient. Plasma bilirubin levels are usually in the range of 35–85 µM/L, although occasionally levels may be as high as 400 µM/L. Plasma bilirubin may further increase in both conditions during intercurrent infection, pregnancy or use of oral contraceptives. Pruritus is absent and serum bile acid levels are normal, as are routine biochemical liver tests, except for serum bilirubin concentration. Bilirubinuria is usually present. No treatment is necessary.

Some distinctive features allow differential diagnosis between the two syndromes.

3.2.1 *DUBIN-JOHNSON SYNDROME*

Patients with the Dubin-Johnson syndrome have a black liver, which results from the accumulation of a melanin-like pigment in lysosomes. Visualization of the gallbladder during oral cholecystography is usually delayed or absent. Urinary excretion of total coproporphyrin is normal, whereas the proportion of isomer I is higher than in normal controls (>80%). Finally, the BSP plasma retention test is normal in its initial phase, but there is a secondary rise in plasma BSP concentration at 90 minutes due to reflux of BSP from the hepatocyte to the plasma.

3.2.2 *ROTOR'S SYNDROME*

In patients with Rotor's syndrome, the appearance and histology of the liver are normal. Oral cholecystography usually visualizes the gallbladder. Total coproporphyrin excretion is greater than normal, as in other hepatobiliary disorders, and isomer I makes a smaller proportion (<80%) than in Dubin-Johnson patients. The plasma disappearance of injected BSP is delayed, with no secondary rise.

4. ACUTE VIRAL HEPATITIS / L.J. Scully and L.J. Worobetz

The term *hepatitis* refers to any inflammatory process of the liver, the most common etiology being viral (Table 3). This is most commonly due to hepatitis A, hepatitis B or hepatitis C infections, and less often due to hepatitis D or E infections. Hepatitis may occur with less common viral infections such as the EB virus, cytomegalovirus, adenovirus, herpes simplex or Coxsackie

TABLE 3.   Causes of acute hepatitis

Viruses
Hepatitis A
Hepatitis B
Hepatitis C
Hepatitis D
Hepatitis E
Herpes simplex
Cytomegalovirus
Epstein-Barr
Adenoviruses
Drugs
Toxins
Alcohol
Ischemia
Wilson's disease
Other

virus. In these cases, however, the clinical picture is usually dominated not by the hepatitis but by other features of the viral illness.

4.1 Types of Viral Hepatitis

4.1.1 *HEPATITIS A*
Previously termed "infectious hepatitis," hepatitis A virus (HAV) is an RNA virus that belongs to the enterovirus family. It is present in the stool of patients during the prodrome or pre-icteric phase until about two weeks after the onset of jaundice. Both IgM and IgG antibodies to the virus (anti-HAV) can be detected. The most helpful sign is the demonstration of an elevated IgM antibody, indicating recent infection (Figure 2).

Hepatitis A is usually transmitted by the fecal–oral route, commonly as a result of food or water contamination, and thus may occur in either sporadic or epidemic forms. Parenteral transmission is also possible but is much less common. Infection can occur at any age but is most common in younger age groups, presenting as a mild gastroenteritis. In North America, we are seeing more symptomatic hepatitis A in older age groups as fewer adults are exposed to hepatitis A in childhood as a result of improved sanitation. The incubation period is about one month, with a range of 20 to 35 days. In children, anicteric or subclinical disease is more frequent, but in older age groups the disease tends to be more severe. The mortality rate – usually from fulminant hepatitis

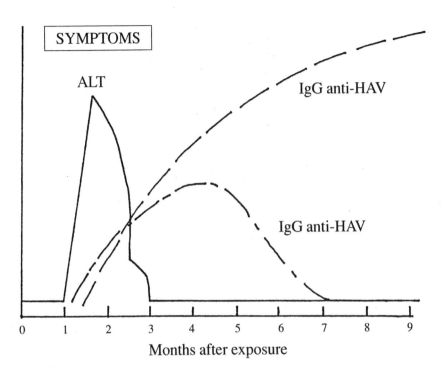

Months after exposure

FIGURE 2.   The serologic course of hepatitis A.

– is very low (0.1%). There is no evidence for a chronic carrier state or the development of chronic liver disease.

4.1.2 HEPATITIS B

In 1965, an antibody in a hemophiliac patient was found to react with an antigen in the serum from an Australian aborigine; the same antigen was subsequently found in patients with viral hepatitis. This antigen was termed the Australian antigen and is now known to be the surface of the hepatitis B virion, now called the hepatitis B surface antigen (HB_sAg).

Three types of particles can be found in hepatitis B serum. The Dane particle is the complete hepatitis B virus (HBV), whereas the small spheres and tubules are excess viral protein (HB_sAg).

The virus consists of a 28 nm central core containing the genome of the hepatitis B virus, a single molecule of partially double-stranded DNA and a specific DNA polymerase with a surrounding double-protein shell. The core is

TABLE 4. Interpretation of hepatitis B markers

Marker	Acute infection	Chronic infection High infectivity	Low infectivity	Past infection
HB$_s$Ag	+	+	+	–
HB$_e$Ag	+ Early, then –	+	–	–
Anti-HB$_c$ IgM	High titer	Low or –	–	–
Anti-HB$_c$ IgG	Moderate to high	High titer	Moderate	Moderate
Anti-HB$_e$	– Early, then +	–	+	+
HBV-DNA/DNA polymerase	+	+	–	–
ALT, AST	Marked elevation	Mild elevation	Normal	Normal

commonly found in the nuclei of infected hepatocytes, with the HB$_s$Ag coat being acquired from the cytoplasm of the hepatocyte. The core of the particle is antigenically distinct from the HB$_s$Ag, allowing techniques to detect separately core antigen (HB$_c$Ag) and HB$_s$Ag along with their respective distinct antibodies (anti-HB$_c$ and anti-HB$_s$). A further antigen, termed HB$_e$Ag, can be detected in the serum of acute hepatitis B, together with DNA polymerase, and consists of subunits of HB$_c$Ag. HB$_e$Ag positivity implies viral replication and is an indicator of high infectivity. The typical course of appearance of the antigens and antibodies is shown in Figure 3. Their significance and importance in interpretation is summarized in Table 4.

Hepatitis B can produce a clinical picture similar to that of hepatitis A but with a longer incubation period (60–110 days). The transmission is parenteral – via skin or mucus membranes, through the administration of blood or blood products, or through inoculation by contaminated needles. Semen, saliva and other secretory products are potentially infectious. Sexual transmission occurs, but the exact mode of transmission is uncertain. Vertical transmission is common in developing countries, passing from mother to fetus or newborn; the infection is acquired at the time of birth or shortly thereafter and results in the vast majority of chronic carriers worldwide. High-risk groups include homosexuals, parenteral drug users and hospital staff who are in contact with

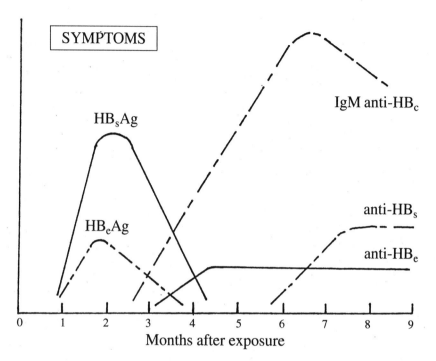

FIGURE 3. The serologic course of self-limited HB$_s$Ag-positive hepatitis B infection.

blood products (e.g., those in renal dialysis units). Hepatitis B infection from transfusion has been minimized by routine screening of donors and blood products and the use of volunteer blood donors.

4.1.3 HEPATITIS C

Hepatitis C virus is a single-stranded RNA virus less than 80 nm in diameter that appears to be a member of the flavivirus family. The virus itself has not been isolated, although the majority of the gene has been cloned and sequenced. Worldwide in distribution, its mode of transmission is parenteral, accounting for at least 80% of cases of post-transfusion hepatitis that were previously labeled as non-A non-B hepatitis. It also accounts for 12–25% of cases of sporadic hepatitis. IV drug use is the main source of hepatitis C infection in Canada. The incubation period is 5–10 weeks, with the acute phase being clinically mild and two-thirds of cases being subicteric. The elevated aminotransferase pattern may be monophasic or multiphasic, with the latter

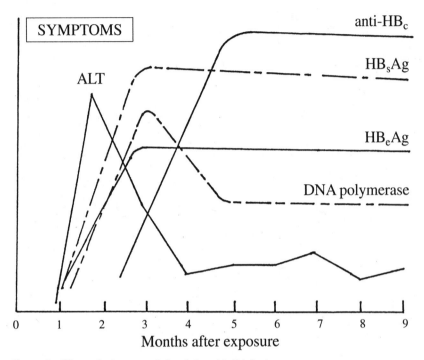

FIGURE 4.   The serologic course of chronic hepatitis B infection.

suggesting chronicity, which develops in 40–60% of cases. Histologically, it is much more difficult to distinguish between progressive and nonprogressive forms of chronic hepatitis C. Even with mild histologic change, up to 20% will progress to cirrhosis. Cirrhosis is a well-known sequela of chronicity; there also is an increased risk of hepatocellular carcinoma. Hepatitis C is also associated with the development of cryoglobulinemia and porphyria cutanea tarda.

Serologic testing for this virus is a rapidly developing field. Two immunoassays identify antibodies to the nonstructural as well as structural epitopes of the virus: ELISA and RIBA (recombinant immunoblotting assay). The ELISA test is very sensitive but not specific. Approximately 50% of individuals donating blood to the Red Cross who have normal liver enzymes and are found to be anti-HCV positive by ELISA will be found negative on subsequent RIBA testing. Hypergammaglobulinemia is a common reason for a false-positive ELISA test. An additional problem with the ELISA test for anti-HCV is the fact that the antibody cannot be detected in the circulation for approximately three to six months following the onset of the illness, as opposed to six to eight weeks for

RIBA testing. Moreover, only 60–70% of patients with acute HCV infection will ever develop anti-HCV ELISA positively.

Studies detecting HCV RNA using the polymerase chain reaction have shown that 80% of antibody-positive individuals are infectious.

4.1.4 HEPATITIS D (DELTA AGENT)

The hepatitis D virus (HDV) is a defective RNA virus that requires the presence of hepatitis B surface antigen for its expression. It is found worldwide, with outbreaks in Italy, the Middle East, Eastern Europe, the South Pacific, South America and Africa. In North America, HDV infection is most common among drug abusers. The delta virus circulates in association with the delta antigen, but until more sensitive assays are developed, this antigen can be detected only during the early phases of infection. The delta virus uses the HB_sAg protein as its external coat to attach itself to and enter hepatocytes; HB_sAg must therefore be present. The serologic marker for acute hepatitis D infection is the IgM antibody to delta antigen.

Hepatitis D infection may present in a number of ways. There may be a simultaneous infection with hepatitis B virus and delta virus, which produces a more severe acute hepatitis than that caused by hepatitis B alone but is usually self-limited. A patient with chronic hepatitis B may develop an acute exacerbation due to acute hepatitis D. This often results in more severe chronic hepatitis. A patient may also present with chronic hepatitis that is due to both chronic B and D viral infections. In the United States, less than 1% of HB_sAg-positive patients have evidence of hepatitis D infection, whereas in parts of Italy 14–50% of HB_sAg-positive patients have evidence of such.

4.1.5 HEPATITIS E

Hepatitis E (epidemic hepatitis) appears to be due to a single-stranded RNA virus of 27–34 nm in size. Previously included in the group labeled non-A non-B hepatitis, hepatitis virus E has now been defined as an enteric virus transmitted by the fecal–oral route. It is the leading cause of acute viral hepatitis in young to middle-aged adults in developing countries and is associated with a high mortality rate (approaching 20%) in infected pregnant women in the third trimester. It is seen only rarely in North America. The incubation period is 10 to 50 days. There are no distinctive clinical features, with secondary cases being rare. Chronicity of infection does not develop. Testing for anti-HE antibodies is available.

Table 5 lists important features of hepatitis types A, B, C, D and E.

4.1.6 HEPATITIS G

Recently a paramyxo-like virus was identified in a small number of patients

TABLE 5. Features of hepatitis A, B, C, D and E

	Type A	Type B	Type C	Type D	Type E
Mode of transmission	Fecal–oral	Percut., venereal	Percut.	Percut.	Fecal–oral
Incubation period (days)	20–35	60–110	35–70	?60–110	10–50
Immune tests					
Early	HAV-IgM	HB_sAg HB_c-IgM	?Anti-HCV	Anti-HD	Anti-HE
Late	HAV-IgG	Anti-HB_sAg	Anti-HCV	Anti-HD	Anti-HE
Chronicity	No	5% adult 90% childhood	10–40%	Common if chronic hepatitis B carrier	No

with severe acute and chronic liver disease who either died of liver failure or underwent a liver transplantation for survival. In some centers, the virus is referred to as hepatitis G virus (HGV). The diagnosis is made by liver biopsy where multinucleated giant cells are present. Paramyxo-like virus particles can also be seen on electron microscopy of the specimen. The epidemiology, response to treatment and forms of prevention have yet to be defined.

4.2 Pathology
In acute viral hepatitis there is acute inflammation of the liver with central lobular necrosis and diffuse cellular infiltration, especially around the portal tracts. More severe cases demonstrate bridging necrosis between central veins and portal tracts (Figures 5–8). Because there is usually preservation of the reticular framework, the liver normally restores itself completely with hepatocyte regeneration. Because of the systemic nature of the infection, inflammation occasionally can be found in other organs, with manifestations including polyarteritis, glomerulonephritis, myocarditis, bone marrow suppression and neurologic features (e.g., meningitis or neuritis).

4.3 Clinical Features
Most viral hepatitis infections are asymptomatic, especially in younger individuals. When infection is symptomatic, initial symptoms are those of any viral infection, beginning with malaise, nausea, vomiting, fatigue and a low-grade fever. More characteristic is severe anorexia, a marked distaste for smoking and a peculiar metallic taste in the mouth. In hepatitis B, about 10% of patients will develop a serum-sickness–like syndrome, with arthral-

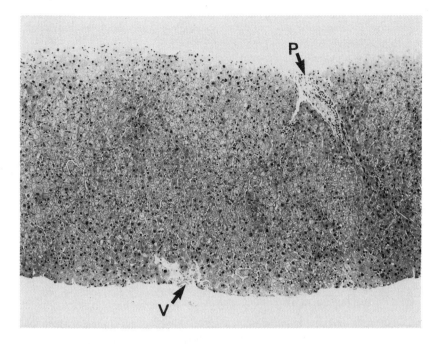

FIGURE 5. Mild hepatitis. There is some increase in inflammatory cells but no obvious hepato-cellular necrosis. P, portal tract; V, central vein. (H & E, original magnification × 92.5)

gia, arthritis, pruritus and rash. Abdominal pain, if present, is mild. Several days later, jaundice appears often preceded by dark urine and light-colored stool, with the fever usually subsiding at this point. The convalescent stage is usually 7 to 10 days, with the total illness lasting 2 to 6 weeks. Physical findings are usually minimal, aside from jaundice and a tender liver on palpation.

4.4 Diagnosis

Acute viral hepatitis can be suspected by the presence of viral prodrome symptoms, which often precede the more classical symptoms (including jaundice, dark urine and pruritus). Of diagnostic importance are the history of exposure to jaundiced persons, recent IV use or transfusions, sexual orientation, travel history and the absence of significant abdominal pain.

After the clinical suspicion of viral hepatitis, laboratory evaluation will help confirm the presence of acute liver injury, may define the etiology and may help monitor the course and prognosis of hepatitis. Classically, the serum ami-

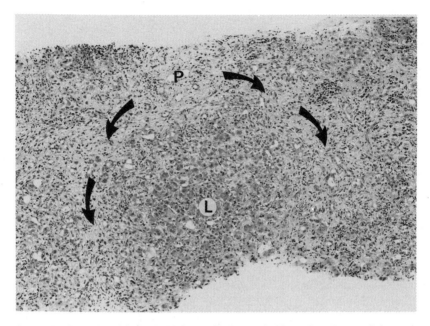

FIGURE 6.   Severe hepatitis. Marked inflammation has resulted in confluent hepatocellular necrosis, termed bridging necrosis (curved arrows), along the portal tracts (P) that surround a residual hepatic lobule (L). (HPS, original magnification × 92.5)

notransferase level is significantly elevated, often to levels >1,000 units, with the alkaline phosphatase only mildly to moderately elevated. This will occur at the end of the prodrome, before jaundice develops. The serum bilirubin is mainly conjugated and reflects the severity of the hepatitis. The prothrombin time defines the extent of liver injury in the acute stage; a prolonged and increasing PT implies a poor prognosis. To determine etiology, one screens for hepatitis A (IgM antibody), hepatitis B (HB_sAg, IgM anti-HB_c), and hepatitis C (anti-HCV), and for hepatitis D (anti-HDV) if the patient is a chronic carrier of hepatitis B.

The differential diagnosis should include other viral infections (such as infectious mononucleosis), cytomegalovirus infection, drug-induced liver disease, autoimmune hepatitis and Wilson's disease. Biliary tract disease (including cholecystitis and cholangitis) is distinguished by the presence of fever and significant abdominal pain. If doubt exists as to the diagnosis of hepatitis, liver biopsy or tests to exclude extrahepatic biliary obstruction may be necessary.

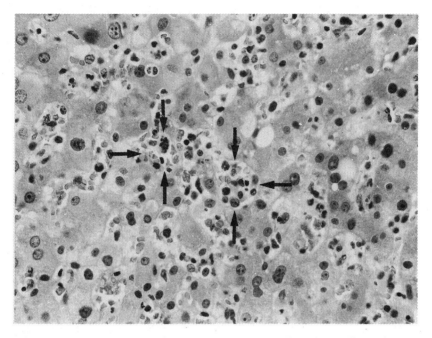

FIGURE 7. Severe hepatitis. High power shows numerous inflammatory cells within the sinusoids as well as foci of hepatocellular necrosis (arrows). Reactive changes, including binucleation and prominent nucleoli, are seen in the viable hepatocytes. (Gomori, original magnification × 370)

4.5 Complications

Most patients with viral hepatitis recover completely. Sequelae can occur more commonly with hepatitis B and C infections.

4.5.1 FULMINANT HEPATITIS

This is the situation of an individual with assumed prior normal liver function developing acute liver cell injury and proceeding to liver failure and hepatic encephalopathy within eight weeks (see Figures 8 and 9). Clinically, the patient suddenly deteriorates, becoming deeply jaundiced, confused and drowsy, and progressing to coma. Because of massive liver failure, there is deficiency of clotting factors, leading to bleeding. At this stage, mortality is greater than 50%. Death may occur from infection, encephalopathy or liver failure itself. Other clinical problems include hypoglycemia, increased intracranial pressure and the hepatorenal syndrome. Histologically, there is mas-

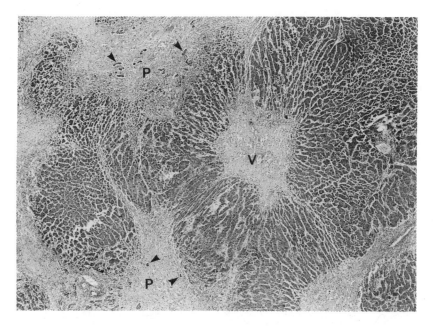

FIGURE 8.   Submassive necrosis. Extensive hepatocellular necrosis is seen, leaving large areas of connective tissue around the central vein (V) and widening of the portal tracts (P), which have become confluent. Residual bile ducts (arrowheads) are seen in the portal tracts. (HPS, original magnification × 370)

sive hepatic necrosis. Yet the reticular framework can be maintained, so if regeneration occurs, complete histologic recovery is the rule.

4.5.2 CHOLESTASIS

Occasionally acute viral hepatitis exhibits a cholestatic phase, in which the patient becomes more pruritic and jaundiced, and the enzyme pattern changes (with a fall in the aminotransferase but with an increased alkaline phosphatase value). Biliary tract disease should be ruled out. Resolution within a few weeks is the rule. This appears more commonly in hepatitis A.

4.5.3 RELAPSING (BIPHASIC) HEPATITIS

Clinically, these patients are improving, only to have a recurrence of the signs and symptoms of their hepatitis, with histology similar to that of the original attack. Resolution is almost always complete. In some cases of hepatitis B, the second phase is due to acute hepatitis D. Hepatitis C is characterized by continued and wide fluctuations in liver aminotransferase values.

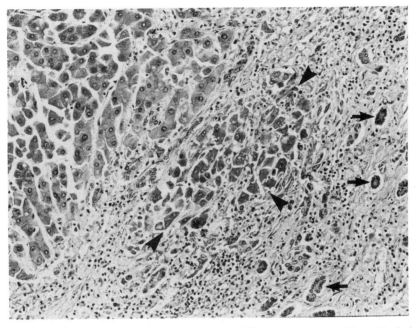

FIGURE 9. Submassive necrosis. High power shows viable hepatocytes on the left, an island of degenerating cells centrally (arrowheads) and residual bile ducts (arrows) in the widened portal tract. (HPS, original magnification × 185)

4.5.4 IMMUNE COMPLEX DISEASE

In hepatitis B, about 5–10% of cases initially develop a serum-sickness–like syndrome (characterized by skin rash, angioedema and arthritis), which is due to circulating immune complexes of viral particles and complement activation. Other immunologic manifestations result from the immunologic response by the host, including pericarditis, aplastic anemia or neurologic abnormalities such as Guillain-Barré syndrome. Chronic hepatitis B may have persisting circulating complex disease and lead to such diseases as proliferative glomerulonephritis with nephrotic syndrome and polyarteritis nodosa.

4.5.5 HEPATITIS B CARRIER STATE

Hepatitis B surface antigen persists in the blood beyond six months in most infected newborns (90%), but only in a minority of adult patients, except for homosexuals (10%) (Figure 4). Persistence of HB_sAg indicates chronic infection. A higher degree of infectivity is indicated by HB_eAg also being present. There are also mutant hepatitis B viruses, which do not produce HB_eAg but are otherwise infectious. Chronic carriers have a higher risk of eventually developing cirrhosis and hepatocellular carcinoma.

4.5.6 *CHRONIC HEPATITIS*
Chronic hepatitis represents continued disease activity beyond six months. This complicates hepatitis B in up to 10% of adult cases and hepatitis C in up to 50%. It does not occur in hepatitis A or E. Chronic hepatitis is suspect if there is persistent symptomatology without resolution, if there are persisting biochemical abnormalities such as increased serum aminotransferase levels after six months, or with the persistence of HB_sAg and HB_eAg (see Section 5).

4.6 Treatment
Most cases of acute viral hepatitis resolve spontaneously and require no specific treatment. Strict bed rest is not necessary. The patient may undertake any activity that does not exacerbate symptoms. Diet can be liberal, encouraging a high calorie intake but excluding alcohol. Hospitalization is not necessary except in cases of uncertain diagnosis or worsening disease, or for socioeconomic reasons. All drugs, especially tranquilizers and sedatives, should be avoided. Corticosteroids do not alter the degree of hepatitis or rate of healing and should be avoided to allow a normal immunologic response, which then can eliminate the virus. Indeed, their use in acute viral hepatitis may increase the risk of a chronic carrier state. Return to work and activity should be guided by the patient's symptoms. Mild elevation of liver enzymes should not prevent mobilization. Prophylaxis should be considered for certain individuals.

4.7 Prophylaxis
Adequate control of hepatitis continues to depend on good sanitation and hygiene, along with screening of blood and blood products. It is important to remember the infectious potential of excreta early in hepatitis A. Potential sources of hepatitis B include blood transfusion, inoculation, high-risk jobs, sexual intercourse (especially in the gay population) and illicit drug use.

For hepatitis A, an attack of hepatitis confers lifelong immunity. A hepatitis A vaccine has been developed, with its use directed mainly at high-risk individuals such as those traveling to areas where the disease is endemic or those working or residing in institutions. Pooled immune serum globulin (ISG) is also available. This should be provided to all household contacts, and is optimally given within one week of exposure at a dose of 0.02 mL/kg IM. Casual school or work contacts are not usually treated prophylactically unless an epidemic is identified. Pre-exposure prophylaxis is used when a susceptible individual (anti-HAV negative) is traveling to an endemic area.

In contrast, hepatitis B has a specific globulin preparation and a vaccine. Hepatitis B immunoglobulin (HBIG) should be given when there has been a clear-cut exposure to an individual who is susceptible, such as inadvertent "needlestick" or nonrecurring sexual contacts. It also should be given, along with hepatitis B vaccine, within 24 to 48 hours to neonates of mothers with acute or chronic hepatitis B. Hepatitis B vaccine, originally manufactured from pooled donor sera, is now synthesized from recombinant DNA. Side effects are minimal with both forms. Several high-risk groups are candidates for the vaccine, including homosexuals, health-care workers, IV drug users, family contacts of chronic carriers, chronic transfusion recipients and dialysis patients. Universal vaccination of all newborns is currently being considered.

There is no vaccine or specific immunoglobulin available for hepatitis C. Pooled gamma globulin may reduce post-transfusion hepatitis C and thus it is reasonable to give following likely exposure such as needlestick, sexual contact with an infected person or transfusion from a known case of hepatitis C.

The value of pooled gamma globulin in the prevention of hepatitis E is uncertain.

5. CHRONIC HEPATITIS / G. Minuk

The term *chronic hepatitis* means active, continuing inflammation of the liver persisting for more than six months that is detectable by biochemical and/or histologic means. It does not imply an etiology. The inflammatory component of chronic hepatitis is manifest by an increase in serum aminotransferase values (AST and ALT) with minimal elevation in cholestatic enzymes (alkaline phosphatase and γ-glutamyl transpeptidase). When the inflammation is severe and/or prolonged, hepatic dysfunction may become apparent with an increase in serum conjugated bilirubin, prothrombin time, and/or a decrease in albumin. Typically, biochemical tests are used to identify and follow patients with chronic hepatitis, while liver biopsies serve to define more precisely the nature of the chronic hepatitis and provide useful information regarding the extent of damage and prognosis.

Three general histologic categories of chronic hepatitis are commonly recognized: nonspecific chronic hepatitis (NSCH), chronic persistent hepatitis (CPH) and chronic active hepatitis (CAH). In NSCH there is a mild increase in the number of inflammatory cells present within the portal tracts and sinusoids of the liver. Hepatocyte necrosis is limited and often confined to zone 1 of the liver lobule. Chronic persistent hepatitis is slightly more severe than

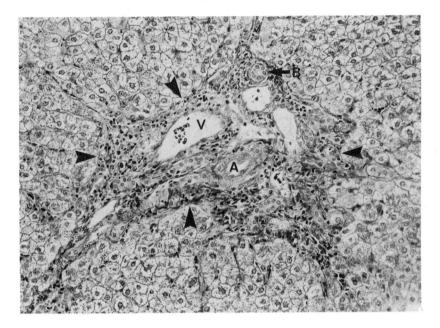

FIGURE 10.   Chronic persistent hepatitis. This portal tract contains a chronic inflammatory infiltrate that is confined to the portal tract and does not extend past the limiting plate. V, vein; A, artery; B, bile duct. (Masson, original magnification × 185)

nonspecific chronic hepatitis. It is characterized by chronic inflammation that is confined to the portal tracts without disruption of the limiting plate that lies between hepatocytes and the portal tract (Figure 10). Both NSCH and CPH are considered benign disorders. They are usually associated with normal or only mildly abnormal serum aminotransferase values and normal liver function tests, and rarely progress to fibrosis or cirrhosis. Chronic active hepatitis is considered a more serious histologic finding than either NSCH or CPH. In CAH lymphocytic and plasma cell infiltration of the portal tracts extends into the liver lobule, causing piecemeal necrosis with erosion of the limiting plate (Figure 11). When the inflammatory process extends from the portal tract to the central vein or adjacent portal tract, then "bridging" is said to be present (portal–central or portal–portal). CAH with bridging necrosis often leads to fibrosis and cirrhosis. A fourth category, called chronic lobular hepatitis, is occasionally identified. Histologically, inflammation and hepatocyte necrosis are seen throughout the liver lobule, but without portal tract involvement. This condition is thought to represent a slow resolution of acute hepatitis and is rarely associated with serious sequelae.

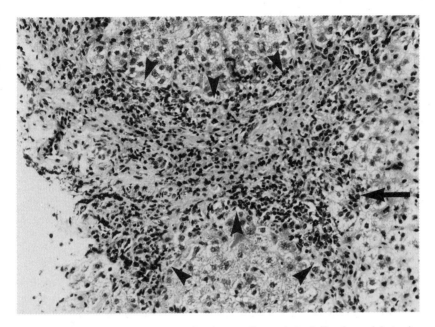

FIGURE 11. Chronic active hepatitis. Inflammatory cells are shown infiltrating and destroying the periportal hepatocytes (arrow) and disrupting the limiting plate (piecemeal necrosis) (arrowheads). (HPS, original magnification × 185)

The three most common causes of chronic hepatitis are viral infections of the liver, drug-induced liver disease and nonalcoholic hepatosteatonecrosis (fatty liver). Other causes include autoimmune chronic active hepatitis ("lupoid hepatitis"), hemochromatosis, Wilson's disease and α_1-antitrypsin deficiency.

5.1 Chronic Viral Hepatitis

5.1.1 GENERAL CONSIDERATIONS
Of the viral infections of the liver, HBV, HCV, HDV and HGV are known to cause chronic liver disease. HFV has not yet been identified, but the term has been reserved for those cases of non-A non-B hepatitis in which anti-HCV results are negative. If a distinct non-HCV virus is responsible for the illness in these patients, then presumably it too is capable of causing chronic liver disease. Epidemiologically, HBV and HCV are the most common causes of chronic viral hepatitis in North America today.

5.1.2 HEPATITIS B VIRUS

5.1.2.1 Evolution to chronic liver disease

There are a number of factors that determine whether an individual will clear an acute HBV infection or progress to a chronic carrier state. Of these, the age at infection is particularly important, with carrier rates of greater than 90% occurring in infected newborns as compared to 5–10% in adults. The immunologic status of the host is also important, with immunocompromised individuals being more likely to become chronic carriers. The severity of the acute disease also correlates with outcome. In general, the milder the acute illness the more likely that it will progress to chronic liver disease. Presumably, individuals with mild acute disease are those with a suboptimal immunologic response to the virus, whereas patients with more severe acute disease are manifesting a prompt and effective immunologic attack on hepatocytes harboring HBV.

5.1.2.2 Presentation

Aside from mild fatigue the majority of patients with chronic type B hepatitis are asymptomatic. During the first 7 to 10 years of their carrier state it is the fatigue or liver enzyme abnormalities that usually attract the attention of the physician to the underlying infection. Beyond 10 years the patient often becomes asymptomatic and liver enzyme tests normalize. During this phase of the illness it is usually a positive hepatitis B surface antigen (HB_sAg) identified at screening that leads to the diagnosis.

5.1.2.3 Diagnosis

By definition, a patient is not a chronic HBV carrier until the HB_sAg test is found to be positive on two testings a minimum of six months apart, or positive when the IgM anti-HB_c is negative. It is important not to be confused by other viral markers of hepatitis B infection. Antibody to HB_sAg (anti-HB_s) usually indicates immunity against HBV, although 30% of chronic carriers will have a transiently positive anti-HB_s during their carrier state that does not reflect immunity. The HB_eAg, HBV-DNA and DNA polymerase findings merely document the amount of virus present in the circulation. When they are strongly positive there is a high viral load, which indicates a high degree of infectivity (all physiologic fluids are potentially infectious), whereas when they are negative or anti-HB_e positive, only blood need be considered potentially infectious to others. Antibodies to the core antigen (anti-HB_c) indicate exposure to the virus. In chronic HBV infection the anti-HB_c is positive but the IgM anti-HB_c is negative, because exposure took place more than six months previously.

5.1.2.4 *Natural history*

The natural history of chronic HBV infection has been well defined. The first six months of the illness represent the acute hepatitis phase of the infection. Thereafter, patients enter the second phase which, based on presence of symptoms and liver enzyme abnormalities, is referred to as the chronic hepatitis phase of the illness. During this period, serologic markers of viral replication (HB_eAg, HBV-DNA and DNA polymerase) are positive and the liver biopsy will have evidence of nonspecific chronic hepatitis, chronic persistent hepatitis or chronic active hepatitis. When present, it is the severity and duration of the chronic active hepatitis in this second phase of the illness that determines whether a patient will end up with cirrhosis. Fortunately, only 20% of patients will progress to cirrhosis. Once the symptoms have resolved, the enzymes have returned to normal and the markers of viral replication have become negative, the patient enters the third phase of the illness, often referred to as the healthy carrier phase. On liver biopsy, a healthy carrier usually has only minor, nonspecific changes or perhaps inactive cirrhosis. The healthy carrier phase is somewhat of a misnomer in that it is during this phase that the complications of cirrhosis and/or hepatocellular carcinoma may arise. The risk of developing hepatocellular carcinoma in chronic HBV carriers is between 200 and 300 times normal, significantly higher than for a chronic smoker developing lung cancer.

5.1.2.5 *Treatment*

There are a number of therapeutic options for the treatment of patients with chronic type B hepatitis. These can be categorized into immunologic approaches, antiviral therapy, cytokines, nucleoside analogues and combination therapy. Of these, only the antiviral agent recombinant interferon has been licensed for use. In most studies, approximately 40% of chronic HBV carriers treated in the chronic hepatitis phase of their illness successfully respond to interferon treatment with a loss of all serologic markers of viral replication (HB_eAg and HBV-DNA moving from positive to negative). Ten percent of these responders will also lose all evidence of infection (seroconverting from HB_sAg positive to negative) during treatment and 50% will become HB_sAg negative during the first five years of follow-up. The relapse rate following discontinuation of therapy is less than 15%.

Given that the majority of patients do not initially respond to interferon therapy, an important question that remains to be resolved is which patients warrant a trial of therapy. Although no firm guidelines exist at present, an argument can be made for treating patients who are markedly symptomatic and incapable of carrying on their employment and/or household responsibilities. Patients who have a high risk of progressing to cirrhosis, such as those with aminotransferase values greater than 2.5 times the upper limit of normal and histologic evidence of severe CAH or early cirrhosis, also warrant consideration for treatment. Of these patients one can predict those most likely to respond. They include patients who acquired their infection during adulthood; females; patients with high pretherapy ALT and low HBV-RNA levels; patients with active histologic disease; those who are HIV antibody negative; those with a heterosexual lifestyle; and patients who are anti-HDV negative.

5.1.2.6 Prevention

The need for immunoprophylaxis to prevent transmission of HBV infection from a chronic carrier is less clear-cut than in the case of acute HBV infection. The argument could be made that if a long-term sexual partner has not acquired the HBV infection from the index case over the course of many years of exposure then it is unlikely that transmission will occur in the future, and therefore immunoprophylaxis with HBIG and/or the HBV vaccine or the use of condoms need not be advocated. The counterargument is that the adverse effects of HBV infection can be so devastating and the safety of the vaccine is so well established that vaccination of susceptible sexual contacts should be offered, at a minimum. For susceptible children living in the house it seems reasonable to suggest both HBIG plus vaccination when the index case is HB_sAg and HB_eAg positive; vaccine alone might be all that is required when the index case is HB_sAg positive but HB_eAg negative.

5.1.3 HEPATITIS C VIRUS

Using sophisticated molecular biological techniques, workers recently identified the hepatitis C virus as the cause of at least 80% of what had been previously referred to as non-A non-B hepatitis. The hepatitis C virus has some genetic homology to pestiviruses.

Currently available for diagnosis are the ELISA and RIBA tests, which detect antibodies to structural and nonstructural epitopes of the virus. Testing is useful in chronic HCV infection, where approximately 90% of infected individuals are positive for this nonprotective antibody.

5.1.3.1 Natural history

The natural history of HCV infection has been better defined with the availability of anti-HCV serologic testing. Widespread application of this test has revealed that approximately 50–60% of patients with acute HCV infection will go on to a chronic carrier state. Of the chronic carriers, 40% will have histologic evidence of CAH and 20% either have or will go on to develop cirrhosis. The mean time to the development of cirrhosis is 20 years. Of much concern is the fact that recent data document an association between chronic HCV infection and hepatocellular carcinoma. The exact relative risk has yet to be determined but appears to be as high as that for HBV and hepatocellular carcinoma. Other disorders that have been described in association with chronic HCV infection are serum-sickness–like illnesses, cryoglobulinemia and porphyria cutanea tarda.

5.1.3.2 Epidemiology

Although HCV infection can be transmitted by the same routes as HBV infection, the majority of cases in which a source of infection has been identified are related to intravenous drug abuse (40% of all cases). Ten percent of patients with chronic HCV infection will have had a history of a previous blood transfusion. The remaining one-half of all patients cannot identify a possible source of infection. Of note is that nonparenteral transmission through sexual or intimate contact and maternal–infant exposure can occur with HCV infection, but much less often than is the case for HBV infection. Transmission through these routes appears to be most likely during the acute phase of the illness in the index case or for a longer period of time in patients who are immunocompromised.

5.1.3.3 Treatment

Recombinant interferon represents the most effective form of therapy available for chronic HCV infection. Numerous studies have identified a 50% response rate (normalization of ALT abnormalities). However, 50% of these responders will relapse, with the majority of relapses occurring within three months of discontinuation of therapy. As is the case for HBV infection, there are no strict guidelines for who should receive interferon treatment for chronic HCV infection. Severely symptomatic patients and those with significant aminotransferase abnormalities and histologic evidence of progression to cirrhosis are the most likely candidates. Unlike those with hepatitis B, subpopulations within this group who are likely to respond have not yet been identified. At the present time, there are insufficient data to advocate the use of immune serum globulin for the prevention of HCV infection, and a vaccine for this virus has not been developed. Condoms should be used during the acute phase of the illness and indefinitely by patients who are immunocompromised.

5.1.4 HEPATITIS D VIRUS

The hepatitis D virus cannot infect the liver in the absence of a HBV infection. Thus, patients can acquire HDV by simultaneous infection with both HBV and HDV, or more commonly when HDV superinfects a chronic HBV carrier.

HDV is cytopathic, often causing fulminant hepatic failure or a rapid progression to cirrhosis, which occurs in 65% of patients with chronic HDV. The annual mortality rate associated with chronic HDV is 1–3%. The diagnosis is most easily made by testing for anti-HDV in the serum; this is present with both acute and chronic HDV infections. HDV antigen and HDV-RNA in serum or liver can also be documented, but only in a limited number of laboratories. In North America this virus is most often transmitted by intravenous drug abuse; in Mediterranean countries nonparenteral transmission may also occur. To date, treatment with interferon for HDV infection has been disappointing. Passive and active immunization against HDV are not yet available.

5.2 Drug-Induced Chronic Hepatitis

Many drugs can cause chronic hepatitis. Whether to discontinue the implicated drug depends to some extent on whether the drug is merely causing persistent enzyme abnormalities or is causing hepatic dysfunction with severe histologic abnormalities. The latter justifies discontinuing the drug, because fibrosis, cirrhosis and death from liver failure or complications of portal hypertension can result. Examples of drugs that are capable of causing liver failure and portal hypertension are oxyphenasitin, isoniazid, nitrofurantoin, alpha methyldopa and dantrolene. On the other hand, if the drug is essential to the health of the patient and there are no unrelated agents that can be substituted, it is reasonable to continue therapy under close clinical supervision as long as the enzyme abnormalities are mild and not associated with symptoms or functional derangements.

5.3 Fatty Liver

Nonalcoholic hepatosteatonecrosis (fatty liver) is a common disorder where symptoms are limited to right upper quadrant discomfort and liver enzyme abnormalities are typically less than 3–4 times normal. The condition tends to occur in patients who are obese, diabetic and, occasionally, hyperlipidemic. Although it was initially considered to be a benign condition, more recent studies suggest that fatty liver can progress to cirrhosis in approximately 10–20% of cases. The diagnosis is easily established by ultrasound (or CT) examination of the liver or histologically where macrovesicular fat is seen. The treatment is that of the underlying condition – weight loss, or correction of the diabetes and/or hyperlipidemia.

5.4 Autoimmune Chronic Active Hepatitis

Autoimmune chronic active hepatitis (A-CAH or lupoid hepatitis) is an immunologically mediated disorder of the liver that often affects young females with a past history or family history of connective tissue diseases or atopic problems such as asthma, hay fever, eczema, etc. This condition differs from classical systemic lupus erythematosus (SLE) with hepatic involvement in that vital organ involvement (CNS, heart) is uncommon. The most common presentation is a young female, with 50% presenting in teenage years. Complaints – which may be fatigue or amenorrhea, or those complaints associated with the accompanying disorders such as arthritis, skin rash, Raynaud's, etc. – often underestimate the severity of the underlying liver lesion. The hepatic presentation can be that of fulminant hepatic failure, acute hepatitis, chronic hepatitis or inactive cirrhosis. Physical findings typically include a large number of spider nevi, hepatosplenomegaly, palmar erythema and those associated with the accompanying disorders. Laboratory investigations reveal pancytopenia, elevated transaminase (>5–10 times normal), polyclonal hypergammaglobulinemia, hypocomplementemia, positive antinuclear factor and antismooth muscle antibody, and HLA-B8 and HLA-Dr3 positivity. Hepatitis B and C serology is typically negative. Liver biopsy is essential to define the diagnosis and severity of the underlying disease. Cirrhosis is present in one-third of cases early in the course.

The decision to treat the underlying liver process is dependent on the presence of symptoms, the extent of the biochemical abnormalities and the severity of the underlying histologic lesion. Particular benefit is seen in the first two years, especially if there is evidence for severe bridging necrosis but without underlying cirrhosis. Treatment is initiated with high-dose corticosteroids (prednisone 40–60 mg/day). The dose is rapidly tapered to a maintenance level just sufficient to keep the liver enzymes within normal values. Often azathioprine is required for its steroid-sparing effect. Following discontinuation of treatment, 50% of patients will relapse, requiring reinitiation of therapy. Untreated A-CAH progresses rapidly to cirrhosis (within 3 to 5 years). In contrast, treatment delays progression (between 15 and 20 years). Ultimately, a liver transplant is often required.

6. ALCOHOLIC LIVER DISEASE / F. Wong and L. Blendis

Liver disease is the fourth commonest cause of death in adults between the ages of 20 and 70 years in Canada. Alcohol is still the commonest cause of chronic liver disease in this country. Not all those who abuse alcohol develop liver damage: the incidence of cirrhosis among alcoholics is approximately 10–30%. The mechanism for the predisposition of certain people to develop cirrhosis is still unknown. The amount of alcohol ingested has been shown in epidemiological studies to be the most important factor in determining the development of cirrhosis. Males drinking in excess of 80 g and females in excess of 40 g of alcohol per day for 10 years are at a high risk of developing cirrhosis. The alcohol content rather than the type of beverage is important, and binge drinking is less injurious to the liver than continued daily drinking.

Women are more susceptible to liver damage than men. They are likely to develop cirrhosis at an earlier age, present at a later stage and have more severe liver disease with more complications. Genetics may play a role in the development of alcoholic liver disease, although no single genetic marker has been identified. Patterns of alcohol drinking behavior are inherited. Genetic pleomorphism of the enzyme systems that metabolize alcohol, leading to different rates of alcohol elimination, also contributes to the individual's susceptibility to alcohol damage. Malnutrition may play a permissive role in producing alcohol hepatotoxicity. However, there is a threshold of alcohol toxicity beyond which no dietary supplements can offer protection.

The spectrum of liver disease covers the relatively benign steatosis to the potentially fatal alcoholic hepatitis and cirrhosis.

6.1 Alcoholic Fatty Liver

Fatty liver is the most frequent hepatic abnormality found in alcoholics. It is a toxic manifestation of ethanol ingestion, appearing within three to seven days of excess alcohol intake. Metabolic changes associated with ethanol ingestion result in increased triglyceride synthesis, decreased lipid oxidation and impaired secretion by the liver. This results in the accumulation of triglycerides in the hepatocytes, mainly in the terminal hepatic venular zone. In more severe cases, the fatty change may be diffuse. The fat tends to accumulate as macrovesicular (large droplets), rather than microvesicular (small droplets), which represents mitochondrial damage. Fatty liver may occur alone or be part of the picture of alcoholic hepatitis or cirrhosis.

Clinically, the patient is usually asymptomatic, and the examination reveals a firm, smooth, enlarged liver. Occasionally the fatty liver may be so severe that the patient is anorexic and nauseated, and has right upper quadrant pain or discomfort. This usually follows a prolonged heavy alcoholic binge. Liver function tests are frequently normal, although the γ-glutamyl transpeptidase (GGT) is invariably elevated while the aminotransferases and alkaline phosphatase may be slightly increased. The patient is never jaundiced, and hepatic synthetic function (albumin and prothrombin time) is preserved. A fatty liver is usually detected by ultrasound. Liver biopsy is required to make a definitive diagnosis. When fatty liver is not associated with alcoholic hepatitis, its prognosis is excellent. Complete abstinence from alcohol and a nutritious diet will lead to disappearance of the fat over four to six weeks.

6.2 Alcoholic Hepatitis

Alcoholic hepatitis may occur separately or in combination with cirrhosis. There are all grades of severity. It is a condition characterized by liver cell necrosis and inflammatory reaction. Histologically, hepatocytes are swollen as a result of an increase in intracellular water secondary to increase in cytosolic proteins. Steatosis, often of the macrovesicular type, is present. Alcoholic hyaline (Mallory's) bodies are purplish red intracytoplasmic inclusions consisting of clumped organelles and intermediate microfilaments. Polymorphs are seen surrounding Mallory's-containing cells and also within damaged hepatocytes. Collagen deposition is usually present. It is maximal in the zone 3 and extends in a perisinusoidal pattern to enclose hepatocytes, giving it a "chicken wiring" effect. Changes in the portal triad are inconspicuous. Marked portal inflammation suggests an associated viral hepatitis such as hepatitis C, whereas fibrosis suggests complicating chronic hepatitis. When the acute inflammation settles, a varying degree of fibrosis is seen, which may eventually lead to cirrhosis.

Clinically, mild cases of alcoholic hepatitis are recognized on liver biopsy only in patients who present with a history of alcohol abuse and abnormal liver function tests. In the moderately severe case, the patient is usually malnourished and presents with a two- to three-week prodrome of fatigue, anorexia, nausea and weight loss. Clinical signs include a fever of <40°C, jaundice and tender hepatomegaly. There may be a bruit over the liver. In the most severe case, which usually follows a period of heavy drinking without eating, the patient is gravely ill with fever, marked jaundice, ascites, and evidence of a hyperdynamic circulation such as systemic hypotension and tachycardia. Florid palmar erythema and spider nevi are present, with or without gynecomastia. Hepatic decompensation can be precipitated by vomiting, diarrhea or intercurrent infection leading to encephalopathy. Hypoglycemia occurs often and can precipitate coma. Gastrointestinal bleeding is common, usually from a local gastric or duodenal lesion, resulting from the combination of a bleeding tendency and portal hypertension. Signs of malnutrition and vitamin deficiencies are common. Intake of moderate doses of acetaminophen in an alcoholic may precipitate florid alcoholic hepatitis.

Laboratory abnormalities include elevations of the aminotransferases, bilirubin, alkaline phosphatase and GGT. The aminotransferase levels rarely exceed 300 IU/L, except in association with acetaminophen ingestion; the

AST/ALT ratio is >2. Hyperbilirubinemia can be quite marked, with levels reaching 300 to 500 μmol/L, and is a reflection of the severity of the illness. The increase in GGT is proportionally greater than that of alkaline phosphatase. There is also leukocytosis of up to 20–25 × 10^9/L and prolongation of the prothrombin time, which does not respond to vitamin K. The serum albumin falls. Serum IgA is markedly increased, with IgG and IgM raised to a lesser extent.

Patients with acute alcoholic hepatitis often deteriorate during the first few weeks in hospital, with a mortality rate of 20–50%. Bad prognostic indicators include spontaneous encephalopathy, markedly prolonged prothrombin time unresponsive to vitamin K and severe hyperbilirubinemia of greater than 350 μmol/L. The condition may take one to six months to resolve, even with complete abstinence. Alcoholic hepatitis progresses to cirrhosis in 25–30% of clinical episodes.

6.3 Alcoholic Cirrhosis

Established cirrhosis is usually a disease of middle age after the patient has had many years of drinking. Although there may be a history of alcoholic hepatitis, cirrhosis can develop in apparently well-nourished, asymptomatic patients. Occasionally the patient may present with end-stage liver disease with malnutrition, ascites, encephalopathy and a bleeding tendency. A history of alcohol abuse usually points to the etiology. Clinically, the patient is wasted. There may be bilateral parotid enlargement, palmar erythema, Dupuytren's contracture and multiple spider nevi. Males develop gynecomastia and small testes. Hepatomegaly is often present, affecting predominantly the left lobe as a result of marked hypertrophy. There may be signs of portal hypertension, which include splenomegaly, ascites and distended abdominal wall veins. At the late stage, the liver may become shrunken and impalpable. There may be signs of alcohol damage in other organ systems, such as peripheral neuropathy and memory loss from cerebral atrophy. Alcoholic cirrhosis is also associated with renal problems, including IgA nephropathy, renal tubular acidosis and the development of hepatorenal syndrome. There is an association between hepatitis B and C and alcoholic cirrhosis.

Histologically, the cirrhosis is micronodular. The degree of steatosis is variable and alcoholic hepatitis may or may not be present. Pericellular fibrosis around hepatocytes is widespread. Portal fibrosis contributes to the development of portal hypertension. There may be increased parenchymal iron deposition. When parenchymal iron deposition is marked, genetic hemochromatosis has to be excluded. With continued cell necrosis and regeneration, the cirrhosis may progress to a macronodular pattern.

Biochemical abnormalities include a low serum albumin, and elevated bilirubin and aminotransferases. AST and ALT levels rarely exceed 300 IU/L and the AST/ALT ratio usually exceeds 2. GGT is disproportionately raised with recent alcohol ingestion and is a widely used screening test for alcohol abuse. With severe disease, the prothrombin time may be prolonged. Portal hypertension results in hypersplenism leading to thrombocytopenia, anemia and leukopenia. Other nonspecific serum changes in acute and chronic alcoholics include elevations in uric acid, lactate and triglyceride, and reductions in glucose and magnesium.

The prognosis of alcoholic cirrhosis depends on whether the patient can abstain from alcohol; this in turn is related to family support, financial resources and socioeconomic state. Patients who abstain have a five-year survival rate of 60–70%, which falls to 40% in those who continue to drink. Women have a shorter survival rate than men. Bad prognostic indicators include a low serum albumin, increased prothrombin time, low hemoglobin, encephalopathy, persistent jaundice and azotemia. Zone 3 fibrosis and perivenular sclerosis are also unfavorable features. Complete abstinence may not improve prognosis when portal hypertension is severe. Hepatocellular carcinoma occurs in 10% of stable cirrhotics. This usually develops after a period of abstinence when macronodular cirrhosis is present. It is usually fatal in six months.

6.4 Management

Early recognition of alcoholism is important. Physicians should have a high index of suspicion when a patient presents with anorexia, nausea, diarrhea, right upper quadrant tenderness and an elevated GGT. The most important therapeutic measure is total abstinence from alcohol. Support groups and regular follow-up can reinforce the need for abstinence. Withdrawal symptoms should be treated with chlordiazepoxide or diazepam. A nutritious, well-balanced diet with vitamin supplements should be instituted.

Alcoholic fatty liver responds to alcohol withdrawal and a nutritious diet. Patients with severe alcoholic hepatitis should be admitted to hospital and complications of liver failure treated appropriately. Specific treatments for alcoholic hepatitis include the use of corticosteroids. A recent meta-analysis of 11 controlled trials showed a significant benefit of steroids for patients with severe alcoholic hepatitis complicated by encephalopathy. Propylthiouracil has been used to dampen the hepatic hypermetabolic state in alcoholic hepatitis, and may reduce the two-year mortality rate. Testosterone and anabolic androgenic steroids have been tried with conflicting results. Intravenous amino acid supplements have been given to the severely protein malnourished with varying degrees of success. Oral supplementation is the preferred route if the patient can tolerate a diet.

Cirrhosis is an irreversible process, and therapy is directed at the complications of liver failure and portal hypertension, although colchicine has been used as an antifibrotic agent without much success. Portacaval shunts will reduce the risk of bleeding from esophageal varices, but the establishment of a shunt is associated with a 30% incidence of hepatic encephalopathy. Hepatic transplantation is a treatment option for patients with end-stage alcoholic cirrhosis, although the ethical issues surrounding the use of such a scarce resource for a self-inflicted disease still need to be settled. In the centers that transplant in cases of alcoholic cirrhosis, the results are comparable to those in patients with other forms of cirrhosis.

7. DRUG-INDUCED LIVER DISEASE / J. Simon

Drugs are an important and common cause of hepatic injury. This is not surprising, as the liver is the predominant site of drug clearance, biotransformation and excretion. Abnormalities cover a wide spectrum from minor nonspecific derangements to fulminant hepatic necrosis. Most common, however, is either acute inflammation or cholestasis, which can closely mimic viral hepatitis and biliary obstruction, respectively. Various other acute and chronic disease patterns also occur (as noted below). Thus drug-induced liver disease is complex, has protean manifestations, and can simulate a wide variety of other hepatic disorders.

The pathogenesis varies with the offending agent, and in most cases is poorly understood. Sometimes the drug or one of its metabolites exerts a direct toxic effect on liver membranes. This type of injury is predictable and dose-related, but is relatively infrequent. Much more commonly, the injury occurs unpredictably in only a tiny fraction of individuals receiving the drug and is independent of dosage. In some such instances genetic predisposition or idiosyncratic metabolism of the drug may be responsible. Immune hypersensitivity is often invoked, but only a minority of cases have concomitant evidence of an allergic reaction such as a rash, arthralgias or eosinophilia. Many instances of putative hypersensitivity may actually be due to toxic intermediate drug metabolites in rarely susceptible individuals. In most situations the reasons for individual susceptibility are unknown, and the precise pathogenesis of the hepatic injury is equally obscure.

Diagnosis requires first and foremost a careful history of drug ingestion, including over-the-counter and illicit agents as well as prescribed medications. A temporal association is also important in cases of acute dysfunction: injury

TABLE 6. Drug-induced liver disease

Type and example	Pathogenesis
Acute hepatocellular injury	
Toxic necrosis (e.g., CCl_4, acetaminophen)	Membrane damage, some via toxic metabolite; dose-related, predictable
Hepatitis-like (e.g., isoniazid, methyldopa)	Idiosyncrasy; ? immune, ? metabolic; unpredictable, not dose-related
Cholestasis	
Inflammatory (e.g., chlorpromazine)	Unknown; unpredictable; periportal inflammation and cholestasis
Pure (e.g., oral contraceptives)	Exaggeration of normal hormonal effect on bile transport; ? genetic idiosyncrasy; pure cholestasis, no inflammation
Miscellaneous acute/subacute	Variable, usually unknown
Chronic liver disease	
Chronic active hepatitis (e.g., isoniazid, methyldopa)	Idiosyncrasy; ? immune, ? metabolic
Chronic cholestasis (e.g., chlorpromazine)	Unknown; rare
Fibrosis/cirrhosis (e.g., methotrexate)	Dose-related, insidious toxic metabolic damage
Tumor: adenomas (oral contraceptives)	Unknown

typically develops within days or a few weeks of starting the drug. Other reactions involve chronic insidious injury and therefore require prolonged drug exposure – e.g., methotrexate fibrosis and oral contraceptive–induced adenomas. Liver biopsy sometimes provides an important clue to certain drug injuries, but more commonly the histologic pattern is nonspecific and/or mimics other primary liver disorders. Thus in many cases the diagnosis of drug injury remains uncertain or unproven even after appropriate patient assessment.

The prognosis is variable. Acute damage usually resolves when the offending agent is withdrawn, but cases of severe acute necrosis can be fatal or result in postnecrotic scarring. In cases of chronic injury, further hepatocellular damage and inflammation will generally cease when the drug is stopped, but any concomitant fibrosis will be irreversible.

No physician can know the innumerable drugs capable of producing liver injury. Rather, it is best to maintain a constant awareness of the possibility, to understand the general types of damage, and to learn the most common agents responsible for each. Table 6 gives an arbitrary classification and examples of drug-induced hepatic injury. A few of the more important examples are briefly discussed below.

7.1 Acute Hepatocellular Injury

This takes at least two distinct forms, both characterized clinically and biochemically by features of acute liver cell destruction.

7.1.1 TOXIC NECROSIS

This involves direct membrane damage by the parent drug or a toxic metabolite. It is therefore dose-related and a predictable occurrence in anyone ingesting a sufficient quantity of the drug. Sometimes the histologic injury is characteristic – e.g., zonal necrosis and fat in carbon tetrachloride toxicity.

Acetaminophen is the most important example. This widely used analgesic is largely excreted as harmless conjugates, but a portion is transformed by hepatic microsomes to toxic intermediate metabolites. Normally these are safely eliminated by conjugation with hepatic glutathione, but a large enough dose of acetaminophen will deplete the available glutathione stores. Once this occurs, cell necrosis results from binding of the toxic intermediates to liver macromolecules. The threshold injurious dose of acetaminophen is usually about 10–15 g acutely; this is far beyond the normal dosage and is generally ingested only in suicide attempts. Alcoholics are susceptible at much lower dosage, however, as a result of heightened microsomal transformation. Acetaminophen should be suspect in an alcoholic with extremely high AST/ALT levels, as values rarely exceed 300 IU in uncomplicated alcoholic hepatitis.

Acetaminophen hepatotoxicity typically becomes apparent only 36 to 48 hours after ingestion; by then it is too late to modify the process. Fortunately, injury is successfully aborted by early therapy with N-acetylcysteine, which repletes hepatic glutathione levels. This should be given within 10 to 16 hours of acetaminophen ingestion to be effective. To guide therapy, nomograms are available relating the probability of liver injury to blood acetaminophen levels and to the amount of time since ingestion.

7.1.2 ACUTE HEPATITIS

This pattern of injury closely mimics acute viral hepatitis clinically, biochemically and histologically. Unlike toxic necrosis, it occurs unpredictably, is not dose-related and affects only rare individuals exposed to the drug. Reasons for the idiosyncratic susceptibility are obscure. Numerous agents can produce this injury pattern; methyldopa, isoniazid and halothane are classic examples, the latter usually producing damage only after repeated exposure to the anesthetic. Acute isoniazid hepatitis occasionally develops only after several months of drug therapy. This is an exception to the general rule of a temporal relationship, and the association may therefore be overlooked.

7.2 Cholestasis
This type of reaction also takes at least two distinct forms.

7.2.1 *INFLAMMATORY TYPE*
Chlorpromazine, other phenothiazines and many other drugs can produce an acute periportal necro-inflammatory reaction. This is characterized clinically and biochemically by a predominant cholestatic disorder with variable features of concomitant inflammation. Differentiation from extrahepatic biliary obstruction is usually required.

7.2.2 *PURE TYPE*
Certain steroid hormonal drugs, most notably oral contraceptives and methyltestosterone, can produce relatively pure impairment of bile flow with little or no associated hepatocellular injury (bland cholestasis). This appears to be due to an idiosyncratic exaggeration of the physiologic effect of sex hormones on bile canalicular transport, and may have a genetic component. The patient typically develops insidiously progressive pruritus, dark urine, and jaundice without associated systemic symptoms. Laboratory tests show high ALP with normal or minimally elevated AST/ALT levels. The liver biopsy is usually unremarkable aside from histologic cholestasis. Women who develop this reaction to oral contraceptives are predisposed to cholestasis of pregnancy, which appears similar or identical in pathogenesis (see Section 17).

Oral contraceptives are also associated with other, less common hepatobiliary effects. These are listed in Table 7.

7.3 Miscellaneous Acute and Subacute Reactions
Many hepatic drug reactions involve a variable mixture of hepatocellular and excretory impairments that do not neatly fit any of the above categories. Laboratory and histologic features are variable and nonspecific. Occasionally granulomatous inflammation occurs (e.g., with sulfonamides), often with acute systemic features. Differentiation from an infective granulomatous disorder may be challenging. A few drugs can produce an alcoholic hepatitis–like picture, including typical histologic features (e.g., amiodarone). Other unusual patterns of drug injury have also been described.

TABLE 7.   Hepatobiliary reactions to oral contraceptives

Cholestasis

Tumors
    Adenomas
    Focal nodular hyperplasia?
    Hepatocellular carcinoma (rare)

Vascular
    Budd-Chiari syndrome ($\uparrow$ clotting tendency)
    Peliosis hepatis (subclinical)

Gallstones ($\uparrow$ lithogenicity of bile)

"Unmasking" of other cholestatic disorders

7.4 Chronic Liver Disease

Though the large majority of drug-induced hepatic injury is acute or subacute, in a few reactions there is an insidious development of chronic disease. These vary in type.

7.4.1 CHRONIC ACTIVE HEPATITIS

A few agents that induce acute hepatitis are also capable of producing chronic inflammation if drug ingestion continues. Methyldopa and isoniazid are the prime examples. Clinically, biochemically and histologically the reaction may be indistinguishable from idiopathic or immune chronic active hepatitis. The disorder typically resolves when the drug intake ceases.

7.4.2 CHRONIC CHOLESTASIS

In rare instances chlorpromazine cholestatic injury becomes prolonged and self-perpetuating even though the drug is discontinued. This can simulate primary biliary cirrhosis, though immunologic features of the latter are lacking.

7.4.3 FIBROSIS/CIRRHOSIS

Insidiously progressive hepatic fibrosis and eventual cirrhosis can occur from methotrexate, some chemotherapeutic agents, and chronic ingestion of arsenicals or vitamin A in megadoses. Scarring typically develops subclinically and with little or no biochemical evidence of hepatic dysfunction. Liver biopsy is therefore the only way to establish the diagnosis. Patients receiving long-term methotrexate therapy for psoriasis or rheumatoid arthritis should generally undergo biopsy after cumulative drug dosage reaches about 1.5 g, and at occasional intervals thereafter.

7.4.4 *TUMORS*

Prolonged intake of oral contraceptives is associated with an increased risk of developing benign hepatic adenomas. These are usually asymptomatic but occasionally produce an acute abdomen due to intraperitoneal rupture and hemorrhage. In rare instances, oral contraceptive–induced adenomas become malignant.

Other unusual drug-related tumors are known to occur as well – e.g., angiosarcoma from chronic exposure to vinyl chloride.

8. INHERITED LIVER DISEASE / P. Adams

8.1 Hemochromatosis

Hemochromatosis is an iron-storage disorder in which there is an inappropriate increase in the absorption of iron from the gut. This leads to iron deposition in various organs with eventual impairment, especially of the liver, pancreas, heart and pituitary. This term should be distinguished from hemosiderosis, which merely describes the appearance histologically of increased stainable iron in the tissue. Hemochromatosis can be divided into inherited and acquired types. In acquired hemochromatosis, the iron overload results from iron accumulation from a hematologic condition such as thalassemia or a sideroblastic anemia.

Genetic hemochromatosis is an inherited disease known to be associated with an abnormal gene tightly linked to the A locus of the HLA complex on chromosome 6. It is one of the most common genetic diseases, inherited as an autosomal recessive trait affecting 1 in 300 of the Caucasian population. The heterozygous individual has normal or minor derangements in iron metabolism that have no clinical significance. The homozygote has continued iron accumulation leading to target organ damage. Normally the body iron content of 3–4 g is maintained such that the absorption of iron is equal to iron loss. In hemochromatosis, the absorption of iron is inappropriate to the needs of the body, resulting in the absorption of 4 mg/day or more. In advanced disease, the total body iron accumulation may be 40–60 g.

Most patients are asymptomatic until the fifth or sixth decade, at which time they may present with nonspecific symptoms of arthritis, diabetes, fatigue or hepatomegaly. Other symptoms include pigmentation of the skin (melanin deposition), impotence and dyspnea secondary to congestive heart failure. The classic triad of skin pigmentation, diabetes and liver disease ("bronze diabetes") occurs in a minority of patients and is a late stage of the disease. It more commonly affects males than females because of the regular menstrual blood loss in women.

A patient with suspected hemochromatosis or unexplained liver disease should be screened for the disease with a serum ferritin and transferrin saturation (serum iron/TIBC). The diagnosis is confirmed by a liver biopsy that demonstrates marked parenchymal iron deposition with iron staining of the tissue. The hepatic iron concentration and the hepatic iron index (hepatic iron concentration/age) are the most helpful in distinguishing genetic hemochromatosis from the increased iron overload that is seen in the alcoholic siderosis of the liver. CT and MRI scanning can detect moderate to marked iron overload in the liver but lack the sensitivity to detect early disease and do not replace the need for liver biopsy.

The treatment of hemochromatosis involves the removal of excess body iron and supportive treatment of the damaged organs. Iron is best removed from the body by weekly or twice-weekly phlebotomy of 500 mL of blood until the body iron stores are within normal limits. The duration of treatment varies with the age and sex of the patient, but older males may require weekly venesections for more than three years. Serum ferritin is measured every three months to assess progress. When the serum ferritin is in the low normal range the frequency of venesections is decreased to three or four per year. The goal of therapy is to prevent any further tissue damage. Unfortunately, many of the symptoms do not improve following iron depletion. The most common cause of death is liver failure and/or hepatocellular carcinoma. The chelating agent deferoxamine is an inefficient, expensive and potentially toxic therapy for hemochromatosis, and is reserved for the patient with iron overload secondary to an iron-loading anemia such as thalassemia. Siblings of the patient with hemochromatosis must be screened with serum ferritin and transferrin saturation, as each sibling has a 1 in 4 chance of being affected. Screening should begin in the teenage years.

8.2 Alpha$_1$-Antitrypsin Deficiency

Alpha1-antitrypsin, a glycoprotein produced by the liver, constitutes the majority of the α_1 globulin fraction seen on protein electrophoresis. Its deficiency is inherited, resulting in pulmonary emphysema and hepatic disease. Various presentations are possible, including neonatal hepatitis, chronic active hepatitis, cirrhosis and hepatocellular carcinoma.

Alpha$_1$-antitrypsin is a protease inhibitor. Its production is controlled by multiple alleles in the Pi system. Normal individuals are PiMM. The inheritance is autosomal codominant. Patients with liver disease most frequently have PiZZ and possess only 20% of the normal amount of serum α_1-antitrypsin.

Diagnosis of α_1-antitrypsin deficiency is suggested by the absence of the α_1 peak on protein electrophoresis and is confirmed by α_1-antitrypsin levels and phenotyping. The characteristic changes seen on liver biopsy include the presence of PAS-positive, diastase-resistant granules in the cytoplasm of the hepatocytes; these granules are α_1-antitrypsin collections within the endoplasmic reticulum. There is an inability to transfer synthesized α_1-antitrypsin from the cytoplasm of the hepatocyte to the serum. Cirrhosis will develop in 10–15% of patients with PiZZ. The risk to heterozygotes of developing liver disease is uncertain. There is no medical therapy for this condition. Patients with advanced forms of liver disease may be candidates for liver transplantation.

8.3 Wilson's Disease

Wilson's disease is an inherited disorder characterized by the pathological accumulation of copper in the liver, central nervous system and other organs. The disease has a prevalence of 1:30,000. It is an autosomal recessive disease; the gene responsible has been localized to the long arm of chromosome 13. It may present as pediatric liver disease or, if it manifests in adulthood, as a set of neuropsychiatric symptoms. The hepatic presentation of the disease is variable, and may include fulminant hepatic failure (often with hemolysis), chronic active hepatitis and cirrhosis. Copper deposition in the central nervous system results in extrapyramidal symptoms of rigidity, choreoathetoid movements and ataxia. Biochemical abnormalities include a low serum ceruloplasmin and high urinary copper concentration. Liver biopsy is often not diagnostic, and copper stains are unreliable. It is often necessary to measure the hepatic copper concentration. A Kayser-Fleischer ring – a copper deposition in Descemet's membrane of the cornea – is characteristic of the disease, although it can appear in other chronic cholestatic liver diseases. Visual inspection may identify the Kayser-Fleischer ring, but a detailed slit lamp examination by an ophthalmologist is recommended when the disease is suspected. The chelating agent d-penicillamine is recommended on a lifelong basis. Patients with advanced disease can be successfully cured of the disease by liver transplantation.

9. CHOLESTASIS / J. Heathcote

Cholestasis simply means failure of flow of bile. The cause of this failure can arise anywhere in the biliary system, from the liver cell down to the ampulla of Vater. For clinical purposes it is easiest to think of cholestasis as being either intra- or extrahepatic (Table 8).

9.1 Intrahepatic Cholestasis

Drug toxicity is the commonest cause of cholestasis occurring at the cellular

TABLE 8. Major causes of cholestasis

Intrahepatic
Common
   Viral hepatitis
   Drugs
   Alcoholic hepatitis ± cirrhosis
Less common
   Primary biliary cirrhosis
   Chronic hepatitis ± cirrhosis
   Metastatic carcinoma
   Cholestasis of pregnancy
   Sepsis, TPN, etc.

Extrahepatic
Common
   Common bile duct stone(s)
   Pancreatic/periampullary cancer
Less common
   Benign biliary stricture
   Sclerosing cholangitis
   Bile duct carcinoma
   Benign pancreatic disease
   Extrinsic duct compression

level. The injury may be predictable, as with estrogens (for example), or unpredictable, as with most idiopathic drug reactions. Histologically and clinically, cholestatic drug reactions can be considered as "bland" or "inflammatory."

Systemic sepsis is often associated with cholestasis. Endotoxins impair canalicular secretory function. If sepsis occurs on a background of cirrhosis, the cholestasis is much more profound.

Most acute and chronic liver diseases exert a cholestatic effect via damage to the small interlobular bile ducts (at least, that is what can be seen within the limits of the regular microscope). Damage to small bile ducts is not at all unusual in acute hepatitis, particularly with hepatitis C. Cholestasis is also a common feature of relapsing hepatitis A.

Several chronic liver diseases specifically target the intrahepatic and sometimes the extrahepatic bile ducts. The diseases of the liver that are associated with paucity of bile ducts are numerous. Primary biliary cirrhosis (PBC) and primary sclerosing cholangitis (PSC) are the best-known examples; other diseases that destroy bile ducts are chronic drug reactions, chronic rejection, graft-versus-host disease and chronic septic cholangitis, to name but a few.

Many infiltrations may cause a biochemical cholestatic pattern of liver disease, generally anicteric – e.g., sarcoidosis, lymphomas, amyloid and granulomas of any etiology.

There is a very rare condition called "benign recurrent cholestasis" whose mechanism is not understood at all. Several rare congenital conditions often associated with abnormal bile acids and/or intrahepatic bile ducts result in severe chronic cholestasis of young children.

9.2 Extrahepatic Cholestasis

Diseases of the large bile ducts are generally due to stones, strictures or tumors. The AIDS epidemic has brought its own forms of cholestatic problems: fungal, protozoal and viral cholangitis. Malignant tumors causing biliary obstruction now include Kaposi's sarcoma, lymphoma, and the more common pancreatic and bile duct carcinomas.

9.3 Primary Biliary Cirrhosis (PBC)

9.3.1 DIAGNOSIS

The more accurate term for this disease is chronic nonsuppurative granulomatous cholangitis. It predominantly affects women in middle age and is frequently associated with autoimmune phenomena outside the liver (renal tubular acidosis, vitiligo, thyroiditis, sicca syndrome, CREST syndrome, rheumatoid arthritis and, less often, glomerulonephritis and vasculitis). It is therefore presumed that PBC is also an autoimmune disease, although the inciting antigen has not been identified.

PBC is rarely diagnosed quickly, because one-third or more of patients are asymptomatic. The biochemical pattern seen in PBC is typically cholestatic: elevated alkaline phosphatase, GGT and 5'NT, with modest elevations of the aminotransferases. An elevated bilirubin is associated with progressive, symptomatic disease, indicating a poor prognosis. The most common symptom of this illness is fatigue, very hard to define yet very distressing to the patient. Other symptoms include pruritus, xanthelasma and, later in the course of the disease, ascites, jaundice and encephalopathy. Portal hypertension occurs early in this disease, as it is presinusoidal in nature; thus, variceal hemorrhage may be a presenting symptom.

The laboratory hallmarks for PBC are a cholestatic serum biochemistry as described above, elevated serum cholesterol, elevated serum IgM and a positive mitochondrial antibody test. Liver histology is diagnostic (Table 9). In men, primary sclerosing cholangitis (PSC) is so much more common than PBC that male patients should have ERCP performed to definitively exclude PSC.

TABLE 9. Diagnostic features of primary biliary cirrhosis

Elevated serum alkaline phosphatase
Elevated serum cholesterol
Antimitochondrial antibody positive
Typical liver histology
Normal ERCP

9.3.2 MANAGEMENT

The management of PBC includes symptomatic, preventive and specific measures.

There is little one can do for the fatigue, although a sympathetic and understanding ear helps. Pruritus, a very disturbing problem, can generally be controlled by using the anion exchange resin, cholestyramine. There are, however, many gastrointestinal side effects of this drug, so rifampin 150 mg b.i.d. or t.i.d. can be tried instead. Ultraviolet light also helps, so that pruritus is less in the summer. A trip down south always helps in the winter!

For the most part, the complications of long-term cholestasis can be prevented, except for the osteoporosis. Once the serum bilirubin is elevated, steatorrhea may occur with subsequent malabsorption of fat-soluble vitamins. Vitamin A and D supplements are available in water-soluble form, and vitamin K is best given parenterally. The fat intake should not be reduced. Although this may reduce the steatorrhea, it will also result in massive weight loss and will not affect the serum cholesterol. Despite the hypercholesterolemia, there is no increase in incidence of ischemic heart disease in PBC. So far nothing has been found to help the osteoporosis, which may cause wedging of the vertebrae, although calcium supplementation of the diet is always recommended.

Many specific therapies for PBC have been tried, none with resounding success. Some are definitely contraindicated – notably prednisone, because it promotes osteoporosis. Treatment with the bile acid ursodeoxycholic acid has very few side effects and causes a dramatic fall in all the biochemical markers for this disease. More complete studies are necessary to see if this drug improves histology and, more importantly, survival. Untreated, the mean survival of symptomatic PBC is 12 years. The survival of those with asymptomatic disease is much longer. The ultimate treatment is liver transplantation; PBC patients do very well.

9.4 Secondary Biliary Cirrhosis

Any disease that permanently and progressively damages bile ducts and is not caused by PBC may lead to secondary biliary cirrhosis, sometimes (although

TABLE 10. Comparison of PBC and PSC

	PBC	PSC
Symptoms	Often none/pruritus	Often none
Biochemistry	Elevated ALP	Elevated ALP
Serum bilirubin	Slow rise	Fluctuates
Non-organ specific Ab	AMA+ve	AMA–ve
Liver histology	Helpful	Not helpful
ERCP	Normal	Abnormal

not usually) in the absence of overt jaundice. The most obvious cause is biliary atresia; other pediatric conditions include the various hypoplastic duct syndromes, other biliary tree abnormalities – Caroli's disease, choledochal cysts, sclerosing cholangitis – and cystic fibrosis, which causes focal biliary cirrhosis. In adults the commonest cause of secondary biliary cirrhosis is probably primary sclerosing cholangitis (PSC), although iatrogenic bile duct strictures also feature.

Primary sclerosing cholangitis affects about 10% of patients with ulcerative colitis or Crohn's colitis, although 30% of patients with PSC have no background of inflammatory bowel disease. Patients are commonly asymptomatic. Just as with PBC, PSC causes presinusoidal portal hypertension, so variceal bleeding may present early – i.e., prior to the onset of jaundice (Table 10). A cholestatic enzyme pattern in any patient with liver problems should prompt the suspicion of PSC. The diagnosis is made only by ERCP, never by liver biopsy. Because liver biopsy is not helpful diagnostically it is performed only to see if the patient is cirrhotic. If PSC is suspected prior to ERCP, then antibiotic coverage should be given at the time of the procedure. Sepsis is the major complication of this disease and needs to be avoided if possible, as infection outside the liver precludes liver transplantation – the treatment of choice for decompensated disease. Prior to transplantation the only treatment available is symptomatic and/or preventive, as described for PBC. As yet there have been no therapeutic trials of any reasonable size performed in PSC and hence there is no standard therapeutic intervention.

9.5 Approach to the Patient with Cholestasis

9.5.1 *DIAGNOSIS*
The history in any patient is always of utmost importance. A complete drug history should be taken, including prescribed and over-the-counter drugs. A past history of cholecystectomy should never be forgotten; common bile duct

stones are not unusual, even in the absence of symptoms and/or dilatated bile ducts on ultrasound. Manifestations of other autoimmune disease should be sought, and inquiry made about chills and fever.

Examination should make special note of the patient's temperature. Signs of chronic cholestasis include scratch marks, shiny nails, increased skin pigmentation, xanthelasma and xanthomatous neuropathy, and jaundice, which in its later stages takes on a greenish hue. Hepatosplenomegaly is common in PBC, PSC and biliary atresia, and with infiltrations like lymphoma.

9.5.2 LABORATORY CONFIRMATION

The standard biochemical tests are most helpful. Liver function tends to remain normal for long periods in cholestasis, but the enzyme markers – alkaline phosphatase, GGT, 5'NT – are always elevated. If the results of these tests confirm the clinical suspicion, then the next step is an ultrasound to look at the bile ducts. If there is jaundice associated with fever or chills, there should be no delay with the ultrasound examination of the abdomen.

9.5.3 FURTHER MANAGEMENT

Further management will depend entirely on whether the patient has dilatated ducts. If the ducts are dilatated, the management will be interventional. If the ducts are not dilatated but there is still a suspicion that the problem lies in the extrahepatic biliary system (common bile duct stones following cholecystectomy, PSC), then an ERCP may still be indicated.

If the history, physical and ultrasound all support a diagnosis of intrahepatic cholestasis, then a liver biopsy is indicated to make a diagnosis, if this is not already obvious at the bedside (e.g., sepsis, drug reactions). Cholestatic drug reactions may take many months to clear after the drug has been withdrawn. A clinical diagnosis of PBC needs to be confirmed by liver biopsy.

There will always be patients in whom no diagnosis can be made immediately. In the absence of jaundice, the physician has time to observe. Granulomas of the liver are the most likely cause of a "missed" diagnosis on biopsy.

10. CIRRHOSIS OF THE LIVER / J. Heathcote

Cirrhosis is a chronic diffuse liver disease that is characterized by fibrosis and nodule formation. Fibrosis is not synonymous with cirrhosis. Nodule formation with disturbed architecture is essential for the diagnosis of cirrhosis. The condition results from liver cell necrosis and the collapse of hepatic lobules, with the liver response being the formation of diffuse fibrous septa and nodular regrowth of hepatocytes. Thus, the ultimate histologic pattern is the same

TABLE 11. Causes of cirrhosis

Alcohol

Viral hepatitis
  Hepatitis B
  Hepatitis C
  Hepatitis D

Metabolic
  Hemochromatosis
  Wilson's disease
  α_1-antitrypsin deficiency
  Galactosemia
  Type IV glycogenosis

Cholestatic
  Sclerosing cholangitis

Autoimmune
  Primary biliary cirrhosis
  Chronic active hepatitis

Drug-induced

Congestive

Cystic fibrosis

---

regardless of etiology. Necrosis is often absent when the liver is ultimately examined either by biopsy or at post mortem.

10.1 Etiology

Known causes of cirrhosis account for about 70% of the cases. Most common etiologies include alcoholism, autoimmune chronic hepatitis and chronic viral hepatitis (Table 11). Less common causes include hemochromatosis, primary biliary cirrhosis, drug-induced liver disease, chronic biliary obstruction and (uncommonly) Wilson's disease. The remaining 30% of patients with cirrhosis of the liver have no known cause, a condition termed *cryptogenic cirrhosis*.

The etiology of the cirrhosis usually cannot be determined by the pathologic appearance of the liver (with some notable exceptions, including hemochromatosis and α_1-antitrypsin deficiency). Terms previously used such as *portal cirrhosis* or *postnecrotic cirrhosis* have been replaced by classifications that include three anatomic categories.

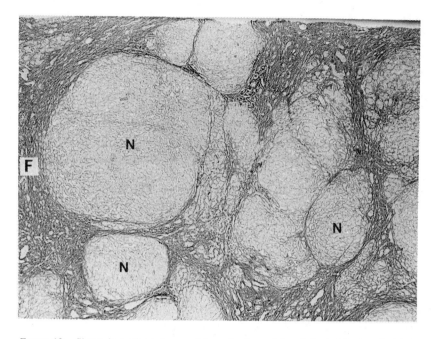

FIGURE 12.   Shown is a mixed macronodular and micronodular cirrhosis. The hepatic lobular architecture has been destroyed and replaced by nodular masses of regenerated cells (N). Fibrous tissue surrounds the nodules. (Retic. stain, original magnification × 37)

10.2 Pathology

Micronodular cirrhosis is characterized by thick, regular septa, by regenerating small nodules of uniform size and by involvement of every lobule. Often associated with the persistence of the injurious agent, this may represent the liver's relative impairment for regeneration, as may be seen in alcoholism, old age, ischemia and malnutrition.

Macronodular cirrhosis is characterized by nodules of variable size, some containing large areas of intact or regenerating parenchyma within each large nodule.

Mixed macronodular and micronodular cirrhosis may result from vigorous regrowth in a previous micronodular cirrhosis (Figure 12).

10.3 Clinical Features

The clinical features of cirrhosis relate to those features that are peculiar to the cause of the cirrhosis but more importantly to the magnitude of the hepatocellular failure and the presence of portal hypertension, along with the ability of the surviving hepatocytes to compensate for the loss. Thus, patients often are categorized as having latent, compensated disease or active, decompensated disease, each having its own clinical pathologic correlations. In the fully compensated state, there may be no symptoms whatever, the disease being suspected by a finding of an enlarged liver or spleen. With progression of the disease, features of hepatocellular failure and portal hypertension emerge.

With hepatocellular failure, patients may complain of weakness, fatigue, weight loss and a general deterioration of health. Physical examination may reveal the stigmata of chronic liver disease (see Section 2).

The ease of diagnosis of cirrhosis is dependent on the degree of liver decompensation. A high index of suspicion is necessary; the condition may be revealed only by a positive history of alcohol ingestion along with the finding of hepatomegaly. In decompensated disease, the diagnosis is much easier; the clinical features of ascites, jaundice and other signs of hepatocellular failure may be present. In severe, acute hepatitis, these signs can be present transiently.

Biochemical tests attempt to identify the specific etiology of the liver disease and to assess the degree of hepatocellular dysfunction. With deteriorating hepatic function, albumin falls, serum bilirubin rises and the prothrombin time becomes prolonged and not correctable by parenteral vitamin K. Liver enzymes, while helpful in assessing ongoing activity, do not reflect function; serum aminotransferases may be only mildly elevated despite severe functional disease. Alkaline phosphatase is usually raised. Commonly a normochromic, normocytic anemia is found. Occasionally a macrocytic anemia presents, but if gastrointestinal bleeding has been occurring, the anemia may be microcytic as a result of iron loss. Depressed leukocyte and platelet counts are found in association with hypersplenism. The urine often contains urobilinogen and bilirubin if the patient is jaundiced. Cases with ascites exhibit a marked reduction in urinary sodium excretion. The radioisotope scan will show patchy uptake by the liver with redistribution to the spleen and bone marrow. Ultrasound and CT scanning will reveal uneven architecture with increased fibrous tissue. These tests do not establish the diagnosis of cirrhosis, which is dependent on liver biopsy with histologic examination. Liver biopsy may also be helpful in establishing an etiology and degree of activity of the underlying process.

Prognosis depends on the degree of hepatocellular function and the etiology, as well as on whether any causative agents can be removed. Clearly the prognosis is improved if the alcoholic patient can abstain, if the patient with hemochromatosis has iron removed by venesection or if excessive copper is

TABLE 12. Criteria for Child-Pugh classification

Group designation	A	B	C
Serum bilirubin$^\alpha$ (mg %)	Below 2.0	2.0–3.0	Over 3.0
Serum albumin (g %)	Over 3.5	3.0–3.5	Under 3.0
Ascites	None	Easily controlled	Poorly controlled
Neurological disorder	None	Minimal	Advanced "coma"
Nutrition	Excellent	Good	Poor, "wasting"

removed in those with Wilson's disease. In addition, vigorous medical care may prolong life and delay or prevent eventual complications such as ascites and GI bleeding. The prognosis is worse with decompensated liver disease, which is characterized by jaundice, ascites, neurologic impairment, hemorrhage and biochemical tests showing severe hypoalbuminemia, hypothrombinemia and hyponatremia.

10.4 Treatment
Clearly, where there is a specific treatment for the underlying etiology of the liver disease this should be offered. All patients should consume a healthy, adequate diet and avoid alcohol. Otherwise the management is that of regular surveillance and early detection of hepatocellular failure. Hepatocellular failure or decompensated cirrhosis may be manifested by any of the following: coagulopathy, jaundice (in noncholestatic liver disease), hepatic encephalopathy, variceal bleeding, ascites. The Child-Pugh classification of cirrhosis, which is a very useful guide to calculate the risk of an invasive procedure, takes into account these variables, plus nutritional status (Table 12). Once decompensation occurs, management includes the control of ascites, avoidance of drugs that are poorly metabolized by the liver and the prompt treatment of infection and variceal hemorrhage. Liver transplantation is now becoming the treatment of choice for many with end-stage decompensated liver disease (see Section 15).

11. PORTAL HYPERTENSION / S.S. Lee

Portal hypertension is defined as increased pressure in the portal vein. With the right atrial pressure as a zero reference, normal portal venous pressure is approximately 4–8 mm Hg. The portal vein is formed by the confluence of the splenic and superior mesenteric veins. Its flow rate normally averages about 1–1.2 L/min. The simple phenomenon of increased pressure in this venous circulation unleashes a wide array of hemodynamic and metabolic consequences,

TABLE 13. Causes of portal hypertension

Prehepatic
  Splenic AV fistula
  Splenic or portal vein thrombosis
  Massive splenomegaly	

Intrahepatic
  Sarcoidosis
  Schistosomiasis
  Nodular regenerative hyperplasia
  Congenital hepatic fibrosis
  Idiopathic portal fibrosis
  Early primary biliary cirrhosis
  Chronic active hepatitis
  Myeloproliferative disorders
  Graft-vs.-host disease
	Presinusoidal

Established cirrhosis Alcoholic hepatitis	Sinusoidal
Alcoholic terminal hyaline sclerosis Veno-occlusive disease	

Posthepatic
  Budd-Chiari syndrome
  Membranous IVC web
  Right heart failure
  Constrictive pericarditis
	Postsinusoidal

including some of the most lethal and distressing complications of chronic liver disease.

11.1 Etiology

The causes of portal hypertension are diverse (Table 13). Since portal pressure is the product of portal blood flow and intrahepatic resistance, any condition causing an increase in flow or resistance will increase portal pressure. An example of a "pure" flow increase is postsurgical or traumatic splenic arterio-venous fistula. The marked increase in splenic and thus portal venous flow leads to the development of portal hypertension. Almost all other causes of portal hypertension are mediated predominantly by increasing resistance, although evidence indicates that most high-resistance syndromes are also accompanied by increases in portal venous flow. In many conditions, the cause of the increased resistance is evident: inflammation and fibrosis lead to vascular distortion, architectural disturbance and impingement of the intravascular spaces. Other less evident factors are predominant in other conditions. For example, in acute alcoholic hepatitis, hepatocyte cell swelling and collagen deposition in the Disse's space lead to narrowing and distortion of sinusoidal spaces. The reasons for the increased mesenteric (and thus portal venous) blood flow in high-resistance states remain unclear. One theory postulates that a circulating vasodilatory humoral factor that would normally be inactivated by the liver escapes into the systemic circulation through shunts or hepatocellular insufficiency.

There are two separate and sometimes overlapping classification systems for the causes of portal hypertension, using either the liver or the hepatic sinusoid as the reference point. The former classifies conditions into prehepatic, intrahepatic and posthepatic causes, while the latter divides conditions into presinusoidal, sinusoidal and postsinusoidal causes (Table 13). However, the exact site of increased resistance in many intrahepatic causes of portal hypertension has recently been questioned, and it is likely that the predominant resistance sites could change according to the stage of some disease processes. For example, early primary biliary cirrhosis is thought to produce mainly presinusoidal hypertension, but as dense cirrhosis supervenes, sinusoidal hypertension becomes more important. Similarly, an early lesion of alcoholic liver disease, the central or terminal hyaline sclerosis, characterized by zone 3 fibrosis, would cause postsinuoidal hypertension, with sinusoidal hypertension predominating as cirrhosis becomes established. In practical terms, there are reasons for trying to correctly classify resistance sites. One is for predicting responses to surgical shunting procedures: presinusoidal conditions generally have well-preserved hepatocellular function and thus respond well to diversion of portal blood, whereas sinusoidal and postsinusoidal conditions tend to be associated with varying degrees of hepatic insufficiency. Another is that ascites generally occurs only with sinusoidal and postsinusoidal hypertension.

11.2 Pathophysiology

Portal pressure can be measured by several methods. A catheter inserted into a hepatic vein and then wedged provides a good estimate of the upstream portal venous pressure, unless the site of resistance is proximal to the intrahepatic portal vein (as in portal vein thrombosis wherein the wedged hepatic vein pressure will be normal in the presence of significant portal hypertension). The spleen, liver or portal vein can be directly percutaneously punctured by small-gauge (19–22 gauge) needles to obtain reliable estimates of portal pressure. Measurement of portal pressure is mostly used for research purposes, as its invasiveness precludes wide clinical use.

Portal hypertension leads to many clinical complications. Ascites is directly

TABLE 14.   Common sites of portal-systemic collateral formation

Location	Portal circulation	Systemic circulation	Clinical consequence
Proximal stomach and distal esophagus	Coronary vein of stomach	Azygos vein	Submucosal gastroesophageal varices
Anterior abdominal wall	Umbilical vein in falciform ligament	Epigastric abdominal wall veins	Caput medusae
Retroperitoneal	Splenic vein branch Sappey's veins (around liver and diaphragm)	Left renal vein Retzius's vein	Usually none Usually none
Anorectal	Middle and superior hemorrhoidal veins	Inferior hemorrhoidal vein	May be mistaken for hemorrhoids

related to the development of sinusoidal or postsinusoidal hypertension. Portal-systemic collateral vessels form in an attempt to decompress the portal hypertension (Table 14). The most troublesome site of collateral formation is around the proximal stomach and distal esophagus (gastroesophageal varices). Bleeding from such varices (or the gastric mucosa) and hepatocellular failure are the two commonest causes of death in cirrhosis. Indeed the mortality rates for variceal bleeding range from 15–50% depending on the degree of hepatic function: Child-Pugh class A, B and C patients have, respectively, 15%, 20–30% and 40–50% mortality rates when their varices bleed.

The risk of bleeding from gastroesophageal varices is related to several factors. First, a threshold minimum level of portal pressure of approximately 12 mm Hg appears necessary for varices to form. However, above this level it is unclear whether absolute height of portal pressure affects the bleeding risk. Factors such as intrathoracic pressure gradients induced by coughing, straining or sneezing, and damage to the variceal wall by acid reflux into the esophagus appear not to play a role. The two factors most important in determining bleeding risk are variceal size and local variceal wall characteristics. Several studies have shown that small varices almost never bleed, while the bleeding risk of medium-sized varices is approximately 10–15% over two years, and that of large varices, approximately 20–30% over the same period. During the past decade, it has become clear that certain varix wall characteristics that are visible through an endoscope are also predictive of high bleeding risk. These are the red and blue color signs. Small localized wall defects such as

TABLE 15. Comparison of portal hypertensive gastropathy and inflammatory gastritis

	Portal hypertensive gastropathy	Inflammatory gastritis
Endoscopic appearance	Mosaic pattern, speckled red spots	Discrete red erosive lesions
Site	Predominantly fundus	Predominantly antrum
Histology	Scant inflammatory cell infiltrate, prominent vascular dilatation, mucosal and submucosal lesions	Heavy inflammatory cell infiltrate, mucosal lesions
Treatment	Surgery, ? beta blockers, ?cytoprotective agents	Acid suppression, cytoprotective agents

thin-walled blebs or sacs in the wall look like red spots or streaks and have variously been termed "red wale markings," "cherry-red spots" or "red streaks," while a diffuse pronounced blue color indicates a large varix (vein) with a stretched mucosa covering it.

Approximately 30–50% of upper GI bleeding episodes in patients with portal hypertension originate from nonvariceal sources. Cirrhotic patients have an increased incidence of acid-peptic disease, mostly erosive gastritis. This is probably due to the alcohol abuse that is common in this population. However, it has recently become clear that the majority of nonvariceal upper GI bleeding in cirrhosis is due to a peculiar form of gastropathy seen in the stomach in portal hypertension. Several features distinguish this portal hypertensive gastropathy from the erosive or inflammatory gastritis seen in nonhypertensive patients (Table 15). The major symptom of portal hypertensive gastropathy is bleeding. Pain or dyspepsia is uncommon as a presenting feature of this type of gastropathy. The appropriate treatment for this condition is still unclear, but it probably responds to measures to decrease portal pressure, although a possible role for cytoprotective agents has also been suggested.

11.3 Diagnosis

Diagnosing portal hypertension is usually easy. The patient often has concomitant ascites and splenomegaly, along with the stigmata of chronic liver disease. However, it should be remembered that all the prehepatic and many of the presinusoidal conditions have well-preserved liver function and no ascites. Abdominal wall collaterals radiate outward from the umbilicus; when they are very prominent, it is easy to see why this condition is termed "caput medusae," after the fearsome creature in Greek mythology with the serpentine hairdo. Rarely, a venous hum over a large caput medusae can be heard with light auscultation – the Cruveilhier-Baumgarten sign. Another diagnostic clue may be the presence of anorectal varices masquerading as hemorrhoids. Gastroesophageal variceal bleeding produces large-volume, brisk bleeding with hematemesis and, later, melena or hematochezia. Portal hypertensive gastropathy may also produce brisk bleeding, but can occasionally cause low-volume oozing manifested only by melena.

11.4 Management

Managing the acute bleeding episode consists of the general resuscitative measures such as volume and blood replacement, and specific measures to stop the bleeding. Various pharmacological, mechanical and surgical modes of arresting hemorrhage are used, usually in that order. Vasoconstrictive drugs to stop bleeding include vasopressin and somatostatin or their longer-acting analogues such as glypressin and octreotide, respectively. Vasopressin infusions induce generalized arteriolar and venous constriction, with resultant decreased portal venous flow and thus pressure, and at least temporary cessation of bleeding in 50–80% of cases. However, the generalized vasoconstriction also may result in peripheral vascular ischemia, myocardial ischemia or infarction and renal tubular damage. Concurrent nitrate administration has been suggested to attenuate some of these side effects, but whether it actually does so is still unproven. A safer alternative may be somatostatin or octreotide. Their mechanism of action is still unclear but probably relates to a suppressive effect on the release of vasodilatory hormones such as glucagon, leading to a net vasoconstrictive effect. Side effects are minimal. Whatever drug is used, it is generally inadvisable to continue drug therapy for more than one to two days.

Mechanical modes of therapy include inflatable balloons for direct tamponade. The Sengstaken-Blakemore tube has both an esophageal and a small gastric balloon; the Linton-Nachlas tube, with only a large gastric balloon, is attached to a small weight to stanch the cephalad flow of blood in the varices. Both tubes carry significant complication rates, especially in inexperienced hands. The Sengstaken tube carries a 15% complication risk, often due to esophageal laceration. Therefore, we prefer the Linton tube.

The most common and probably the most effective nonsurgical therapies are endoscopic variceal sclerotherapy and ligation. Highly irritant solutions such as ethanolamine, polidocanol or even absolute ethanol are injected through endoscopic direct vision into and around the bleeding varix. The subsequent inflammation leads to eventual thrombosis and fibrosis of the varix lumen. Possible complications include chest pain, dysphagia, and esophageal ulceration and stricturing. The injection of irritant solutions that eventually lodge in the pulmonary circulation can result in lung function abnormalities, although these tend to be subclinical. A newer and probably safer method of endoscopic therapy is ligation or banding, similar to the rubber band ligations used to fibrose anorectal hemorrhoids. This technique has been used only since the 1990s, and initial studies suggest that its efficacy is similar to sclerotherapy, with fewer esophageal complications. The combination of endoscopic therapy and either balloon tamponade or drug therapy to control actively bleeding varices is successful in 80–95% of cases.

When all the above measures fail, emergency surgery may be tried. Emergency portacaval shunt surgery has been abandoned because of a 30–50% operative mortality rate. The simplest and probably best choice in the emergency situation is esophageal transection, in which a mechanical device transects and removes a ring of esophageal tissue, and then staples the ends together. Another type of "surgery" is the transjugular intrahepatic portalsystemic shunt (TIPS). In this procedure, an intrahepatic shunt between a hepatic and portal vein branch is made by balloon dilation of liver tissue, and then an expandable metal stent of approximately 1 cm diameter is lodged into the fistula. The procedure can be done by a radiologist using fluoroscopyguided catheterization, and requires only light sedation and local anesthesia.

Once the acute bleeding episode has been treated, how do we reduce the risk of future rebleeding? Before considering any other therapy, some obvious common-sense measures should be taken. For example, patients with cirrhosis caused by alcohol (the cause of approximately 50–60% of cirrhosis in Canada) absolutely must stop drinking; the rebleeding and mortality rates in patients who continue their alcohol use are much higher than in those who remain abstinent.

Prophylactic therapy to prevent bleeding may be divided into primary (to prevent the first bleed in a patient with varices who has never bled) and secondary prophylaxis (to prevent rebleeds). There is still much conflicting literature on these two topics, but for now, the following preliminary recommendations can be made. First, patients with large varices that have never bled should be started on beta blocker therapy at doses sufficient to reduce the resting heart rate by 20–25%. Beta-adrenergic antagonists are thought to produce arteriolar and venous constriction and significantly reduce blood flow through portal-systemic collaterals while modestly reducing portal pressure. Endoscopic sclerotherapy/banding, TIPS or surgery should not be used for primary prophylaxis.

The appropriate secondary prophylaxis regimes remain controversial. There is probably a minority subgroup who respond favorably to beta blocker therapy, but they cannot be easily identified. One approach is to perform enough endoscopic sclerotherapy/banding sessions (usually 3–6) to obliterate varices or reduce them to small size. Treatment failures on this regime (e.g., those with recurrent bleeding) could be considered either for TIPS or surgery. TIPS should not be done in patients with a history of, or active, encephalopathy.

Prehepatic causes of portal hypertension such as portal vein thrombosis generally respond well to some type of portal-mesenteric diversion procedure such as mesocaval or portacaval shunting. In these cases, normal liver function protects against the development of encephalopathy or hepatic insufficiency when portal blood is diverted away from the liver.

Of course the definitive treatment for most of the complications of end-stage liver disease, including recurrent GI bleeding due to severe portal hypertension, is orthotopic liver transplantation. Since the presence of a surgical portacaval or mesocaval shunt greatly complicates the transplantation procedure, we have generally abandoned these types of shunting operations in patients with cirrhosis.

12. ASCITES / F. Wong and L. Blendis

Ascites is a detectable collection of free fluid in the peritoneal cavity. Ascitic fluid is derived from the vascular compartment subserving the hepatosplanchnic viscera. Two factors are important in the formation of ascites: the plasma colloidal osmotic pressure, which tends to retain fluid in the vascular compartment, and the portal venous pressure, which tends to force fluid into the tissue space. In cirrhosis, hepatocellular dysfunction leads to decreased albumin synthesis and a reduced colloidal osmotic pressure, while the portal hypertension serves to localize excess fluid to the peritoneal cavity rather than the periphery. Portal hypertension alone without hepatic dysfunction rarely results in ascites.

The pathogenesis of ascites formation remains controversial. The "underfill" theory proposes that ascites occurs as a primary event when a critical imbalance of Starling's forces is present. Sequestration of fluid into the peritoneal cavity results in a reduction of the circulatory volume. This in turn leads to stimulation of the sympathetic nervous and renin-angiotensin-aldosterone systems, which promote renal sodium and water retention. The "overfill" (or "overflow") theory, on the other hand, proposes that renal sodium retention occurs as a primary event. This may be due to the increased production of a sodium-retaining factor or the reduced synthesis of a natriuretic factor by the diseased liver. The circulatory volume is expanded. In the presence of abnormal Starling's forces in the splanchnic circulation, the retained fluid is preferentially localized to the peritoneal cavity as ascites. More recently, the peripheral arterial vasodilatation hypothesis, which encompasses features of both the underfill and overflow theories, was put forward. It proposes that in cirrhosis, arterial vasodilatation leads to a decrease in splanchnic and systemic vascular resistance with pooling of blood in the splanchnic circulation, leading to a reduction in the effective arterial blood volume. This in turn activates neurohumoral pressor systems, promoting renal sodium and water retention in an attempt to restore the effective arterial blood volume and maintain blood pressure. When increased renal sodium reabsorption cannot compensate for the arterial vasodilatation, arterial underfilling occurs. Then the cascade of further activation of various neurohumoral pressor systems leading to increased sodium retention begins, and ultimately ascites is formed (Figure 13).

Arterial vasodilatation is also responsible for the hyperdynamic circulation that is often evident in cirrhosis. This clinically manifests as an increased cardiac output, bounding pulse, wide pulse pressure and systemic hypotension. Locally produced vasodilators may be responsible. More recently, it has been proposed that chronic endotoxemia associated with cirrhosis may stimulate the synthesis and release of a potent endothelial-derived relaxing factor, nitric oxide, resulting in splanchnic and systemic vasodilatation.

Clinically, the first evidence of ascites is an increase in abdominal girth accompanied by weight gain. Peritoneal fluid of less than 2 L is difficult to detect clinically, and ultrasound is useful in defining small amounts of ascites. The patient is sallow and intravascularly depleted. Muscle wasting is profound. The abdomen is distended, often with fullness in the flanks and an everted umbilicus. Scrotal edema is frequent. Distended abdominal wall veins that radiate from the umbilicus represent the presence of portal-systemic collaterals. The earliest sign of ascites is dullness to percussion in the flanks. Shifting dullness and a fluid thrill mean that more fluid is present.

A pleural effusion is found in a small percentage of patients with ascites, usually on the right side. This is due to the presence of a diaphragmatic defect that allows ascitic fluid to pass into the pleural cavity.

Examination of ascitic fluid by diagnostic paracentesis should be performed at first presentation, or when there is alteration of the patient's clinical state, such as a sudden increase in the amount of ascitic fluid, worsening of encephalopathy or presence of fever. The purpose of the examination is to rule out other complications such as spontaneous bacterial peritonitis, tuberculosis and hepatocellular carcinoma. Ascitic fluid analysis should include a total polymorph count, protein and albumin concentrations and direct inoculation of at least 10 mL of ascitic fluid each into blood culture bottles at the bedside, as

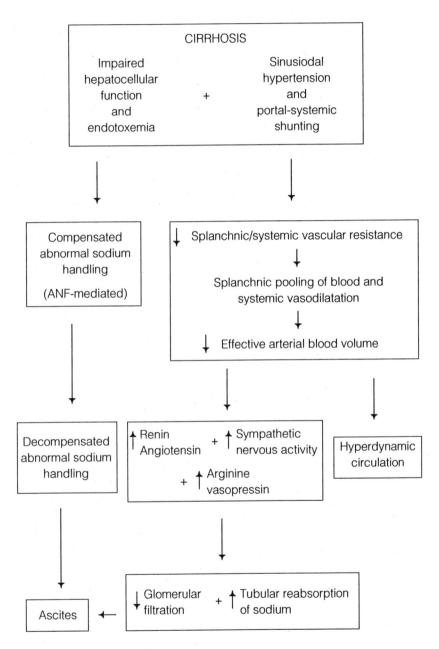

FIGURE 13. Pathogenesis of ascites.

this increases the positive culture yield. A serum–ascitic fluid albumin gradient of less than 11 g/L represents cirrhotic rather than malignant ascites. A high protein content may be associated with Budd-Chiari syndrome or seen in pancreatic ascites. A total polymorph count of greater than 250/μL is diagnostic of spontaneous bacterial peritonitis..

Although bed rest will result in a redistribution of body fluid, fluid and salt restriction is required to mobilize the ascites. The patient is usually prescribed a no-added-salt diet containing 2 g (100 mmol) sodium, and monitored carefully with daily weights. Measurement of abdominal girth is unreliable, as gaseous distention is common. Too rapid mobilization of fluid will result in worsening of renal function; one should aim at a weight loss of 0.5 kg/day. Patients with peripheral edema can have their fluid mobilized more rapidly, as the edema fluid can easily be absorbed to replenish the intravascular volume.

Diuretic therapy is usually required in addition to salt and fluid restriction. The potassium-sparing diuretic spironolactone, starting at a dose of 100 mg/day, may be increased by 100 mg per week up to 400 mg/day if the response is inadequate. Spironolactone has a slow onset of action, and therefore frequent dose adjustments are unnecessary. Its half-life in cirrhotic patients can be as long as 10 days; therefore, it also has a slow offset of action and patients should still be monitored after spironolactone is discontinued. One of its unacceptable side effects is painful gynecomastia. Other potassium-sparing diuretics, such as amiloride and triamterene, are less potent but acceptable alternatives. If there is no diuretic response and the patient is compliant with the sodium intake, a loop diuretic such as furosemide is added. Electrolyte abnormalities are common with diuretic therapy and should be monitored regularly. Hypokalemia and hypochloremic alkalosis can precipitate encephalopathy. Too rapid diuresis can lead to azotemia and the hepatorenal syndrome.

Refractory ascites is defined as ascites unresponsive to 400 mg of spironolactone or 30 mg of amiloride plus up to 120 mg of furosemide daily for two weeks. Noncompliance with sodium restriction is a major and often overlooked cause of resistant ascites, and careful questioning of the patient and the patient's relatives is often required to confirm this. Other causes of resistant ascites include the development of spontaneous bacterial peritonitis, hepatocellular carcinoma and intrinsic renal pathology. Refractory ascites without any underlying cause usually indicates advanced cirrhosis associated with a grave prognosis, with only a 50% survival at two years. Large-volume paracentesis is now recognized as a safe and effective therapy for the treatment of refractory ascites. Removal of ascitic fluid volume of up to 5 L without the simultaneous infusion of plasma expanders such as concentrated albumin is safe in non-edematous patients. Larger volumes can be removed in edematous patients. However, repeated paracenteses may not be practical for all patients with refractory ascites, and a peritoneovenous (LeVeen) shunt should be considered in selected patients with good liver reserve. It may be dramatically effective in resolving the ascites, but in patients with decompensated liver disease it is followed by higher morbidity and mortality. Previous abdominal surgery, spontaneous bacterial peritonitis and large varices are relative contraindications to the procedure. Early complications include pulmonary edema and disseminated intravascular coagulopathy. Late complications include thrombosis of the superior vena cava, infection and blockage or dislodgement of the shunt, all of which require its immediate removal. In suitable patients, the LeVeen shunt, in addition to improved management of ascites, can significantly enhance well-being and nutritional status. Liver transplantation should always be considered as a treatment option in these patients.

12.1 Spontaneous Bacterial Peritonitis

Spontaneous bacterial peritonitis (SBP) is a common and often fatal complication of cirrhosis. In this clinical syndrome, ascites becomes infected in the absence of a recognizable cause of peritonitis. Its increased incidence over the past decade may be due to greater recognition. It is particularly frequent if the patient has severely decompensated cirrhosis with jaundice. In most cases, the infection occurs after admission into hospital. About one-third of cases of SBP are asymptomatic; therefore, the clinician should not hesitate in performing a diagnostic paracentesis. Typically, it presents with fever and/or abdominal pain. It may also present atypically, solely as a worsening of the encephalopathy. Diagnosis of SBP is made by paracentesis. Positive culture results may take 48 hours and Gram's stains of ascitic fluid are positive in only 10–50% of infected patients. The "gold standard" for diagnosis of SBP is a polymorphonuclear (PMN) count of >250 cells/μL. A variant of SBP known as *culture-negative neutrocytic ascites* occurs as culture-negative cases of suspected SBP with an ascitic fluid PMN count of >250 cells/μL. The patients with culture-negative neutrocytic ascites have the same clinical presentation and carry the same unfavorable prognosis as those with SBP. Therefore, treatment for suspected SBP should start immediately after the diagnostic PMN count rather than waiting for positive culture results. Gram-negative bacilli account for 70% of cases of SBP. E. coli is the most common pathogen isolated. Other gram-negative organisms include Klebsiella species, Citrobacter freundii, Proteus and Enterobacter. Gram-positive organisms are responsible for 25% of cases; these include Streptococcus pneumoniae, Streptococcus vir-

TABLE 16. Differentiation between secondary and spontaneous bacterial peritonitis

	Secondary bacterial peritonitis	Spontaneous bacterial peritonitis
Organisms	Multiple	Single
Ascitic protein count	>1 g/dL	<1 g/dL
Response to treatment		
PMN count	Continues to rise despite treatment	Falls exponentially
Ascitic culture	Remains positive	Rapidly becomes sterile

idans, group D streptococci and Staphylococcus aureus. Anaerobic organisms are uncommon causes of SBP, as the oxygen tension in the ascitic fluid is too high for their survival. Among these, Bacteroides species appear to be more common than other anaerobes. Cefotaxime, a new broad-spectrum, third-generation cephalosporin, is now recognized as the treatment of choice for SBP. Its spectrum includes most organisms responsible for SBP and it is not nephrotoxic in the therapeutic range. A 5-day course of cefotaxime 2 g intravenously every 8 hours has been shown to be as effective as a 10-day course. The ascitic fluid PMN count should decrease rapidly, normalizing within 48 hours in response to treatment together with a parallel clinical improvement. Aminoglycosides should not be used since cirrhotic patients are particularly sensitive to their nephrotoxic effects, and monitoring serum levels of aminoglycosides is no guarantee against aminoglycoside-induced nephrotoxicity. Secondary bacterial peritonitis should be considered as a differential diagnosis if the following features are present: (1) multiple organisms are grown from the ascitic fluid; (2) ascitic fluid protein concentration >1 g/dL; or (3) PMN count remains high despite antibiotic therapy (Table 16). Radiographic examinations are required to exclude perforation of the gastrointestinal tract, with emergency surgery only where perforation is confirmed. Despite successful treatment of SBP, the prognosis of these patients remains poor. SBP recurs frequently in cirrhotic patients. Selective intestinal decontamination to eliminate aerobic gram-negative bacilli with oral nonabsorbable antibiotics has proved effective in reducing the recurrence of SBP. Norfloxacin 400 mg daily is the drug of choice as it also has the advantages of rarely causing bacterial resistance and having a low incidence of side effects when administered chronically. Despite decreased SBP recurrence rates with prophylactic antibiotics, no change in mortality has been demonstrated as yet. All patients who have experienced one episode of SBP should be considered for liver transplantation.

TABLE 17. Grading of hepatic encephalopathy

Grade	Level of consciousness	Intellectual function	Neurological findings	EEG
1	Lack of awareness Personality change Day/night reversal	Short attention	Incoordination Mild asterixis	Slowing (5–6 cps) Triphasic
2	Lethargic Inappropriate behavior	Disoriented	Asterixis Abnormal reflexes	Slowing Triphasic
3	Asleep Rousable	Loss of meaningful communication	Asterixis Abnormal reflex	Slowing Triphasic
4	Unrousable	Absent	Decerebrate	Very slow (2–3 cps), delta

13. HEPATIC ENCEPHALOPATHY / L.J. Worobetz

Hepatic encephalopathy is a complex, potentially reversible neuropsychiatric condition that occurs in patients with acute and chronic liver disease. It is characterized by changes of personality, consciousness, behavior and neuromuscular function (Table 17). Early features include reversal of sleep pattern, hypersomnia, irritability and personal neglect. In later stages, delirium and coma may occur. Neurologic signs may include hyperreflexia, rigidity, myoclonus and asterixis. Asterixis is not specific to hepatic encephalopathy and may be present in other causes of metabolic encephalopathy. Seizures and lateralizing signs are uncommon and are more commonly seen in acute than chronic liver failure. Clinically, a number of encephalopathic patterns can be observed: acute, acute recurrent, chronic recurrent and chronic permanent encephalopathy (the latter often forms part of the spectrum of acquired hepatocerebral degeneration).

There is no specific biochemical test for hepatic encephalopathy. Blood tests should help to rule out other causes of encephalopathy and detect precipitating factors such as hypoglycemia or electrolyte imbalance. An elevated serum ammonia level is characteristic but not essential, and correlates poorly with the level of encephalopathy. The cerebrospinal fluid is usually normal or occasionally shows increased protein. Lumbar puncture and CT scan may be necessary to rule out other concomitant CNS pathology. The EEG shows slow, triphasic wave activity found mainly over frontal areas, but this pattern is not specific.

Factors of importance in the pathogenesis of encephalopathy are the shunting of blood around the hepatocytes into the systemic circulation and the pres-

TABLE 18. Common precipitants of hepatic encephalopathy

Increased nitrogen load
  Gastrointestinal bleeding
  Excess dietary protein
  Azotemia
  Constipation

Electrolyte imbalance
  Hypokalemia
  Alkalosis
  Hypoxia
  Hypovolemia

Drugs
  Narcotics, tranquilizers, sedatives

Miscellaneous
  Infection
  Surgery
  Superimposed acute liver disease
  Progressive liver disease

---

ence of hepatocellular dysfunction. Encephalopathy probably results from one or more toxic products of gut origin that are usually metabolized by the liver entering this systemic circulation and reaching the brain. Abnormalities of ammonia metabolism are most frequently incriminated in the pathophysiology. The normal gut flora produce a urease that enzymatically cleaves NH_3 from protein in the lumen. Nonionized ammonia is then absorbed into the portal circulation. It reaches the systemic circulation because of shunts and the inability of the liver to metabolize the ammonia. Other hypotheses relate to the findings of increased levels of aromatic amino acids and decreased levels of branched-chain amino acid, the possibility of false neurotransmitters and the concept of increased γ-aminobutyric acid (GABA) neurotransmission. It is likely that hepatic encephalopathy results from the complicated interplay of many factors, not just one.

Hepatic encephalopathy may arise spontaneously but more commonly will develop as a result of some precipitating factor in the course of acute or chronic liver disease (Table 18). The most important aspect of management is prompt recognition and treatment of these precipitating factors. Exogenous factors include increased dietary protein, administration of certain drugs (such as sedatives), gastrointestinal bleeding, azotemia, electrolyte imbalance from diuretic therapy, hypoxia and infection. Also important is the necessity to provide meticulous care of the confused and often comatose patient. Otherwise, the goal of therapy is to lower the level of toxic substances by reducing or excluding protein from the diet and by cleaning nitrogenous materials from the gut. To this end, constipation is avoided by the use of laxatives and, in more urgent cases, cleansing of the gut with enemas or colonic lavage. Lactulose, a synthetic disaccharide that is degraded by intestinal bacteria to produce acidification and an osmotic fermentative diarrhea, is commonly used acutely. Its chronic use can reduce the frequency of episodes of encephalopathy. Alternatively, antibiotics such as neomycin or metronidazole may be used; these inhibit urea splitting and deaminating bacteria, reducing the production of ammonia and other potential toxins.

Other experimental therapeutic approaches exist, particularly when the encephalopathy becomes refractory. On the basis of increased aromatic amino acids and decreased branched-chain amino acids found in encephalopathy (and the resulting effect on neurotransmitter synthesis), branched-chain amino acids given orally or intravenously have a potentially therapeutic role in improving encephalopathy. Some of the new benzodiazepine-receptor antagonists may be of value. These drugs, which block the benzodiazepine/GABA-receptor complex, may lead to a decrease in inhibitory GABA-mediated transmission in the brain and lessen the encephalopathy. Based on the possible relationship of a defect in dopaminergic neurotransmission and encephalopathy, both L-dopa and bromocriptine have been tried, with controversial results. Orthotopic liver transplantation should entirely reverse the hepatic encephalopathy. Thus, this should be considered in all patients with hepatic encephalopathy whose liver disease makes them suitable for liver transplantation.

14. HEPATORENAL SYNDROME / L.J. Worobetz

The hepatorenal syndrome is a syndrome of advancing renal failure in a patient with severe hepatocellular failure, usually advanced cirrhosis. In most instances, the uremia and oliguria that characterize this syndrome arise either spontaneously or in response to changes in blood volume or fluid shifts within body compartments. Patients are seldom admitted with this diagnosis; its development is usually precipitated by events in the hospital, which may include overly vigorous diuretic therapy, diarrhea or GI bleeding. The histology of the kidneys is virtually normal, with the renal failure being a functional failure. Such kidneys have been successfully transplanted and have functioned normally. Conversely, if hepatic function is restored by liver transplantation, kidney function may return to normal. In this syndrome there are abnormali-

TABLE 19. Diagnosis of hepatorenal syndrome

Chronic liver disease with ascites
Azotemia/oliguria

Tubular function maintained
  Urine:plasma osmolarity ratio >1.0
  Urine:plasma creatinine ratio >30
  Urine [Na$^+$] <10 mEq/dL

No sustained benefit by intravascular volume expansion

ties in renal blood flow, including active renal vasoconstriction, thus decreasing effective renal circulation, especially to the renal cortex. The cause of this is unknown, but is best thought of as an imbalance between systemic vasodilators and renal vasoconstricting mechanisms.

In the early stages, renal dysfunction is characterized by failure to excrete a water load, a reduction in the urinary sodium to <10 mEq/L and a progressive hyponatremia (Table 19). Ascites is usually present. As the syndrome progresses there is increasing azotemia, usually with hepatic failure and increasing difficulty controlling the ascites. Sodium is avidly reabsorbed with increasing urinary osmolality. The patient becomes drowsy, nauseated and thirsty. Terminally, the patient's blood pressure drops, coma deepens and urine volume falls further. The terminal stages may last a few days to weeks.

Clinically, it is important to distinguish hepatorenal syndrome from other causes of renal failure. Iatrogenic renal failure must be ruled out, including drug-induced disease from aminoglycosides and nonsteroidal anti-inflammatory medication. Hepatorenal syndrome must also be distinguished from prerenal azotemia and acute tubular necrosis. Acute tubular necrosis has a high urinary sodium. Although prerenal azotemia may show similar tubular function, this is ruled out by the clinical setting in which hepatorenal syndrome occurs and the lack of sustained benefit by expansion of intravascular volume. In addition, cirrhosis, especially alcoholic cirrhosis, may leave glomerular mesangial deposits of IgA, which is diagnosed by the presence of proteinuria with microhematuria and casts.

Treatment of established hepatorenal syndrome is difficult. Thus, emphasis is toward prevention by avoiding diuretic overdose, treating ascites slowly and recognizing complications early, including electrolyte imbalance, hemorrhage and infection. Conservative management includes the restriction of fluids, sodium and potassium. All potentially nephrotoxic drugs should be withdrawn and a septic workup should be carried out. Volume expansion with albumin results in only transient improvement. Isotonic saline is usually avidly retained, worsening the ascites and possibly precipitating pulmonary edema. Mannitol is not used, as this may lead to intracellular acidosis. Dialysis does not improve survival. The final combination of azotemia, hyponatremia and hypotension is terminal. Liver transplantation should be considered, but presumably would have been offered to the patient earlier in the course of the hepatic illness.

15. LIVER TRANSPLANTATION / I. Altraif and G.A. Levy

In 1963, Thomas Starzl and associates in Denver, Colorado, reported the first liver transplant in a human, a 3-year-old boy with biliary atresia. The first successful transplant was performed in 1967, in a 1½-year-old girl with primary hepatocellular carcinoma who lived for 13 months, but died of recurrent tumor. Reported one-year survival in the early years was 25–35% using steroid and azathioprine as immunosuppressives.

With the introduction of cyclosporine in the early 1980s, one-year graft survival improved to 70%, making liver transplantation an effective and safe form of therapy for patients with end-stage liver disease. This led to a dramatic increase in the number of liver transplant centers in North America to more than 130 in 1993, and there are now over 3,000 liver transplants performed annually in the United States alone. In Canada, there are now active centers in Halifax, Nova Scotia; Montreal, Quebec; Toronto, Ontario; London, Ontario; Edmonton, Alberta; and Vancouver, British Columbia. Over 200 liver transplants are performed yearly in Canada. Survival rates of 80–90% have recently been reported by many centers, demonstrating that liver transplantation is the most effective form of therapy for patients with end-stage liver disease.

15.1 Operative Assessment
A patient is considered a suitable candidate for liver transplantation when the diagnosis of end-stage, irreversible liver disease is made. The indications for liver transplantation in adults and children are listed in Table 20 (although this is not an inclusive list). The selection of appropriate candidates from a large number of patients with liver disease requires a strict individual assessment. Exclusion of patients with contraindications to liver transplantation results in selection of patients who are likely to survive and therefore will benefit from the procedure (Table 21).

15.2 Preoperative Workup
The principles behind the liver transplant workup are to firmly establish the

TABLE 20.   Indications for liver transplantation

Adult
Irreversible advanced chronic liver disease
  Predominantly cholestatic liver disease
    Primary biliary cirrhosis
    Primary sclerosing cholangitis
    Secondary biliary cirrhosis
    Drug-induced biliary cirrhosis and cholestasis

  Predominantly hepatocellular liver disease
    Chronic viral hepatitis
      Hepatitis B
      Hepatitis B with hepatitis D
      Hepatitis C
    Drug-induced liver disease
    Cryptogenic cirrhosis
    Autoimmune chronic active hepatitis with cirrhosis
    Alcoholic liver disease
    Wilson's disease
    Congenital hepatic fibrosis
    α_1- antitrypsin deficiency

Vascular diseases that lead to hepatic dysfunction or portal hypertension or both
  Budd-Chiari syndrome
  Veno-occlusive disease

Hepatic malignancies not resectable without hepatic replacement but confined to the liver
  Hepatocellular carcinoma
  Intrahepatic cholangiocarcinoma
  Isolated hepatic metastases – carcinoid tumor

Fulminant hepatic failure
  Viral hepatitis (A, B, C, B+, D)
  Wilson's disease
  Drug or toxin induced
  Others

Inherited metabolic disorders
  Hemophilia A
  Homozygous familial hypercholesterolemia
  Primary hyperoxaluria type I
  Others

Pediatric
Biliary atresia

Metabolic abnormalities
  Tyrosinemia
  Glycogen storage disease
  Others

(cont'd)

TABLE 20.   Indications for liver transplantation (cont'd)

Cirrhosis

Fulminant hepatitis

Retransplantation
Primary dysfunction
Recurrent hepatitis
Arterial thrombosis
Chronic rejection

---

etiology of the liver disease, identify contraindications and determine the patient's ability to withstand surgery (Table 22). Assessment by a multidisciplinary team, which includes medical, surgical, social and psychiatric specialists, is done in patients to ensure the success of the transplantation process.

Once the patient is declared a candidate for liver transplantation, he or she goes onto a liver transplant list awaiting a suitable donor. Preoperatively, transplant candidates may present with complications that require urgent attention such as gastrointestinal bleeding, spontaneous bacterial peritonitis, hepatic encephalopathy or other complications related or unrelated to their underlying liver disease.

15.3 Timing of Transplantation
With improving results of liver transplantation, patients who once were transplanted only for treatment of life-threatening complications are now being transplanted earlier in the course of their disease. Today many patients undergo liver transplantation because of quality of life issues such as extreme fatigue, pruritus and inability to hold employment or participate in the activities of daily living. It is clear that transplantation should be considered prior to catastrophic complications and the need for life support.

15.4 Operative Procedure
A bilateral subcostal incision with an upper midline extension is used. The recipient liver is dissected free from its attachment to the diaphragm, the inferior vena cava is mobilized from the retroperitoneum and the structures of the portal triad – i.e., the hepatic artery, portal vein and common bile duct – are dissected. During the anhepatic phase of the operation, the patient may be

TABLE 21.   Contraindications for orthotopic liver transplantation

---

Advanced cardiopulmonary diseases, life-limiting
Disorders of any other organ system that are not correctable by liver transplantation
Active infection outside the hepatobiliary system
HIV positivity
Inability to accept the procedure, understand its nature, and cooperate in the medical care
  required following transplantation
Primary malignant disease outside the hepatobiliary system
Active alcohol and/or substance abuse
Metastatic hepatobiliary malignancy
Option of alternative effective medical or surgical therapy
HB_sAg positivity (HBV-DNA positive)
Advanced age

---

placed on venovenous bypass to maintain hemodynamic stability. This is performed by directing flow from the iliac vein (via a saphenous vein cutdown) and the portal vein through a vortex pump back into the axillary vein without systemic heparinization. This prevents splanchnic and intestinal congestion, decreases third space losses and reduces the incidence of renal failure by decompression of the renal vein outflow. The suprahepatic and infrahepatic cava anastomoses are performed, followed by anastomosis of the portal vein. The patient is taken off the bypass, if it was used at this point. The hepatic artery anastomosis at the gastroduodenal junction is then performed. Lastly, the common bile duct is reconstructed. A choledochojejunostomy to a Roux-en-Y loop is used in patients with inadequate or diseased recipient ducts. The patient is then brought to the surgical intensive care unit, intubated with lines and catheters in place.

15.5 Postoperative Management
Issues that must be addressed in the postoperative period include management of fluid and electrolytes, respiratory function, monitoring of neurologic status, immunosuppression and graft function.

In most cases patients are quickly extubated within 24 hours of surgery. However, ventilatory support may be needed for an extended period, particularly when there is delayed graft function, presence of pleural effusion, pulmonary infiltrate and diaphragmatic dysfunction or paralysis.

15.5.1 COAGULATION
Abnormalities of coagulation are sensitive markers of hepatic dysfunction.

TABLE 22.   Liver transplantation workup

Bloodwork
Hematology
    CBC, group and reserve; PT; PTT
Renal
    Electrolytes, blood glucose, BUN, creatinine, magnesium, phosphate, calcium
Liver
    AST, ALT, ALP, bilirubin, proteins (A/G), amylase

Other
Serum Fe/TIBC; ferritin; transferrin; sickle cell (only if patient is black); serum copper;
    ceruloplasmin; immunoelectrophoresis; α_1-antitrypsin; α-fetoprotein; antimitochondrial
    antibody; rheumatoid factor; antinuclear factor; antismooth muscle

Serology
HB_sAg; anti-HB_sAg; HB_eAg; anti-HB_eAg; anti-HB_cAg; anti-HCV; anti-HAV; IgM, IgG; EBV
    titers; CMV titers; varicella titers

If patient has hepatitis B+ HBV-DNA
HIV

Tissue typing
HLA tissue typing

24-hr urine collection
Creatinine clearance, Ca, Mg, PO_4

Other tests
Chest x-ray PA and lateral
Abdominal ultrasound with Doppler hepatic vessels
Abdominal angiogram (if nonvisualization of hepatic and portal
    veins and hepatic artery on ultrasound)
Upper endoscopy ± colonoscopy (patients >50 years of age)
Pulmonary function test
ECG
2-D echo of heart
Transjugular liver biopsy with hepatic vein pressures

Consults

Anesthesia	Pharmacist
Dentistry	Dietician
Hematology	Social worker
Psychiatry	

These are routinely assessed by measurement of prothrombin time, partial thromboplastin time and/or assay of coagulation factors V or VII. Following successful liver transplantation, coagulation parameters should return to normal levels within 48 hours in most patients. Failure of coagulation parameters to normalize is an ominous sign of graft failure and suggests the need for retransplantation.

15.5.2 RENAL FUNCTION
Renal insufficiency, occasionally requiring dialysis, is not uncommon postoperatively in liver transplant patients. This may be due to a combination of factors including pre-existing renal insufficiency (hepatorenal syndrome), intraoperative blood loss and hypotension leading to tubular necrosis, drug-induced nephrotoxicity, poor liver function and sepsis.

15.5.3 NEUROLOGIC FUNCTION
Most patients wake up within several hours of liver transplantation, whereas patients with fulminant hepatic failure (FHF) may require one to three days to return to normal neurologic status after liver transplantation. In patients with FHF, monitoring of intracranial pressure may help in perioperative management. Narcotics and sedatives are kept to a minimum in the immediate postoperative period. During this period confusion and seizures can be seen. They are usually related to metabolic disturbances (low serum magnesium levels), but are known complications of cyclosporine and FK506. It has been recommended that all patients be placed on a continuous infusion of magnesium sulfate for the first 72 to 96 hours postoperatively.

15.5.4 MEDICATIONS

15.5.4.1 Antibiotics
Prophylactic antibiotics are usually given preoperatively and continued for 24 hours. The use of broad-spectrum antibiotics has resulted in a decrease in perioperative bacterial infection, but increased incidence of antibiotic-induced enterocolitis and fungal infections.

15.5.4.2 Anticoagulation
Dipyridamole and low-dose heparin are used in patients in the immediate postoperative period to minimize the risk of deep vein thrombosis and thrombosis of blood graft vessels. This is discontinued within seven days once the patient is fully ambulatory.

TABLE 23. Drug interactions with cyclosporine A

Decreased metabolism	Increased metabolism	Increased nephrotoxicity
Erythromycin	Phenytoin	Amphothericin B
Ketoconazole	Rifampicin	Aminoglycosides
Corticosteroids	Isoniazid	Melphalan
Cimetidine	Sulfonamides/	Trimethoprim
Verapamil	trimethoprim,	Cotrimoxazole
	sulfadimidine	Nonsteroidal anti-inflammatory agents

15.5.4.3 Antacids

H_2 blockers and/or liquid antacids are used routinely to keep the gastric pH above 4 to prevent stress ulceration.

15.5.4.4 Immunosuppression

The introduction of cyclosporine is considered one of the most important causes of improvement in the results of liver transplantation. Since its early introduction in late 1978, the survival of liver transplant recipients has increased from 30 to 70%. Cyclosporine is an antibiotic isolated from the fungus Tolypocladium inflatum gans. It binds to a specific receptor, cyclophillin, and through a complex series of intracellular events prevents activation of T cells and production of interleukin-2. The drug is given preferably by the oral route or by slow intravenous infusion. The dosage of cyclosporine is adjusted to maintain a trough cyclosporine whole blood level of 300–400 ng/mL (monoclonal radioimmunoassay). Cyclosporine A is lipid soluble, and absorption is dependent upon the availability of bile. Therefore, until adequate bile flow is restored, adequate cyclosporine levels are difficult to obtain with the current oral preparations.

Close monitoring of cyclosporine levels on a daily basis in the immediate postoperative period is mandatory, as the compound has a narrow therapeutic index (efficacy versus toxicity). Cyclosporine is metabolized by the cytochrome P-450 oxidase system. Any drug that enhances P-450 activity will decrease cyclosporine levels, whereas P-450 inhibitors will result in enhanced cyclosporine levels. Caution must be exercised in giving any drug that may interfere with cyclosporine metabolism to patients who are taking cyclosporine. Table 23 represents known common drugs that interact with cyclosporine.

TABLE 24. Side effects of cyclosporine A

Major	(%)	Minor	(%)
Renal dysfunction	51.7	Hypertrichosis	32.9
Hypertension	38.6	Tremor	20.7
Lymphoma	0.2	Paresthesias	5.2
Malignant tumor	0.6	Headaches	0.8
Infection		Gum hyperplasia	14.8
Bacterial	18.3		
Viral	12.6		
Fungal	3.2		

Side effects of cyclosporine A are noted in Table 24. Other less common side effects include confusion, seizure, agitation, headache, hearing loss, anorexia, diarrhea, nausea/vomiting, abdominal discomfort and gynecomastia.

15.5.4.5 *Steroids*
All patients receive 100 mg of methylprednisolone preoperatively. Subsequently, this is reduced rapidly to a dose of 0.3 mg/kg/day. Side effects include an increased incidence of infections (bacterial and fungal), hyperglycemia and impaired wound healing.

15.5.4.6 *Polyclonal antilymphocyte globulin*
Polyclonal antilymphocyte products are potent and effective both in the induction of immunotherapy and the treatment of acute rejection episodes. Induction therapy with antilymphocyte products has been reported to reduce both the incidence and severity of postoperative rejection; however, it is associated with an increased incidence of lymphoproliferative disorders and cytomegalovirus (CMV) infections. The therapy is monitored by keeping absolute lymphocyte counts <200 cells/mm tubes. Side effects of antilymphocyte products include fever, thrombocytopenia, leukopenia, anaphylaxis, joint pain and increased susceptibility to infections and malignancy.

15.5.4.7 *Monoclonal antilymphocyte product (OKT3)*
OKT3 is a murine, monoclonal antibody to the CD3 antigen of human T cells. It has been used both in induction of immunosuppressive therapy as well as in the treatment of steroid-resistant severe rejection. OKT3, being a mouse immunoglobulin, is extremely antigenic, and usually its use results in antibody formation. To prevent formation of these antibodies, azathioprine is used concomitantly. Despite this, life-threatening side effects have been

TABLE 25. Early postoperative complications in liver transplantation

Complication	Incidence (%)
Hemorrhage	3–18
Primary dysfunction	2–23
Hepatic artery thrombosis	10–20
Portal vein thrombosis	< 5
Biliary tract	13–34
Allograft rejection	60–80
Infections	
Bacterial	30–40
Viral	30
Fungal	20

observed with its use. High fever, tremor, diarrhea, vomiting and nausea, chest pain and rigors are common side effects. Prior to being given an initial dose of OKT3, patients are usually given a bolus dose of Solu-Medrol®, antihistamine, acetaminophen and diuretics to prevent side effects. These adverse effects are related to the release of tumor necrosis factor and interleukin-1.

15.5.4.8 New immunosuppressive agents
FK506 has been shown to be approximately 100 times more potent than cyclosporine. However, a number of studies have shown that this agent is at least as toxic as cyclosporine. Recent studies have suggested that FK506 may be a useful immunosuppressive agent, particularly as rescue therapy to reverse ductopenic rejection – i.e., unresponsiveness to conventional immunosuppression.

15.6 Postoperative Complications (Tables 25 and 26)

15.6.1 HEMORRHAGE
The incidence of postoperative hemorrhages that necessitate an exploratory laparotomy is 8.4%. This appears to correlate with previous upper abdominal surgery, portal hypertension and the degree of coagulation disturbances prior to transplant. Postoperative hemorrhage is associated with high mortality. Thus, patients are monitored in the immediate postoperative period for hematocrit, hemodynamic instability and abdominal distention that are suggestive of ongoing intra-abdominal bleeding.

15.6.2 HEPATIC ARTERY THROMBOSIS
This is a devastating complication seen in 10–20% of adults; even higher inci-

TABLE 26.   Causes of graft dysfunction

Rejection (cellular or ductopenic)
Opportunistic
    Viral: CMV, EBV, HSV, VZV and adenovirus
    Bacterial, fungal
Vascular thrombosis
Biliary tract complications
Drug-induced hepatoxicity
Recurrent disease
Parenteral nutrition
De novo viral hepatitis

dence is seen in children. Factors thought to be associated with hepatic artery thrombosis include the size of the vessels, type of vascular anastomosis and nontechnical factors including the presence of rejection, infection, hemoconcentration or dehydration. Acute hepatic artery thrombosis in the immediate postoperative period is characterized by a dramatic increase in liver enzymes (AST, ALT) associated with coagulopathy and encephalopathy. Subacute thrombosis may lead to bile leaks, biliary strictures (secondary to ischemia in the donor anastomosis) and intrahepatic abscesses resulting in relapsing bacteremia. The diagnosis of hepatic artery thrombosis is made by Doppler ultrasonography and confirmed by angiography. Hepatic artery thrombosis may be treated by thrombectomy and revision of the hepatic artery if diagnosed early. Occasionally it may be left untreated, but patients usually require retransplantation either semi-electively or on an emergency basis.

15.6.3 PORTAL VEIN THROMBOSIS
This is a rare complication, occurring in 1.8% of patients. Presentation depends on the timing of the thrombosis. Early postoperative portal vein thrombosis resembles hepatic artery thrombosis. When thrombosis occurs four to five weeks following the transplant, patients may have a nonspecific rise in liver enzymes or may present with evidence of portal hypertension or ileus. Diagnosis is often made by Doppler ultrasonography and confirmed by angiography. Treatment consists of emergency thrombolytic therapy or surgery if it is recognized early. Otherwise, retransplantation is done.

15.6.4 BILIARY TRACT COMPLICATIONS
Biliary tract complications following orthotopic liver transplantation are reported to be in the range of 13–34%. Factors that are felt to contribute include inadequate blood supply causing ischemic damage to the bile ducts;

local infection; graft rejection; change in bile secretion; drug toxicity; preservation injury; and operative techniques. Bile leaks may be localized and may present with no or minimal symptomatology, only to be discovered on routine cholangiography. However, bile leakage may present as an intra-abdominal abscess or as frank bile peritonitis.

Treatment depends on the timing and presentation of the leak. Early leakage with intra-abdominal peritonitis requires exploration with repair and drainage. Continued leaks in the stable patient have been managed by percutaneous drainage, endoscopic techniques and conservative therapy, or any combination of the above.

15.6.5 PRIMARY GRAFT DYSFUNCTION

Primary graft dysfunction is defined as initial poor function following orthotopic transplantation. Evidence of deterioration includes minimal bile production, uncorrectable coagulopathy, rapid rise of transaminases, acidosis, hypoglycemia and mental deterioration. The incidence of primary dysfunction is reported to be in the range of 2–23% and carries with it a significant mortality rate. Most patients die if retransplantation is not performed within 48 to 72 hours of diagnosis. Prostaglandin E_1 treatment of primary graft dysfunction appears promising and may change this approach.

15.6.6 ALLOGRAFT REJECTION

Acute allograft rejection occurs in 60–80% of transplant patients, usually in the first three months after transplantation. Rejection is suspected in patients with rising liver enzymes that may be accompanied by fever, malaise and right upper quadrant discomfort. Diagnosis is confirmed by liver biopsy. Histologic findings are periportal inflammation with mononuclear cells and eosinophils, bile duct injury and endophlebitis. Episodes of cellular rejection usually respond to high-dose steroid therapy. Those patients whose rejection fails to respond to steroids are usually treated with a 7- to 14-day course of antithymocyte globulin (monoclonal or polyclonal). Failure to respond to immunosuppressive therapy may result in ductopenic rejection (chronic rejection) and lead to biliary cirrhosis, which may result in the need for retransplantation in 5–10% of all transplanted patients.

15.6.7 INFECTION

The major cause of death following liver transplantation is infection. Immunosuppressed patients are at risk for bacterial, viral and fungal infections. Bacterial infections with nonopportunistic organisms are usually seen in the early postoperative period. Opportunistic bacterial infections develop one to two months or more after transplantation. Wound infection and intra-abdominal sepsis account for the majority of bacterial infections seen in transplanted patients.

Viral infections are seen frequently in immunosuppressed patients, and usually occur at six weeks or later. Cytomegalovirus (CMV) is present in over half of the population and in nonimmunosuppressed persons is virtually nonpathogenic. However, CMV infection in transplanted patients may account for 30% of the infections seen and is a source of morbidity and some mortality. CMV infection is characterized by high fever, usually associated with anorexia, malaise and arthralgias. Laboratory tests that are suggestive of CMV infection include leukopenia and a mild elevation of liver enzymes. In 13% of patients with CMV, pulmonary manifestation may develop. Liver biopsy findings in patients with CMV hepatitis include polyclusters of neutrophils surrounding CMV nuclear inclusion bodies. The therapy for CMV infection includes reduction of immunosuppression and the use of antiviral agents such as ganciclovir. Other viral infections seen in the transplanted patients include herpes simplex, Epstein-Barr virus, varicella zoster and adenovirus. Fungal infections have been noted in up to 20% of patients and carry with them a 20–100% mortality rate. Infections in general are usually proportional to the degree of immunosuppression.

15.7 Results of Liver Transplantation

The one-year survival after liver transplantation is now 80%. Most mortality occurs within the first 90 days. After one year, few patients or grafts are lost. Furthermore, 60% of patients return to gainful employment, demonstrating that this procedure is not only of benefit to the patient but to society as a whole. Though there are few reports of cost-effectiveness studies, in the Pittsburgh experience liver transplantation was less expensive than caring for similar patients treated for the complications of cirrhosis. Patients with diseases such as cholestatic liver disease, which tend not to recur after liver transplantation, have an excellent long prognosis (greater than 80% five-year survival). In contrast, patients transplanted for viral hepatitis, and in particular hepatitis B, have a poor long-term outlook (less than 30% five-year survival). Highly selected patients with asymptomatic small hepatocellular carcinomas can have an excellent long-term survival rate if they do not have coexistent viral hepatitis B infection.

15.8 Future Directions

Induction of tolerance is under experimental investigation. This seems to be possible in animal models. If tolerance can be induced in humans, it will obviate the need for long-term immunosuppression and its complications.

Liver transplantation in the pediatric age group is limited by the shortage of pediatric donors. As a result, reduced liver grafts are performed routinely with great success nowadays. Split liver transplantation, whereby a donor liver is given to two recipients, has been performed with success. However, improvements in surgical techniques are required before this procedure can become routine. Liver transplantation is now performed routinely in some centers with greater than 80% one-year survival. Xenograft transplantation remains experimental at present. Isolated hepatocyte transplantation has been performed in animals for treatment of metabolic liver diseases. Finally, artificial support systems that may help patients with fulminant hepatic failure are now being studied in large controlled trials which, if successful, may reduce the need for transplantation in this condition.

16. NEOPLASMS OF THE LIVER / G. Minuk

In adults, most primary tumors occur in cirrhotic livers. Fortunately, primary liver tumors are uncommon in North America, representing only 2% of all malignancies. Of the primary tumors, 30–40% are hepatocellular carcinoma, while the rest are gallbladder or bile duct tumors. A much higher incidence of primary liver tumors in other countries makes hepatocellular carcinoma the most common tumor worldwide. Liver cancers can be caused by a variety of toxic substances and infectious agents, including chronic hepatitis B and C.

A number of benign tumors can develop in the liver. Hemangioma is the most common type, and is often detected by ultrasound performed for unrelated reasons. Approximately 10% of the general population has hemangioma of the liver. Liver cell adenoma is a benign tumor that may develop as the result of hormonal stimulation by oral contraceptives and other hormonal agents. This tumor has a higher risk of rupture and bleeding than the others and may also have malignant potential. Focal nodular hyperplasia, another benign tumor of the liver, does not appear to be hormonally sensitive. The most common tumor in liver tissue is one that has metastasized from elsewhere. The sites from which metastases occur frequently include lung, colon, pancreas, breast, stomach and ovary. The presence of multiple tumors in the liver is suggestive of metastatic disease, but multifocal hepatocellular carcinomas can also occur in some world populations. Often a liver biopsy is required to distinguish primary from metastatic malignancy of the liver.

16.1 Primary Hepatocellular Carcinoma
Hepatocellular carcinoma or hepatoma arises from areas of long-standing liver injury with liver necrosis and repair, as in cirrhotic livers. The risk of

developing hepatocellular carcinoma is greatest in patients with chronic hepatitis B and C infections, hemochromatosis and cirrhosis from α_1-antitrypsin deficiency. Hepatitis B virus can predispose to hepatoma in either a cirrhotic or noncirrhotic liver. The basis for this appears to be integration of the HBV-DNA into portions of the human genome where growth-modulating genes are present. Hepatocellular carcinoma is not often seen in patients with alcoholic cirrhosis who continue to drink, unless the alcoholic has coexisting viral hepatitis. Hepatic co-carcinogens that appear to play a role in hepatocellular carcinoma include aflatoxins and the radiocontrast agent thorotrast.

Hepatocellular carcinoma should be considered whenever a patient with known cirrhosis deteriorates with rapid weight loss, enlarging liver, abdominal pain or bloody ascites. A hepatic bruit may be present. Patients may present with one of many paraneoplastic syndromes including erythrocytosis, hypercalcemia or dysproteinemia. Hypoglycemia can also occur. Serum α-fetoprotein levels are elevated in the majority of cases. Ultrasound or CT scan imaging is often used to identify the mass, but occasionally radionuclear scanning (using gallium) or x-ray angiography may help further define the nature of the mass lesion and provide important operative details. A biopsy of the mass or examination of ascites fluid for cytology may yield a conclusive diagnosis.

Treatment is disappointing. Radiation and chemotherapy have little impact. Surgical resection represents the only opportunity for cure, but resection is often complicated by the presence of underlying cirrhosis, the occasional multicentric nature of the tumor and the presence of micrometastases. Up to 70% of patients already have metastatic disease at the time of diagnosis. The mean survival from the time of diagnosis is approximately 6 to 12 months. Screening strategies include ultrasound and/or α-fetoprotein determinations every 6 months in high-risk patients. This approach clearly identifies tumors at an earlier stage but has not yet been shown to improve morbidity or mortality rates.

17. LIVER DISEASE IN PREGNANCY / R.J. Hilsden and E.A. Shaffer

17.1 Normal Pregnancy
The pregnant state is mildly cholestatic from the increase in endogenous estrogens. This changes several biochemical tests, but primary liver disease is an uncommon complication. When features of liver disease do occur during pregnancy, prompt evaluation is essential as some conditions, such as acute fatty liver of pregnancy, rapidly progress to become fatal to both mother and fetus.

The anatomic and physiologic changes that accompany pregnancy alter physical findings and liver biochemistries. Yet normal pregnancy does not significantly affect liver metabolism or function.

Pregnancy does not change liver size. In the third trimester, the enlarging uterus displaces the liver superiorly and posteriorly. Therefore, a palpable liver suggests significant hepatomegaly and underlying liver disease. A small amount of peripheral edema is also common during pregnancy, as are some findings that usually connote chronic liver disease, such as spider angiomas and palmar erythema.

Total blood volume and cardiac output increase with pregnancy, but hepatic blood flow remains unchanged. The expanded blood volume and deviation of venous return through the azygous system (due to pressure of the gravid uterus on the inferior vena cava) elevate portal venous pressure. This engorges the esophageal veins, resulting in small, clinically insignificant esophageal varices in late pregnancy.

Pregnancy does not alter the expected values for serum bilirubin, aminotransferases, γ-glutamyl transpeptidase or 5'-nucleotidase, or the prothrombin time. Dilution from the expanded plasma volume causes a 10 g/L fall in serum albumin and in total protein. Alkaline phosphatase, primarily of placental and skeletal origin, increases 1.5 times normal after the fifth week. Alkaline phosphatase may remain elevated for up to six weeks after delivery. There is an increase in serum globulin, total cholesterol and triglyceride.

Liver diseases occurring during pregnancy can be divided into three categories: (1) acute liver disease coincident with pregnancy; (2) pregnancy occurring in a patient with established chronic liver disease; and (3) liver diseases unique to pregnancy.

17.2 Acute Liver Disease Coincident with Pregnancy

Any liver disease that can afflict young women may arise during pregnancy. Of these, viral hepatitis is the most common cause of jaundice in pregnancy. Pregnancy does not affect the course of viral hepatitis, except for hepatitis E, which occurs as epidemics in underdeveloped countries. In such settings, the combination of pregnancy and hepatitis plus the indigenous malnutrition results in a significant mortality rate (10–40%). In developed areas, hepatitis B poses a high risk of neonatal infection. Neonates born to mothers who are hepatitis B surface antigen (HB_sAg) positive must receive immunoprophylaxis to prevent the long-term sequelae of chronic hepatitis B: cirrhosis and hepatocellular carcinoma.

Viral hepatitis due to herpes simplex or cytomegalovirus can occur in pregnant women who are otherwise immunocompetent, and may lead to fulminant hepatic failure. Acyclovir therapy is extremely effective for herpes simplex.

17.3 Pregnancy Occurring in Chronic Liver Disease

Pregnancy is unusual in patients with chronic liver disease. Fertility becomes nearly normal when cirrhosis is well compensated or the active liver disease improves with appropriate therapy (e.g., chronic hepatitis on steroids). The degree of hepatic impairment determines the risk for the mother during the pregnancy. Hemorrhage from esophageal varices is the most significant complication of cirrhosis in pregnancy. The increased blood volume and flow through the azygous system raises the pressure in the esophageal veins; in established cirrhosis this increases variceal size and the likelihood of bleeding.

17.4 Liver Diseases Unique to Pregnancy

Liver diseases unique to pregnancy are acute fatty liver of pregnancy; intrahepatic cholestasis of pregnancy; toxemia of pregnancy and the HELLP syndrome (hemolysis, elevated liver enzymes, low platelets); and spontaneous rupture of the liver.

17.4.1 ACUTE FATTY LIVER OF PREGNANCY

Acute fatty liver of pregnancy is characterized by fatty infiltration of the liver. It may rapidly progress to hepatic failure and death. Acute fatty liver may be uncommon (1 in 13,328 deliveries), but is important, having a maternal mortality of 18% and fetal mortality of 23%. The etiology is unknown, but the microvesicular fat that accumulates in hepatocytes probably represents disordered intermediary fat metabolism, perhaps related to mitochondrial injury.

Acute fatty liver of pregnancy almost invariably presents in the third trimester, with a peak frequency around 36–37 weeks gestation. Occasionally, it will become apparent only after delivery. There is an association with nulliparity, twin gestations, male fetus and pre-eclampsia or eclampsia. Presentation can vary from nonspecific symptoms to fulminant hepatic failure. Nausea and vomiting with or without abdominal pain are common. Examination may reveal a tender liver. Pruritus is uncommon and would suggest the possibility of a different liver problem such as intrahepatic cholestasis of pregnancy. Progressive hepatic failure then rapidly supervenes, with the development of jaundice, generalized bleeding from coagulopathy, hypoglycemia, hepatic encephalopathy and renal failure. Such severe cases have an inexorable downhill course unless the fetus is delivered; even then, deterioration may continue for a further 48 to 72 hours.

Laboratory features include a moderately elevated aminotransferase, which is usually around 300 IU/L but may range from normal to 1,000 IU/L. Alkaline phosphatase and serum bilirubin are elevated. Liver biopsy reveals tiny droplets of fat (microvesicular fat) inside hepatocytes. Some cholestasis may be present, but only minimal inflammation or necrosis. The same microvesicular fatty change also affects the heart, kidneys and pancreas.

To diagnose acute fatty liver of pregnancy requires a high degree of suspicion, as the presentation is often nonspecific. Consider it whenever marked nausea and vomiting develop in the third trimester of pregnancy. Suspicion increases with a twin pregnancy, nulliparity or signs of toxemia. Ultrasound or CT scans may detect the increased fat in the liver and help exclude complications such as a subcapsular hematoma or another entity such as choledocholithiasis. Liver biopsy is diagnostic. Biopsy even via the transvenous route (necessary when a coagulopathy makes percutaneous liver biopsy hazardous) should be done if the results will alter management. For example, differentiation of acute viral hepatitis from acute fatty liver is important to determine whether rapid delivery is indicated. Delivery can be life-saving in acute fatty liver.

Management involves aggressive supportive care, even in an intensive unit. Correct any hypoglycemia or bleeding tendencies. The only definitive treatment for the condition is prompt delivery. Acute fatty liver of pregnancy will not recur with subsequent pregnancies; only one case has been reported.

17.4.2 INTRAHEPATIC CHOLESTASIS OF PREGNANCY

Intrahepatic cholestasis of pregnancy accounts for 20–25% of cases of jaundice during pregnancy. The etiology is unknown. There is a clear genetic predisposition, with an increased frequency in women of Scandinavian or Chilean descent. It is often familial. Even some male family members given estrogens have demonstrated a cholestatic tendency. Dominant inheritance is suggested. The cholestasis (failure of bile formation) represents an exaggerated response of the liver to the normal increase in endogenous estrogens during pregnancy.

Presentation typically is in the third trimester. Pruritus onsets insidiously; in half of these patients, jaundice follows. Other cholestatic features include dark urine and, occasionally, pale stool. Women generally feel well, apart from the pruritus. They do not have significant nausea, vomiting or abdominal pain; if these are present, other diagnoses should be sought. Although a benign condition for the mother (other than the inexorable pruritus), intrahepatic cholestasis may decrease fetal survival, being associated with an increased risk of stillbirth and prematurity. Serum alkaline phosphatase and cholesterol rise, but aminotransferases are only modestly elevated. Ultrasound and cholangiography are normal. Liver biopsy shows cholestasis. The evaluation of the pregnant woman with cholestasis involves excluding other causes of jaundice and pruritus including viral hepatitis, primary biliary cirrhosis and biliary tract disease by the appropriate laboratory and ultrasound investigations. Liver biopsy may be necessary in some atypical cases.

Treatment is supportive. The pruritus can be severe and disabling, preventing sleep and normal activities.

Antihistamines are unhelpful, but bile salt–binding agents such as cholestyramine are useful. Ursodeoxycholic acid therapy, theoretically replacing other "toxic bile acids" and perhaps improving bile formation (washing out pruritogenic agents), also is effective. S-adenosylmethionine, which alters membrane fluidity, also appears to work. Rifampin may reduce pruritus by increasing the excretion of pruritogenic agents. Treatment for cholestasis and pruritus, however, generally is unsatisfactory. Many recommend that delivery occur as soon as fetal lung maturity is documented, to prevent the increased risk of stillbirth. Parenteral vitamin K may be needed to correct a prothrombin deficiency, especially if cholestyramine administration has worsened the associated fat malabsorption.

Symptoms usually abate within two weeks of delivery. There is a significant risk of recurrence with subsequent pregnancies and with the use of oral contraceptives or other estrogens.

17.4.3 PREGNANCY TOXEMIAS AND THE HELLP SYNDROME

In severe pre-eclampsia or eclampsia, liver involvement is evident by abdominal tenderness and abnormal liver biochemistry. Focal and diffuse hepatocellular necrosis can occur from endothelial damage and platelet and fibrin deposition in the sinusoids. Subcapsular hematoma and hepatic rupture rarely develop.

The HELLP syndrome (hemolysis, elevated liver enzymes, low platelets) is usually associated with pre-eclampsia; occasionally, it may arise in the absence of either hypertension or proteinuria. Liver complications are similar to those in pre-eclampsia. Differentiation of acute fatty liver of pregnancy from the HELLP syndrome may be clinically difficult, but the treatment – prompt delivery and supportive care – is identical for both.

18. VASCULAR DISORDERS OF THE LIVER / L.J. Worobetz

The most frequent abnormality of circulation to affect the liver is congestive heart failure, which leads to reduced outflow of blood from the liver. Thus, common causes of hepatic congestion include constrictive pericarditis, obstruction of the inferior vena cava and hepatic veins (Budd-Chiari syndrome) and occlusion of the small hepatic veins (veno-occlusive disease).

Increased resistance to hepatic venous outflow results in congestive hepatomegaly, dilatation of hepatic venules and sinusoids, and hypoxia. The hypoxia in turn leads to hepatocyte damage with possible fibrosis and cirrhosis, the latter termed cardiac cirrhosis.

18.1 Congestive Heart Failure

The clinical features of congestive heart failure include tender hepatomegaly and abdominal discomfort. In tricuspid insufficiency, the liver may be pulsatile. Ascites, which may be present, often involves exudate with a high protein content. Characteristic biochemical abnormalities are mild hyperbilirubinemia with a moderate elevation of aminotransferases (<300) and a mild elevation of alkaline phosphatase, especially in acute congestion. In ischemic liver damage, aminotransferase can be quite high (from the necrosis), simulating hepatitis – hence the term ischemic hepatitis. The prognosis is directly related to the severity and the response to therapy of the underlying heart failure.

18.2 Hepatic Vein Thrombosis (Budd-Chiari Syndrome)

Hepatic vein thrombosis is a rare disorder that may occur alone or in association with inferior vena cava thrombosis. It may be associated with polycythemia vera, paroxysmal nocturnal hemoglobinuria, hypercoagulability, use of oral contraceptives or neoplasia, or it may be secondary to obstruction by a membranous web. The presentation may be acute, with rapidly developing hepatomegaly, ascites, and abdominal pain leading to liver failure and coma. The chronic presentation is usually that of progressive ascites. The degree of aminotransferase elevation is variable, depending on the rapidity of the onset. The liver biopsy shows large hemorrhagic areas with congestion, atrophy and necrosis around the center of the lobule. Diagnosis may be assisted by liver-spleen colloid scan showing decreased uptake in areas that are otherwise normally drained by the hepatic vein. The caudate lobe demonstrates a normal uptake in that it has a different drainage, that being directly into the vena cava. Hepatic vein Doppler studies clarify the impaired venous blood flow. The conclusive study is IVC hepatic venography revealing blocked hepatic veins. Assuming absence of a correctable lesion such as a membranous web, treatment by anticoagulants and streptokinase is rarely successful. With acute thrombosis, most patients die of liver failure and hepatic coma. Occasionally helpful is a portacaval or mesocaval shunt to allow decompression.

18.3 Veno-occlusive Disease

Veno-occlusive disease means the obstruction of small and medium-sized intrahepatic veins. Causal factors include pyrroline alkaloids, hepatic irradiation, azathioprine and graft-versus-host disease related to bone marrow transplantation. The presentation mimics the Budd-Chiari syndrome. In the acute form, presentation may include hepatomegaly, ascites and liver failure. The chronic form leads to cirrhosis and portal hypertension with esophageal varices. The liver biopsy characteristically shows intense congestion around the hepatic venule with thickened obstructive hepatic veins. There is no effective therapy available. Control of the ascites may be required. Some patients have a spontaneous recovery, while others develop cirrhosis with sequelae of portal hypertension, varices and ascites. Liver transplantation may be the only hope for many.

18.4 Portal Vein Thrombosis

Thrombosis of the portal venous system may result from trauma, pancreatitis, neoplasia (e.g., hepatoma), neonatal umbilical sepsis, pylephlebitis or a complication of cirrhosis, or may be idiopathic. Patients usually present with massive hematemesis that is recurrent. Splenomegaly is present. Biochemical tests of the liver are normal or only mildly elevated. Because liver function is usually normal, ascites and encephalopathy are uncommon and bleeding episodes are better tolerated. Diagnosis may be confirmed by special Doppler ultrasound studies of the portal vein, splenoportogram and/or a venous phase of hepatic angiography. If treatment is required for recurrent hematemesis from esophageal varices, sclerotherapy may be necessary. Because of normal liver parenchyma, surgical approaches such as mesocaval shunt may be considered and are generally better tolerated than by patients with chronic liver disease.

SUGGESTED READING LIST

General
Schiff L, Schiff ER (eds.). Diseases of the liver. 6th ed. Philadelphia: JB Lippincott, 1987.
Sherlock S, Dooley J (eds.). Diseases of the liver and biliary system. 9th ed. Oxford: Blackwell Scientific Publications, 1993.

Section 2 Approach to the Patient with Liver Disease
Frank BB. Clinical evaluation of jaundice. JAMA 1989; 262:3031–3034.
Gollan JL (ed.). Pathobiology of bilirubin and jaundice. Semin Liver Dis 1988; 8:105–199.
Reichling JJ, Kaplan MM. Clinical use of serum enzymes in liver disease. Dig Dis Sci 1988; 33:1601–1614.

Section 3 Congenital Hyperbilirubinemia
Sorrentino D, Anthony JE, Berk PD. Familial hyperbilirubinemia syndromes: kinetic approaches. Baillieres Clin Gastroenterol 1989; 3:313–336.

Watson KJ and Gollan JL. Gilbert's syndrome. Baillieres Clin Gastroenterol 1989; 3:337–355.

Section 4 Acute Viral Hepatitis
Alter HJ, Purcell RH, Shih JW, et al. Detection of antibody to hepatitis C virus in prospectively followed recipients with acute and chronic non-A, non-B transfusion hepatitis. N Engl J Med 1989; 321:1494–1500.

Hollinger FB, Lin HJ. Community-acquired hepatitis C virus infection. Gastroenterology 1992; 102:1426–1429.

Hoofnagle JH, Di Bisceglie AM. Serologic diagnosis of acute and chronic viral hepatitis. Semin Liver Dis 1991; 11:73–84.

Krugman S, Overby LR, Mushahwar IK, et al. Viral hepatitis, type B: studies on natural history and prevention re-examined. N Engl J Med 1979; 300:101–106.

Section 5 Chronic Hepatitis
Autoimmune Chronic Hepatitis
Johnson PJ, McFarlane IG, Eddleston AL. The natural course and heterogeneity of autoimmune-type chronic active hepatitis. Semin Liver Dis 1991; 11:187–196.

Ludwig J. The nomenclature of chronic active hepatitis: an obituary. Gastroenterology 1993; 105:274–278.

Viral Hepatitis
Aagh RD, Stevens CE, Hollinger FB, et al. Hepatitis C virus infection in post-transfusion hepatitis: an analysis with first- and second-generation assays. N Engl J Med 1991; 325:1325–1329.

Alter MJ, Margolis HS, Krawczynski K, et al. The natural history of community-acquired hepatitis C in the United States. N Engl J Med 1992; 327:1899–1905.

Hoofnagle JH, Di Bisceglie AM, Shindo M. Antiviral therapy of hepatitis C – present and future. J Hepatol 1993; 17:130–136.

Katkov WN, Dienstag JL. Prevention and therapy of viral hepatitis. Semin Liver Dis 1991; 11:165–174.

Perrillo RP. Antiviral therapy of chronic hepatitis B: past, present, and future. J Hepatol 1993; 17:56–63.

Rizzetto M, Verme G. Delta hepatitis – present status. J Hepatol 1985; 1:187–193.

Seeff LB, Koff RS. Evolving concepts of the clinical and serologic consequences of hepatitis B virus infection. Semin Liver Dis 1986; 6:11–22.

Fatty Liver
Powell EE, Cooksley WG, Hanson R, Searle J, Halliday JW, Powell LW. The natural history of nonalcoholic steatohepatitis: a follow-up study of forty-two patients for up to 21 years. Hepatology 1990; 11:74–80.

Section 6 Alcoholic Liver Disease
Fleming KA, McGee JO. Alcohol induced liver disease. J Clin Pathol 1984; 37:721–733.

Lieber CS. Alcoholic liver disease: a public health issue in need of a public health approach. Semin Liver Dis 1993; 13:105–107.

Mendenhall CL: Alcoholic hepatitis. In: Schiff L, Schiff ER (eds.), Diseases of the liver. 6th ed. Philadelphia: JB Lippincott, 1987:669–685.

Section 7 Drug-Induced Liver Disease
Kaplowitz N (ed.). Recent advances in drug metabolism and hepatotoxicity. Semin Liver Dis 1990; 10 (special issue): 234–338.

Ludwig J, Axelsen R. Drug effects on the liver: an updated tabular compilation of drugs and drug-related hepatic diseases. Dig Dis Sci 1983; 28:651–666.

Zimmerman HJ. Update of hepatotoxicity due to classes of drugs in common clinical use: non-steroidal drugs, anti-inflammatory drugs, antibiotics, antihypertensives, and cardiac and psychotropic agents. Semin Liver Dis 1990; 10:322–338.

Section 8 Inherited Liver Disease
Hemochromatosis

Adams PC, Kertesz AE, Valberg LS. Clinical presentation of hemochromatosis: a changing scene. Am J Med 1991; 90:445–449.

Adams PC, Speechley M, Kertesz AE. Long-term survival analysis in hereditary hemochromatosis. Gastroenterol 1991; 101:368–372.

Crosby WH. Hemochromatosis: current concepts and management. Hosp Pract 1987; 22:173–177, 181–192.

Edwards CQ, Kushner JP. Screening for hemochromatosis. N Engl J Med 1993; 328:1616–1620.

Alpha$_1$-Antitrypsin Deficiency

Fisher RL, Taylor L, Sherlock S. Alpha-1-antitrypsin deficiency in liver disease: the extent of the problem. Gastroenterol 1976; 71:646–651.

Wilson's disease

Brewer GJ, Yuzbasiyan-Gurkan V. Wilson's disease: an update, with emphasis on new approaches to treatment. Dig Dis 1989; 7:178–193.

Nazer H, Ede RJ, Mowat AP, et al. Wilson's disease: clinical presentation and use of prognostic index. Gut 1986; 27:1377.

Scheinberg IH, Sternlieb I. Wilson's disease. Major problems in internal medicine, vol. 23. Philadelphia: WB Saunders, 1984.

Tanzi RE, Petrukhin, K, Chernov I, et al. The Wilson disease gene is a copper transporting ATPase with homology to the Menkes disease gene. Nature Genetics 1993; 5:344–350.

Section 9 Cholestasis
Favrant M, Williams R. Natural history and prognosis in primary sclerosing cholangitis. Eur J Gastroenterol Hepatol 1992; 4:272–275.

Kaplan MM. Primary biliary cirrhosis. N Engl J Med 1987; 316:521–528.

Lester R (ed.). The pathogenesis of cholestasis: past and future trends. Semin Liver Dis 1993; 13 (special issue): 219–316.

Vierling JM. Immune disorder of the liver and bile duct. Gastroenterol Clin North Am 1992; 21:427–449.

Section 10 Cirrhosis of the Liver
D'Amico G, Morabito A, Pogliaro L, et al. Survival and prognostic indicators in compensated and decompensated cirrhosis. Dig Dis Sci 1986; 31:468.

MacSween RNM, Anthony PP, Scheuer PJ. Pathology of the liver. 2d ed. Edinburgh: Churchill Livingstone, 1987.

Section 11 Portal Hypertension

De Franchis R, Primignani M. Why do varices bleed? Gastroenterol Clin North Am 1992; 21:85–96.

Hilsden RJ, Lee SS. Suspecting variceal bleeding in portal hypertensive patients. Can J Diag 1993; 10:91–103.

Polio J, Groszmann RJ. Hemodynamic factors involved in the development and rupture of esophageal varices: a pathophysiologic approach to treatment. Semin Liver Dis 1986; 6:318–331.

Stiegmann GV, Goff JS, Michaletz-Onody PA, et al. Endoscopic sclerotherapy as compared with endoscopic ligation for bleeding esophageal varices. N Engl J Med 1992; 326:1527–1532.

Triger DR, Hosking SW. The gastric mucosa in portal hypertension. J Hepatol 1989; 8:267–272.

Sections 12 and 14 Ascites/Hepatorenal Syndrome

Epstein M (ed.). The kidney in liver disease. 3d ed. Baltimore: Williams and Wilkins, 1988:3.

Epstein M. The sodium retention of cirrhosis: a reappraisal. Hepatology 1986; 6:312.

Henriksen JH, Ring-Larsen H. Ascites formation in liver cirrhosis: the how and the why. Dig Dis 1990; 8:152.

Section 13 Hepatic Encephalopathy

Butterworth RF. Pathogenesis and treatment of portal-systemic encephalopathy: an update. Dig Dis Sci 1992; 37:321–327.

Ferenc P, Puspok A, Steindl P. Current concepts in the pathophysiology of hepatic encephalopathy. Eur J Clin Invest 1992; 22:573–581.

Section 15 Liver Transplantation

Kirby RM, McMaster P, Clents D, et al. Orthotopic liver transplantation: postoperative complications and their management. Br J Surg 1987; 74:3–11.

Krom RAF, Wiesner RH, Rettke SR, et al. The first 100 liver transplantations at the Mayo Clinic. Symposium on liver transplantation part 1. Mayo Clinic Proc 1989; 64:84–94.

Maddrey WC, Van Thiel DH. Liver transplantation: an overview. Hepatology 1988; 8:948–959.

Sheiner PA, Greig PD, Levy GA. Perioperative management of the liver transplant patient. In: Vincent JL (ed.), Update in intensive care and emergency medicine, update 1990. Berlin: Springer-Verlag, 1990:706–717.

Section 16 Neoplasms of the Liver

Okuda K. Diagnosis and nonsurgical treatment of hepatocellular carcinoma. Hepato-Gastroenterology 1990; 37:155–270.

Rustgi VK (ed.). Hepatic carcinoma. Gastroenterol Clin North Am 1987; 16: 545–649.

Section 17 Liver Disease in Pregnancy

Riely CA, Abell TL (eds.). Gastrointestinal and liver problems in pregnancy. Gastroenterol Clin North Am 1992; 21:873–921, 937–958.

Section 18 Vascular Disorders of the Liver
Gibson PR, Dudley FJ. Ischemic hepatitis: clinical features, diagnosis and prognosis. Aust NZ J Med 1984; 14:822.
Klein AS, Sitzmann JV, Coleman J, et al. Current management of the Budd-Chiari syndrome. Ann Surg 1990; 212:144.

ACKNOWLEDGMENT

The authors would like to acknowledge the assistance of Dr. Emma Lew, Department of Pathology, University of Saskatchewan, in the preparation of the pathology pictures.

OBJECTIVES

Jaundice/Ascites/Hepatic Encephalopathy/Liver Failure
1. Describe normal bilirubin metabolism.
2. Describe pathophysiologic mechanisms of jaundice.
3. Outline the diagnostic tests used in approaching patients with jaundice and discuss liver function tests.
4. Define jaundice.
5. Describe mechanisms of ascites formation.
6. List five conditions that associate with ascites.
7. Describe the techniques and diagnostic tests used to detect ascites.
8. Discuss the indication of abdominal paracentesis and interpret the findings.
9. Recognize the complications of ascites.
10. Outline the management of ascites.
11. Give indications for LeVeen's shunt.
12. Interpret serum and urinary electrolytes in patients with ascites.
13. Discuss the mechanisms of action and side effects of drugs used in the treatment of ascites.
14. Demonstrate clinical skills in approaching patients with hepatic encephalopathy and hepatic failure.
15. List the stigmata of chronic liver disease.
16. List neurotransmitters that possibly have pathogenetic roles in hepatic encephalopathy.
17. List precipitating factors of hepatic encephalopathy.
18. Discuss the use of ammonia blood level in hepatic encephalopathy.
19. Outline the management of hepatic encephalopathy.
20. Discuss the mechanisms of action of lactulose, neomycin, and metronidazole in the treatment of hepatic encephalopathy.

21. Discuss the role of liver transplantation.
22. Differentiate between hepatorenal failure and prerenal azotemia.
23. Discuss the management of hepatorenal failure.

Cirrhosis

1. List underlying causes of cirrhosis.
2. List complications of cirrhosis.
3. List major mechanisms contributing to portal hypertension.
4. Discuss diagnostic methods used in patients with cirrhosis.
5. Describe complications of liver biopsy.
6. Classify portal hypertension.
7. List the consequences of portal hypertension.
8. Describe the management of patients with bleeding esophageal varices.
9. Discuss the use of Sengstaken-Blakemore tube in patients with bleeding esophageal varices.
10. Discuss the efficacy, mechanisms of action and side effects of vasopressin used in treating bleeding esophageal varices.
11. Discuss the role of sclerotherapy in patients with bleeding esophageal varices.
12. List major complications of sclerotherapy.
13. Discuss the surgical management of portal hypertension.

Hepatitis

1. List causative agents for acute hepatitis.
2. Discuss serologic tests used in hepatitis.
3. Discuss the significance of delta agent.
4. Give indications of hepatitis B vaccination.
5. Discuss the clinical manifestations of hepatitis A and hepatitis B infections.
6. Discuss the clinical manifestations of non-A non-B hepatitis.
7. List causes of chronic liver disease.
8. Describe histologic features of chronic active hepatitis and chronic persistent hepatitis.
9. Discuss the role of corticosteroids and/or azathioprine in the treatment of chronic liver disease.
10. List possible complications of corticosteroids.
11. Describe major drug-metabolizing pathways of the liver.
12. List five drugs that cause chronic liver disease.
13. Describe alcohol metabolism.
14. Give the spectrum of alcohol-related liver diseases.

15. Discuss clinical manifestations of alcoholic hepatitis.
16. Discuss the management of alcoholic hepatitis.

Cholestasis/PBC/Hemochromatosis/Wilson's Disease

1. Define cholestasis.
2. List conditions associated with cholestasis.
3. Discuss the approach to neonatal jaundice.
4. Discuss diagnostic tests used in patients with cholestasis.
5. Define primary biliary cirrhosis.
6. Discuss the clinical manifestations of primary biliary cirrhosis and diagnostic tests.
7. Give histologic staging of primary biliary cirrhosis.
8. Discuss the treatment of PBC.
9. List the complications of PBC.
10. Discuss normal iron metabolism.
11. Describe salient clinical features of hemochromatosis.
12. Discuss diagnostic tests used in hemochromatosis.
13. Differentiate first-degree idiopathic hemochromatosis from second-degree hemochromatosis.
14. Discuss the management of hemochromatosis.
15. Define Wilson's disease.
16. Describe clinical manifestations of Wilson's disease.
17. Discuss the diagnostic tests for Wilson's disease.
18. Discuss the use and side effects of penicillamine in treating Wilson's disease.
19. List the diagnostic methods that differentiate liver abscesses, neoplasms and cysts.

Jaundice and Liver Disease in Children

1. Understand bilirubin metabolism in the neonate. Understand the significance of bilirubin metabolism in the fetus, and the changes that occur during the first 72 hours after birth.
2. Understand "physiologic jaundice of the newborn."
   a. Why does it occur?
   b. What brings it to an end?
   c. Under what circumstances will it be "unphysiologic"?
   d. What treatment modalities are available to modify and treat this disorder?
3. Understand the importance of careful choice of drugs in the newborn and in the nursing mother.

4. Understand the significance of unconjugated versus conjugated bilirubin in the plasma.
5. Be aware of kernicterus and its various manifestations.
6. Be aware of "hydrops fetalis," "RhoGAM®," Rh and ABO immunization.
7. Be aware of "neonatal hepatitis syndrome," and understand that it is a spectrum of specific and nonspecific disorders of the liver.
8. Know the normal age presentation.
9. Be aware of "giant cell hepatitis," including its histologic abnormality.
10. Be aware of "biliary atresia," including its pathology.
11. Be aware that a number of metabolic disorders may present as "neonatal hepatitis syndrome," including galactosemia; α_1-antitrypsin deficiency; tyrosinemia; cystic fibrosis.
12. Be aware that a number of perinatal infections may present as "neonatal hepatitis syndrome," including first-degree cytomegalovirus infection and rubella.
13. Understand the significance in investigation of:
    a. HIDA scan
    b. Liver biopsy
    c. Mini lap and operative cholangiogram
    d. Alpha-fetoprotein
14. Know the prognosis of giant cell hepatitis and biliary atresia.
15. Be aware of the Kasai procedure and liver transplantation.

14

Manifestations of Gastrointestinal Disease in the Child

R.B. Scott, M.R. Oliver, D.J. Morrison, H. Machida and
S.R. Martin

1. RECURRENT ABDOMINAL PAIN / R.B. Scott

1.1 Definition

Recurrent abdominal pain (RAP) is defined as at least three episodes of pain occurring over a period of at least three months in children 3 years or more of age, and which are of sufficient severity that the discomfort interferes with their activities. The overall incidence of recurrent abdominal pain is 10.8%, with 12.3% of girls and 9.5% of boys being affected. The prevalence of RAP at any given age is quite constant in school-age boys, but in girls prevalence reaches a peak between the ages of 8 and 10.

1.2 History

The discomfort of RAP is typically localized in the periumbilical region and is nonradiating. In almost all other respects it is variable in character from patient to patient – often vague and ill-defined, a dull ache or a crampy feeling, but occasionally a sharp and colicky pain. It is generally mild to moderate in intensity; the child will stop playing, sit or lie down, but in a minority of affected children the pain will be sufficiently severe to cause crying. The temporal occurrence, frequency and duration of pain are also highly variable. Pain may occur at any time of the day, be reported upon awaking, or be present until the child falls asleep. However, the discomfort will only rarely awaken the child from sleep at night. The occurrence of pain generally bears no consistent relation to the ingestion of specific foods or to meals, physical activity, defecation, urination or (in girls) menstruation. Episodes may occur infrequently or several times a day, and last from a few minutes to several hours at a time. Although aggravating factors are frequently absent, a relationship between recurrent attacks of abdominal pain and stressful situations is reported in approximately one-third of affected children. A brief rest is often cited as a relieving factor. Characteristically, treatment with antacids, anticholinergics, H_2 antagonists, barbiturates and analgesics provides no consistent relief. Episodes of RAP are commonly associated with nonspecific symptoms: pallor, nausea, headaches, limb or "growing" pains and drowsiness after attacks. Sporadic vomiting may occur, but repetitive or bilious emesis should suggest the possibility of an organic disorder. Diarrhea and documented elevation of temperature are occasionally reported but are atypical, and should also suggest an alternative etiology. Characteristically, the children are otherwise well and active between episodes.

There is nothing specific or diagnostic with respect to the past or family history of the child who presents with RAP. However, as a group, the parents and siblings of children with RAP are much more likely than those of unaffected children or those with organic disease to experience somatization of stress and to provide a history of recurrent abdominal pain/irritable bowel syndrome, peptic ulcer, severe headaches and disorders that were in the past very loosely labeled as "nervous breakdown."

1.3 Physical Signs

Except for subjective abdominal tenderness, the physical examination of children with RAP is striking in its normality. Plots of the previous and currently measured heights and weights demonstrate a normal growth velocity, and objective physical signs of disease are absent.

1.4 Psychosocial Factors

The intellectual abilities of children with RAP are identical to those of unaffected children, but certain personality traits are more commonly recognized in children with RAP than in those without. These children have been described as overachievers, overconscientious, high-strung, fussy or particular, anxious, and timid or apprehensive – generalizations that do not always apply in the individual case, however.

There is a close association between emotional status and function of the gastrointestinal tract, and the literature contains numerous anecdotal reports of children presenting with recurrent abdominal pain in whom there is (1) no organic cause, (2) a temporal relationship between discomfort and a specific stress, and (3) resolution of the pain in response to measures that relieve the stress. However, objective evidence of psychological difficulties – and not just the absence of an organic etiology – is necessary before a "psychogenic" label is applied. Using these criteria, psychological or emotional disturbance will be a primary diagnosis in only a very small number of children presenting with RAP.

1.5 Differential Diagnosis and Approach to Investigation

Although the differential diagnosis of abdominal pain is extensive, a complete history and physical examination with limited laboratory investigations should enable the physician to make a positive diagnosis of recurrent abdominal pain. In 90–95% of affected children, RAP is functional; organic disease is identified in only 5–10%. The approach to diagnosis should not be one of extensive investigation to exclude organic disease. In the majority of cases of recurrent abdominal pain, the extent of appropriate investigation should be limited to a complete blood count, urinalysis, and perhaps a stool occult blood test. Comprehensive lists of organic causes of chronic abdominal pain are available but need be referred to only when features of the history and physical examination, or the CBC and urinalysis, strongly suggest an organic problem that is not readily apparent. Specific aspects of the history that should signal concern on the part of the physician include significant recurrent pain in a child under the age of 3; consistent localization of pain away from the umbilicus; frequently being woken from sleep by pain; repetitive or bilious emesis; and any constellation of symptoms and signs that are typical of a specific organic etiology.

Urogenital and alimentary disorders are the most common organic causes of RAP. Genitourinary diseases such as recurrent infection and hydronephrosis or obstructive uropathy can present with abdominal pain. In patients with these disorders who present without urinary tract symptoms, an abnormal urinalysis and pyuria will frequently bring attention to the underlying problem.

Constipation is a common disorder and patients may experience crampy abdominal discomfort in association with the urge to defecate. A suggestive history and the demonstration on physical examination of bulky stool retained in the rectum should initiate a trial of appropriate treatment.

A history of abdominal pain, bloating, flatus and watery diarrhea that occurs with heavy ingestion of "sugarless" gums or confections suggests the possibility of malabsorption of nonabsorbable carbohydrates. The same history occurring with milk intake in individuals whose ethnic background might predispose to lactase deficiency (oriental, black or peri-Mediterranean) suggests lactose malabsorption.

Pernicious vomiting or bilious emesis in the presence of abdominal pain should always alert the clinician to the possibility of an intestinal obstruction. Malrotation or incomplete rotation of the mid-gut is a disorder that may present as a bowel obstruction and also predisposes to intestinal volvulus.

Whenever malrotation is suspected an upper gastrointestinal series should be performed to determine the position of the duodenojejunal flexure, and a barium enema may be required to ensure proper location of the cecum in the lower right quadrant.

Primary peptic ulcer disease is much less common in children than in adults and frequently lacks the typical meal-related characteristics that are common with the adult presentation. A family history of peptic ulcer disease, vomiting, nighttime awakening with pain, hematemesis or melena, or unexplained anemia should suggest the diagnosis.

1.6 Pathophysiology and Treatment

A thorough history, careful physical examination and a minimum of laboratory examinations are essential to provide the data that allow a physician to reach a positive diagnosis of RAP. This care and thoroughness are crucial to the success of subsequent management because they demonstrate that the complaint has been seriously evaluated by the physician and lend credibility to the diagnosis that is subsequently rendered. Having made a positive diagnosis, it is then important to cease investigation and to educate and reassure the patient and parents. If this is not done the parents' perception that there is a significant probability of an underlying organic problem may be reinforced. On the other hand, reassurance in the absence of explanation (i.e., simply saying "Don't worry") is of little value.

It must be made clear that the discomfort of RAP is genuine, not imagined or manufactured for gain or manipulation. It is important to point out that this is a common complaint. Identify for the parent those criteria upon which you based the diagnosis of RAP: the periumbilical location of the discomfort, the absence of any constellation of historical or objective physical findings that suggest underlying organic disease, continued normal growth and development (show the parents the growth chart), continued general well-being between episodes, and a family history of similar functional complaints, if that exists. In those cases where they can be identified note the positive association of RAP with stressful situations or events and any characteristics of the child's personality that might serve to exaggerate the stress. Try to elicit and allay any specific concerns on the part of the child or parents (e.g., "Does my child have appendicitis?").

Encourage the parents to discuss potential stressful contributing events with the child, and recommend a positive approach to coping that includes a return to all normal activities. Insist on attendance at school. Discuss the prognosis of this condition with the parents and provide reassurance by offering to reassess the child should there be any change in the symptoms.

Patient education is generally very effective in relieving the parents' anxiety. Drugs, and specifically analgesics or sedatives, are not considered effective or appropriate. However, a recent prospective, double-blind, randomized control trial demonstrated a significant decrease in RAP in children given additional dietary fiber as compared to placebo.

1.7 Prognosis

Many children and their parents experience considerable immediate relief at having organic disease excluded. In the long term one-third of patients managed in this fashion are completely free of pain as adults, one-third experience continuing abdominal pain, and one-third develop alternative symptomatology such as headaches. Almost all lead unrestricted lives. The goal of management should be to develop, through education, the increased understanding and constructive coping mechanisms that will prevent symptoms from generating dysfunctional behavior.

2. REGURGITATION AND VOMITING / M.R. Oliver and R.B. Scott

2.1 Definitions

Regurgitation is the apparently effortless reflux of gastric contents (from a zone of positive intra-abdominal pressure) into the esophagus (a zone of negative intrathoracic pressure) or oropharynx that occurs whenever the antireflux mechanism at the gastroesophageal junction is impaired. In contrast, vomiting is a complex, coordinated reflex that may occur in response to a variety of stimuli, and results in the forceful expulsion of gastric contents through the mouth. Retching, which often precedes vomiting, is characterized by repeated spasmodic inspiratory efforts involving both the chest wall and diaphragm made against a closed glottis. Retching culminates in a powerful sustained contraction of the abdominal muscles, accompanied by increased descent of the diaphragm. In the gastrointestinal tract, reverse peristalsis in the duodenum is followed by contraction of the pylorus and antrum, relaxation of the fundus and esophagus, and opening of the mouth. All this activity is under significant central nervous system control and is often preceded by an autonomic prodrome.

2.2 Gastroesophageal Reflux Disease (GERD) and Regurgitation

2.2.1 INTRODUCTION

The symptom of recurrent effortless regurgitation is present to a variable extent in roughly 50% of newborn infants. Gradual, spontaneous resolution of this condition occurs over the first year of life in the majority of affected infants. In children and adults occasional reflux remains a normal physiological phenomenon that is most often seen postprandially. Pathological reflux occurs when an underlying disorder predisposes to reflux or when reflux is complicated by failure to thrive, respiratory problems or esophagitis.

2.2.2 PATHOGENESIS
The etiology of GERD is multifactorial and dependent on factors that affect the competency of the antireflux mechanism, volume and potency (pH, digestive enzymes, bile acids) of refluxed gastric contents, esophageal clearance (effectiveness of peristalsis and neutralization of refluxed acid), esophageal mucosal resistance and pulmonary protective reflexes. Recently it has been shown that transient inappropriate relaxation of the lower esophageal sphincter (i.e., relaxation not associated with a voluntary swallow and primary peristalsis) is a major pathological factor in the development of gastroesophageal disease. The mechanism and mediators of this event are not yet understood.

2.2.3 CLINICAL FEATURES AND DIFFERENTIAL DIAGNOSIS
A comprehensive history and physical examination should be conducted and the following points elucidated:

1. If possible distinguish between effortless regurgitation and forceful emesis. (Forceful vomiting may be indicative of another underlying disorder; see Table 1.)
2. Search for symptoms and signs suggestive of a disorder predisposing to regurgitation or vomiting (Table 1).
3. Document the frequency and volume of reflux episodes.
4. Search for symptoms or signs to suggest complications of the regurgitation (Table 2).

2.2.4 MANAGEMENT
The majority of well infants presenting with reflux do not require additional invasive investigations. Management consists of observation and conservative measures (Table 3, phase 1) including posturing and avoidance of overfeeding.

Infants in whom reflux is persistent, severe or associated with symptoms and signs suggestive of a predisposing disorder require further investigation appropriate to the presentation. Initial hematologic and biochemical screening tests in these infants should include a complete blood count. Esophagitis may be associated with a hypochromic, microcytic anemia. Urinalysis is helpful in

TABLE 1. Causes of vomiting in infancy and childhood

Gastrointestinal disorders
Malformations and obstructions
  Pyloric stenosis
  Malrotation
  Volvulus – gastric, small intestinal or sigmoid
  Atresias
  Duplications
  Intussusception

Food intolerances
  Cow's and soy milk protein intolerance
  Celiac disease

Peptic ulcer disease – gastric and duodenal ulcers, gastritis
Pancreatitis
Hepatobiliary – stones, hepatitis, Reye's syndrome

Nongastrointestinal disorders
Infections – urinary tract, gastroenteritis, respiratory tract, appendicitis
Neurological – meningitis, hydrocephalus, tumor
Metabolic – inborn errors of metabolism, adrenal hyperplasia, hypercalcemia
Drugs – digoxin, theophylline, antibiotics
Cardiopulmonary disease – bronchopulmonary dysplasia, pneumonia, cystic fibrosis,
  congestive cardiac failure
Psychological – anorexia nervosa, bulimia

TABLE 2. Complications of gastroesophageal reflux

Systemic
Failure to thrive

Esophageal
Pain
Hematemesis
Anemia
Hypoproteinemia
Dysphagia secondary to stricture or dysmotility
Sandifer's syndrome

Respiratory
Apnea
Bronchospasm
Laryngospasm
Aspiration pneumonia

TABLE 3. Summary of treatment for GERD

Medical

Phase 1 – Conservative measures
  Posturing prone, head up 30°
  Avoidance of overfeeding
  Avoidance of precipitating factors such as infant seats

Phase 2 – Prokinetic agents
  Cisapride 0.2 mg/kg/dose po qid (can cause diarrhea and abdominal pain)
  Metoclopramide 0.1 mg/kg/dose po qid (CNS side effects)
  Bethanechol 0.2 mg/kg/dose po tid (respiratory side effects)

Phase 3 – H_2 blockers
  Ranitidine 2 mg/kg/dose po bid
  Cimetidine 7.5 mg/kg/dose po qid

Surgical

Nissen fundoplication ± pyloric drainage procedure in the presence of severe delay in gastric emptying

excluding a urinary tract disorder predisposing to gastroesophageal reflux. Electrolytes, urea, creatinine and anion gap should be assessed since renal dysfunction, disorders of intermediary metabolism and urea cycle defects may be suggested by uremia, acidosis or a low urea. Additional investigations are dictated by the differential diagnosis.

An upper gastrointestinal barium study lacks both sensitivity and specificity as an indicator of reflux; however, it *is* an appropriate initial investigation to exclude predisposing anatomic abnormalities. If malrotation is suspected, a barium enema may be required to ascertain the position of the cecum. In this more symptomatic group of patients treatment consists of phase 1 and 2 measures (Table 3). We currently advocate the use of cisapride, because metoclopramide and bethanechol may have significant central nervous system and respiratory side effects.

Infants and children with suspected complications of GERD usually require more extensive investigation appropriate to their symptoms. In addition to the aforementioned studies, investigations at a tertiary referral center might include 24-hour pH probe monitoring of the distal esophagus to document reflux frequency and pattern (postprandial, nocturnal), total daily duration of esophageal acid exposure, and whether the reflux has a temporal relationship with respiratory symptoms. Manometric studies may be useful to exclude motor defects of the esophagus. Biopsy of the distal esophagus permits histological assessment of tissue and grading of the degree of esophagitis. This can be done either via a suction biopsy or endoscopically. Scintigraphy after ingestion of a radiolabeled meal has been employed to detect aspiration, but negative studies are common and do not exclude the possibility of previous or subsequent episodes of aspiration related to reflux. In addition to phase 2 therapy, patients with esophagitis require an H_2 blocker (Table 3, phase 3). Symptoms of esophagitis often recur after the cessation of treatment and intermittent or prolonged use of the H_2 blocker may be needed. Omeprazole, the proton pump inhibitor, is a much more effective antagonist of acid secretion and in clinical trials in adults has healed esophagitis.

Surgical treatment in the form of a Nissen fundoplication should be reserved for infants or children in cases of failed aggressive medical management for complicated GERD (failure to thrive, respiratory dysfunction or esophagitis). Surgery is beneficial in over 90% of cases. The rate of major postoperative complications such as bowel obstruction secondary to adhesions is less than 5%; minor postoperative complaints such as gas bloat occur in 30–40% of patients.

2.3 Vomiting

The approach to the investigation and management of vomiting is based on a complete medical history and physical examination, which should focus on the exclusion of important etiologic factors, especially life-threatening gastrointestinal and nongastrointestinal disorders (Table 1). Vomiting can lead to complications such as the Mallory-Weiss syndrome, aspiration of gastric contents, failure to thrive, dehydration and the electrolyte abnormality of hypokalemic, hypochloremic metabolic alkalosis. Therefore, these complicating conditions should be considered in the clinical assessment since they often require attention and treatment.

The following sections provide a general approach to the common clinical problem of vomiting and then highlight two important causes of this symptom in the pediatric age group: hypertrophic pyloric stenosis and intussusception.

2.3.1 HISTORY

A complete history should detail the age of the patient and the frequency and content of the vomitus. In infants who present in the first weeks of life one needs to consider disorders more common to this age, including metabolic disease and structural bowel obstruction resulting from a developmental anomaly of the gut. In older children one needs to place more emphasis on other potential causes such as gastroenteritis, otitis media, pneumonia and accidental drug ingestion. The contents of the vomitus can be of significant importance. The presence of bile is suggestive of a proximal intestinal obstruction, and blood suggests esophageal, gastric or proximal duodenal disease such as peptic ulcers.

Note the clinical setting, pattern of vomiting and any potential precipitating factors. Review associated gastrointestinal and/or systemic symptoms. Assess the patient for the presence of dehydration or other complications of recurrent vomiting. Consideration should be given to medications that might have been ingested and that, in toxic dosage, can produce vomiting (e.g., digoxin, theophylline). The family history may also suggest an etiology (inherited metabolic disorders, peptic ulcer disease, etc.).

2.3.2 PHYSICAL EXAMINATION

A complete physical assessment should evaluate the overall appearance of the infant or child to determine whether the child is well or sick. Document all vital signs and the level of hydration. Plot somatic growth parameters, including height, weight and head circumference; include past measurements to allow assessment of the pattern of growth. A fall in height and weight over time might suggest an underlying chronic disease, while a head circumference greater than the 98th percentile can be suggestive of hydrocephalus or other causes of raised intracranial pressure that can lead to vomiting. A complete ear, nose and throat, cardiopulmonary and neurological examination will help exclude important differential diagnoses. Examine the abdomen for the presence of distention and palpate for evidence of localized signs, including masses that can be present with intussusception or pyloric stenosis.

2.3.3 INVESTIGATION AND MANAGEMENT

It should be emphasized that not all the investigations listed and discussed below may be necessary. The ones used by the clinician will depend on the conclusions drawn following clinical assessment. The first major aim in the management of a child or infant with recurrent vomiting is to stabilize the patient's condition. This may require intravenous rehydration. The next goal is to delineate the cause of symptoms and exclude potential life-threatening diseases. Initial investigations should include a urinalysis for protein, glucose, leukocytes and reducing substances. Further to this a culture of the urine is often necessary to exclude infection of the urinary tract.

Blood should be drawn for a complete blood count and differential if infection is suspected. Electrolytes, urea, creatinine and anion gap provide information regarding fluid balance and metabolic status. Vomiting will usually lead to alkalosis resulting from loss of both hydrogen and chloride; therefore, the presence of acidosis in someone with persistent emesis should suggest a metabolic cause for the symptoms. Liver enzymes should be measured if hepatitis is a potential diagnosis. Amylase and lipase should be measured if eating precipitates both increased pain and emesis. A plain radiograph of the abdomen in supine and erect position helps exclude a bowel obstruction.

Additional investigations may be necessary if the etiology is unclear. A barium meal with follow-through exam is indicated to exclude structural lesions of the gut such as a malrotation. Abdominal ultrasound is helpful in the diagnosis of pyloric stenosis and biliary and urinary tract diseases. Upper gastrointestinal endoscopy will aid in the diagnosis of suspected peptic ulcer disease, gastritis and duodenitis. Other more diverse tests such as urine drug and metabolic screen, plasma amino acids and organic acids, and cerebral computerized tomography should be reserved for cases where the clinician suspects a specific metabolic disease or a space-occupying central nervous system lesion. Psychiatric assessment may be required if behavioral abnormalities are present and the history is suggestive of anorexia nervosa or bulimia.

2.3.4 HYPERTROPHIC PYLORIC STENOSIS
In this condition the grossly thickened circular muscle of the pylorus leads to partial obstruction, projectile vomiting and poor weight gain. The abnormality is not present at birth and develops in the first two to eight weeks of life. It is inherited in a polygenic manner, with the highest incidence in firstborns and males. Though the etiology remains unclear it is thought to be due to an acquired lesion involving the local enteric innervation of this region. It can occur in association with congenital anomalies of the gut, including esophageal and duodenal atresia and anorectal abnormalities.

2.3.4.1 Clinical features
These infants present with vomiting that is projectile and never bile-stained. Symptoms begin in the second to third week of life. As the severity of obstruction increases, the infant loses a significant amount of weight. Visible peristalsis can be seen through the anterior abdominal wall of these infants and a pyloric tumor is often palpable.

2.3.4.2 Investigations
A complete blood count, electrolytes, urea and creatinine should be obtained. These infants will often have a hypochloremic metabolic alkalosis and are dehydrated. If there is doubt about the diagnosis, ultrasound or barium swallow will help demonstrate the stenosis.

2.3.4.3 *Management*

Initial therapy is aimed at correcting dehydration and metabolic alkalosis with intravenous fluids. Nasogastric suction with appropriate replacement fluids is appropriate to prevent further emesis. Following this, a pyloromyotomy is performed to relieve the obstruction.

2.3.5 *INTUSSUSCEPTION*

This is a prolapse (or "telescoping") of a segment of the intestine into a more distal segment. It is the second most common cause of intestinal obstruction in children, after pyloric stenosis. It is most common in infancy but can occur in newborns and in older children. Most cases are labeled as being idiopathic, but some may be due to the lead point provided by a polyp, Meckel's diverticulum or lymph node. The most common type of intussusception is ileocolic in position, with more than 90% occurring near the ileocecal valve. The phenomenon leads to obstruction and impairs blood flow to the intussuscepted bowel, which can result in infarction and perforation.

2.3.5.1 *Clinical features*

The typical history is of a previously well infant who presents with the sudden onset of severe abdominal colic, drawing up his or her legs and screaming at 15- to 20-minute intervals. Bouts of colic are separated by periods of lethargy, and as time passes these symptoms are followed by vomiting and the passage of bloody stools. Often a sausage-shaped mass can be palpated in the abdomen. Older children may present with only the typical pain.

2.3.5.2 *Diagnosis and treatment*

If intussusception is suspected the initial step is to resuscitate those patients who require it with intravenous fluids, drain the stomach with a nasogastric tube, and confirm the diagnosis with a barium enema. Treatment can then be divided into nonoperative and operative approaches. In the former, a contrast barium enema is performed under fluoroscopic guidance and reduction of the intussusception is achieved through the hydrostatic pressure of a column of barium. A surgeon should be available in case of perforation or failed reduction. The risk of perforation with this method is greatest for infants less than 6 months of age or in whom there is a history of symptoms lasting longer than 48 hours. This barium enema allows reduction in 75% of cases; however, there is a 10% recurrence rate. Surgical treatment includes laparotomy and manual reduction, and is reserved for patients with signs of perforation or if nonoperative methods fail to reduce the intussusception.

3. COLIC / D.J. Morrison

The term *colic* is used to describe intense or excessive crying or fussiness in an otherwise healthy infant. This typically starts in the first month of life and resolves by three to four months (although it certainly can persist longer). A variety of definitions of excessive crying have been used. Perhaps the most useful is "more than three hours per day for more than three days per week." The commonest time of day seems to be early evening. In extreme cases the crying may occur throughout daytime and nighttime hours. Prospective studies have shown that colic is common, occurring in 13–49% of infants (depending on the definition used).

The etiology of colic is unknown. The fact that it occurs in healthy babies and resolves without later sequelae has prompted its description as a disorder of development.

It has been speculated that colic represents a variation in normal crying behavior, and thus in a number of studies parents have been asked to keep diaries of crying in their infants. Dr. T. Berry Brazleton's studies are the most commonly quoted. He found that 35% of infants met the criteria of more than three hours of crying per day at 6 weeks of age.

Intestinal immaturity with delayed development of normal patterns of intestinal motor activity and resulting poor propulsion has been proposed as an etiology. Many infants with colic appear uncomfortable, draw their legs up and pass wind. This may be secondary to air swallowing with crying. Antispasmodics and antiflatulents have not been shown to help in colic and are not recommended.

The question of milk intolerance as a possible cause of colic is frequently raised, and formula changes are a commonly tried intervention. Good double-blind studies have been conducted looking at the role of cow's milk formulas in colic. It appears that cow's milk protein and whey may play a role in the etiology of colic in a subgroup of patients. This is, however, an infrequent explanation. The incidence of lactose or carbohydrate malabsorption does not appear to be any different in patients with colic compared to those without.

Colic was once blamed on "overanxious mothers," but there is no scientific confirmation of this etiology. Certainly, prolonged crying in an infant can itself give rise to anxiety in parents.

In the evaluation of a patient with colic it is first essential to take a thorough history to rule out pathological causes of crying. Inquire about feeding practice, formula preparation, burping procedure and soothing techniques. Determine the infant's growth and development as well as any illnesses. For an accurate description of the duration of crying it is useful to have the mother keep a diary over a few days, as crying can often seem to last longer than it actually does. A thorough physical examination must be performed to rule out illness, particularly infection or intestinal obstruction.

If no apparent cause is found for the crying it is first essential to relieve the parents' feelings of guilt and explain to the parents that they do not cause the colic. Explaining the natural history of colic (frequency and duration) can be very helpful. Advising parents on obtaining relief (babysitting or even a weekend away) is often the best intervention. Trials of soothing techniques (e.g., car rides or automatic rockers) may help. One prospective study looked at the preventive practice of carrying infants in body carriers several hours daily, and found that this decreased crying. A trial of casein-hydrolyzed formula for the infant or a milk-free diet for the breastfeeding mother may be useful. It is, however, essential to ensure that this is not misinterpreted by parents as a diagnosis of milk allergy.

4. CHRONIC CONSTIPATION, ENCOPRESIS AND SOILING / R.B. Scott

4.1 Definition
Constipation is a symptom indicative of an abnormality in stool or its elimination: the stool is too large or too hard; passage is too infrequent, painful or incomplete. There is an extremely wide range in what constitutes normal bowel habit, and this changes markedly between birth and adolescence. As a generalization, stool frequency is less in the formula-fed than in the breastfed infant. The formula-fed infant tends to pass 3 to 5 bowel motions per day; breastfed infants, however, can be very well and pass soft stool without difficulty with a frequency that may range from 10 stools per day to 1 stool every 10 days. At 2 to 3 years of age the modal frequency of defecation is 2 bowel motions per day. From age 3 to adulthood bowel motions are passed between 3 times per day and 3 times per week in 96% of individuals. One-quarter of all cases of chronic constipation begin during the first year of life, but the majority of children affected develop problems in the preschool years. Chronic constipation is a very common cause of referral to pediatric gastroenterology practices and tends to affect males slightly more often than females (by a ratio of 1.5:1).

Encopresis is a term that has become synonymous with a voluntary or involuntary passage of stool in an inappropriate place (usually the underclothing). *Soiling* refers to the constant involuntary seepage of stool associated with fecal impaction. Chronic constipation complicated by encopresis or soiling is reported to make up 3% of referrals to large teaching hospital clinics. It occurs in 1–2% of 7-year-old primary school children, and is more prevalent in males than females (by a ratio of 5:1).

4.2 Pathophysiology

The colon absorbs water and electrolytes, and collects and packages indigestible residue as a formed stool for later evacuation. Colonic motor function is specialized to perform these functions. Repeated ring contractions or haustral contractions cause to-and-fro shuttling of luminal contents, delaying their transit and enhancing absorption. One to three times a day mass movements transport colonic contents distally, and stool passing into and distending the rectum initiates an urge to defecate. Normal defecation is a combination of autonomic and voluntary functions. The rectum ends in the pelvic floor, passes through the levator ani muscle and continues as the anal canal. The latter is surrounded by internal (smooth muscle) and external (striated muscle) sphincters. The basal tone of these sphincters creates a high-pressure area within the canal, which constitutes a continence mechanism. Voluntary contraction of the puborectalis muscle is another important mechanism relating to fecal incontinence, as it creates an angle (usually greater than 90°) between the axis of the rectum and the axis of the anal canal (anorectal angle). Distention of the rectum is the stimulus that initiates reflex defecation. When the fecal bolus distends the rectum, sensory receptors in the rectal wall are stimulated, leading to conscious perception of rectal distention and involuntary relaxation of the internal anal sphincter. In the absence of voluntary contraction of the puborectalis muscle and the external anal sphincter, the fecal bolus is expelled.

Intestinal transit time is closely related to defecation frequency. The reduction of frequency of defecation with age is associated with an increase in intestinal transit time. In the first month of life transit time is 8 hours, at age 2 it is 16 hours, between 3 and 13 years it is 26 hours and in an adult it is 48 hours or more. Transit time is largely influenced by the amount of fiber in the diet. Fiber-rich diets favor the retention of water and result in increased stool weight and volume, shorter transit time and more frequent defecation. Normal stools have a water content of 60–85% of mass. An increase or decrease in volume of stool water of as little as 100 mL in the adult can represent diarrhea or constipation, respectively. In constipation the increased desiccation of colonic contents is due to increased duration of mucosal contact rather than an alteration of mucosal absorptive function.

4.3 Differential Diagnosis

In the child who presents as having a difficulty with elimination, the physician must determine whether the problem is functional, organic or a parental misinterpretation of symptoms. Examples of the latter include the healthy, breastfed infant who passes a soft stool without difficulty once every 10 days and the normal infant who passes soft stools on a regular basis but frequently becomes fussy, cries or turns red and grunts while defecating. Similarly, 1- to 2-year-old children will interrupt their other activities, become flushed, stand in a rigid posture, and appear to be concentrating on the passage of a bowel motion that is difficult to pass. Often there is no difficulty and these children are in fact attempting to utilize a newly acquired skill and withhold passage of a bowel movement.

Organic constipation may be the result of mechanical obstruction, perianal difficulties causing painful defecation, metabolic or medical disorders, neuromuscular disorders or medications that favor the development of constipation. Mechanical obstruction may occur as a result of congenital, postsurgical or inflammatory stenosis at the level of the anal canal; obstruction by an intrinsic mass such as adenocarcinoma in the adult; or obstruction by an extrinsic mass such as neoplasia or pregnancy. Painful defecation may result from trauma or surgery to the anorectal region, anal fissures, thrombosed hemorrhoids or a perianal abscess/infection. Metabolic and medical disorders that have been associated with organic constipation include hypercalcemia, hypokalemia, hypothyroidism, porphyria and conditions leading to polyurea and dehydration, including diabetes insipidus, diabetes mellitus and chronic renal failure. Organic constipation can result from dysfunction at all levels of the neuromuscular axis: central nervous disorders such as cerebral palsy or stroke; abnormalities of the peripheral nervous system, including myelomeningocele, trauma, polio or diabetic nephropathy; conditions affecting the enteric nervous system such as Hirschsprung's disease; and skeletal or smooth muscle myopathies. Medications known to predispose to constipation include the opiates, anticholinergics, tricyclic antidepressants and phenothiazines, aluminum-containing antacids, diuretics, iron and vincristine.

Precipitants of functional constipation include decreased fluid intake or increased fluid losses; decreased physical activity; a diet that is low in fiber, contains excessive milk or is nutritionally insufficient; and anything that leads to chronic involuntary inhibition of defecation. Imposed schedules and some children's reluctance to use different facilities are examples of the latter; children may also be simply too busy to attend to the urge to defecate.

In the child who presents with encopresis, the physician must consider whether the incontinence of stool is due to a congenital or acquired neuromuscular disorder, or a behavioral disturbance. However, most of these children have soiling secondary to chronic fecal impaction and overflow. In such cases children may have secondary behavioral disturbance but their primary problem is one of gross rectal distention with loss of the rectal–anorectal angle and the continence function of the puborectalis sling. Whenever there is a mass movement the only residual continence mechanism in these children is the external voluntary anal sphincter, which rapidly fatigues, leading to involuntary soiling. It is not unusual for younger children to deny any knowledge that this is occurring, because if they admit to awareness their parents often expect them to be able to prevent soiling. Such children will regain continence only if their gross rectal distention is relieved.

4.3.1 DIFFERENTIATION OF CHRONIC FECAL RETENTION FROM HIRSCHSPRUNG'S DISEASE

The most frequently considered organic problem in the differential diagnosis of patients presenting with functional constipation is Hirschsprung's disease. These two conditions can frequently be distinguished by significant differences in the history and physical examination. These are detailed in Table 4.

4.4 Treatment

If an organic cause of constipation is suspected, it should be investigated and treated; however, most patients with constipation have no underlying organic abnormality. In patients with mild constipation, dietary modification with an increase in fluid or fiber intake, establishment of a regular bowel habit with a prompt response to the urge to defecate, and appropriate physical activity may be a sufficient remedy. Many individuals will require a laxative in addition. Patients whose constipation is complicated by fecal impaction and soiling require very aggressive management, including education, clearing of the impaction, establishment of a regular bowel habit, laxative therapy titrated to achieve the passage of a soft bowel motion daily, appropriate diet and exercise, and (in younger children) positive reinforcement for appropriate behavior. Therapy must be aggressive and persist for three to six months until the distended and dysfunctional colon has an opportunity to return to normal caliber, tone and sensitivity.

The fecal impaction can generally be cleared by administration of Fleet® enemas at intervals of 12 hours (generally 2–4 are sufficient). There is a variety of laxatives on the market whose mechanism of action includes hydrophilic (dietary fiber), lubricant (mineral oil), osmotic (glycerin suppositories, lactulose, magnesium citrate/sulfate and sodium phosphate/biphosphate), secretory (ricinoleic acid, free hydroxy fatty acids, dihydroxy bile acids, and

TABLE 4. Differentiating features of functional constipation and aganglionic megacolon (Hirschsprung's disease)

	Constipation	Hirschsprung's disease
Age of onset	Acquired sometime after birth	Present from birth
Growth	Normal	Poor
History	Coercive bowel training Colicky abdominal pain Rarely abdominal distention Periodic voluminous stools Soiling	Lack of coercive bowel training Rarely abdominal pain Abdomen distended Pellet-like or ribbon-like stools No soiling
Past history	No episodes of intestinal obstruction	Frequent episodes of intestinal obstruction
Physical exam	Well child Feces-packed, capacious rectum	Nutritional status poor Empty rectum
Barium enema	Absence of transition zone and a distended distal colon	Presence of transition zone
Manometry	Rectoanal inhibitory reflex intact	Absent rectoanal inhibitory reflex
Biopsy	Normal	Absence of ganglia in myenteric plexus and hypertrophy of nerve trunks
Course	Negligible mortality Variable morbidity	High mortality, depending on promptness of diagnosis, and variable morbidity, depending on type and outcome of surgical management

dioctyl sodium sulfosuccinate) and motor stimulants (anthraquinones and diphenylmethene derivatives). Natural bran, methylcellulose, polycarbophil and psyllium are all forms of fiber that by virtue of their ability to bind water within their structure lead to an increase in stool bulk and weight, and are associated with more rapid transit and more frequent bowel motions. These are safe and effective in children if sufficient amounts are taken, but children's compliance is often poor. Mineral oil is the lubricant laxative of choice in the pediatric age group because of better compliance. It is an indigestible, tasteless oil that adds bulk, softens and lubricates the stool and exerts an additional osmotic effect. Its aspiration can lead to lipoid pneumonia; therefore this form of treatment should be avoided in patients known to aspirate or with a history of reflux. Taken with meals mineral oil will result in a degree of fat-soluble vitamin malabsorption. This problem can be addressed by giving it as a single dose several hours after the evening meal. Properly used, mineral oil is an inexpensive, well-tolerated, effective and safe children's laxative. In those children who refuse mineral oil the osmotic agent lactulose is a more expensive but effective alternative.

Constipation in the very young infant can often be managed by adding prune juice to the diet or brown sugar to the formula, or by feeding the infant purées with a natural laxative action (containing prunes, for example). Mineral oil is frequently not a good choice in this age group because of the frequency of gastroesophageal reflux.

5. MALABSORPTION / R.B. Scott

5.1 Definition
Well-being depends not only upon an adequate dietary intake of essential nutrients (water, carbohydrate, protein, lipid, vitamins and minerals), but upon the normal digestion and absorption of those nutrients across the intestinal mucosa. Malabsorption is a clinical condition characterized by disruption of the normal digestive, absorptive sequence of any dietary constituent across the intestinal mucosa.

5.2 Pathophysiologic Approach to Investigation
Different nutrients are absorbed at widely different sites and through a variety of specific and intricate mechanisms. Figure 1 summarizes the contribution of (1) pancreatic and (2) hepatic secretion; (3) mucosal brush-border enzymes and transport proteins; (4) intracellular enzymes, and synthetic and packaging mechanisms; and (5) the delivery of triglycerides into the lymphatic system, and of amino acids and monosaccharides into capillaries for delivery through the portal circulation to the liver and the rest of the body. The absorption of electrolytes, minerals and vitamins is similarly varied and complex. Each step in the digestion and absorption of these nutrients is vulnerable to disease; this accounts for the large number of disorders that could theoretically result in malabsorption. In practice, malabsorption may be a very selective defect and result in a specific nutrient deficiency, or be a more generalized disorder leading to a wide spectrum of nutrient deficiencies. To complicate matters even further, the spectrum of signs and symptoms of deficiency is wide, and each disorder has its own characteristic array. However, the signs and symptoms are generally not specific for a given nutrient deficiency or malabsorptive disorder.

In the face of this complexity the clinician requires a conceptual framework that will facilitate the evaluation and diagnosis of children suspected of suffer-

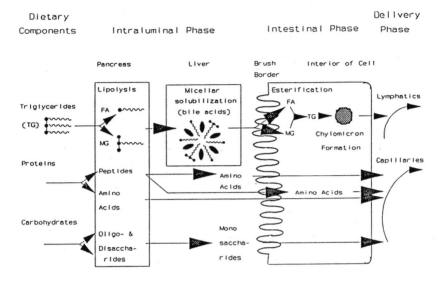

FIGURE 1.   Digestion and absorption of triglycerides, proteins and carbohydrates.
SOURCE: Adapted from Silverman A, Roy CC. Pediatric clinical gastroenterology. 3d ed. St. Louis: CV Mosby, 1983:250.

ing from malabsorption. The diagnosis of malabsorption requires:

1. recognition of malnutrition;
2. evaluation of alternative etiologies for the development of malnutrition;
3. conclusive demonstration of malabsorption, if it is strongly suspected; and
4. appropriate investigations to determine a specific pathophysiology.

5.2.1 RECOGNITION OF MALNUTRITION

Recognition of malnutrition requires that the clinician identify the clinical symptom or sign consistent with malnutrition and suggestive of malabsorption. Protein deficiency is suggested by muscular wasting, growth failure, edema, leukonychia, parotid gland enlargement, hepatomegaly (fatty liver) and hair that is depigmented, dull and easily plucked. Caloric deficiency in the child is characterized by lethargy, reduced adipose tissue stores, muscle wasting and growth failure. Diarrhea is often present in patients with malabsorption. Carbohydrate malabsorption is characterized by an osmotic diarrhea; fat malabsorption (steatorrhea) is characterized by pale, bulky, foul and oily stools. Fat malabsorption is usually a more serious metabolic and clinical abnormality, since fat is the most highly concentrated form of food energy, and because fat absorption is the source of dietary sterols required for hormonal synthesis and absorption of fat-soluble vitamins and essential fatty acids. The symptoms and signs characteristic of fat-soluble and water-soluble vitamin malabsorption are itemized in Table 4 in Chapter 2, "Nutrition in Gastrointestinal Disease." Although the serum value of a particular protein, lipid, vitamin or mineral may ultimately be necessary to make a diagnosis of specific nutrient deficiency, a carefully performed history and physical examination is usually sufficient to provide a reproducible and clinically valid nutritional assessment. The history and physical examination should emphasize a detailed dietary history, a review of growth parameters, a clinical assessment of adipose tissue and lean body mass and the features of edema, anemia, rickets, bleeding diathesis, stomatitis, glossitis or dermatitis.

5.2.2 ALTERNATIVE ETIOLOGIES OF MALNUTRITION

Once malnutrition is suspected or recognized, the mechanism of its etiology must be identified. The clinician must determine whether the nutritional deficiency is most likely related to decreased intake, maldigestion/malabsorption, increased losses, increased requirements or impaired utilization. One of the commonest causes of failure to thrive in gastroenterology outpatient clinics continues to be inadequate caloric intake, frequently secondary to the implementation of "therapeutic" diets that are nutritionally inadequate. One of the more important tests in the evaluation of a child with protein-calorie malnutrition is a careful evaluation of the response to a calorically adequate diet, which may sometimes require hospitalization. One must not forget, however, that the protein-calorie malnutrition of a variety of malabsorptive disorders (e.g., celiac disease) may be due in large part to disease-related anorexia. Crohn's disease is an example of a chronic intestinal illness that can result in increased intestinal losses of blood and protein and present clinically with anemia, edema and failure to thrive without any significant component of malabsorption. Patients with chronic inflammatory bowel disease may also exhibit the anemia of chronic disease where utilization is impaired and iron deficiency anemia persists in the face of adequate iron intake, absorption and stores. The increased activity of the athlete and hyperthyroidism are examples of conditions that give rise to increased caloric requirements.

5.2.3 CONFIRMATION OF MALABSORPTION

Many disorders affecting intestinal absorption, with the notable exception of carbohydrate malabsorption, alter lipid absorption and produce steatorrhea. For this reason the initial approach to the diagnosis of noncarbohydrate malabsorption usually rests with accurate measurement of 72-hour fecal fat excretion and determination of the coefficient of fat absorption. An excretion

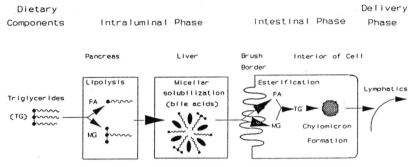

FIGURE 2.   Phases in the digestion of lipids.
SOURCE: Adapted from Silverman A, Roy CC. Pediatric clinical gastroenterology. 3d ed. St. Louis: CV Mosby, 1983:250.

greater than 7% of intake is generally considered indicative of steatorrhea in the child or adult. Determination of the specific etiology of steatorrhea then depends on the systematic consideration of what can go wrong at each step of fat absorption.

5.2.4 DETERMINATION OF THE SPECIFIC PATHOPHYSIOLOGY
If malabsorption is the suspected mechanism underlying malnutrition, what approach should be taken to determine a specific physiologic defect? In patients who present with a history of surgical resection, an anatomic approach to the diagnosis may be sufficient, because there is some specialization of the gut with respect to the site of absorption of specific nutrients. Iron and calcium are absorbed principally in the duodenum, folate in the jejunum, and bile acids and vitamin B_{12} in the terminal ileum. In normal individuals, fat, carbohydrate and protein are almost completely absorbed within the first 100 cm of small intestine. The colon serves an important function in the reabsorption of water and electrolytes. Infants with malabsorption secondary to congenital or surgically acquired short bowel can be a particularly difficult management problem, and it is not uncommon for them to spend months in hospital receiving parenteral nutrition to supplement very gradual increments in their enteral intake. In time, gradual adaptation of the gut will occur. If an awareness of the anatomic specialization of the gut is not a useful approach, then one can utilize the physiology of lipid digestion and an examination of stool character and microscopic appearance as a framework to guide further investigation (Figure 2).

The first major step in lipid digestion is lipolysis of dietary triglycerides by pancreatic enzymes and the release of free fatty acids and monoglycerides.

The most common cause of pancreatic insufficiency of childhood is of course cystic fibrosis, which presents classically as the triad of elevated sweat chloride, neutral fat malabsorption and chronic obstructive pulmonary disease. Microscopic examination of a single stool specimen stained with Oil red O provides a quick, qualitative screening test for the presence of undigested or neutral fat in the stool. Other disorders that are less frequent causes of pancreatic insufficiency and neutral fat steatorrhea include Shwachman's syndrome, severe malnutrition, chronic pancreatitis and deficiency of specific pancreatic enzymes.

The second major step in lipid digestion is the micellar solubilization of the products of triglyceride lipolysis, by bile acid secreted into the intestinal lumen by the liver. The micelle is a water-soluble vehicle that transports water-insoluble fatty acids from the oil droplets from which they are released by lipase and colipase, bringing them through the luminal fluid to the mucosal surface for absorption. Severe cholestatic liver disease or obstruction of the biliary tree, such as occurs in the infant with biliary atresia, interferes with excretion of bile into the lumen. Jaundice from partial or complete obstruction of biliary outflow is a clinical clue to the cause of neutral fat steatorrhea in these patients. Bacterial overgrowth is a condition where (in the absence of jaundice) an unusual proliferation of bacterial organisms within the gut lumen causes deconjugation of bile acids and interferes with normal micellar solubilization.

The absorption of fatty acids and ß-monoglycerides across the mucosa is the next step in digestion and absorption of lipids. Any condition that decreases mucosal surface area can interfere with the absorption of digested triglycerides. Celiac disease is the most common of the malabsorptive disorders characterized by the decrease in mucosal surface area. In this condition, gluten ingestion results in atrophy of the normal villus pattern of the intestinal mucosa, and as a result there is insufficient surface area for the absorption of fatty acids and ß-monoglycerides. Once again the stool smear can serve as a subjective screen for the presence of numerous crystalline or needle-shaped structures that are birefringent under polarized light and represent malabsorbed free fatty acid soaps. Although the diagnosis should never depend solely on the stool smear this can be a useful technique in indicating whether a sweat chloride or jejunal biopsy is more likely to be diagnostic in a child presenting with malabsorption. Congenital short bowel, mucosal injury secondary to cow's milk protein or soy protein intolerance, bacterial overgrowth or immunodeficiency can also result in a reduction in mucosal surface area.

Once fatty acids and ß-monoglycerides have been absorbed, they are re-esterified to triglyceride within the jejunal mucosal cell and packaged with lipoproteins to form chylomicrons. Abetalipoproteinemia is a relatively uncommon malabsorptive syndrome caused by an inability of the jejunal mucosal cell to synthesize beta-lipoproteins. Without the lipoproteins, chylomicrons cannot be formed and fat cannot be transported out of the cell into the lymphatics. Once the lipids and lipoproteins have been packaged they must be transferred out of the cell by microsomal triglyceride transfer protein, and absence of this protein will also prevent delivery of chylomicron into the lymphatics. The jejunal biopsy can be diagnostic of this disorder, as the mucosal cells can be stained with Oil red O (a lipophilic stain), which shows the cells to be choked with resynthesized triglycerides that cannot be excreted from the basal aspect of the cell wall into the lymphatics.

The last stage of lipid digestion is the transport of chylomicrons from the mucosal cell into the intestinal lymphatics, eventually to drain through the thoracic duct into the superior vena cava. Congenital or acquired obstruction of the intestinal lymphatic system results in leakage of lymph into the bowel lumen. Loss of the lymph results in steatorrhea through the loss of chylomicrons, protein-losing enteropathy through the loss of albumin, and lymphopenia from the loss of lymphocytes. Occasionally the diagnosis may be suggested by the presence of localized external lymphedema. Confirmation of intestinal lymphangiectasis may be difficult, as the condition can be very localized and biopsy may not always be appropriately placed to show the characteristic dilatated lacteals within the villi.

5.3 Physiologic Approach to Watery Diarrhea

Watery diarrhea is usually indicative of an osmotic diarrhea (carbohydrate malabsorption) or of a secretory diarrhea (intestinal secretion of electrolytes is greater than absorption). Patients with an osmotic diarrhea (carbohydrate malabsorption) tend to complain of gas cramps, excessive flatus production, and frequent watery stools that burn their buttocks. The etiology of these symptoms is as follows. In these patients the nonabsorbed carbohydrate exerts an osmotic force with the increased delivery of carbohydrate-rich fluid to the colon. In the colon, the plentiful bacterial flora ferment the carbohydrate to release large amounts of hydrogen and carbon dioxide gas and short-chain acids. Osmotic diarrhea may occur in a variety of situations or disorders. Excessive intake of nonabsorbable carbohydrates in the form of gum, candies or confections is an occasional cause of this syndrome. Congenital glucose-galactose malabsorption and congenital sucrase-isomaltase deficiency are rare causes. Late-onset inherited lactase deficiency is uncommon in Caucasians of northern European heritage, more common in peoples of peri-Mediterranean origin and nearly universal in black and Asian populations. The pediatrician and family practitioner are quite familiar with the common secondary disaccharidase (sucrase and lactase) deficiencies that occur transiently in response to viral gastroenteritis. Such infections may occasionally be sufficiently severe, particularly in young infants, to cause secondary monosaccharide malabsorption as well. Illness with acute onset, characterized by low-grade fever, 24 hours of vomiting and explosive watery diarrhea that burns the infant's buttocks but resolves on a non–disaccharide-containing formula, is typical of viral gastroenteritis. Laboratory investigations that support the diagnosis of osmotic diarrhea include evaluation of the watery stool for the presence of pH below 5.5 and reducing substances (tested with the Clini-test® tablet). Greater than 0.5% reducing substances is indicative of carbohydrate malabsorption. The lactose, sucrose or glucose breath hydrogen tolerance test is predicated on the fact that hydrogen gas is not produced by the human and can be excreted in expired air only when colonic fermentation has produced high concentrations of hydrogen gas that diffuse into the blood and then the lungs. If a specific defect of carbohydrate absorption (e.g., lactase deficiency) is suspected a fasted child is made to ingest 2 g/kg (up to a maximum of 50 g) of the suspect sugar in a solution, and samples of end expiratory gases are obtained every 30 minutes for 3 hours and tested for H_2 gas using a gas chromatograph. A rise in breath H_2 of more than 20 ppm is diagnostic of malabsorption and fermentation of that sugar by the enteric bacterial flora.

Profuse watery diarrhea that is demonstrated to be secretory (osmolality of the stool water is approximately equal to the sum of sodium and chloride concentrations) is discussed in Chapter 7, "The Small Intestine." In the context of this discussion of malabsorption, it is important to remember that congenital defects in both chloride and sodium absorption have been reported. In addition, bile acid malabsorption and fatty acid malabsorption are important stimulants of colonic secretion.

5.4 Summary
Intestinal malabsorption can arise from a multitude of differing and intricate mechanisms. A useful framework to guide investigation in patients with suspected malabsorption is provided by a knowledge of gastrointestinal pathophysiology – particularly a knowledge of the anatomic specialization of absorption in the gut and the physiology of lipid digestion.

6. CYSTIC FIBROSIS / H. Machida

Cystic fibrosis (CF) is an autosomal recessive disease that causes chronic morbidity and decreases the life-span of most affected individuals. Because of a defect at a single gene locus that encodes a protein, the cystic fibrosis transmembrane regulator (CFTR), individuals with cystic fibrosis have defective cyclic adenosine monophosphate–regulated chloride transport in epithelial cells of exocrine organs. Although the exact pathophysiology remains to be clarified for each involved organ, there is an accumulation of viscous secretions associated with progressive obstruction and subsequent destruction of excretory ducts.

Chronic pulmonary disease is the major cause of morbidity in the majority of patients. These individuals have progressive bronchiectasis and associated bacterial endobronchial infections, most often secondary to Pseudomonas species.

Although the pulmonary disease is most prominent, the GI manifestations of cystic fibrosis are extensive and contribute to significant morbidity and even mortality. This section will review the clinical problems related to the gastrointestinal tract, particularly the pancreatic insufficiency and hepatic disease in cystic fibrosis.

6.1 Pancreatic Insufficiency

Approximately 80% of patients with cystic fibrosis are born with pancreatic insufficiency, and another 5–10% develop pancreatic insufficiency in subsequent years. These patients have marked impairment of pancreatic exocrine function, including decreased secretion of water, bicarbonate, lipase, amylase and proteinases from the pancreas into the duodenum. In the very young, the endocrine function of the pancreas is usually normal, but many gradually develop evidence of glucose intolerance; a small number develop clinical diabetes requiring insulin therapy. Patients with pancreatic insufficiency may present with any of the following clinical entities with or without pulmonary disease.

6.1.1 MECONIUM ILEUS

Meconium ileus is partial or complete obstruction of the intestine, commonly the ileum, with thick inspissated meconium. This occurs in approximately 15% of infants with cystic fibrosis. Any infant with meconium ileus must have cystic fibrosis excluded. These infants may present with delayed passage of meconium, abdominal distention, vomiting or other signs of obstruction. Meconium ileus may be complicated by antenatal or postnatal volvulus, atresia, perforation of the bowel and meconium peritonitis. In cases with complications, infants may require surgery shortly after birth. Extensive bowel resection may leave them with the short bowel syndrome.

These infants are investigated initially with a plain abdominal x-ray for evidence of obstruction or perforation. If the bowel perforates in utero the perforation often seals, and the x-ray may show calcifications from the meconium in the peritoneum. If meconium ileus is a possibility, surgery should be considered immediately. As long as the x-ray shows no evidence of free air (implying a perforation), most infants are given a gentle water-soluble contrast enema to attempt to relieve the obstruction or at least outline the obstruction for the surgeon. These enemas can cause significant fluid shifts in small neonates, so an IV must be running during the procedure. If the procedure is unsuccessful, surgery is required. The majority of infants with meconium ileus also have pancreatic insufficiency, but this condition can occur in pancreatic-sufficient patients as well.

6.1.2 CHRONIC DIARRHEA

After the neonatal period, chronic diarrhea with or without failure to thrive is common. These infants have loose stools essentially from birth, and one may obtain a history of delay in the passage of meconium. The parents may describe the diarrheal stools as being pale, foul smelling, fatty and/or soupy. The diarrhea is primarily secondary to fat malabsorption because of the pancreatic insufficiency. However, infants who have had small bowel resection, such as for bowel atresia secondary to meconium ileus, may have mucosal disease secondary to bacterial overgrowth. This will contribute significantly to the diarrhea and may cause it to become more watery. Initially, if they do not have respiratory problems, infants with cystic fibrosis tend to have a relatively good appetite and can in some cases compensate for the extreme loss of nutrients by increasing their intake. As they develop pulmonary symptoms or become gradually malnourished, however, their appetite will decrease.

6.1.3 FAILURE TO THRIVE

In cystic fibrosis, failure to thrive is usually a result of a combination of decreased intake, loss of fat in the stools and increased metabolic requirements. The requirements of the average cystic fibrosis patient have been reported to be 120% of normal. Nevertheless, some patients have essentially normal caloric requirements, and others may have requirements in excess of 150% of normal. Many in the early childhood years are able to maintain their nutritional status well with pancreatic enzyme supplementation and good nutrition. Unfortunately, the increased caloric requirements of puberty coupled with deteriorating lung function often make it impossible for the most severely affected patients to maintain their nutrition and normal growth. In addition, CF patients may have anorexia of chronic disease and difficulty eating due to chronic cough. They present with a gradual decrease in growth percentiles, first of the weight and subsequently of the height. Puberty may be delayed or arrested in the early stages. At this time, nutritional supplementation becomes extremely important. Pancreatic enzyme supplementation must be maximized, and nutritional supplementation given either orally or by enteral tube feeding. Total parenteral nutrition is rarely required. If enteral feeds are needed, we use nasogastric tubes in all our patients except those who have nasal polyps. These patients are taught to put their nasogastric tubes down five to six nights a week to obtain 10 hours of nocturnal supplementary feedings. We have had patients as young as 4 years of age who are able to put their own tubes down. The optimal supplement to use is still being debated. We have been most successful with regular high-calorie formula such as Ensure® with fiber, particularly in patients who have evidence of glucose intolerance. Some centers do not give pancreatic enzyme supplements with the tube feeding; others give enteric-coated enzymes at the initiation of tube feeds; still others add pancreatic enzyme powder to the feeds. We have had the most success with the latter approach. With infants, we use the enteral tube feeds in those who present with significant failure to thrive and are unable to take enough calories for catch-up growth, and also in those who have had small bowel resections. Generally, these infants will require the tube feeding only for several weeks to months. We have had only two children between the ages of 2 and 9 who have needed enteral tube feeding. In the adolescent group who require enteral feeding supplementation, we find that about 50% require the supplementation for only a transient period of six months to two years while they are experiencing the significant growth of puberty. A small number of our patients have had to remain on the enteral tube feeding program for years in order to maintain their weight and nutritional status.

6.1.4 FAT-SOLUBLE VITAMIN DEFICIENCY

As a result of significant malabsorption prior to treatment, patients may present with overt evidence of bruising or bleeding due to vitamin K deficiency. We have seen one infant female who presented with this condition as well as evidence of xerophthalmia, apparently due to vitamin A deficiency. The clinical effects of vitamin E deficiencies in cystic fibrosis are not well documented, but this vitamin must be given to patients in a supplement and in adequate doses. We also supplement with vitamin D, although vitamin D deficiency, particularly evidence of rickets, is very uncommon in patients with cystic fibrosis.

6.1.5 HYPOALBUMINEMIA AND EDEMA

In spite of their pancreatic insufficiency, most patients with cystic fibrosis do not have difficulty with hypoalbuminemia secondary to protein malabsorption. Protein malabsorption, however, is a problem in infants who are fed a soy protein formula, and sometimes in those who are breastfed. These infants will present with significant hypoalbuminemia, edema and usually a history of diarrhea. We have had at least one infant who presented with heart failure secondary to severe hypoalbuminemia. Feeding with soy formula must be discontinued, but often those who are receiving breast milk may have their albumin corrected with pancreatic enzyme supplementation. Older patients with severe malnutrition or cor pulmonale may also develop hypoalbuminemia.

6.1.6 RECTAL PROLAPSE

An infant with untreated pancreatic insufficiency becomes increasingly malnourished and continues to pass numerous stools, and thus may begin to have regular rectal prolapse. This is not infrequently the complaint that brings the infant to medical attention. In these cases, a diagnosis of cystic fibrosis must be made quickly and the child renourished. The prolapse will resolve with appropriate nutrition and pancreatic enzyme supplementation to decrease the stooling. In most of these infants the rectal prolapse reduces spontaneously. If it does not, it must be gently reduced manually.

6.1.7 DISTAL INTESTINAL OBSTRUCTION SYNDROME

The distal intestinal obstruction syndrome (DIOS), also known as meconium ileus equivalent, is partial or complete obstruction of the bowel resulting from fecal masses, usually in the cecum. This can occur in any age of child with cystic fibrosis, but we find it most often in the older child. Younger children with DIOS present with decreased appetite, decreased stooling, distention and often vomiting. Older patients complain of grumbling or crampy abdominal pain and a gradual decrease in stooling. In most patients, the fecal masses are easily palpated and an x-ray is not always required. If the diagnosis is made early, most can be treated with N-acetylcysteine given orally. We give a loading dose in a cola drink and 3 subsequent doses (1 dose every 6 hours over 24 hours). Fluids must be encouraged during this time. If there is evidence of marked obstruction, we admit the patients to hospital and give them polyethylene glycol–salt solution (GoLYTELY^{TM}) orally or by nasogastric tube. This completely clears the obstructive fecal masses. It is essential to ensure that patients with DIOS get adequate enzymes, as the syndrome seems to occur most often in patients who are not getting enough enzymes or in whom the duodenal pH is too low for optimal efficacy of the enzymes.

6.1.8 *PANCREATITIS*
Five to 10% of patients with cystic fibrosis will remain pancreatic-sufficient throughout their life. Unfortunately, some pancreatic-sufficient patients develop pancreatitis, which may present with vomiting and acute pain that radiates to the back or with recurrent low-grade abdominal pain and perhaps a change in appetite. Those who present with acute pancreatitis should be treated as any other patient with pancreatitis. The bowel is rested until the enzymes return essentially to normal and the patient is asymptomatic. In patients who are found to have mild abdominal pain and only slight increase in enzymes, management is less definitive. We have treated these patients with pancreatic enzymes to try to decrease the amount of stimulation of the pancreas. Unfortunately, the pancreatitis tends to be a recurrent problem in some individuals.

6.2 Hepatobiliary Disease
Hepatobiliary disease in cystic fibrosis is well documented. Fortunately, although a significant number of patients have subtle manifestation of hepatobiliary abnormalities, only a small number have severe liver disease. Given the increasing life expectancy of patients with cystic fibrosis there may be an increasing need to manage patients with severe liver problems. The following briefly outlines the clinical features of some of the hepatobiliary problems associated with cystic fibrosis.

6.2.1 *NEONATAL JAUNDICE*
Prolonged conjugated hyperbilirubinemia is reported to occur in neonates with cystic fibrosis. In some cases, the hypobilirubinemia may be secondary to a problem unrelated to the cystic fibrosis; nevertheless, any infant with conjugated hypobilirubinemia of unknown origin should be investigated for cystic fibrosis.

6.2.2 *ELEVATED LIVER ENZYMES*
A significant portion of patients with cystic fibrosis have mildly elevated liver enzymes, including alkaline phosphatase, γ-glutamyl transferase (GGT), aspartate aminotransferase (AST) and alanine aminotransferase (ALT). This is not uncommon in patients who had a meconium ileus as a neonate and are pancreatic-insufficient. In most of these patients, the enzymes either normalize or remain slightly elevated throughout their life. A small proportion develop serious liver disease.

6.2.3 *HEPATOSPLENOMEGALY*
Many patients with cystic fibrosis have a slightly large liver secondary to fatty

infiltration, probably because of poor nutrition. In these patients, the liver is smooth and soft. In those who develop progressive liver disease, the liver is initially large; it gradually begins to feel hard and often nodular. Splenomegaly is usually not detected until the patient is aged 6 or older. On histologic examination, these patients have multinodular or biliary cirrhosis. The liver disease tends to progress slowly and the prominent clinical problems are secondary to hypersplenism. It can be years before there are changes in the albumin, PT or PTT, or an elevation of the bilirubin. With the significant portal hypertension, the patients are at risk for bleeding from esophageal or small bowel varices. As the life-span of patients with cystic fibrosis increases, one would expect to see increasing morbidity and mortality from liver failure.

In very recent years, ursodeoxycholic acid has been used to try to improve the liver disease in cystic fibrosis. Short-term studies report that patients treated with ursodeoxycholic acid show improvement in their liver enzymes and, in some cases, in liver function studies. It has yet to be determined whether long-term treatment will actually prevent progression of the liver disease and perhaps protect some children from developing cirrhosis.

6.3 Management of Pancreatic Insufficiency

As there are numerous gastrointestinal problems in cystic fibrosis and their interrelationship can be quite complex, it is beyond the scope of this section to discuss the management in detail. In the majority of cases, the problem must be identified, assessed and managed as in patients without cystic fibrosis. Nevertheless, because the pancreatic insufficiency causes most of the gastrointestinal problems, an approach to its management will be outlined.

There are several indirect methods that assess pancreatic insufficiency, but the only direct measurement of pancreatic function is a pancreatic stimulation test. Unfortunately, this test requires intubation of the duodenum, it is invasive and uncomfortable for the patient, and generally it will not contribute significantly to the patient's management. Therefore, this test is usually reserved for complicated cases. We usually assess the pancreatic insufficiency by a 72-hour fecal fat collection, which measures the percentage of fat lost in the stools daily. If possible, this test is done before the patient is placed on pancreatic enzyme supplementation and post-enzyme supplementation.

Once the pancreatic insufficiency is diagnosed, it is treated with supplementary pancreatic enzymes. The aim of treatment is to control the fat malabsorption so that the patient has normal growth and good nutrition. (In the majority of cases it is impossible to reduce fecal fat loss to less than 12%, even on optimal enzyme supplementation.) Commonly, the enzymes given are in capsule form and contain enteric-coated spheres of lipase, amylase and proteinases. These enteric-coated spheres are released in the alkaline environment of the duodenum. The strength of these preparations varies; usually the dosage is expressed in lipase units. We find that the appropriate dosage of lipase is best determined empirically.

We begin giving infants under 6 months of age at diagnosis 1 enteric-coated capsule with 4,000 units of lipase per feed. By 1 year of age, the majority will be on 8,000 to 10,000 lipase units per feed and 4,000 per small snack. Subsequently, the enzymes are evaluated and increased as the patient grows and whenever there is evidence of increasing malabsorption. By age 8 the majority of patients with pancreatic insufficiency will require 80,000 to 100,000 lipase units per meal. In most cases an increase in lipase above this level does not improve their absorption. In older children, we generally use capsules containing 20,000 lipase units each, so that the child can take fewer capsules per meal. The disadvantage with this is that the child may be taking more enzymes than required for small meals or snacks.

With the lack of bicarbonate secretion from the pancreas, the duodenal pH may be too low for optimal activity of the pancreatic enzyme supplements. In patients in whom the number of enzymes seems maximal for age and weight, ranitidine is started at 2 mg/kg b.i.d. to enhance the efficacy of the enzymes.

6.4 Summary

The gastrointestinal effects of cystic fibrosis are extensive. Most of the prominent problems are secondary to the pancreatic disease. Once this is treated adequately with enzymes, vitamin replacement and adequate nutrition, many problems will resolve. Severe liver disease is less common; it can be devastating in the patients in whom it occurs and may be of more concern as the lifespan of the patients increases. Research into the pathophysiology of the liver disease and into pharmacologic agents such as ursodeoxycholic acid is ongoing. Because failure to thrive and liver disease can present insidiously, it is essential to monitor these patients on a regular basis, including documentation of height and weight, a complete physical examination and a regular biochemical evaluation.

7. APPROACH TO THE JAUNDICED NEONATE / S.R. Martin

Jaundice is caused by the deposition of bile pigment in the skin and other tissues as a result of an elevated serum bilirubin concentration. Bilirubin is formed from the degradation of hemoglobin as well as other heme-containing proteins, mainly within cells of the reticuloendothelial system. Bilirubin is carried in the circulation bound to albumin and taken up in the liver by the

TABLE 5. Factors contributing to physiological jaundice in the neonate

Absence of placental bilirubin metabolism
Reduced hepatic blood flow via ductus venosus shunting
Decreased red blood cell survival
Increased red blood cell mass
Reduced enteric bacterial flora
Presence of intestinal β-glucuronidase
Immature liver function
Delayed oral feeding

hepatocytes, where it is conjugated with glucuronic acid before being secreted into bile. Conjugated bilirubin is then converted to urobilirubins by intestinal bacteria, preventing its reabsorption and permitting its excretion in the feces. Jaundice in the neonatal period (<1 month) is present in up to 60% of full-term and 80% of premature infants; usually it is a physiological phenomenon related to the developmental nature of bilirubin metabolism. Infants of certain racial background (oriental, Greek, North American native) may be particularly susceptible.

7.1 Physiological Jaundice

Physiological jaundice generally appears around the third to fifth day, rises by no more than 85 μmol/L/day and resolves by the end of the second week of life. Hyperbilirubinemia is always of the unconjugated fraction. Peak levels rarely exceed 150 μmol/L in full-term infants, although in premature infants levels of 200 μmol/L are not uncommon and the resolution may be slower. Several mechanisms that contribute to the development of physiological jaundice, including increased bilirubin load and decreased capacity to process bilirubin, are shown in Table 5.

After birth the placenta is no longer available for bilirubin metabolism and the immature liver has a limited capacity for uptake of bilirubin from plasma and for its binding, conjugation and secretion into bile. Blood flow may not immediately favor hepatic perfusion (shunting via the ductus venosus). An increased bilirubin load derives from the neonate's elevated hematocrit combined with a reduced red blood cell life-span. Delayed feedings result in retention of meconium containing significant amounts of bilirubin within the intestine, which initially has reduced bacterial flora. This limits the conversion of conjugated bilirubin into urobilinogens. Also present is ß-glucuronidase, which converts conjugated bilirubin into a reabsorbable form.

7.2 Pathological Jaundice

Jaundice is quantified by measuring the serum bilirubin composed, in general, of unconjugated and conjugated fractions. Because it is impossible to differentiate visually between jaundice caused by unconjugated hyperbilirubinemia and that caused by conjugated hyperbilirubinemia, each of which has different etiologies, therapies and prognosis, the first step in evaluating a jaundiced baby is to determine the total and conjugated bilirubin concentrations. Potentially life-threatening illnesses may present with neonatal jaundice, so it is important that the initial evaluation distinguish between physiological and pathological causes of jaundice in order to start any therapy without delay. Pathological jaundice is suggested and requires investigation when any of the following conditions arises:

1. jaundice appearing within the first 24 hours;
2. a rate of rise of more than 85 μmol/L/24 hours;
3. total bilirubin >250 μmol/L in breastfed infants, or >200 μmol/L in formula-fed infants;
4. persistence of jaundice beyond 2 weeks of age; or
5. a conjugated fraction >34 μmol/L, or >15% of the total bilirubin concentration.

7.2.1 UNCONJUGATED HYPERBILIRUBINEMIA

In practice, jaundice is caused either by increased production or decreased clearance of bilirubin by the liver. The pathological causes of unconjugated hyperbilirubinemia are shown in Table 6.

7.2.1.1 Increased bilirubin production

Any process that presents a greater bilirubin load to the liver than can be processed will result in hyperbilirubinemia. Thus, red blood cell hemolysis from a variety of causes, including maternal–infant blood group incompatibility (Rh, ABO, minor groups), membrane defects, red cell enzyme deficiencies and toxic effects of drugs, increases the load of unconjugated bilirubin presented to the liver. Hemoglobinopathies rarely present in the neonatal period because of the presence of a large proportion of the relatively stable fetal hemoglobin (Hgb F). Massive hemolysis may occasionally also raise *conjugated* bilirubin levels to 25–30% of the total, possibly resulting from the toxic effects of bilirubin secretion into bile. Conditions resulting in increased red cell breakdown, especially hematomas, elevate the serum bilirubin; these are relatively more important in smaller premature infants. Finally, some conditions accentuate the normally high neonatal hemoglobin, resulting in polycythemia. Examples are maternal–infant transfusion, delayed umbilical cord

TABLE 6. Causes of unconjugated hyperbilirubinemia in the neonate

---

Increased bilirubin production
Hemolytic disease
  Blood group incompatibility (Rh, ABO, minor groups)
  Membrane defects (spherocytosis, elliptocytosis, infantile pyknocytosis)
  Enzyme deficits (G6-PD, hexokinase, pyruvate kinase)
  Drugs (oxytocin, vitamin K)
Increased breakdown
  Infection
  Hematoma, swallowed maternal blood
Increased RBC mass
  Polycythemia (maternal diabetes, delayed cord clamp, small for gestational age, altitude)

Decreased bilirubin metabolism
Reduced uptake
  Portacaval shunt, hypoxia, sepsis, acidosis, congenital heart disease
Decreased conjugation
  Crigler-Najjar type I, II
  Gilbert's syndrome
  Lucey-Driscoll syndrome
  hypothyroidism
  panhypopituitarism

Altered enterohepatic circulation
Breastfeeding
  Free fatty acids, steroids, breast milk β-glucuronidase
Intestinal hypomotility
  Retained meconium
Reduced intestinal flora
  Newborn, antibiotic use

---

clamping at birth, and conditions that result in relative intrauterine hypoxia (maternal diabetes mellitus, high altitude, newborn small for gestational age).

7.2.1.2 Altered bilirubin metabolism

At any stage in the processing of bilirubin – uptake, transport, conjugation, excretion – abnormalities may affect the unconjugated bilirubin concentration. The Crigler-Najjar syndrome is an inherited disorder characterized by absent or low hepatic glucuronyl transferase activity. Type I is associated with very high levels of bilirubin and with kernicterus, whereas type II has lower bilirubin levels and is responsive to enzyme induction with phenobarbital to lower the serum bilirubin. Gilbert's syndrome, an autosomal dominant condition, is a mild form of elevated bilirubin with reduced glucuronyl transferase activity, in which jaundice (which is rarely observed in the newborn) is often provoked by stress or fasting. It requires no treatment. Lucey-Driscoll syndrome is a transient form of acquired reduction in glucuronyl transferase activity in the newborn, caused by a factor in maternal serum. Endocrine disorders such as panhypopituitarism and hypothyroidism affect bile conjugation by unclear mechanisms.

7.2.1.3 Altered enterohepatic circulation

Jaundice induced by breast milk occurs in approximately 1 in 200 infants. Jaundice may present in the first week in the early form or after the first week in the late form, which is associated with higher bilirubin levels. The degree of hyperbilirubinemia is quite variable (171–462 µmol/L) and may last from 3 to 10 weeks. Despite the occasional presence of very elevated unconjugated bilirubin levels, kernicterus has not been reported in normal term newborns with breast milk–induced jaundice. Several breast milk components have been implicated, including free fatty acids, an isomer of naturally occurring steroids and ß-glucuronidase. Hyperbilirubinemia may also be caused by antibiotic-induced reductions in intestinal flora that increase the level of intestinal conjugated bilirubin, the preferred substrate for ß-glucuronidase, whose action produces unconjugated bilirubin that is readily absorbed.

7.2.1.4 Kernicterus

The importance of determining an etiology for unconjugated hyperbilirubinemia lies in directing appropriate treatment to prevent kernicterus. Severe unconjugated hyperbilirubinemia is associated with brain toxicity possibly secondary to cellular hypoxia induced by bilirubin. Early symptoms are non-specific – e.g., lethargy, vomiting, poor feeding and loss of the Moro reflex. Progressive injury leads to respiratory difficulties, bulging fontanelles, a high-pitched cry, loss of deep tendon reflexes and opisthotonos, finally resulting in gaze paresis, convulsions and death. In survivors long-term sequelae include choreoathetosis, spasticity, seizures and sensorineural hearing loss.

Although the lowest level of bilirubin predictive of kernicterus is not known, it is almost universal at levels >500 µmol/L, present in one-third of full-term infants >342 µmol/L, and rare below this latter level. However, numerous factors play a role in increasing bilirubin toxicity at lower levels. Some concern exists that more subtle long-term effects may occur in any infant with raised unconjugated bilirubin concentration; motor development may be affected by levels greater than 255 µmol/L. Bilirubin toxicity may be increased by factors that reduce binding to albumin, such as hypoproteinemia, acidosis, hypothermia, hypoglycemia-induced elevations of plasma free fatty acids and drugs (sulfa, salicylates, heparin, hematin, ceftriaxone, sodium benzoate), or by factors affecting the permeability of the blood–brain barrier, such as prematurity, asphyxia, hyperosmolarity, infection, respiratory distress syndrome, acidosis and intraventricular hemorrhage. Such factors are frequent in very low birth weight infants, in whom kernicterus may occur at unconjugated bilirubin levels as low as 255 µmol/L.

7.2.1.5 Management
In contrast to cholestatic infants, those with unconjugated hyperbilirubinemia have normal colored stools, the urine is not dark and the liver is only rarely enlarged and is not firm or nodular. When unconjugated hyperbilirubinemia is confirmed, initial management should identify maternal and infant risk factors according to the causes shown in Table 6. Correction of underlying illnesses (sepsis, hypothermia, acidosis, hypoxia) should be initiated. Specific investigations should include maternal and infant blood group, Coombs' test, hemoglobin or hematocrit, red cell indices and morphology to identify polycythemia, hemolysis or red blood cell disorders. Early feedings should be instituted where possible. For high-risk infants with early jaundice (appearing within the first 24 hours), rapidly rising levels of bilirubin (>85 µmol/L/24 hours) or elevated levels of bilirubin (>250 µmol/L in breastfed or >200 µmol/L in formula-fed infants), specific therapy usually includes phototherapy, exchange transfusion or occasionally oral administration of bilirubin binding agents such as charcoal or agar. Phenobarbital may be given to stimulate the enzymes responsible for bilirubin conjugation. Inhibition of bilirubin formation from its heme precursors may in the future be achieved with agents like tin-protoporphyrin, an inhibitor of heme oxygenase. Breast milk jaundice usually does not require treatment other than maintaining good hydration of the infant with more frequent feedings and occasionally supplemental water or formula, as well as periodic serum bilirubin determinations. Cessation of breast milk feedings for 36 to 48 hours will significantly reduce bilirubin levels that are of concern.

7.2.2 CONJUGATED HYPERBILIRUBINEMIA IN THE NEONATE
Conjugated hyperbilirubinemia in the newborn is a sign of cholestasis and always requires further investigation. Because cholestasis implies impairment of bile flow at any point from its formation in the hepatocyte to its excretion from the common bile duct, the causes of neonatal cholestasis are many. However, therapeutic interventions that will significantly affect the outcome are relatively few. For certain conditions, notably infections, some metabolic and endocrine disorders and biliary atresia, early intervention is associated with

better outcome. The goal, therefore, is to identify treatable causes as early as possible.

The more common causes of cholestatic jaundice in the neonate are outlined in Table 7. Although several groups of illnesses are recognized (infectious, metabolic/endocrine, disorders of the bile ducts, cholestatic syndromes), in practice the diagnostic approach consists initially of differentiating biliary obstruction (which requires surgical intervention) from intrahepatic causes of cholestasis. Idiopathic neonatal cholestasis is commonly, but less precisely (because true hepatitis is not often present), referred to as neonatal hepatitis. Neonatal hepatitis is used as a general name for a wide variety of different disorders that present similarly and together with biliary atresia account for 70–80% of all neonatal cholestasis. As specific diseases are elucidated the proportion accounted for by true idiopathic neonatal hepatitis appears to be diminishing. A possible diagnostic approach is shown in Figure 3.

A maternal history of unexplained illness, rash, exposure to cats or uncooked meat may provide clues to infectious causes. A history of blood transfusion or intravenous drug abuse should be sought, although cholestasis is unusual in the neonate with vertically transmitted hepatitis B or C, or human immunodeficiency virus. The family history is especially important for metabolic disorders such as galactosemia, fructosemia, tyrosinemia, Niemann-Pick, α_1-antitrypsin deficiency, peroxisomal disorders or cystic fibrosis as well as familial disorders such as Alagille's syndrome or familial progressive intrahepatic cholestasis (Byler's disease). A history of previous infant deaths in the family due to unexplained liver disease may be important now that previously lethal familial diseases (such as bile acid synthesis defects) can be successfully treated.

The infant's presentation may also suggest a particular etiology. Lethargy, poor feeding or vomiting may signify sepsis or hypoglycemia associated with pituitary dysfunction. Forceful vomiting may indicate intestinal obstruction, but may also occur with galactosemia and fructosemia. While the normal neonate usually does not have fructose in the diet, several medications have a sucrose-based vehicle that is metabolized to fructose. Jaundice with acholic stools in the first 24 hours of life may suggest a bile duct lesion (stone, stricture, perforation). A well appearing infant of full-term gestation and normal birth weight with gradual onset of persistently acholic stools is likely to have extrahepatic biliary atresia.

The physical examination frequently may guide subsequent investigations. The particular facies and high-pitched cry associated with the murmur of peripheral pulmonic stenosis may suggest Alagille's syndrome. A small for gestational age infant with petechiae, rash, retinal lesions, hepatosplenome-

TABLE 7.   Causes of conjugated hyperbilirubinemia in the neonate

---

Infection
Bacterial urinary tract infection/sepsis
Cytomegalovirus
Rubella
Herpes viruses: simplex; type 6
Toxoplasmosis
Syphilis
Other viruses: adenovirus, Coxsackie virus, echovirus, parvovirus B19

Metabolic
Galactosemia
Fructosemia
Tyrosinemia
Peroxisomal disorders
Bile acid synthesis disorders
α_1-antitrypsin deficiency
Cystic fibrosis
Niemann-Pick disease
Endocrine disorders: hypopituitarism, hypothyroidism
Neonatal hemochromatosis

Bile duct disorders
Extrahepatic
   Biliary atresia
   Bile duct perforation, stenosis
   Neonatal sclerosing cholangitis
   Choledochal cyst
   Cholelithiasis
   Intra/extrahepatic masses
   Inspissated bile/bile plug
Intrahepatic
   Alagille's syndrome
   Byler's disease (familial progressive cholestasis)
   Nonsyndromic bile duct paucity

Miscellaneous
Parenteral nutrition
Intestinal obstruction
Shock
Trisomy 21

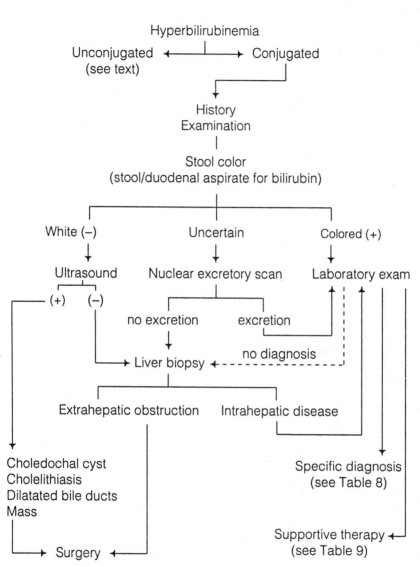

FIGURE 3. Algorithm for diagnostic evaluation of neonatal cholestasis.

galy and adenopathy portrays the clinical appearance of congenital viral infection. An enlarged, firm and/or nodular liver suggests fibrosis, most commonly due to biliary atresia. Biliary atresia also may be associated with situs inversus and a murmur of congenital heart disease. A palpable right upper quadrant mass may signify a choledochal cyst. A micropenis in the male, optic disk atrophy or midline facial defects such as cleft lip may be a clue to hypopituitarism. Severe hypotonia is associated with peroxisomal disorders. Finally the rectal examination may provide stool to determine the presence or absence of bile.

7.2.2.1 Management

If the stool is persistently white, investigations should be directed toward possible extrahepatic biliary obstruction. Although acholic stools may occasionally occur with severe intrahepatic disease, Alagille's syndrome and cystic fibrosis, additional clinical features and laboratory investigations usually are diagnostic. An abdominal ultrasound will detect a choledochal cyst, cholelithiasis, dilatated bile ducts from obstruction or stenosis, and intrahepatic or extrahepatic masses. Elements of the polysplenia syndrome (preduodenal portal vein, situs inversus, abnormal inferior vena cava), associated with biliary atresia, may also be detected. At this stage it would be appropriate to refer to a pediatric surgeon for surgery and intraoperative cholangiogram. Sometimes the color of the stool is uncertain and tests for bilirubin in the stool (Ictotest®) are equivocal. (Confusion may arise because yellow secretions or urine will color otherwise acholic stools. This often can be avoided by obtaining stool by rectal examination or by breaking open the stool to reveal its true color.) In such cases hepatobiliary scintigraphy using a ^{99m}Tc-labeled iminodiacetic acid derivative, following five days of treatment with phenobarbital to enhance excretion, may demonstrate patency of the biliary tree. If excretion into the intestine is demonstrated, further diagnostic laboratory investigations are indicated. The absence of excretion is less specific and may arise with intrahepatic cholestasis, as previously mentioned.

A percutaneous liver biopsy will usually differentiate extrahepatic biliary obstruction, particularly biliary atresia, from intrahepatic causes of cholestasis. Typically, biliary atresia is associated with fibrous expansion of the portal tracts, bile ductular proliferation and portal bile plugs. Idiopathic neonatal cholestasis is characterized by disorganization of the structure of the lobule, mononuclear cell infiltration, focal hepatocyte necrosis and more diffuse presence of giant cells than found with other disorders. Bile duct paucity is suggested by absence of intralobular bile ducts, but an adequate number of portal spaces must be present to confirm the diagnosis. Early biopsies may suggest idiopathic cholestasis, requiring clinical suspicion and repeat biopsy to arrive at the correct diagnosis. The less common nonsyndromic forms of bile duct paucity may ultimately be shown to be secondary forms because the list of diseases associated with this histological picture appears to be increasing with time.

TABLE 8. Laboratory evaluation of conjugated hyperbilirubinemia

---

Total and direct serum bilirubin
Alkaline phosphatase, aminotransferases, γ-glutamyl transpeptidase
Prothrombin time, serum albumin (factor V levels, if available)
Complete blood cell count, differential
Urine culture (blood/cerebrospinal fluid, if indicated)
Serology for cytomegalovirus, rubella, herpes simplex, herpes type 6, toxoplasmosis, syphilis
    (adenovirus, Coxsackie virus, reovirus III, parvovirus B19, if available)
Urine for reducing substances, serum galactose-1-phosphate uridyltransferase, serum/urine
    amino acids and organic acids
Sweat chloride
α_1-antitrypsin level and Pi phenotype
Urine for bile acid metabolites
Ophthalmologic examination
Radiograph of vertebral column, long bones, skull
Serum ferritin

Laboratory investigations useful in the evaluation of the cholestatic neonate are outlined in Table 8. Serum bilirubin measures the degree of cholestasis. Alkaline phosphatase and γ-glutamyl transpeptidase (GGT) are greatly elevated with biliary obstruction. However, with prolonged cholestasis alkaline phosphatase may be elevated on the basis of the effects of vitamin D malabsorption on bone; γ-glutamyl transpeptidase is normally elevated in the neonatal period. A measure of hepatic synthetic function is provided by prothrombin time, serum albumin and, where available, factor V levels. The most urgent investigations search for possible bacterial infection and certain metabolic/endocrine disorders for which prompt therapy will reverse the cholestasis as well as treat the underlying disease state. Thus, bacterial cultures of the urine and/or blood; urine for reducing substances (while the infant is ingesting lactose in the form of breast milk or lactose-based formula) or serum galactose-1-phosphate uridyltransferase to diagnose galactosemia; and tests of pituitary function (thyroxin, thyroid stimulating hormone, cortisol and growth hormone levels), in the appropriate clinical setting, are indicated. Serum for very long chain fatty acids may aid in the diagnosis of peroxisomal disorders. Recently, bile acid synthesis defects have been described that respond to specific bile acid replacement therapy if begun early in the course. The presentation and liver biopsy resemble idiopathic neonatal cholestasis (neonatal hepatitis), although the GGT is normal. The diagnosis requires bile acid metabolite analysis of the urine, a technique available in only a few tertiary pediatric centers. The only other cause of neonatal cholestasis with nor-

TABLE 9.   Management of chronic cholestasis

Malnutrition
Increase caloric intake, if necessary by enteral feedings
Supplement with medium-chain triglycerides
Supplement with water-soluble vitamins and minerals

Fat-soluble vitamin deficiency
Vitamin A 5,000–25,000 IU po qd as Aquasol® A, or 50,000 IU IM/month where available
Vitamin E 50–100 IU po qd (polyethylene glycol–based form)
Vitamin K$_1$ 2.5–5.0 mg po qd, or 10 mg IM twice monthly
Vitamin D$_2$ 5,000–8,000 IU po qd, or preferably 5 mg IM/3 months where available, or 3,000
   IU IV/1–4 weeks with crystalline cholecalciferol IV

Pruritus
Hydroxyzine
Ursodeoxycholic acid
Rifampin
Cholestyramine
Ultraviolet B light therapy
Biliary diversion

---

mal or low GGT is progressive familial intrahepatic cholestasis (Byler's disease). The diagnosis of many infections is made serologically, particularly with specific IgM antibody titers. Maternal titers may be required to interpret elevated IgG titers in the face of possible placental transfer. The sweat chloride test is specific for cystic fibrosis but requires a sufficient collection of sweat to be interpretable. Ophthalmologic evaluation may detect the chorioretinitis common in congenital infections, cataracts that develop with galactosemia or the posterior embryotoxon of Alagille's syndrome. Vertebral radiographs may demonstrate the butterfly vertebrae of Alagille's syndrome and long bone radiographs may be abnormal in some congenital infections. Intracranial calcifications that accompany congenital infections may be detected with skull films, ultrasound or CT scan.

7.2.3 TREATMENT

Treatment for many of these disorders is supportive. Ensuring optimal caloric intake for growth may at times require nasogastric tube feeding to supplement a poor intake. Fat malabsorption is common as a result of lack of intestinal luminal bile acids; it may be treated with supplemental medium-chain triglycerides, which can be absorbed in the absence of luminal bile acids. Supplemental fat-soluble vitamins are required to prevent rickets (vitamin D), coagulopathy (vitamin K), peripheral neuropathy (vitamin E) or xerophthalmia (vitamin A). Only vitamin E is available in a well-absorbed oral form (d-alpha-tocopheryl polyethylene glycol succinate); intramuscular administration of other fat-soluble vitamins is frequently necessary. Pruritus is treated with variable success with the agents and procedures listed in Table 9. Progression of cholestasis requires monitoring the child for the development of cirrhosis and treating its complications of ascites, portal hypertension and liver failure.

OBJECTIVES

Abdominal Pain
1. Review anatomy/neuroanatomy regarding:
   a. Source of pain perceived in the abdomen
   b. Referral of pain from intra-abdominal organs
2. Understand the significance of acute versus chronic pain.
3. Understand the type of pain from specific organs and conditions: e.g.,
   a. Hollow viscus – e.g., bowel – e.g., colitis
   b. Solid organ – e.g., liver, pancreas – e.g., hepatitis, pancreatitis
   c. Peritoneum – e.g., peritonitis
4. Understand the concept of nonspecificity of pain in the infant.
5. Be able to recognize acute appendicitis in an 8-year-old child ("typical" signs and symptoms) versus a 1-year-old infant (nonspecific signs and symptoms).
6. Be able to review a history for pain in or related to:
   a. Upper bowel (gastroesophageal reflux, peptic ulcer)
   b. Mid- and lower bowel (gastroenteritis, colitis)
   c. Urinary tract (pyelitis, cystitis)
   d. Liver (hepatitis)
   e. Pancreas (pancreatitis)
   f. Bowel (nonspecific recurrent abdominal pain in childhood)
   g. Lung – lower lobe (pneumonia)
   h. Other organs – muscle, bone, spine
   i. Metabolic and toxic conditions (diabetic precoma, lead poisoning, lactase deficiency, celiac disease)
7. Understand the following concepts:
   a. Careful history
   b. Careful examination
   c. Minimum required laboratory tests/examination

    d. Careful explanation to parent *and child* about your findings and expectations
8. Be able to describe those features of abdominal pain that suggest it may be of functional versus organic etiology.

Constipation

1. Understand the definition of constipation.
2. Differentiate constipation from infrequent pasty stools (e.g., in breastfed infants).
3. Understand and be able to give an example of various basic reasons for constipation:
   a. Slow motility (e.g., endocrine)
   b. Slow motility (e.g., visceral colonic myopathy)
   c. Renal or other metabolic disorder
4. Understand the signs and symptoms of bowel obstruction for congenital versus acquired lesions.
5. Understand Hirschsprung's disease – its pathogenesis and the various types of signs and symptoms it may produce.
6. Understand functional megacolon and fecal soiling.
7. Understand the short- and long-term significance of anal fissure in infancy.
8. Understand the basis for management of simple constipation in children.

Diarrhea

1. Review and understand the definition of diarrhea.
2. Understand that diarrhea is a *symptom*, not a disease. Therefore, one investigates and treats the *disease* whenever possible, and expects the symptom to clear.
3. Understand broadly the causes of diarrhea (review physiology notes):
   a. Intake of excessive/unabsorbable solute
   b. Maldigestion
   c. Malabsorption
   d. Secretion
   e. Dysmotility
   Be able to give two examples of each.
4. Understand the importance of water balance in young children, and the significance of vomiting and diarrhea in disturbing this balance.
5. Be able by history to suggest that diarrhea is being caused by:
   a. Pancreatic insufficiency
   b. Celiac disease
   c. Acute rotaviral gastroenteritis

    d. Acute infectious colitis (Shigella)

    e. Dysfunctional bowel syndrome in infancy (toddlers' diarrhea, irritable bowel syndrome of infancy)

6. Be aware of and understand how to interpret:

    a. Screening tests for malassimilation (e.g., serum carotene, folate, iron):
        D-xylose absorption test
        72-hour stool fat assessment

    b. Radiologic studies of bowel:
        Barium enema
        GI swallow
        Small bowel follow-through

7. Be aware of use of:

    a. Cultures of bowel content

    b. Examination of ova and parasites

    c. Sigmoidoscopy

    d. Jejunal biopsy (small bowel biopsy)

8. Understand the significance, in relation to a history of diarrhea, of:

    a. "Failure to thrive"

    b. Bloating, cramps

    c. Fever

    d. Blood in/on stool

    e. Family history

    f. Anorexia, nausea, vomiting

List of Contributors

ADAMS, P., University Hospital, 339 Windermere Rd., P.O. Box 5539, London, ON N6A 5A6. Tel: (519) 663-3513, Fax: (519) 663-3232.

ALTRAIF, I., c/o Dr. G.A. Levy, Toronto Hospital, 200 Elizabeth St., GWE 3-538, Toronto, ON M5G 2C4.

ARCHAMBAULT, A., Université de Montréal, Hôpital Maisonneuve-Rosemont, 5415, boul. de l'Assomption #305, Montréal, PQ H1T 2M4. Tel: (514) 252-3430, Fax: (514) 252-3894.

BLENDIS, L., Toronto Hospital, 200 Elizabeth St., Toronto, ON M5G 2C4. Tel: (416) 340-3834 Fax: (416) 595-5826.

BURNSTEIN, M., Associate Professor of Surgery, University of Toronto; Staff Surgeon, St. Michael's Hospital, 30 Bond St., Toronto, ON M5B 1W8. Tel: (416) 864-6050.

CHAMPION, M.C., Division of Gastroenterology, Ottawa Civic Hospital, 1053 Carling Ave., Ottawa, ON K1Y 4E9. Tel: (613) 761-4674, Fax: (613) 761-5269.

FEDORAK, R.N., University of Alberta, 519 Newton Research Building, 11315-87 Ave., Edmonton, AB T6G 2C2. Tel: (403) 492-6941, Fax: (403) 492-3744.

FREEMAN, H.J., Rm. F-274, Vancouver Hospital & Health Sciences Centre, U.B.C. Pavilion, 2211 Wesbrook, Vancouver, BC V6T 1W5. Tel: (604) 822-7216, Fax: (604) 822-7897.

GILLIES, R.R., Division of Gastroenterology, Ottawa Civic Hospital, 1053 Carling Ave., Ottawa, ON K1Y 4E9. Tel: (613) 761-4603, Fax: (613) 761-5269.

GREGOIRE, S., Ottawa General Hospital, 311 McArthur Rd., Ste. 203, Vanier, ON K1L 6P1. Tel: (613) 744-8180.

HABAL, F., Toronto Hospital, General Division, 200 Elizabeth St., EN9 229, Toronto, ON M5G 2C4. Tel: (416) 340-5023, Fax: (416) 595-5251.

HALLÉ, P., Hôpital du Saint-Sacrement, Service de Gastro-entérologie, 1050, chemin Ste-Foy, Québec, PQ G1S 4L8. Tel: (418) 682-7623.

HEATHCOTE, J., Toronto Western Hospital, 399 Bathurst St., 4th Floor, West Wing, Room 828, Toronto, ON M5T 2S8. Tel: (416) 369-5914, Fax: (416) 369-5553.

HILSDEN, R.J., Dept. of Gastroenterology, University of Calgary Health Sciences Centre, 3330 Hospital Dr. NW, Calgary, AB T2N 4N1. Tel: (403) 220-6536, Fax: (403) 283-3028.

HUNT, R.H., Chedoke-McMaster Hospitals, Box 2000, Hamilton, ON L8N 3Z5. Tel: (905) 521-2100 ext. 6404, Fax: (905) 521-5072.

LEE, S.S., Dept. of Medicine, University of Calgary Health Sciences Centre, 3330 Hospital Dr. NW, Calgary, AB T2N 4N1. Tel: (403) 220-4500, Fax: (403) 283-4740.

LEMOYNE, M., Hôpital Saint-Luc, 1058, rue Saint-Denis, Montréal, PQ H2X 3J4. Tel: (514) 281-2121, Fax: (514) 281-3564.

LEVY, G.A., Toronto Hospital, 200 Elizabeth St., GWE 3-538, Toronto, ON M5G 2C4.

MACHIDA, H., Alberta Children's Hospital, 1820 Richmond Rd. SW, Calgary, AB T2T 5C7. Tel: (403) 229-7211, Fax: (403) 229-7221.

MARTIN, S.R., Hôpital Sainte-Justine, Université de Montréal, 3175, Côte Sainte-Catherine, Montréal, PQ H3T 1C5. Tel: (514) 345-4931, Fax: (514) 345-4999.

MEBAN, S., Division of General Surgery, Ottawa Civic Hospital, 1053 Carling Ave., Ottawa, ON K1Y 4E9. Tel: (613) 761-4660.

MINUK, G., Health Sciences Centre, Liver Disease Unit, Rm. GF-407, 820 Sherbrook St., Winnipeg, MB R3A 1R9. Tel: (204) 787-4662, Fax: (204) 787-4826.

MORRISON, D.J., Alberta Children's Hospital, 1820 Richmond Rd. SW, Calgary, AB T2T 5C7. Tel: (403) 229-7211.

OLIVER, M.R., Alberta Children's Hospital, 1820 Richmond Rd. SW, Calgary, AB T2T 5C7. Tel: (403) 220-4556.

PARÉ, P., Hôtel-Dieu de Québec, 11, Côte du Palais, Québec, PQ G1R 2J6. Tel: (418) 691-5252, Fax: (418) 691-5331.

PATEL, D.G., Division of Gastroenterology, Ottawa Civic Hospital, 1053 Carling Ave., Ottawa, ON K1Y 4E9. Tel: (613) 761-4501, Fax: (613) 761-5269.

PATERSON, W.G., GI Division, Hotel Dieu Hospital, 166 Brock St., Kingston, ON K7L 5G2. Tel: (613) 544-3310 ext. 2332 or 3376, Fax: (613) 544-3114.

SALENA, B.J., Chedoke-McMaster Hospitals, Box 2000, Hamilton, ON L8N 3Z5. Tel: (905) 521-2100 ext. 6782, Fax: (905) 521-5072.

SCOTT, R.B., Alberta Children's Hospital, Dept. of Paediatrics; Faculty of Medicine, University of Calgary Health Sciences Centre, 3330 Hospital Dr. NW, Calgary, AB T2N 4N1. Tel: (403) 220-4556.

SCULLY, L.J., Division of Gastroenterology, GI Unit A1, Ottawa Civic Hospital, 1053 Carling Avenue, Ottawa, ON K1Y 4E9. Tel: (613) 761-4830, Fax: (613) 761-5269.

SEKAR, A.S.C., Division of Gastroenterology, Ottawa Civic Hospital, 1053 Carling Avenue, Ottawa, ON K1Y 4E9. Tel: (613) 729-3179, Fax: (613) 761-5269.

SHAFFER, E.A., Director, Dept. of Medicine, Foothills Hospital, 1403-29 Street NW, Rm. C210, Calgary, AB T2N 2T9. Tel: (403) 670-1500, Fax: (403) 670-1095.

SIDOROV, J.J., Professor of Medicine, Dalhousie University, 5991 Spring Garden Rd., Ste. 645, Halifax, NS B3H 1Y6. Tel: (902) 423-8239, Fax: (902) 443-7909.

SIMON, J., Queen's University, 78 Barrie St., Kingston, ON K7L 3J7. Tel: (613) 544-3310, Fax: (613) 544-2490.

STEINBRECHER, U.P., Rm. F-137, Vancouver Hospital & Health Sciences Centre, U.B.C. Pavilion, 2211 Wesbrook, Vancouver, BC V6T 1W5. Tel: (604) 822-7727, Fax: (604) 822-7897.

THOMPSON, W.G., Division of Gastroenterology, Ottawa Civic Hospital, 1053 Carling Ave., Ottawa, ON K1Y 4E9. Tel: (613) 761-4147, Fax: (613) 761-5269.

THOMSON, A.B.R., University of Alberta, 519 Newton Research Building, 11315-87 Ave., Edmonton, AB T6G 2C2. Tel: (403) 492-6490, Fax: (403) 492-7964.

TURNBULL, G.K., Camp Hill Medical Centre, 1335 Queen St., Halifax, NS B3J 2H6. Tel: (902) 496-3620, Fax: (902) 425-8222.

VAIR, B., Camp Hill Medical Centre, 2nd Floor Halifax Infirmary, 1335 Queen St., Halifax, NS B3J 2H6. Tel: (902) 428-3242.

WHITTAKER, J.S., St. Paul's Hospital, 1081 Burrard St., Vancouver, BC V6Z 1Y6. Tel: (604) 631-5034, Fax: (604) 631-5338.

WONG, F., Toronto Hospital, 200 Elizabeth St., Toronto, ON M5G 2C4. Tel: (416) 340-3834, Fax: (416) 595-5826.

WOROBETZ, L.J., Dept. of Medicine, Royal University Hospital, Saskatoon, SK S7N 0W8. Tel: (306) 966-7964, Fax: (306) 966-8021.

Index

The bold letter **t** following a page reference indicates a table. The bold letter **f** indicates a figure.

564 INDEX